ESSENTIALS OF

DOMESTIC ANIMAL EMBRYOLOGY

Commissioning Editor: Robert Edwards, Joyce Rodenhuis
Development Editor: Nicola Lally
Project Manager: Nancy Arnott
Designer/Design direction: Charles Gray
Illustration Manager: Merlyn Harvey
Illustrator: Oxford Illustrators

ESSENTIALS OF

DOMESTIC
ANIMAL
EMBRYOLOGY

By

Poul Hyttel
University of Copenhagen, Denmark

Fred Sinowatz
LMU Munich, Germany

Morten Vejlsted
University of Copenhagen, Denmark

With the Editorial Assistance of

Keith Betteridge
Ontario Veterinary College, University of Guelph, Canada

Foreword by
Eric W. Overström, Ph.D.
Professor and Head
Department of Biology & Biotechnology
Director, Life Sciences & Bioengineering Center
Worcester Polytechnic Institute
Worcester, Massachusetts

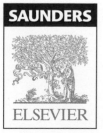

SAUNDERS

ELSEVIER

Edinburgh London New York Oxford Philadelphia St Louis Sydney Toronto 2010

SAUNDERS
ELSEVIER

First published 2010, © Elsevier Limited. All rights reserved.

ISBN 978-0-7020-2899-1

British Library Cataloguing in Publication Data
A catalogue record for this book is available from the British Library

Library of Congress Cataloging in Publication Data
A catalog record for this book is available from the Library of Congress

Notice
Neither the Publisher nor the Editors assume any responsibility for any loss or injury and/or damage to persons or property arising out of or related to any use of the material contained in this book. It is the responsibility of the treating practitioner, relying on independent expertise and knowledge of the patient, to determine the best treatment and method of application for the patient.

The Publisher

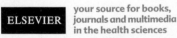

ELSEVIER your source for books, journals and multimedia in the health sciences

www.elsevierhealth.com

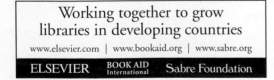

Working together to grow libraries in developing countries

www.elsevier.com | www.bookaid.org | www.sabre.org

ELSEVIER   BOOK AID International   Sabre Foundation

The publisher's policy is to use **paper manufactured from sustainable forests**

Printed in China

CONTENTS

Several highly qualified scientists have demonstrated their willingness to contribute to the book project.

Keith J. Betteridge BVSc MVSc PhD FRCVS

University Professor Emeritus

Department of Biomedical Sciences
Ontario Veterinary College
University of Guelph, Ontario
Canada

Gry Boe-Hansen DVM Phd

Lecturer

School of Veterinary Science
University of Queensland, Australia

Henrik Callesen DVM PhD DVSc

Research Professor

Department of Genetics and Biotechnology
Faculty of Agricultural Sciences, Aarhus University,
Denmark

Ernst-Martin Füchtbauer PhD Dr.habil

Associate Professor

Department of Molecular Biology
Aarhus University
Denmark

Vanessa Hall PhD

Post Doc

Department of Basic Animal and Veterinary Sciences
Faculty of Life Sciences, University of Copenhagen
Denmark

Poul Hyttel DVM Phd DVSc

Professor

Department of Basic Animal and Veterinary Sciences
Faculty of Life Sciences, University of Copenhagen
Denmark

Palle Serup Phd

Director of Research

Department of Developmental Biology
Hagedorn Research Institute
Denmark

Fred Sinowatz Dr.med vet. Dr.med Dr.habil

Professor

Institute of Veterinary Anatomy, Histology and
Embryology
LMU Munich,
Germany

Gábor Vajta MD PhD DVSc

Scientific Director

Cairns Fertility Centre
Australia
Adjunct Professor, University of Copenhagen,
Denmark
Adjunct Professor, James Cook University, Australia

Morten Vejlsted DVM Phd

Assistant Professor

Department of Large Animal Sciences
Faculty of Life Sciences, University of Copenhagen,
Denmark

For me, some of the most exciting and glorious moments in teaching gross anatomy of the domestic animals have occurred during days shared with open-minded students surrounded by steel tables full of pregnant uteri and fetuses in the dissection room. To examine those fetal specimens is to open an anatomy book; a book in which each organ and structure is perfectly defined and its developmental history is perfectly retained – truly the optimal situation for memorable anatomical "Aha-Erlebnishen" for students and teachers alike!

Embryology has always been a prerequisite for a real understanding of gross anatomy and of the teratology that results from development going awry. Today, however, it is that and much more besides; contemporary biomedical research requires embryology (or, rather, developmental biology) to play a central role in its progress – a role with important societal implications. Assisted reproduction technologies, for example, are as much applied to domestic animals as to humans in which vitro fertilization has become a common step *ex soma* to bridge one generation of mankind to the next. In the domestic animals, techniques such as cloning by somatic cell nuclear transfer have made possible genetic modifications that offer the prospects of modifying animals so that they produce valuable proteins, serve as models of human diseases, or provide organs for xenotransplantation in the future. All of these prospects depend upon a thorough knowledge of embryology and many of them are contentious. They put the discipline in an ethical spotlight that, in my view, obliges contemporary embryologists to participate in scientifically based societal debates.

For a while, ever more sophisticated assisted reproduction technologies moved the "cutting edge" of embryological research out of the body and into the in-vitro environment. However, the expansion of this field to encompass embryonic stem cells has refocused us on the embryo *per se*; the control of stem cell differentiation in vitro will depend absolutely on fundamental knowledge of the molecular regulation of developmental processes in vivo. The embryo itself has become the key to success – the circle is closed!

"Cutting edges" are these days fashioned from an amalgam of conventional embryology, genomics, transcriptomics and epigenomics applied to the investigation of the molecular mechanisms of developmental biology. Information is growing exponentially, and to combine in-depth molecular understanding with overall holistic embryology is a challenge – a challenge that becomes crystal clear when writing a textbook on the essentials of domestic animal embryology! For years, teaching the subject has been hampered by the lack of such a textbook and medical embryology textbooks were used as a poor compromise. By 2006, when McGaedy et al published their welcome textbook on veterinary embryology, we had already embarked on the present book with the goal of making our own research material, collected over several decades, palatable and stimulating for students. Working towards this goal has been a great experience for us and we hope that you the reader will find that we have accomplished at least part of what we intended. Future improvements, of course, will depend largely on feedback and I would much appreciate receiving constructive criticism.

In the meantime, it is my sincere wish that reading this book may lead you into at least one "Aha-Erlebnis" in the wondrous world of embryology!

Poul Hyttel
Vidiekjaer
Valby, Denmark
June 3, 2009

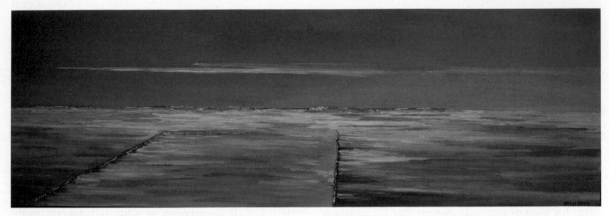

My painting (2003) of the open horizon of Skagen, Denmark, where I grew up and was 'imprinted'. I see embryology in the same light: a vista with infinite potentials that are just waiting to be realized.

Over the last 20 years, modern life science research efforts have rapidly advanced our knowledge of the normal and abnormal processes of domestic animal development. As our depth of understanding of the cellular and molecular mechanisms has grown, so too has the recognition of the potential for, and successful application of, this knowledge to enhance animal-based food and fiber production. It is during embryo and fetal development, from the formation of competent gametes to parturition, that powerful advancements in molecular genetic manipulation and assisted reproductive technologies are employed, and these efforts have had profound impact on animal production worldwide. As a result of these advances, there remains an unmet need for a contemporaneous text of domestic animal development to support education and training of today's veterinarians, animal scientists and developmental biologists. *Essentials of Domestic Animal Embryology* fulfills this need by providing the student, the instructor and the veterinary practitioner with an in depth presentation of the elaborate, chronological processes that culminate in formation of functional embryonic structures from the development of gametes through the peri-partum period. As our understanding of the precisely orchestrated processes of animal development advances, and animal genomes are further unveiled and analyzed, the importance of animal development becomes central to understanding and enhancing animal growth, sustaining health and determining the underlying causes of disease.

Although there continues to be available a number of quality texts of human embryology (for example *Langman's Medical Embryology*), focus on a single species remains a serious limitation for veterinary and animal science audiences and prevents a thorough view of the wide and distinct variations that exist among domestic animal species, with particular reference to processes of blastogenesis, implantation and placentation. Certainly, Bradley

Patton's 1927 benchmark publication in English, *Embryology of the Pig*, provided a wonderfully illustrated, descriptive account of this often utilized example of mammalian embryonic development. A concise descriptive publication of development in the pig, *The Embryonic Pig: A Chronological Account*, was later published by A.W. Marrable in 1971. In 1984, Drew Noden and Alexander de Lahunta, similarly recognizing the lack of an adequate text on domestic species embryology that would be useful for veterinary students, published *The Embryology of Domestic Animals: Developmental Mechanisms and Malformations*. An important contribution to veterinary curricula for many years to follow, this book presented traditional system-by-system descriptive material on the developmental anatomy of domestic species including birds, and the authors also included many relevant experimental and clinical case references throughout the book. Unfortunately, a revised edition was not forthcoming, and is not currently available. More recently, the finely detailed German text, *Lehrbuch der Embryologie der Haustiere (1991)*, was published by Imogen Russe and Fred Sinowatz (current co-author). Excellent illustrations and micrographs characterize this comprehensive embryology reference text of domestic species. Printed only in German, broad international adoption has been limited. In 2006, McGaedy and colleagues published *Veterinary Embryology*, a text targeting the particular needs of the veterinary student. Accordingly, the publication of *Essentials of Domestic Animal Embryology* is particularly timely as it fills a resource void for those students keen to study and understand the fundamental processes of animal development, be they students, instructors, research scientists or veterinary practitioners.

On reflection, this book project was conceived following from a discussion Poul and I had during a scientific meeting in 2000. As we shared and compared our experiences teaching animal embryology and anatomy to veterinary students, there was mutual recognition that a modern text in domestic animal development was sorely needed to contribute to the essential academic underpinnings for 21st century veterinary and animal science curricula. To appeal to a more global audience, contributions were solicited from established co-authors recognized internationally as experts in the field. Their chapters have been seamlessly woven into a very readable and informative text book. Of particular note are the inclusion of Chapters 1, 2, 20 and 21, each of which provides a distinguishing topic perspective, and include a historical account of the study of animal embryology, a discussion of current cell and molecular-based regulatory mechanisms that govern key developmental processes, comparative embryology of the chicken and mouse, and a succinct summary of the advent, development and broad application assisted reproductive technologies (ARTs) to enhance production of domestic animals, respectively.

Lead author, professor Poul Hyttel is recognized internationally as a distinguished research scientist, and a passionate educator and student mentor of animal reproduction and cell biology at the Royal Veterinary and Agricultural University, and most recently the University of Copenhagen. He has directed both the veterinary anatomy and histology/cell biology courses for many years in Copenhagen,

and has received formal awards and recognition, as well as continuous accolades from students for his passion and dedicated commitment to teaching. Under his direction, Poul has assembled a distinguished international group of contributing co-authors including professor Fred Sinowatz (Munich) and Dr. Morten Vejlsted (Copenhagen), among others. Keith Betteridge, distinguished professor of animal reproduction at the University of Guelph, has provided thorough editorial review of the text, This first edition presents a logical, contemporaneous and comprehensive view of the current state of knowledge in the field. The format provides succinct text information that is well supported by quality illustrations, photographs and micrographs. I believe that the student, instructor and practitioner alike will embrace this text as it will prove to be an invaluable resource to further both their education and their knowledge in the field of domestic animal embryology.

May 2009   Worcester, Massachusetts, USA

Eric W. Overström, Ph.D.
Professor and Head
Department of Biology & Biotechnology
Director, Life Sciences & Bioengineering Center
Worcester Polytechnic Institute
Worcester, Massachusetts

ACKNOWLEDGEMENTS

Writing this embryology textbook set the authors on a long and winding road. The project was initially proposed by Eric Overström in 2000. At that time Eric taught a course on developmental biology at Tufts University, Boston, US, and held a Fulbright stipend allowing regular trips to Copenhagen, Denmark. I am indebted to Eric for his enthusiasm in initiating the book project which resulted in many happy hours together in Copenhagen.

I feel enormously privileged to have been able to undertake this book project with cutting edge scientists who share my passion for scholarly university life. My co-authors, Fred Sinowatz and Morten Vejlsted, have both made extraordinary efforts in writing their many chapters. In particular, Fred's astonishing embryological breadth, ranging from the molecular to the gross anatomical levels, has been indispensable to the setting of our goals, and I am truly grateful that we were allowed to use high quality drawings from the previous embryology textbook that he produced with Imogen Rüsse and published in German. Other highly qualified contributors, Gry Boe-Hansen, Henrik Callesen, Ernst-Martin Füchtbauer, Vanessa Hall, Palle Serup and Gábor Vajta, have each brought their particular expertise to bear on other chapters to ensure that the text is as up-to-date as possible. I am greatly indebted to all these colleagues who have so generously shared their time and ideas with me.

As non-native English speakers the authors are extremely grateful for the willingness of Keith Betteridge, one of the pioneers of embryo transfer, to undertake a thorough linguistic edit of the completed text. Due to the breadth of Keith's scientific view, the linguistic affair developed into an inspiring dialogue about many conceptual subjects of embryology. It has been a pleasure to learn from the extreme precision with which Keith has tackled each step in the process.

Several qualified persons have devoted time and given extremely valuable comments to the text. I would like to thank Marie Louise Grøndahl, Vibeke Dantzer and Kjeld Christensen for their highly appreciated efforts.

Images have been an important issue in the production of the book. I would like to thank Jytte Nielsen and Hanne Marie Moelbak Holm for their skilled contribution to the preparation of thousands of sections for light and electron microscopy over the years as well as for digital processing of the micrographs.

Finally, I would like to thank Danish Pig Production for a very fruitful collaboration enabling the collection of thousands of porcine embryos over the years. The data generated from these resources have contributed significantly to the book and many of the photographs are taken from these embryos.

Poul Hyttel
Vidiekjaer
Valby
Denmark
June 3, 2009

CHAPTER 1

Poul Hyttel and Gábor Vajta

History of embryology

Embryology, the study of development from fertilization to birth, has always intrigued philosophers and scientists. Universal fascination with the way in which 'life' unfolds has led to spirited discussion of the complexities of the process amongst embryologists over the years. In 1899, **Ernst Haeckel** (1834–1919) considered that 'Ontogeny is a short recapitulation of phylogeny'. In other words, **ontogeny** (the development of an organism from the fertilized egg to its mature form) reflects, in a matter of days or months, the origin and evolution of a species (**phylogeny**), a continuing process that is measured in millions of years. Although this is not entirely true, one has only to look at a 19-day-old sheep embryo to understand Haeckel's viewpoint; the gill-like pharyngeal arches and the somites, for example (Fig. 1-1) are common to embryos of all chordates. Although trained as a physician, Haeckel abandoned his practice after reading *The Origin of Species* by **Charles Robert Darwin** (1809–1882) published in 1859 (and available at that time for fifteen shillings!). Always suspicious of teleological and mystical explanations of life, Haeckel used Darwin's theories as ammunition for attacking entrenched religious dogma on the one hand and elaborating his own views on the other. However, in projecting phylogeny into ontogeny, Haeckel made one mistake: his mechanism of change required that formation of new characters, diagnostic of new species, occur through their addition to a basic developmental scheme. For example, because most metazoans pass through a developmental stage called a gastrula (a ball of cells with an infolding that later forms the gut) Haeckel thought that at one time an organism called a '*gastraea*' must have

existed, looking much like the gastrula stage of ontogeny. This hypothesized ancestral metazoan, he thought, gave rise to all multi-celled animals. Such a 'single straight line' conception of phylogeny, with all creatures standing on the shoulders of predecessors in one trajectory, has now been abandoned; phylogeny divides into a multitude of lines.

Many of the ancient Greek philosophers were interested in embryology. According to Democritus (ca. 455–370 BC), the sex of an individual is determined by the origin of the sperm: males arising from the right testicle (of course!) and females from the left. This hypothesis was somewhat modified by Pythagoras, Hippocrates and Galen. However, gender bias was always evident, for science was the privilege of men; philosophers mostly positioned females between man and animals, so males were supposed to originate from the stronger sperm of the right testicle.

The first real embryologist that we know about was the Greek philosopher **Aristotle** (384–322 BC). In *The Generation of Animals* (ca. 350 BC) he described the different ways that animals are born: from eggs (oviparity, as in birds, frogs and most invertebrates), by live birth (viviparity, as in placental animals and some fish) or by production of an egg that hatches inside the body (ovoviviparity, which occurs in certain reptiles and sharks). It was Aristotle who also noted the two major patterns of cell division in early development: holoblastic cleavage in which the entire egg is divided into progressively smaller cells (as in frogs and mammals) and the meroblastic pattern in which only that part of the egg destined to become the embryo proper divides, with the remainder serving nutritive

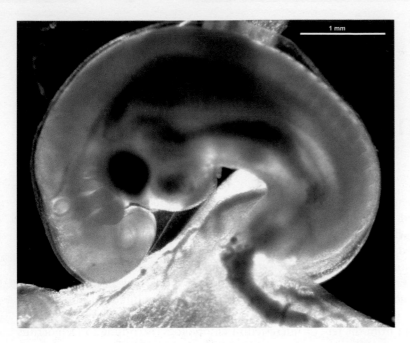

Fig. 1-1: Sheep embryo at Day 19 of development.

purposes (as in birds). The fetal membranes and the umbilical cord in cattle were described by Aristotle and he recognized their importance for fetal nutrition. By sequential studies of fertilized chick eggs, Aristotle made the very important observation that the embryo develops its organ systems gradually – they are not preformed. This concept of *de novo* formation of embryonic structures, which is referred to as **epigenesis**, remained enormously controversial for more than 2000 years before becoming fully accepted; Aristotle was way ahead of his time. The enigma of sexual reproduction also intrigued Aristotle. He realized that both sexes are needed for conception but felt that the male's semen did not contribute to conception physically, but by providing an unknown form-giving force that interacts with menstrual blood in the womb of the female to materialize as an embryo. In this case Aristotle was wrong. Ironically, in contrast to the non-acceptance of his correct views on epigenesis, his error about conception prevailed for about 2000 years, and it took a battle of almost a hundred years to correct it!

During those 2000 years, the science of embryology developed very slowly along descriptive ana-

tomical lines. One of the first anatomical descriptions of the pregnant uterus of the pig was by **Kopho** (years of birth and death unknown) in the early 13th century in his work *Anatomio Porci*. Kopho worked at the famous medical school of Salerno using pigs as models because human cadavers could not be dissected for religious reasons. During the early Renaissance, the famous and incomparably artistic anatomical studies of **Leonardo da Vinci** (1452– 1519) included investigation of the pregnant uterus of a cow. His drawings of a pregnant bicornuate uterus and of the fetus and fetal membranes released from the uterus are reproduced in Fig. 1-2. In an accompanying drawing, Leonardo depicted a human uterus cut open to 'reveal', not a human placenta but a multiplex, villous, ruminant placenta (see Chapter 9)! Clearly it had not been possible for him to actually study a human pregnancy. The structures are described in the characteristic mirrored writing of Leonardo, who worked mostly in Florence.

The Renaissance, from the 13th to the 15th century, was a great time for anatomical studies and, happily, coincided with the invention of book printing by Johann Gutenberg. Thus, the first major publication

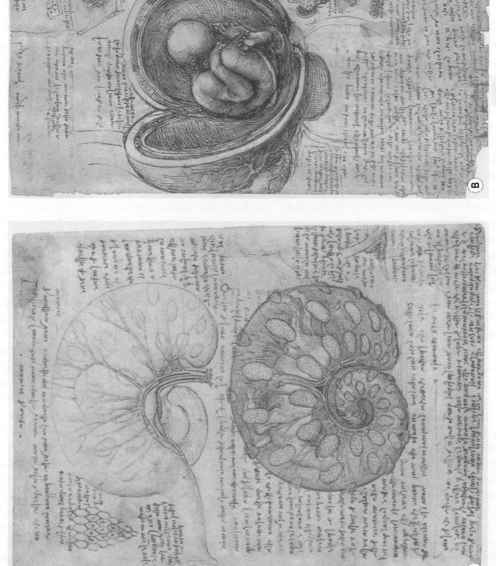

Fig. 1-2: Drawings of Leonardo da Vinci. A: Top: A pregnant bicornuate uterus of the cow. Bottom: Fetus and fetal membranes showing the cotyledons of the placenta (see Chapter 9). B: Opened simplex uterus of human showing the fetus with the umbilical cord. Note that the placenta is of the ruminant multiplex type with several placentomes drawn on the cut wall of the uterus and, at the right top, a single cotyledon drawn at a higher magnification displaying its villous surface.

on comparative embryology was *De Formato Foetu* in 1600 by the Italian anatomist **Hieronymus Fabricius of Acquapendente** (1533–1619). Fabricius described and illustrated the gross anatomy of embryos and their membranes in that book, but was not actually the first to do so; another Italian anatomist, **Bartolomeo Eustachius** (1514–1574), had previously published illustrations of dog and sheep embryos in 1552. We now recognize the names of Fabricius, in the term *bursa Fabricii* (the immunologically competent portion of the bird gut), and of Eustachius in the Eustachian tube.

The work of Eustachius, Fabricius and others gave insight into how organs develop from their immature to mature forms, but left unanswered the basic enigma of how and where the mammalian embryo originates. However, the development of the microscope by Zacharias Janssen, a Dutch eyeglass maker, in 1590 ushered in a new era of embryological science to tackle that 2000-year-old question. The Dutch dominance in the optical field at that time may not be just a coincidence; the naval ambitions of their new empire required excellent telescopes and lens systems. Janssen's microscope in its original form, however, was not really appropriate for cell and tissue research; it was approximately 2 metres long, achieved only 10 to 20 times magnification, and its principal use was to attract an audience at country fairs! In 1672, the Italian medical doctor **Marcello Malpighi** (1628–1694) published the first microscopic account of chick development, identifying the neural groove, the somites, and circulation of blood in the arteries and veins to and from the yolk. Malpighi also observed that even the unincubated chick egg is considerably structured, leading him to think that a preformed version of the chicken resided in the egg. Later (in 1722), the French ophthalmologist **Antoine Maître-Jan** (1650–1730) pointed out that although the egg examined by Malpighi was technically 'unincubated', it had been left sitting in the Bolognese sun in August and so was certainly not 'unheated'. Nevertheless, Malpighi's notion of a preformed chicken initiated one of the great debates in embryology that was to last throughout the 17th and 18th centuries. The question was: are the organs of the embryo formed *de novo*

(**epigenesis**), or they are already present in a miniature form in the egg (or the sperm when this cell was discovered), a concept referred to as **preformation**. We will return to this debate in a moment.

The new microscopic techniques also prompted a vigorous search for the **mammalian gametes**. The chicken egg and its initial transformation into a chick were obvious, as Aristotle had described, but what mediated the formation of the embryo in mammals? Where was the mammalian egg to be found?

One of the earliest and most influential names in the fascinating story of the discovery of the mammalian egg was that of **William Harvey** (1578–1657), personal physician to the English kings James I and Charles I, and famous for his description of the circulation of the blood. In 1651, Harvey published *De Generatione Animalium* (Disputations touching the Generation of Animals) with a famous frontispiece showing Zeus freeing all creation from an egg bearing the inscription *Ex ovo omnia* (All things come from the egg). However, it should be realized that, far from advancing 17th century knowledge of reproduction and embryology, Harvey's observations in some ways impeded progress. From having studied with Fabricius, Harvey was imbued with Aristotle's view that the semen provided a force that interacted with the menstrual blood to materialize as an embryo. Harvey set out to understand this process by looking for the earliest products of conception in female deer killed during the breeding season in the course of King Charles I's hunts in his Royal forests and parks over a 12-year period. In the red and fallow deer that he studied, the male's rut begins in mid-September and so Harvey dissected uteri throughout the months of September to December. Believing, wrongly, that copulation coincides with the onset of the rut, Harvey was mystified to find nothing that he recognized as an embryo until mid-November, some two months later. This forced him to the erroneous, but entirely logical conclusion that 'nothing after coition is to be found in [the] uterus for many days together'. When he did find a conceptus, that, for Harvey, was the egg: 'Aristotle's definition of an egg applies to it, namely, an egg is that out of a part of which an animal is begotten and the remainder is the food for that which is begotten'.

Three factors of veterinary interest had led this brilliant man astray. First, he did not appreciate that the females did not come into oestrus until early October and so his estimates of breeding dates were wrong. Second, he dismissed the ovaries ('female testicles') as making no contribution to conception because they failed to swell up as the testes of males do during rut. Third, expecting to find an egg-shaped conceptus, he failed to recognize the 'purulent matter … friable … and inclining to yellow', which he observed much earlier after mating and describes quite vividly, as being the filamentous blastocyst so characteristic of ruminants. Had Harvey used a lens, or conducted his studies on species (like rabbits or horses) with spherical early conceptuses, discovery of the real egg might have been advanced considerably!

It is easy to be critical with hindsight of course, and we should remember that Harvey made important contributions to embryology: his descriptions of early development were impeccable; he was the first to observe the blastoderm of the chick embryo (the small region of the egg containing the yolk-free cytoplasm that gives rise to the embryo proper) and to indicate that blood islands form before the heart does; and he was aware of the gradual development of the embryo, subscribing to the school of epigenesis as did Aristotle.

The observations by Harvey and the search for the mammalian egg were extended by **Regnier de Graaf** (1641–1673) who performed detailed studies of the female reproductive organs, especially the ovary. De Graaf, like his friend Leeuwenhoek, worked in Delft. From a comparison of mammalian ovaries with those of chicken, de Graaf considered mammalian antral ovarian follicles to be the eggs; an assumption he confirmed by tasting! His contribution to science was later acknowledged by the German medical doctor **Theodor Ludwig Wilhelm Bischoff** (1807–1882) who introduced the nomenclature 'Graafian follicle'. De Graaf also noted some connection between follicular maturation and the development of oocytes but, without an appropriate microscope, he could not substantiate this and his observations

were for a long time forgotten. Had he lived a little longer (he died tragically early, at the age of 32), the discovery of the mammalian egg could probably have avoided a delay of about 150 years!

As it was, the first scientist to actually see the mammalian egg (which everyone believed to exist, but no one had seen) was the Estonian medical doctor **Karl Ernst von Baer** (1792–1876). He opened the 'Graafian egg', as the follicle was known at that time, and saw with his naked eye a small yellow point which he released and examined under the microscope (Baer, 1827). There, upon a first glance, Baer was stunned and could hardly believe that he had found what so many famous scientists including Harvey, de Graaf, Purkinje and others had failed to find. He was so overcome that he had to work up courage to look into the microscope a second time. The mammalian egg had been identified.

How about the spermatozoa? **Anton van Leeuwenhoek** (1632–1723), a Dutch tradesman and scientist from Delft, was the first to report having seen moving **spermatozoa**. He constructed a single lens microscope that magnified up to about 300 times. Technically, this microscope was an amazing achievement – no bigger than a small postage stamp and resembling a primitive micromanipulator. It was used close to the eye like a magnifying glass. Using this, Leeuwenhoek drew spermatozoa from different species. Initially, Leeuwenhoek was reluctant to study sperm and he questioned the propriety of writing about semen and intercourse. When he first focused his microscope on semen, Leeuwenhoek discovered what he then took to be globules. However, he so disliked the prospect of having to discuss his findings that he quickly turned to other matters. Three or four years later, however, in 1677, a student from the medical school at Leiden brought him a specimen of semen in which he had found small animals with tails, which Leeuwenhoek now observed as well. Consequently, Leeuwenhoek resumed his own observations and, in his own semen (acquired, he stressed, not by sinfully defiling himself but as a natural consequence of conjugal coitus), observed a multitude of *animalcules,* less than a millionth the size of a coarse grain of sand

and with thin, undulating, transparent tails. A month later, Leeuwenhoek described these observations in a brief letter to Lord Brouncker, president of the Royal Society in London. Still uneasy about the subject matter, he begged Brouncker not to publish it if he thought it would give offence. Leeuwenhoek's observations prompted vivid discussions and controversies on the significance of these living objects. At first, it was commonly held that the tadpole-like creatures were parasites. Leeuwenhoek may have been biased towards that view as he was actually engaged in parallel studies of parasites and was the first to see *Giardia*, a protozoan parasite that infects the gastrointestinal tract. *Giardia* are flagellated and may, at poor microscopical resolution, resemble spermatozoa. Other scientists considered that the whirling action of the objects was meant to prevent solidification of the semen. In the preformation school, however, Leeuwenhoek's observations encouraged the thought that the sperm head contained preformed miniatures of babies, foals, calves etc. and so these scientists became known as the spermists.

The two mammalian gametes had been identified. Instead of forming a common platform for further endeavours, however, this knowledge prompted a bitter dispute, as to whether the embryo arose from the egg or from the sperm!

In parallel with the search for the mammalian gametes, the combat between the schools of epigenesis and preformation became more and more intense. The latter had the backing of 18th century science, religion and philosophy for several reasons. First, if the body is prefigured and just needs to be unrolled, no extra mysterious force is needed to initiate embryonic development. This was a religiously convenient point of view, paying proper respect to God's creation of mankind. Second, if the body is prefigured in the germ cells, a further generation will already exist prefigured in the germ cells of the next, rather like Russian nested Matryoshka dolls. This concept was also convenient, ensuring that the forms of species would remain constant. The fact that at a certain point Matryoshka dolls cannot get any smaller would seem like an obvious objection to the concept today. However, there was no biological size scale at the time of these arguments because the cell theory of **Theodor Schwann** (1810–1882) was not proposed until 1847. Thus preformationists could claim, as formulated in 1764 by the Swiss naturalist and philosophical writer **Charles Bonnet** (1720–1793), that 'Nature works as small as it wishes'. Basically, preformation was a conservative theory, and it was unable to answer some of the questions raised by the limited knowledge of genetic variation at that time. It was, for example, known that matings between black and white parents resulted in babies of intermediate colour, an outcome incompatible with preformation in either gamete.

In the late 18th century, **Caspar Friedrich Wolff** (1734–1794), a German embryologist working in St. Petersburg, made detailed observations on chick embryos that resulted in the first strong case for epigenesis. He demonstrated how the gut arises from the folding of an originally indifferent flat tissue and interpreted his findings as evidence of epigenesis when, in 1767, he wrote that 'When the formation of the intestine in this manner has been duly weighed, almost no doubt can remain, I believe, of the truth of epigenesis'. Wolff's name lives on in the term 'Wolffian duct' for the mesonephric duct.

In spite of Wolff's contribution, the preformation theory persisted until the 1820s when new techniques for tissue staining and microscopy allowed a further advance in the science of embryology. Three friends, **Christian Pander** (1794–1865), Karl Ernst von Baer, and **Martin Heinrich Rathke** (1793–1860), all of whom came from the Baltic region and studied in Germany, formulated concepts of great relevance for contemporary embryology. Pander expanded the observations made by Wolff and also, despite studying the chick embryo for only some 15 months before becoming a palaeontologist, discovered the germ layers (Pander, 1817). The overall term 'germ layers' is derived from the Latin *germen* ('bud' or 'sprout') whereas the three individual layers are of Greek origin: ectoderm from *ectos* ('outside') and *derma* ('skin'), mesoderm from *mesos* ('middle'), and endoderm from *endon* ('within'). Pander also noted that organs were not formed from a single germ layer. A remarkable feature of Pander's book from 1817 is the quality of the illustrations drawn by the German anatomist and artist **Eduard Joseph d'Alton** (1772–1840); they beautifully depict details that had not yet been defined (Fig. 1-3). This classical work underlines the necessity for precise observational skills in embryology.

Rathke studied comparative embryology in frogs, salamanders, fish, birds, and mammals and pointed out the similarities in development among all these vertebrate groups. He described for the first time the

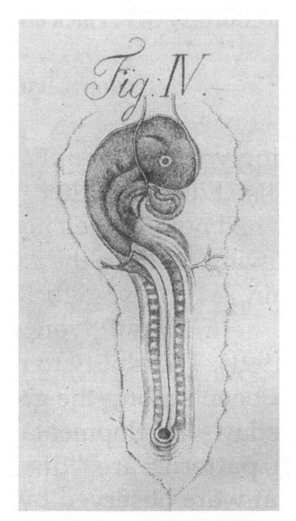

Fig. 1-3: Drawing of a Day 2 chick embryo by Eduard Joseph d'Alton displayed in Pander (1817).

pharyngeal arches common to the development of these animals. 'Rathke's pouch' – the ectodermal contribution to the pituitary gland – commemorates him.

In addition to identifying the mammalian ovum, von Baer extended Pander's observations on chick embryos and described the notochord for the first time. Moreover, von Baer again appreciated the common principles that direct initial embryological development regardless of species; in 1828 he wrote 'I have two small embryos preserved in alcohol that I forgot to label. At present I am unable to determine the genus to which they belong. They may be lizards, small birds, or even mammals'.

Staining and microscopy techniques continued to improve during the 19th century and allowed for more detailed observations on the initial cleavage stages by the German biologist **Theodor Ludwig Wilhelm von Bischoff** (1807–1882) in the rabbit, and by the Swiss anatomist and physiologist **Rudolph Albert von Kölliker** (1817–1905) in man and various domestic animals. Kölliker also published the first textbook on embryology in man and higher animals in 1861.

Thanks to the contributions of Pander, von Baer and Rathke, the preformation school in its radical form ceased in the 1820s. However, the concept survived for another 80 years in the sense that a certain group of scientists regarded the cells of the early cleavage stage embryo to represent right and left halves of the body as it took form. This implied that the information for building the body is segregated regionally in the egg. In 1893, **August Weismann** (1834–1914) proposed his germ cell plasm theory as an extension of this idea. Based on the sparse knowledge of fertilization available at that time, he was far-sighted enough to propose that the egg and the sperm provided equal chromosomal contributions, both quantitatively and qualitatively, to the new organism. Moreover, he postulated that chromosomes carried the inherited potentials of this new organism, which was remarkable at that time considering that the chromosomes had not yet been identified as the carriers of inherited matter. However, Weismann thought that not all information on the chromosomes passed into every cell of the embryo. Rather, different parts of information went to different cells, explaining their **differentiation**. Weismann clearly understood the principle of how traits are inherited through fertilization, but he was wrong about the mechanisms of differentiation. Weismann's differentiation theory was put to the test practically by the German embryologist **Wilhelm Roux** (1850–1924) who had already, in 1888, published the results of experiments in which individual cells of 2- and 4-cell frog embryos were destroyed by a hot needle. As predicted by Weismann's theory, Roux observed the formation of embryos in which only one side developed normally. These results inspired another German embryologist, **Hans Adolf Eduard Driesch** (1867–1941) to perform experiments using cell separation instead of Roux's cell destruction technique. To his enormous surprise, Driesch obtained results that were quite different from those of Roux. Using separated cells from early cleavage stage sea urchin embryos he demonstrated that each of the cells was able to develop into a small but complete embryo and larva (Driesch, 1892). He repeated the same experiment with 4-cell embryos and obtained similar results; the larvae were smaller but otherwise looked completely normal.

The final evidence against the Roux-Weismann theory was provided by the elegant experiments published by yet another German embryologist, **Hans Spemann** (1869–1941). Originally, just like Driesch, he had set out to support the theory with his experiments on salamanders. However, by separating the cells of early cleavage stage embryos with a ligature (a hair taken from his newborn son's head), he soon found that the separated cells were each able to form a small embryo – they were **totipotent**. In 1928, Spemann conducted the first nuclear transfer experiment, transferring the nucleus of a salamander embryo cell into a cell without a nucleus. Using a hair as a noose, as he had done in his 1902 splitting of the salamander embryo, Spemann tightened the noose around a newly fertilized egg cell, forcing the nucleus to one side and cytoplasm to the other. Next, he waited as the side with the nucleus divided and grew into a 16-cell embryo. Then he loosened the noose, and allowed

the nucleus from one of the embryo cells to slip over into the egg cytoplasm on the other side. Spemann then promptly tightened the noose completely, physically breaking the ball of cytoplasm and its new nucleus away from the remains of the 16-cell embryo. From this single cell grew a normal salamander embryo, proving that the nucleus from an early embryonic cell was able to direct the complete growth of a salamander. Spemann had created the first clone by nuclear transfer. Spemann published his results in his 1938 book 'Embryonic Development and Induction' in which he called for the 'fantastical experiment' of cloning from differentiated or adult cells and theoretically paved the way for the cloning by somatic cell nuclear transfer that we know today. Unfortunately, Spemann saw no practical way of realizing such an experiment at that time. Spemann was awarded the Nobel Prize for Physiology or Medicine in 1935 for his discovery of the effect now known as **embryonic induction** – the influence exercised by various parts of the embryo that directs the development of groups of cells into particular tissues and organs. The works of Driesch and Spemann finally put an end to the concept that inherited information is divided among the cells of the developing embryo.

The whereabouts of inherited materials had still not been determined in the late 19th and early 20th century when a group of American embryologists set out to discover whether inheritance resided in the cytoplasm or the nucleus of the fertilized egg. **Edmund Beecher Wilson** (1856–1939) was of the opinion that the nucleus is the carrier while **Thomas Hunt Morgan** (1866–1945) thought the cytoplasm to be responsible. Wilson allied himself with the German biologist **Theodor Heinrich Boveri** (1862–1915) working at the Naples Zoological Station. Boveri had produced major support for the chromosomal hypothesis of inheritance by fertilizing sea urchin eggs with two spermatozoa. At first cleavage, such eggs produced four mitotic poles and divided into four cells instead of two. Subsequently, Boveri separated the cells and demonstrated that they developed abnormally, each in its own particular way, due to the fact that they carried different chromosomes. Hence, Boveri claimed that each chromosome is distinct and controls different vital processes. Wilson and **Nettie Maria Stevens** (1861–1912), one of the first American women to be recognized for her contribution to science, extended the work of Boveri. They demonstrated the relationship between chromosomes and sex: XO or XY embryos developed into males and XX embryos into females (Wilson, 1905; Stevens, 1905a,b). For the first time a particular phenotypical characteristic was clearly correlated with a property of the nucleus. Eventually, Morgan found mutations that correlated with sex and with the X chromosome. This persuaded him that his earlier view that inheritance was through the cytoplasm was wrong and that genes are physically linked to one another on the chromosomes. Consequently, a group of embryologists had laid a cornerstone to the discovery that the chromosomes in the cell nucleus are responsible for the development of inherited characteristics.

In the early 20th century, embryology and genetics were not considered separate sciences. They diverged in the 1920s when Morgan redefined genetics as the science studying the transmission of inherited traits, distinguishing it from embryology, the science studying the expression of those traits. This division did not occur without hostility; geneticists considered the embryologists old-fashioned while embryologists looked upon geneticists as being uninformed about how organisms actually develop! Fortunately, we nowadays see a rapprochement of genetics and embryology in a very fruitful symbiosis. Two of the scientists who advocated synergism between embryology and genetics in the early days were **Salome Gluecksohn-Schoenheimer** (now Gluecksohn-Waelsch; 1907–2007) and **Conrad Hal Waddington** (1905–1975). Gluecksohn-Schoenheimer received her doctorate in Spemann's laboratory, but fled Hitler's Germany for the United States. Her far-sighted research demonstrated that mutations in the *Brachyury* gene of the mouse caused aberrant development of the posterior portion of the embryo, and she localized the defect to the notochord (Gluecksohn-Schoenheimer, 1938, 1940), providing another example of the close link between embryology and genetics. Interestingly, it took 50 years for her results to be confirmed by DNA hybridization after cloning

of the *Brachyury* gene (Wilkinson et al., 1990). Waddington, on the other hand, addressed the causal link between embryology and genetics by isolating several genes that caused wing malformations in fruit flies. Moreover, his interpretation and visual conception of 'the epigenetic landscape' affecting initial cell differentiation in the embryo still surfaces during contemporary presentations on embryonic stem cells and their differentiation (Waddington, 1957, Fig. 1-4).

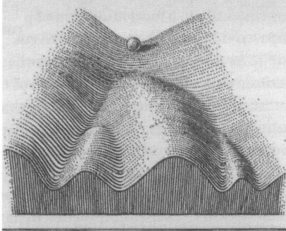

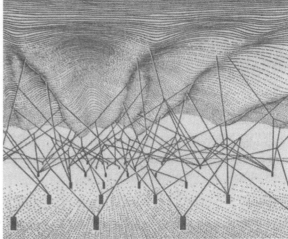

Fig. 1-4: Top: CH Waddington's depiction of the epigenetic landscape with the ball representing a cell and the valleys representing different avenues of differentiation. Bottom: A less commonly depicted view behind the epigenetic landscape illustrating how the tension of different genes control the fate of the ball. From Waddington (1957)

The question of totipotency, initially addressed by Driesch and Spemann, was later revisited at a finer level. Thus, whereas Driesch and Spemann had proved the totipotency of the *cells* of the early cleavage stage embryo, experiments in the 1950s by **Robert Briggs** (1911–1983) and **Thomas King** (1921–2000) tested the totipotency of the *nucleus* or rather the genome. Their nuclear transfer model was an exact realization of the 'fantastic experiment' proposed by Hans Spemann, although they had never heard about his suggestion. To accomplish their objective they had to develop methods by which they could remove the genome of an egg without destroying it (enucleation), pick up a donor nucleus of another cell, and transfer that nucleus to the enucleated egg. As their approach was extremely unorthodox, their first grant application to the National Cancer Institute was refused as a 'hare-brained' idea. However, they eventually obtained some support, and after months of experimentation they produced the first blastocyst from nuclear transfer. Their initial success was short-lived. In their enthusiasm, they gathered the complete staff of the institute to show them the blastocyst. After numerous looks into the microscope, followed by applause and congratulations, they re-checked the dish and found only a completely destroyed embryo. Fortunately, although the first embryo died, the nuclear transfer system worked; in 1952, Briggs and King successfully demonstrated that donor nuclei from frog blastula stages could direct the development of complete tadpoles when transferred into enucleated eggs. This research further paved the way for the somatic cell nuclear transfer that is nowadays used for cloning of mammals. Briggs and King also discovered that when cells from later stages (tailbud-stage tadpoles for example), were used as nuclear donors, normal development did not occur unless the nuclei came from the germ cells. Thus, somatic cells appeared to lose their ability to direct development as their degree of differentiation increased. This point was later pursued by **John B. Gurdon** who worked with another frog species, *Xenopus*, rather than Briggs and King's *Rana*. Gurdon et al. (1975) found that when nuclei of cultured skin cells from adult frogs were transferred into enucleated eggs, development of the clones never progressed beyond the formation of the neural tube. However, when serial nuclear transfers were made from the cloned embryos to other enucleated eggs, it was possible to generate numerous tadpoles; the genomic totipotency of somatic cells had been proven. It should be noted though that the frog experiments never managed to close the developmental circle by producing an adult organism by transferring a somatic cell nucleus from another adult organism.

Closing the circle did not happen until the nuclear transfer technique was transposed to mammals by the Danish veterinarian **Steen Malte Willadsen** working in Cambridge during the 1980s. Willadsen (1986) succeeded in transferring not just the nucleus, but the entire cell from sheep morula-stage embryos to enucleated eggs by electrical cell fusion. His work resulted in the first mammal to be born after cloning by nuclear transfer. In 1996, this technology was taken one step further by **Keith H Campbell**, working at the Roslin Institute in Scotland in a research group headed by **Ian Wilmut**. Campbell et al. (1996) succeeded in producing lambs following transfer of nuclei of cultured cells, harvested from the inner cell mass, to enucleated eggs. Key to this success was Campbell's meticulous cell cycle experimentation that demonstrated the need for a certain degree of synchrony of cell cycle between the donor nucleus and the recipient cytoplasm. The ability to clone mammals from cultured cells represented a major breakthrough in biomedical science, facilitating genetic manipulation of the cells prior to nuclear transfer and opening an avenue for production of transgenic animals (animals in which a foreign gene, the transgene, has been added). Consequently, **Angelika Schnieke**, working in the same group of researchers, was able to announce the birth of the transgenic sheep Polly, a lamb cloned from cultured fetal sheep fibroblasts into which the gene for human clotting factor IX had been inserted with a promoter that would allow for expression of the transgene in the mammary gland (Schnieke et al., 1997). It was from that event that the concept of 'biopharming' (production of valuable proteins in transgenic animals) emerged. The report on Polly, however, was preceded by another from the Roslin group; a publication that stunned not only the scientific community, but all layers of society, world-wide. That was the report of the birth of the cloned lamb Dolly (Wilmut et al. 1997). Dolly was created by Wilmut and his group by transferring cultured mammary gland cells from a 6-year-old ewe into enucleated eggs. Again, the success depended on control of the cell cycle; the mammary gland nuclear donor cells were kept under culture conditions that suppressed their mitotic activity, provoked a state of cellular senescence, and locked them at the G1 state of the cell cycle, or G0. Research since then has resulted in the cloning of many animals of many species (including cattle, mice, goats, pigs, cats, rabbits, horses, dogs, and rats) and has also demonstrated that bringing the nuclear donor cells into quiescence is not a necessity.

In its combination with genetics, embryology is an exponentially developing science; how it will continue to develop, only time can tell. As a subject, embryology made its way into the curriculum of veterinary medicine in the mid 19th century when it became incorporated into the teaching of anatomy. In 1924, the first textbook on veterinary embryology was published by **Zeitzschmann** and others (though not many) have appeared since. *Embryology of the Pig* by **Bradley M Patten** deserves special mention as it has been an admirable resource and inspiration for the authors of this book. Likewise, the 'bible' of comparative embryology *Developmental Biology* by **Scott F. Gilbert** we have found admirable for its breadth of coverage and for its inimitable style.

Because embryology was originally based upon the anatomical descriptive tradition and also entered the curricula of medicine and veterinary medicine as part of anatomy, its nomenclature is Latin- and Greek-based. For ease of reading, however, we have anglicized some terms rather than use their strict Latin or Greek forms.

FURTHER READING

Aristotle (ca. 350 BC): The generation of animals. A.L. Peck (trans.). eBooks@Adelaide, 2004 (see http://etext.library. adelaide.edu.au/a/aristotle/generation/).

Baer, K.E.V. (1827): De ovi mammalium et hominis genesi. Voss, Leipzig.

Bonnet, C. (1764): Contemplation de la Nature. Marc-Michel Ray, Amsterdam.

Briggs, R. and King, T.J. (1952): Transplantation of living nuclei from blastula cells into enucleated frogs' eggs. Proc. Natl. Acad. Sci. USA 38:455–464.

Campbell, K.H., McWhir, J., Ritchie, W.A. and Wilmut I. (1996): Sheep cloned by nuclear transfer from a cultured cell line. Nature 380:64–66.

Darwin, C. (1859): On the Origin of Species by Means of Natural Selection, or the Preservation of Favoured Races in the Struggle for Life. John Murray, London.

Fabricius, H. of Aquapendente (1600): De formato foetu. Pasquala, Padova.

Gilbert, S.F. (2003): Developmental biology. 7th edn. Sinauer Associates, Sunderland, Massachusetts.

Gluecksohn-Schoenheimer, S. (1938): The development of two tailless mutants in the house mouse. Genetics 23:573–584.

Gluecksohn-Schoenheimer, S. (1940): The effect of an early lethal (t^0) in the house mouse. Genetics 25:391–400.

Gurdon, J.B., Laskey, R.A. and Reeves, O.R. (1975): The developmental capacity of nuclei transplanted from keratinized cells of adult frogs. J. Embryol. Exp. Morphol. 34:93–112.

Harvey, W. (1651): Excitationes de generatione animalium. Elzevier, Amsterdam.

Kölliker, A. (1881): Entwiklungsgeschichte des Menschen und der höhere Thiere. Engelmann, Leipzig.

Maître-Jan, A. (1722): Observations sur la formation du poulet. L. d'Houdry, Paris.

Malpighi, M. (1672): De formatione pulli in ovo (London). Reprinted in HB Adelmann 'Marcello Malpighi and the evolution of embryology'. Cornell University Press, Ithaca, NY, 1966.

Pander, H.C. (1817/18): Beitrage zur Entwiklungsgeschichte des Hühnchens in Eye. Brönner, Wüzburg.

Patten, B.M. (1948): Embryology of the pig. 3rd edn. Blakiston Company, New York, Toronto.

Roux, W. (1888): Contributions to the developmental mechanisms of the embryo. On the artificial production of half embryos by destruction of one of the first two blastomeres and the later development (postgeneration) of the missing half of the body. In B.H. Willier and J.M. Oppenheimer (eds.) 1974 'Foundations of experimental embryology', Hafner, New York, pp. 2-37.

Schnieke, A., Schnieke, A.E., Kind, A.J., Ritchie, W.A., Mycock, K., Scott, A.R., Ritchie, M., Wilmut, I., Colman, A. and Campbell, K.H. (1997): Human factor IX transgenic sheep produced by transfer of nuclei from transfected fetal fibroblasts. Science 278:2130–2134.

Schwann, T. and Schleyden, M.J. (1847): Microscopical researches into the accordance in the structure and growth of animals and plants. London: Printed for the Sydenham Society.

Stevens, N.M. (1905a): Studies in spermatogenesis with special reference to the 'accessory chromosome'. Carnegie Institute of Washington, Washington. D.C.

Stevens, N.M. (1905b): A study of the germ cells of *Aphis rosae* and *Aphis oenotherae*. J. Exp. Zool. 2:371–405, 507–545.

Waddington, C.H. (1957): The strategy of the genes. Geo Allen & Unwin, London.

Weismann, A. (1893): The germ-plasm: A theory of heredity. Translated by W. Newton Parker and H. Ronnfeld. Walter Scott Ltd., London.

Wilkinson, D.G., Bhatt, S. and Herrmann, B.G. (1990): Expression pattern of the mouse *T*-gene and its role in mesoderm formation. Nature 343:657–659.

Willadsen, S.M. (1986): Nuclear transplantation in sheep embryos. Nature 320:63–65.

Wilmut, I., Schnieke, A.E., McWhir, J., Kind, A.J. and Campbell, K. (1997): Viable offspring from fetal and adult mammalian cells. Nature 385:810–814.

Wilson, E.B. (1905): The chromosome in relation to the determination of sex in insects. Science 22:500–502.

Wolf, K.F. (1767): De formatione intestorum praecipue. Novi Commentarii Academine Scientarum Imperialis Petropolitanae 12:403–507.

CHAPTER 2

Cellular and molecular mechanisms in embryonic development

Morten Vejlsted

INITIAL EMBRYONIC DEVELOPMENT AND GESTATIONAL PERIODS

Embryonic development encompasses all the processes whereby a single cell – the fertilized egg or **zygote** – gives rise to first an embryo, then a fetus which at birth has the capacity to adapt to post-natal life. These processes occur as a continuum but, for convenience, they may be arbitrarily divided into successive periods. Thus, intra-uterine development is often divided into an **embryonic period,** where all major organ systems are established, and a **fetal period,** which consists primarily of growth and organ refinement (see Chapter 18). Development of the organism does not stop with birth, however; organs continue to grow and mature at least until puberty and many tissues need continuous replenishment throughout life. Aging and death may therefore also be included the natural developmental process of the organism.

The embryonic period is initiated at **fertilization** when the **oocyte**, covered by the zona pellucida, is penetrated by the fertilizing spermatozoon resulting in the formation of the one-celled **zygote**, in which a **maternal pronucleus** (from the oocyte) and a **paternal pronucleus** (from the spermatozoon) develop (Fig. 2-1; see Chapter 5). At the first post-fertilization mitosis the zygote develops into the 2-cell **embryo**. These two, and subsequent early embryonic cells, are for a period referred to as **blastomeres**. During the initial mitotic divisions of blastomeres, the increase in the number is not accompanied by any increase in the volume; the overall volume of the embryo remains constant as

the size of the blastomeres halves with each division. Such unique cell divisions are referred to as **cleavages** (Chapter 6). Then, coincident with the cells having reached a certain minimal size through cleavage divisions, a phase of cell growth is introduced into the cell cycles, with daughter cells growing to approximately the size of the mother cell. This more constant cell size, together with abundant cell proliferation and deposition of extracellular material, then leads to an increase in the size of the embryo as a whole. Both cell proliferation and cell growth are principles of general cell biology and will not be dealt with in further detail in this book.

The blastomeres eventually form a small mulberry-like cluster of cells referred to as the **morula** (Fig. 2-1; see Chapter 6). Initially, the morula is characterized by bulging individual blastomeres; later, outer cells will adhere tightly to each other and form a more uniform surface of the morula. This process is referred to as compaction. The outer cells develop into the **trophectoderm**. Subsequently, during the process of **blastulation**, a fluid-filled cavity, the **blastocyst cavity**, develops inside the trophectoderm, and the inner cells, forming the **inner cell mass (ICM)**, gather at one pole of the embryo which is now known as a **blastocyst**. The trophectoderm will participate in placenta formation (see Chapter 9) while the ICM gives rise to the embryo proper. The blastocyst expands, hatches from the zona pellucida, and later, towards the end of blastulation, the ICM forms an internal and external cell layer, referred to as the **hypoblast** and **epiblast**, respectively, to establish the **bilaminar embryonic disc**. Formation of the disc is, in

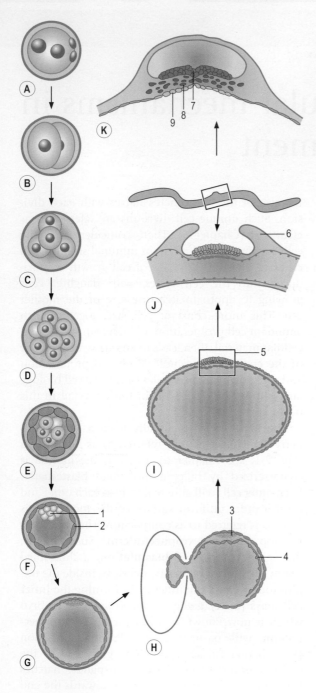

Fig. 2-1: Initial development of the mammalian embryo. A: Zygote; B: 2-cell embryo; C: 4-cell embryo; D: Early morula; E: Compact morula; F: Blastocyst; G: Expanded blastocyst; H: Blastocyst in the process of hatching from the zona pellucida; I: Ovoid blastocyst with embryonic disc; J: Elongated blastocyst; K: Embryonic disc in the process of gastrulation. 1: Inner cell mass; 2: Trophectoderm; 3: Epiblast; 4: Hypoblast; 5: Embryonic disc; 6: Amniotic folds; 7: Ectoderm; 8: Mesoderm; 9: Endoderm.

domestic animal species, associated with the removal of the trophectoderm covering the epiblast (see Chapter 6). Along with this, the overall shape of the embryo changes from spherical to ovoid and further to tubular and filamentous except in the horse. The time period from fertilization to completion of blastulation lasts about 10 to 12 days in pigs, sheep, goat, and cat, 14 days in cattle and horses, and 16 days in the dog.

During the subsequent phase of the embryonic period, the bilaminar embryonic disc is transformed into a **trilaminar embryonic disc**, through the process of **gastrulation** (Fig. 2-1; see Chapter 7). Gastrulation leads to formation of the three somatic germ layers, **ectoderm**, **mesoderm** and **endoderm**, and formation of the **primordial germ cells**, the progenitors of the germ cell lineage. Early during the process of gastrulation, a portion of the trophectoderm located around the embryonic disc, together with its underlying extra-embryonic mesoderm, forms amniotic folds that finally fuse and enclose the disc in the **amniotic cavity**.

Following gastrulation, the three somatic germ layers further differentiate into various cell types and finally form the outline of most organ systems, thereby defining the end of the embryonic period (Fig. 2-2). The increasing number of cell types derived from the initial three somatic cell lineages formed during the process of gastrulation obviously requires intricate regulation of cell behaviour and organization of cells in order to create a complete organism with its many different, but interdependent, tissues and organs. Different mechanisms

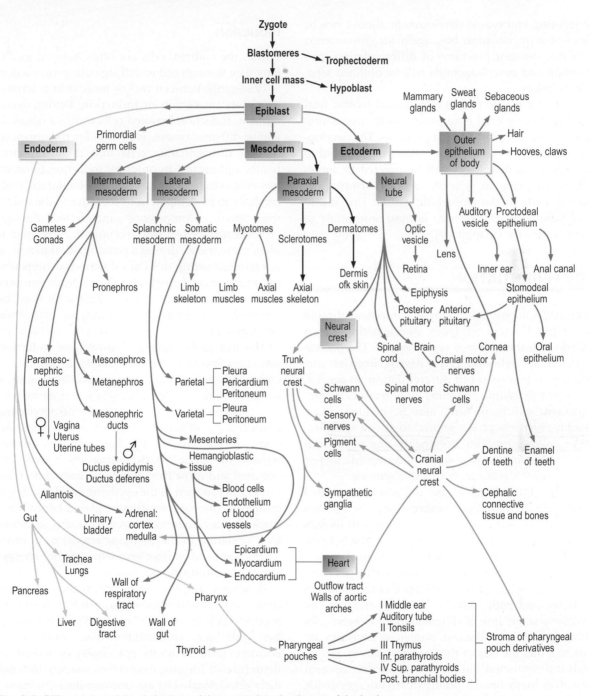

Fig. 2-2: Differentiation of the derivatives of the zygote into the tissues of the body.

regulating embryonic development should not be looked at in isolation but, again for convenience, the concomitant processes of **differentiation**, **patterning** and **morphogenesis** will be outlined separately below.

The embryonic period is followed by the **fetal period**, lasting until term, with growth, maturation and remodelling of the organ systems. The development of each organ system, collectively referred to as 'special embryology', will be covered in subsequent chapters. In general, most embryonic loss occurs early in the embryonic period. This is also the time when the embryo is most susceptible to teratogens (see Chapter 19).

DIFFERENTIATION

The adult mammalian body is composed of more than 230 different cell types, all originating from a single cell, the fertilized egg or zygote. The process whereby specialized cell types develop from less specialized is known as **cell differentiation**. In general, an event preceding cell differentiation is **cell commitment** which, in turn, may be divided into a labile, reversible phase referred to as **cell specification** followed by an irreversible one called **cell determination**. Once a cell is 'determined', its fate is fixed and it will irrevocably differentiate.

Cell differentiation is ultimately regulated through **differential gene expression**. Like a stream running down the side of a mountain with its flow branching many times before it reaches the bottom, so do embryonic cells differentiate from common origins to gradually form specialized cell types (Figs. 1-4, 2-2). And just as a leaf dropped onto the stream follows one path only, so does a particular cell follow a single line of differentiation. However, for both the leaf and the cell, numerous decisions are taken along the way to the final destination. Hence, cell differentiation during embryonic development involves many branch points where lineages divide and sequential decisions on differentiation are taken. As outlined above, these decisions are at first reversible (cell specification), but later become irreversible (cell determination).

Induction

Within the embryo, cells are often induced to differentiate through cell-to-cell signalling. Interaction at close range between two or more cells is termed proximate interaction or **induction**. During development, induction between cells within a tissue, or within different tissues, is pivotal for the organization of differentiating cells into their respective tissues and organs. In order for induction to occur, however, cells to be induced (the potential responders) have to be **competent** or receptive to the inductive signals. Competence, manifested through expression of cell-surface receptors for example, is often present only during a certain critical period. If not induced within this critical period, a competent cell may undergo programmed cell death, **apoptosis,** instead of differentiation. Apoptosis is to be regarded as a normal mechanism of embryonic development.

The first embryologist to investigate induction was Hans Spemann (see Chapter 1). In amphibian embryos, he noted that lens formation in the surface ectoderm was achieved only when a close interaction between the optic vesicle from the developing brain and the surface ectoderm was allowed to occur (Fig. 2-3; see Chapter 11). Spemann was able to remove the optic vesicle before this interaction occurred and show that, as a consequence, no lens-formation was seen in the overlying ectoderm. Interestingly, if the optic vesicle was placed beneath the trunk surface ectoderm, it was not possible to induce lens formation in the overlying ectoderm. In other words, the trunk surface ectoderm was not competent for lens induction.

Another example of induction is the generation of the nervous system through the induction of neuroectoderm (Fig. 2-4, see Chapter 8). Early ectodermal cells may either differentiate into surface ectoderm (and thence the epidermis), or neuroectoderm (thence forming the nervous system). Initially, early ectodermal cells are uncommitted (or naïve) and competent to differentiate in either direction. However, signals from the notochord (an important midline structure in vertebrate species appearing during gastrulation; see Chapter 7) induce overlying

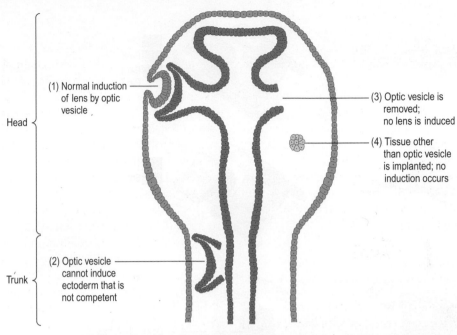

Fig. 2-3: Induction of lens formation as studied by Hans Spemann. Under normal circumstances, the neural ectoderm of the optic vesicle induces lens formation in the competent surface ectoderm of the head (1). An ectopically placed optic vesicle cannot induce lens formation in incompetent ectoderm of the trunk (2). If the optic vesicle is removed, no lens formation is induced (3). Other tissues transplanted beneath the competent surface ectoderm of the head do not induce lens formation (4).

ectodermal cells to differentiate into neuroectoderm. In particular the signalling molecule known as Sonic hedgehog (Shh) is pivotal in this process. Ectodermal cells outside the embryonic midline receive no inductive signals and form surface ectoderm by default. Experiments have shown that: if the notochord is removed, only surface ectoderm will form; placing notochordal tissue outside the embryonic midline will induce the formation of neuroectoderm instead of surface ectoderm; and midline ectoderm removed from the influence of underlying notochord will form surface ectoderm. This example illustrates the fact that during cell specification the fate of cell differentiation can be altered by changing the position of the cell within the embryo. Once cell determination has occurred, this plasticity is lost.

Signalling molecules, such as Sonic hedgehog, that act between cells within a close range are referred to as paracrine factors or **morphogens**. Many of these, involved in induction, are also involved in embryonic cell patterning (see below). Four major families of these signalling molecules are particularly important:

- The **Fibroblast Growth Factor (FGF) family**, which includes more than 20 related proteins.
- The **Hedgehog family**, including proteins encoded by the *Sonic hedgehog (Shh), Desert hedgehog (Dhh),* and *Indian hedgehog (Ihh)* genes.
- The **Wingless (Wnt) family**, containing at least 15 members, all of which interact with transmembrane receptors known as Frizzled proteins.
- The **Transforming Growth Factor-β (TGF-β) superfamily**, which includes at least 30 molecules with members such as the **TGF-β**, **Activin**, and **Bone Morphogenetic Protein (BMP)** families as well as the proteins **Nodal, Glial-Derived Neurotrophic Factor (GDNF), Inhibin,** and **Müllerian Inhibitory Substance (MIS).**

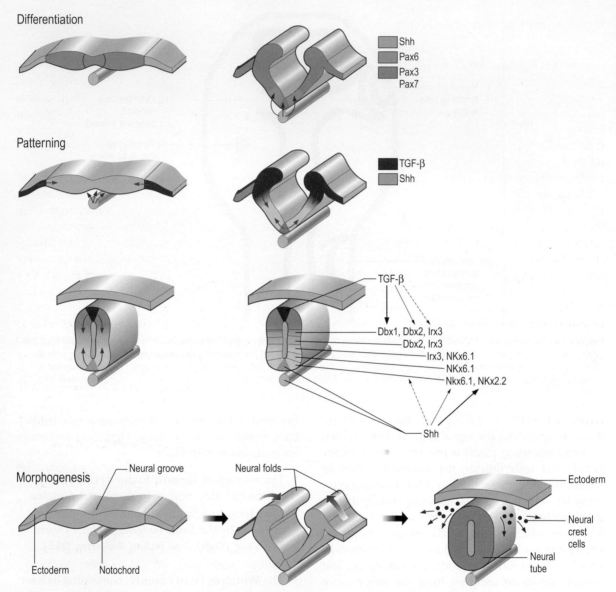

Differentiation

	Shh
	Pax6
	Pax3
	Pax7

Patterning

| | TGF-β |
| | Shh |

TGF-β

Dbx1, Dbx2, Irx3
Dbx2, Irx3
Irx3, NKx6.1
NKx6.1
Nkx6.1, NKx2.2

Shh

Morphogenesis

Neural groove

Neural folds

Ectoderm

Neural crest cells

Ectoderm   Notochord

Neural tube

Fig. 2-4: The initial development of the nervous system as an example of differentiation, patterning, and morphogenesis. **Differentiation**: Sonic hedgehog (Shh) secreted from the notochord induces formation of the overlying neuroectoderm. Already during induction, a gradient of this molecule is involved in determining the structure of the neural tube by a rough **patterning** into dorso-ventral zones by expression of the transcription factors Pax 6 (ventrally) and Pax 3 and 7 (dorsally). **Patterning**: Shh from the notochord (as already mentioned) and TGF-β from the surface ectoderm is involved in the rough dorso-ventral patterning of the neural tube resulting in further generations of transcription factors controlling the finer patterning of different layers of afferent (dorsal) and efferent (ventral) neurons. **Morphogenesis**: The change in shape from the flat neural plate into a neural tube is caused by the formation of hinge points where cells become apically constricted and proliferation of the surface ectoderm at the margins of the neural plate pushes the sides together. Neural crest cells leave the neural tube at the hinge point to form other structures. Modified from Strachan and Read (2004).

Cellular and genomic potency

The zygote and the first few generations of blastomeres have equal **developmental potential**, or **potency**. In fact, each of these cells is individually able to give rise to all cells of the embryo proper as well as the cells forming extra-embryonic membranes and the embryonic part of the placenta. This cell characteristic is referred to as **cellular totipotency**. In domestic animal species, cellular totipotency was first shown in sheep by the Danish scientist, Steen Willadsen. He isolated blastomeres of early cleavage stage ovine embryos and from them was able to produce twins and quadruplets upon transfer to surrogate mothers. In a figurative sense, cellular totipotency corresponds to the beginning of the stream in Fig. 1-4. Soon, however, branching begins and the embryonic cells become more and more restricted in their developmental potential (i.e. they lose potency). As described earlier in this chapter, subpopulations of embryonic cells, i.e. the ICM and the epiblast, retain the ability to form all tissues of the embryo proper, but lose the competence to form extra-embryonic tissues. This restricted characteristic is referred to as **pluripotency**. Embryonic stem (ES) cell experiments, though, have challenged this concept by indicating that ES cells, which are in vitro descendants of the ICM, can actually form trophectoderm.

The production by Wilmut and colleagues in 1996 of the cloned sheep, Dolly, by introduction of a differentiated mammary gland cell into an oocyte from which the genome had been removed, demonstrated that even a differentiated cell possesses some kind of totipotency (see Chapter 21). In this context it is important to distinguish between **cellular totipotency** and **genomic totipotency**. Thus, the zygote and the early blastomeres possess cellular totipotency because they are each able in themselves to give rise to both the embryo proper and all extra-embryonic tissues. The mammary gland cell, on the other hand, possessed genomic totipotency; the cell could form all the tissues but only with the aid of the cytoplasmic apparatus and genomic reprogramming provided by the oocyte cytoplasm.

Following gastrulation (see Chapter 7), pluripotency remains in the germ line only, as the remaining embryonic cells differentiate into one of the three principal germ layers: the ectoderm, mesoderm or endoderm. Cells within each of these somatic germ layers are considered **multipotent** and, in general, have different developmental potentials. Eventually, cells within each germ layer give rise to **unipotent** tissue-specific progenitor or precursor cells (in classical histology known by the suffix: -blasts) capable of producing single types of differentiated cells only. The male germ line, at least in mice, may, however, harbour pluripotent stem cells as long as spermatogenesis continues. In general, though, the cells within a given lineage eventually reach a stage of differentiation where they have fully matured and no longer divide; they are **terminally differentiated**. In order to maintain some regenerative capacity in organs and tissues, however, a few cells have been found to stay plastic, forming a pool of unipotent (or even multipotent) **somatic stem cells** from which cells can be recruited. The haematopoietic stem cells and the mesenchymal stem cells in adult bone marrow provide examples of somatic stem cells.

Molecular control of differentiation

At the molecular level, many complex pathways are involved in the decisions taken during cell differentiation. A couple of the key components operating during the process are:

- **Epigenetic (chromatin) changes.** Epigenetic changes result in stable (i.e. heritable) patterns of gene expression within descendant cells of any given lineage. As mentioned above, the genetic make-up (i.e. the combination of DNA sequences) is not changed during differentiation; all descendants of the zygote arise through mitotic divisions and are therefore expected to carry the same genomic information. One exception is development of lymphocytes where genetic rearrangements occur. However, several epigenetic mechanisms rigidly, and in a well-orchestrated manner, control how genes are sequentially expressed during embryonic development in order to control the differentiation pathways. The three most important mechanisms are: **DNA methylation**, by which the chromatin of some genome regions becomes highly condensed and transcriptionally inactive (see below); **histone modifications** including acetylation of histone proteins generally inducing a more open chromatin conformation allowing for transcription; and **Polycomb-trithorax gene regulation** (operating, for example, on the Hox genes described below), changing the chromatin structure into transcriptionally repressed (Polycomb) or active (trithorax) conformations. At least the processes of DNA methylation and histone modifications are linked, providing a powerful mechanism for long-term gene silencing.

- **Transcription factors.** The presence of a new, stable transcription factor activates expression of developmentally important genes. Throughout most of this book, some of the major transcription factors operating in various aspects of embryonic development are presented in molecular boxes. These include the master Hox genes described below.

PATTERNING

Patterning is the process whereby embryonic cells organize into tissues and organs. While differentiation gives rise to cells with specialized structure and function, this process alone does not form an organism; the differentiated cells need to be spatially organized in three dimensions and in well-defined relationships to each other. All mammalian embryos tend to follow basic body plans providing cranio-caudal, dorso-ventral and proximo-distal axes. The dorso-ventral axis is already present in the blastocyst with the ICM being positioned at one pole (see Chapter 6). Formation of the cranio-caudal axis comes with gastrulation (see Chapter 7), whereas the proximo-distal axis is delayed until limb formation (see Chapter 16).

Patterning is the consequence of **regional gene expression** which may be installed through the action of **gradients of signalling molecules**. Target cells closer to the signalling source receive signals in a higher concentration than do those located more distally. Signalling molecules working in this way are known as **morphogens**. At least the embryonic cranio-caudal and proximo-distal body axes are patterned using more or less known morphogenetic fields.

An example of patterning by regional gene expression controlled by gradients of signalling molecules is the formation of the neural tube (Fig. 2-4). Thus, Sonic hedgehog from the notochord (which is also active during the induction of the neuroectoderm) and TGF-β from the surface ectoderm are involved in a rough dorso-ventral patterning of the neural tube resulting in sequential generations of transcription factors controlling the finer patterning of different layers of afferent (dorsal) and efferent (ventral) neurons.

Homeobox genes

Another good example of regional gene expression resulting in patterning is provided by fruit fly homeotic genes, known as the **Homeobox (or Hox) genes** in mammals. In the fruit fly, *Drosophila melanogaster*, these genes were originally shown to provide cells a positional identity along the cranio-caudal axis. Artificially manipulating these genes resulted in altered development of whole body segments. In the Antennapedia mutant, for example, legs instead of antennae were observed to grow out of the head. Thus, homeotic genes were acting as high-level executives in the differentiation of cells within a whole region or segment. Analysing *Drosophila* mutants revealed two clusters of homeotic genes located on one chromosome encoding what are now known as homeodomain (referring to the DNA-binding motif) transcription factors. These genes were found to be expressed along the cranio-caudal axis, dividing the body into discrete zones (Fig. 2-5). Similar genes are found in mammals. In the mouse and humans, these Hox genes are grouped in four clusters, known as *Hox-A*, *Hox-B*, *Hox-C*, and

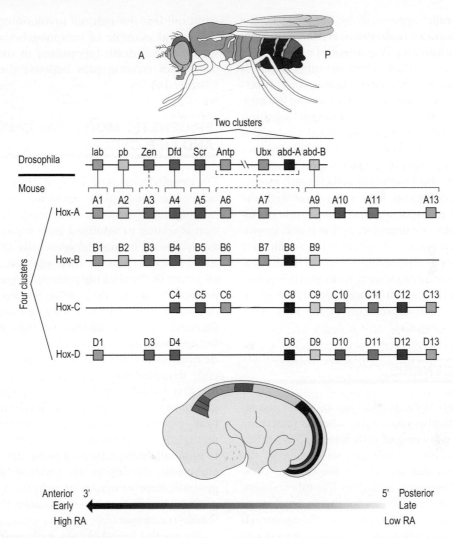

Fig. 2-5: Arrangement of the homeotic genes in *Drosophila* and the Hox genes in the mouse. Homology between the *Drosophila* genes and those in each cluster of the mouse is indicated by the colour code. A gradient of retinoic acid (RA) is involved in the definition of the 'Hox code'. Modified from Sadler (2006).

Hox-D, each located on its particular chromosome. It has turned out, in mice at least, that the Hox genes located in the 3′ end of each cluster are expressed first during development and control patterning of the anterior body parts, whereas genes located towards the 5′ end are expressed later and control formation of more posterior body parts. The earliest expression of Hox genes in mammals occurs during gastrulation starting with 3′ genes. Thus, in time and space, Hox genes appear to control the segmental development of the embryo from anterior to posterior. In contrast to what happens in *Drosophila*, the Hox genes in mammals are expressed in an overlapping pattern. Importantly, though, a particular combination of Hox genes from the four clusters expressed within each region along the body axis provides cells with a specific positional identity. This identity is known as the '**Hox code**'.

The 'Hox code' appears to be inducible by the exposure of pluri- or multipotent cells to a gradient of signalling molecules. A gradient of retinoic acid, or some of its immediate down-stream products, is likely involved in this process. During the process of gastrulation, involution of cells forming the mesoderm and endoderm occurs through organizer regions within the primitive streak extending forward from the posterior end of the epiblast (see Chapter 7). Each such organizer region imposes a 'Hox code' on the involuting cells. In the mouse, three organizer regions have been identified: the early-gastrula, mid-gastrula, and late-gastrula organizer regions. The late organizer region is also known as the primitive node. Together with an anterior signalling centre, the anterior visceral endoderm (AVE), the gastrula organizers form anterior-posterior gradients of signalling molecules. These gradients induce certain expressions of the Hox genes defining the 'Hox code'.

MORPHOGENESIS

Morphogenesis is the mechanism by which tissues and organs are shaped. Hence, whereas patterning results in the gathering of cells into regions for formation of organs, morphogenesis results in the overall and internal shaping of the organs. Thus, during morphogenesis, structures like tubes, sheets, and dense clumps of cells are formed in response to differential rates of cell proliferation, changes in cell size and/or shape, cell fusions and/or changes in cell adhesion properties, for example. The formation of the neural tube during neurulation is one example where local changes in cell shape and cell proliferation bring groups of distant cells together to form a new structure (Fig. 2-4; see Chapter 8). The change from a flat neural plate to a closed neural tube is caused by both formation of hinge points, where cells become apically constricted due to changes in cell shape, and by cell proliferation in the margins pushing the sides together. Another example of morphogenesis is found within the epiblast during the process of gastrulation: a single sheet of cells is converted into the three somatic germ layers and the

germ cell line through cell involution (see Chapter 7). A final example of morphogenesis is the programmed cell death (apoptosis) in the hand- and foot-plates creating gaps between the digits (see Chapter 16).

EPIGENETIC MODIFICATIONS AND LIFE CYCLES

DNA methylation is probably the best characterized epigenetic mechanism operating during animal development (Fig. 2-6). In general, DNA methylation is related to inhibited gene expression. In the newly formed primordial germ cells, DNA is highly methylated as it is in their epiblast progenitors. However, by the time the primordial germ cells have entered the genital ridge, DNA has become largely devoid of methylation. During subsequent gametogenesis, when oocytes and spermatozoa are formed from the primordial germ cell derivatives, **de novo methylation** of DNA occurs. This genome-wide demethylation and remethylation represents the **first round** of the so-called **epigenetic reprogramming** preparing for the development of the next generation. Importantly, sex-specific DNA methylation of particular loci occurs (later leading to monoallelic expression of particular genes during embryonic development), forming the basis of **genomic imprinting**. Apparently, the male gamete's genome becomes more methylated than does its female counterpart.

The **second round** of **epigenetic reprogramming** occurs following fertilization. In species such as the mouse, rat, pig and cattle, the paternal genome appears to be more labile than the maternal one and starts its active genome-wide DNA demethylation as early as in the zygote. Apparently, this does not apply to the sheep and rabbit. However, around the morula and early blastocyst stage, both parental genomes have become equally demethylated. Interestingly, and of importance for embryonic development, the methylated imprinted genes appear to escape this round of demethylation and remain methylated. Imprints are only erased and redefined during gametogenesis. The fact that the methylated

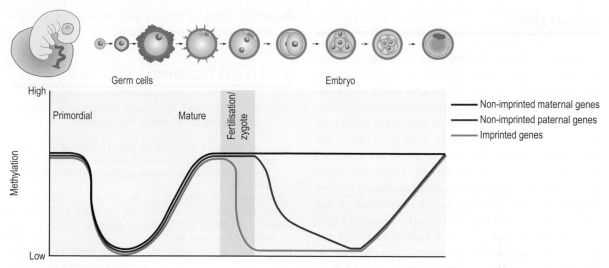

Fig. 2-6: Overall DNA methylation pattern. A first round of DNA demethylation and remethylation is seen during the development of gametes from the primordial germ cells in the embryo including the imprinted genes. A second round of demethylation and remethylation is seen after fertilization when the paternal genome is actively demethylated. At this second round of epigenetic reprogramming, the methylated imprinted genes escape demethylation. By the time of blastocyst development, the genome is remethylated. Modified from Dean et al. (2003).

imprinted genes maintain their sex-specific methylation allows for sex-specific monoallelic expression of these genes, which is of great significance for embryonic and, in particular, placental development. The second round of demethylation is soon followed by de novo methylation coinciding roughly with the blastomeres' differentiating into trophectoderm and the ICM. Curiously, the extent of methylation is, at least in some species, more pronounced in the pluripotent cells forming the ICM (and later the epiblast) than it is in those forming trophectoderm.

X-chromosome inactivation denotes the selective inactivation of alleles on one of the two X-chromosomes in females providing a mechanism for **dosage compensation** or functional hemizygosity for X-linked genes. Inactivated X-chromosomes may be visible as **Barr bodies**, condensed chromatin lying along the inside of the nuclear envelope in female mammals. The silencing process appears to be initiated by a single gene, *XIST*, being expressed on the inactivated X-chromosome only. *XIST* is one of the few known imprinted X-linked genes. The inactivation process starts during the period of de novo methylation in the second round of epigenetic reprogramming at the blastocyst stage. Within the ICM, inactivation of either the paternally- or maternally-derived X-chromosome occurs at random. However, in the trophectoderm the maternally-inherited allele of the *XIST* gene is preferentially repressed leading to inactivation of the paternal X-chromosome. This illustrates a general phenomenon known as the **parental genome conflict** or 'the battle of the sexes': there is a preference for expression of paternal genes in the trophectoderm and other extra-embryonic tissues and a preference for expression of maternal genes in the embryo-forming cells.

In primordial germ cells, which pass genes on to the next generation, genomic imprints have to be erased and inactivated X-chromosomes have to be reactivated to allow for activated X-chromosomes to be passed on to all gametes.

SUMMARY

Gestation includes **embryonic** and **fetal periods**. During the embryonic period, the **zygote** is produced at fertilization and cleavages result in the formation of the **morula**. Subsequently, the outer **trophectoderm** and the **inner cell mass (ICM)** are formed in the **blastocyst**. The ICM gives rise to the **hypoblast** and **epiblast** that establish the bilayered embryonic disc after hatching from the **zona pellucida**. The epiblast then embarks on the process of **gastrulation** resulting in the formation of the trilaminar disc with the three somatic germ layers (**ectoderm, mesoderm, and endoderm**) and the **primordial germ cells**. The germ layers combine in formation of organs. During the fetal period, which lasts until term, the organ systems grow, mature and become remodelled. Development is a gradual process regulated by several different processes including the general principles of **cell proliferation** and **growth** as well as the more developmentally-specific processes of cell differentiation, patterning and morphogenesis. **Cell differentiation** may be envisioned as involving sequential lineage decisions guiding the cells through reversible **specification** to irreversible **determination**. Cells may be induced to differentiate through cell-cell contact or through signalling molecules, morphogens. The differentiated cells are brought together in a three-dimensional interaction to form **tissues** and **organs** through the process of **patterning**. During patterning, morphogens may act in a more complex manner, producing gradients that result in differentiation of functionally different zones. Patterning operates through the activation of regional gene expression of which the mammalian Hox genes defining the cranio-caudal axis of the embryo is a good example. Final changes in overall form of tissues and organs are accomplished through **morphogenesis**.

FURTHER READING

Allegrucci, C., Thurston, A., Lucas, E. and Young, L. (2005): Epigenetics and the germline. Reproduction 129:137–149.

Dean, W., Santos, F. and Reik, W. (2003): Epigenetic reprogramming in early mammalian development and following somatic cell nuclear transfer. Cell Dev. Biol. 14:93–100.

Garcia-Fernàndez J. (2005): The genesis and evolution of the homeobox gene clusters. Nat. Rev. Gen. 6:881–892.

Gilbert, S.F. (2003): Developmental Biology, 7th edn. Sinauer Associates, Inc.

Gjørret, J.O., Knijn, H.M., Dieleman, S.J., Avery, B., Larsson, L.-I. and Maddox-Hyttel, P. (2003): Chronology of apoptosis in bovine embryos produced in vivo and in vitro. Biol. Reprod. 69:1193–1200.

Gjørret, J.O., Fabian, D., Avery, B.M. and Maddox-Hyttel, P. (2007): Active caspase-3 and ultrastructural evidence of apoptosis in spontaneous and induced cell death in bovine in vitro produced pre-implantation embryos. Mol. Reprod. Dev. 74:961–971.

Noden, D.M. and de Lahunta, A. (1985): The Embryology of Domestic Animals. Williams & Wilkins.

Pearson, J. C., Lemons, D. and McGinnis, W. (2005): Modulating Hox gene functions during animal body patterning. Nat. Rev. Gen. 6:893–904.

Robb, L. and Tam, P.P.L. (2004): Gastrula organiser and embryonic patterning in the mouse. Seminars in Cell & Developmental Biology 15:543–554.

Sadler, T.W. (2006): Langman's Medical Embryology, 10th edn. Lippincott Williams & Wilkins.

Strachan, T. and Read, A.P. (2004): Human Molecular Genetics, 3rd edn. Garland Science.

Swales, A.K.E. and Spears, N. (2005): Genomic imprinting and reproduction. Reproduction 130:389–399.

Wilmut, I., Schnieke, A.E., McWhir, J., Kind, A.J. and Campbell, K. (1997): Viable offspring from fetal and adult mammalian cells. Nature 385:810–814.

Young, L. and Beaujean, N. (2004): DNA methylation in the preimplantation embryo: The different stories of the mouse and sheep. Anim. Reprod. Sci. 82–83:61–78.

CHAPTER 3

Morten Vejlsted

Comparative reproduction

This chapter provides an introduction to the regulatory systems involved in reproduction, with a particular focus on the female and on the hormones of pregnancy that have such a direct bearing on embryology. For further details on more general reproductive physiology, especially in the male, readers are referred to textbooks listed at the end of the chapter.

PUBERTY AND THE OESTROUS CYCLE

The **endocrine** and **nervous systems** play interwoven roles in the cascade of events leading to the formation of mature gametes, fertilization, establishment and maintenance of pregnancy, birth and, finally, rearing of offspring. These processes begin at puberty. In the female, puberty is marked by the onset of regular cyclic activity in the ovary affecting behaviour and the entire genital system: the **oestrous cycle** in domestic animals.

The female reproductive system consists of the paired **ovaries**, in which the oocytes develop, and the **tubular genital tract** comprising the oviducts, uterus, vagina, and vestibulum (Fig. 3-1). The **oviduct** is divided into a wide funnel-shaped portion, the **infundibulum**, that receives the oocyte(s) at ovulation, a wide tubular portion, the **ampulla**, and a longer thin portion, the **isthmus**, connecting to the uterine horn. Fertilization is thought to occur at the transition between the ampulla and isthmus. The ovary, except in the mare, is found in the **ovarian bursa** – a cavity formed mainly by the mesosalpinx. In domestic animals

the **uterus** is bicornuate, comprising two **uterine horns**, the **uterine body**, and the **uterine cervix**. The uterine body is short in most species but relatively long in the mare. The cervix presents an **internal orifice** (or os) to the uterine body and an **external orifice** (os) to the **vagina**. The external orifice forms a prominent **portio vaginalis** in the ruminants and the mare. The **cervical canal** is bordered with longitudinal folds. Additional circular folds are found in ruminants and protrusions, the pulvini cervicales, lock into each other in the cervix of the sow. The opening of the urethra marks the transition between the vagina and the **vestibulum**, which is demarcated externally by the **vulva**. In the adult cow and mare, the ovaries and the uterus can easily be manipulated by rectal palpation, a method widely used for assessment of the reproductive status of the ovaries, particularly in cattle. In the mare, and to a lesser extent in other species, ovarian status and initiation of pregnancy can be readily assessed using transrectal ultrasound scanning.

Before puberty, the initial development of the female gametes, the **oocytes**, enclosed in their **ovarian follicles**, is regulated more or less autonomously. However, as will be explained in Chapter 4, such pre-pubertal oocytes never reach a stage of development at which they are ready for fertilization. After the onset of puberty, however, signals provided by certain regions in the brain, including the pineal gland, hypothalamus and the pituitary gland, allow for production of fertilizable oocytes. From the anterior pituitary gland, the gonadotropins (i.e. hormones stimulating cells within the gonads) **FSH** (follicle-stimulating hormone) and **LH** (luteinizing hormone) are released. This release

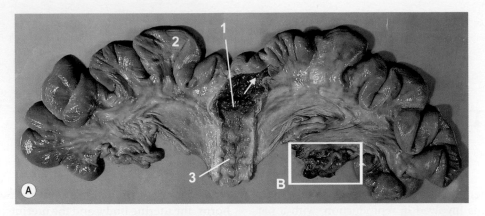

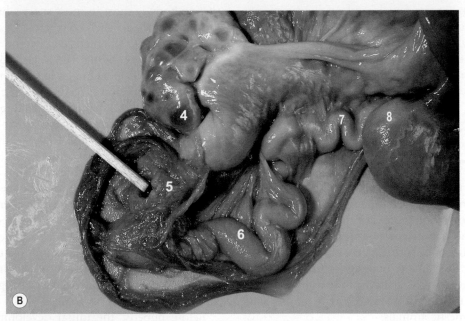

Fig. 3-1: Dorsal aspect of the genital organs of the sow. The box 'B' in A is presented at a higher magnification in B. 1: Uterine body; 2: Uterine horn; 3: Pulvini cervicales; 4: Ovary with antral follicles; 5: Infundibulum; 6: Ampulla; 7: Isthmus; 8: Tip of uterine horn. The wooden stick points to the abdominal opening of the oviduct.

is controlled by **GnRHs** (gonadotropin-releasing hormones) that are secreted from the hypothalamus and conveyed to the anterior pituitary gland through the hypothalamo-hypophyseal portal blood circulation. Secretion of GnRHs, and thus of FSH and LH, is influenced by visual, olfactory, auditory and tactile stimuli from the environment and also by

homeostatic feedback systems within the animal. It is not until puberty that the central nervous system has matured sufficiently to allow the complex integration of all these inputs.

The onset of puberty precedes the development of physical maturity. Therefore, although the pubertal female is fertile (sexually mature and able to

Table 3-1: Age at puberty in common domestic animal species

Species	Age at puberty
Cattle	8–18 months
Horse	10–24 months
Swine	6–8 months
Sheep	6–15 months
Goat	4–8 months
Dog	6–20 months
Cat	5–12 months

Table 3-2: Characteristics of the different phases of the oestrous cycle and anoestrus.

Phase[1]	Characteristics
Prooestrus	The phase immediately preceding oestrus. The main hormones being produced in the ovary are oestrogens.
Oestrus	The period (under natural conditions) of acceptance of the male. Ovulation occurs during this phase in all domestic species, with the exception of the cow where it occurs shortly afterwards. The main hormones being produced in the ovary, in response to FSH and LH, are oestrogens.
Metoestrus	The phase succeeding oestrus when the male is no longer accepted. Period of corpus luteum formation. The main hormone being produced in the ovary is progesterone.
Dioestrus	The period of the mature, functional corpus luteum. The main hormone being produced in the ovary is progesterone.
Anoestrus	The prolonged phase of sexual rest interrupting oestrous cyclicity in some species. The reproductive system is mainly quiescent.

[1]*The phases of prooestrus and oestrus may collectively be referred to as the follicular phase and the phases of metoestrus and dioestrus may be referred to as the luteal phase.*

reproduce), her fecundity has not yet reached its maximum. Factors influencing the onset of puberty include age, body weight, breed, nutrition, disease and, in some species, season of the year and proximity of a male. The ages at which the common domestic species reach puberty are listed in Table 3-1.

FSH released from the pituitary gland reaches the ovary by the systemic circulation. In the ovary, it stimulates a pool of growing follicles to develop further (see Chapter 4). **Oestrogens**, which are produced in the granulosa and theca cells lining the follicle and surrounding the oocyte, exert a positive feedback on the hypothalamic GnRH secretion. Another principal effect of the oestrogens is to induce oestrous symptoms, and so puberty is often signalled by the occurrence of the first period of **oestrus** or **heat** (sexual receptivity). After puberty, the animal enters a phase of life characterized by repeated **oestrous cycles**. The oestrous cycle is subdivided into prooestrus, oestrus, metoestrus, and dioestrus (Tables 3-2, 3-3).

In most species, the increasing levels of oestrogens produced in the ovarian follicles during **prooestrus** reach a certain threshold level that leads to a major surge of GnRH being secreted by the hypothalamus during oestrus. On reaching the anterior pituitary gland, the GnRH stimulates a secretory **surge of mainly LH** (Fig. 3-2; Table 3-4). In the ovary, LH is needed to bring about the final maturation of the oocyte(s) (see Chapter 4) and their release through the process of **ovulation**. Among the domestic animal species, the cat (and the camel) is unique in that the GnRH surge leading to ovulation is induced by copulation. Furthermore, the queen may continue displaying oestrous behaviour and accept the male even after having entered metoestrus (see below).

Following ovulation, the cells that lined the follicle before its rupture become transformed into a **corpus luteum** (plur. corpora lutea), under the

Table 3-3: Characteristics of the oestrous cycle and time of ovulation in domestic animal species.

Species	Cycle length	Duration of oestrus	Time of ovulation
Cattle	21 (18–24) days[1]	4–24 hours	12 (10–15) hours after end of oestrus
Horse	21 (18–24) days[2]	3–9 days	24–48 hours before end of oestrus
Swine	21 (18–24) days[1]	2–3 days	38–48 hours after onset of oestrus
Sheep	17 (14–19) days[2]	18–72 hours	18–20 hours after onset of oestrus
Goat	19–21 days[2]	22–60 hours	Near the end of oestrus
Dog	Monocyclic (up to 2 months)	9 days	1–2 days after onset of oestrus
Cat	14–21 days[2]	4–10 days[3]	Induced ovulation

[1]Non-seasonal polycyclic; [2]seasonally polycyclic; [3]4 days if ovulation is induced.

continued influence of LH, during **metoestrus**. The development of the corpus luteum (or corpora lutea) begins gradually a few hours before ovulation and is marked by the synthesis of progesterone, instead of oestrogens, by the follicular cells. The corpus luteum formed by these cells after ovulation is a well-defined, sometimes slightly cavitated, spherical structure, named for its yellowish colour in cattle. During **dioestrus**, the production of progesterone by the corpus luteum reaches its maximum. The principal roles of progesterone are: first, to exert a negative feedback on the hypothalamus, inhibiting GnRH release and, therefore, new recruitment of oocytes for ovulation; and, second, to prepare the endometrium for pregnancy. If insemination and conception occur, progesterone is the principal hormone responsible for the maintenance of pregnancy. In the non-pregnant animal (excluding the cat and the dog) the life span of the corpus luteum is relatively short; in the absence of an embryo within the uterus, the endometrium releases prostaglandin-$F_{2\alpha}$ leading to **luteolysis** (regression of corpus luteum). The consequent decline in progesterone results in removal of the progesterone block on the hypothalamic GnRH secretion and allows for resumption of the oestrous cycle.

In the pregnant uterus, endometrial prostaglandin-$F_{2\alpha}$ release into the blood stream is blocked, leading to persistence of the corpus luteum. This inhibition of prostaglandin release is a component of '**maternal recognition of pregnancy**' which depends on species-specific signals produced by the embryo(s) and recognized by the endometrium (Table 3-5; see Chapter 9). In the dog and cat, the uterus appears to have no effect on the lifespan of corpus luteum and the mechanisms leading to its regression in these species are not yet elucidated. In the dog, the corpus luteum may remain functional for up to two months. Later in pregnancy, progesterone is also produced in the placenta (see Chapter 9), rendering the corpus luteum more or less superfluous in some species.

The domestic breeds of pigs and cattle are **non-seasonal polycyclic** animals, meaning that sows and cows experience recurring cyclic activity throughout the year, interrupted only by pregnancy, lactation or pathological conditions.

In contrast, the mare, ewe, doe and queen are **seasonally polycyclic**; their cyclicity is profoundly influenced by the amount and timing of light. Perception of altering daylight is mediated by the pineal gland which, through the synthesis of melatonin and other hormones, influences hypothalamic GnRH release. The mare is a 'long-day' breeder, meaning that the period with the highest cyclic activity is from spring to autumn in most individuals. During the winter, the mare will normally become anoestrous. Likewise, the queen is

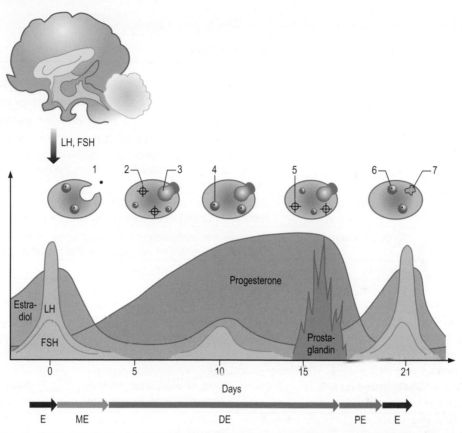

Fig. 3-2: Ovarian events and blood plasma concentrations of reproductive hormones through the oestrous cycle in the cow. During oestrus (E), the production of oestrogens from the developing follicles result in the release of a surge of LH and, to a minor extent, FSH from the pituitary gland which stimulate ovulation of the oocyte (1). The non-ovulated follicles undergo atresia (2) whereas the follicle cells of the ovulated follicle develop into the corpus luteum (3) secreting progesterone. A new wave of follicles develops (4), but undergoes atresia (5). Yet another wave of follicles produces the ovulatory follicle (6) for the next oestrus. If the ovulated oocyte does not result in pregnancy, prostaglandin released from the endometrium causes regression of the corpus luteum and eventual formation of a corpus albicans (7). The oestrous cycle is divided into oestrus (E), metoestrus (ME), dioestrus (DE), and prooestrus (PE).

anoestrous in the autumn and begins her cyclic activity with increasing daylight. Small ruminants, on the other hand, are 'short-day' breeders, exhibiting cyclic activity during autumn and early winter, followed by a period of anoestrus.

The bitch is **monocyclic** and experiences long periods of anoestrus between single periods of oestrus. Normally, one or two (sometimes three) oestrous periods are seen per year separated by longer anoestrous periods with no obvious seasonality.

HORMONAL MAINTENANCE OF PREGNANCY

The source of progesterone, the main hormone responsible for maintenance of pregnancy, varies between the species. In cattle the main source is the corpus luteum during the first half of gestation, but the placenta from around Day 120–150 up to Day 250. In the horse, several accessory corpora lutea form during the second month of pregnancy and,

Table 3-4: Important reproductive hormones, their origin and main function

Hormone	Origin	Main function
Melatonin	Pineal gland	Responsible for seasonality in the horse, sheep, goat and cat.
GnRH	Hypothalamus	Stimulates FSH and LH release from the anterior pituitary gland.
FSH	Anterior pituitary gland	Stimulates development of the follicles within the ovary.
LH	Anterior pituitary gland	Stimulates development and maturation of the follicles and oocytes, induces ovulation, and sustains formation and maintenance of corpus luteum within the ovary. Induces oestrous symptoms.
Oestrogen	Ovarian follicle	Stimulates the GnRH secretion of the hypothalamus and the number of GnRH receptors in the anterior pituitary gland.
Progesterone	Corpus luteum	Prepares the endometrium for pregnancy, maintains pregnancy, and decreases GnRH release from the hypothalamus.
Prostaglandin $F_{2\alpha}$	Uterus	Induces regression of corpus luteum.

Table 3-5: Gestational length, time of maternal recognition of pregnancy, and average number of offspring in domestic animal species

Species	Gestational length	Time of maternal recognition of pregnancy	Average number of offspring
Cattle	9 months (279–290 days)	Days 16–17	1
Horse	11 months (310–365 days)	Days 6–17	1
Swine	115 days	Day 12	8–16
Sheep	5 months (144–152 days)	Days 12–13	1–3
Goat	5 months (144–151 days)	Day 17	1–3
Dog	63 (58–68 days)	[1]	3–12
Cat	62 (58–65 days)	[1]	3–6

[1]Mechanisms underlying maternal recognition of pregnancy in the dog and cat are poorly understood, but probably do not depend on signals from the conceptus.

together with the original or 'primary' corpus luteum, produce progesterone until the end of the third month. Thereafter, the placenta takes over until term. In the ewe, corpora lutea are the major source during the first one-third of pregnancy, but are replaced by the placenta thereafter. In pigs, goats, dogs and cats, corpora lutea are the major source of progesterone throughout gestation.

Production of progesterone by the corpus luteum in the absence of pregnancy is most pronounced in the queen and the bitch where, as explained above, the non-pregnant uterus does not induce prostaglandin-mediated luteolysis. Most bitches experience pseudopregnancy with (overt) or without (covert) clinical signs during the metoestrous and dioestrous periods. Another pituitary gland hormone, prolactin, is probably responsible for this phenomenon. In the queen, corpora lutea also persist for a prolonged period in the absence of pregnancy. However, during the season of cyclic activity, the queen returns to oestrus. Mechanisms regulating the lifetime of the corpora lutea in the dog and cat are not clear.

SUMMARY

The **female genital organs** comprise the **ovaries**, **oviducts**, **uterus** (subdivided into horns, body and cervix), **vagina** and **vestibulum**. At **puberty** the female enters the **oestrous cycle** consisting of **prooestrus**, **oestrus**, **metoestrus** and **dioestrus**. The cow and the sow are **non-seasonal polycyclic**, the mare, ewe, doe, and queen are **seasonal polycyclic**, and the bitch is **monocyclic**. In seasonal polycyclic and monocyclic species, the cyclicity is interrupted by longer periods of **anoestrus**. In prooestrus, developing antral follicles synthesize **oestrogens** that stimulate release of a preovulatory surge of **LH** (luteinizing hormone) and to some degree **FSH** (follicle stimulating hormone) during the subsequent oestrus, which is characterized by acceptance of the male. The LH surge stimulates maturation of the oocyte and follicle, culminating in one or several **ovulations**, depending on the species. During the subsequent metoestrus, the ovulated follicle(s) develop into one or more **corpora lutea** that synthesize **progesterone**, the hormone responsible for preparing the uterus for pregnancy. Progesterone production reaches its maximum during dioestrus. If pregnancy is established, the corpus luteum/corpora lutea remain(s) functional, but if conception fails, release of **prostaglandin-$F_{2\alpha}$** from the endometrium causes regression of the corpus luteum/corpora lutea (luteolysis) and a return to prooestrus.

FURTHER READING

Allen, W.R. (2005): Maternal recognition and maintenance of pregnancy in the mare. Anim. Reprod. 2:209–223.

Arthur's Veterinary Reproduction and Obstetrics 2001, 8th edn. Noakes, D.E., Parkinson, T.J. and England, G.C.W. eds. W. B. Saunders.

Concannon, P., Tsutsui, T. and Shille, V. (2001): Embryo development, hormonal requirements and maternal responses during canine pregnancy. J. Reprod. Fert. Suppl. 57:169–179.

Denker, H.-W., Eng, L.A. and Hammer, C.E. (1978a): Studies on the early development and implantation in the cat. II. Implantation: Proteinases. Anat. Embryol. 154:39–54.

Denker, H.-W., Eng L.A., Mootz, U. and Hammer, C.E. (1978b): Studies on the early development and implantation in the cat. I. Cleavage and blastocyst formation. Anatomischer Anzeiger 144:457–468.

Engel, F., Klein, R., Baumgärtner, W. and Hoffmann, B. (2005): Investigations on the expression of cytokines in the canine corpus luteum in relation to dioestrus. Anim. Reprod. Sci. 87:163–176.

Evans, H.E. and Sack, W.O. (1973): Prenatal development of domestic and laboratory mammals: Growth curves, external features and selected references. Anat. Histol. Embryol. 2:11–45.

Holst, P.A. and Phemister, R.D. (1971): The prenatal development of the dog: Preimplantation events. Biol. Reprod. 5:194–206.

Patten, B.M. 1948. Embryology of the pig. 3rd edn. Blakiston, New York.

Rüsse, I. and Sinowatz, F. (1998): Lehrbuch der Embryologie der Haustiere. 2. Auflage. Parey Buchverlag.

Senger, P. (2003): Pathways to pregnancy and parturition, 2nd edn. Current Conceptions, Inc.

CHAPTER 4

Gametogenesis

Poul Hyttel

At fertilization, the maternal and paternal genomes are united in the one-cell fertilized ovum, forming the **zygote**. In order to carry the two genomes to the site of unification in the oviduct, specialized cells known as the gametes have developed. The maternal gamete, the **oocyte**, is the largest cell of the body and has an inherent competence to initiate embryonic development once it has undergone a process known as activation, described under fertilization in Chapter 5. This particular ability of the oocyte is used biotechnologically, especially in cloning by nuclear transfer. Cloning involves removing the oocyte's own genome and then having its remaining cytoplasm initiate embryonic development based on the genome of a nuclear donor cell fused to the oocyte (see Chapter 21).

The paternal gamete, the **spermatozoon**, on the other hand, has developed an ability for motion and penetration of the oocyte's investments; it is these dynamic qualities of the spermatozoon that enable it to transport the paternal genome from the male to the female.

In the following we will focus on how these specialized gametes develop, how their genome is prepared for fertilization, and how the particular architecture of the cells is achieved. The first phase in this process involves the population of the developing gonad by **primordial germ cells** from which the germ cells develop. The subsequent process, by which the maternal and paternal gametes are produced from the primordial germ cells, is referred to as **gametogenesis.** Gametogenesis includes **meiosis**, to allow for recombination of genetic material and for reduction of the number of chromosomes from the diploid to the haploid complement, and **cytodifferentiation**, to achieve the cellular structure characteristic of the female or male gamete.

PRIMORDIAL GERM CELLS

The primordial germ cells are the predecessors of the female and male gametes. When the embryo differentiates into the somatic germ layers (ectoderm, mesoderm and endoderm) during the process of gastrulation (see Chapter 7), most cells lose their pluripotency (the ability to develop into all cell types of the mammalian body). However, one set of cells remains pluripotent. These are the **primordial germ cells** which, at least in the pig, first become recognizable in the posterior rim of the embryonic disc at gastrulation. From here they move into the newly formed mesoderm and endoderm (Fig. 4-1). A few days later, the primordial germ cells are found in the visceral mesoderm surrounding the yolk sac and the allantois outside the embryo proper. Presumably, the primordial germ cells are brought to this location outside the forming embryo in order to 'rescue' them from the differentiation signals driving gastrulation within the embryo proper. By the time the first somites are formed, the primordial germ cells can be found in the mesoderm of both the yolk sac and the allantois, but also in the mesoderm of the incipient genital ridge where they are ready to populate the developing gonad (Figs 4-2, 4-3, 4-4). Thus, actively

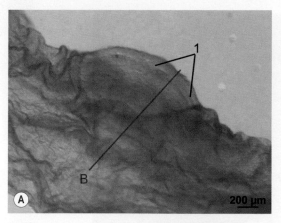
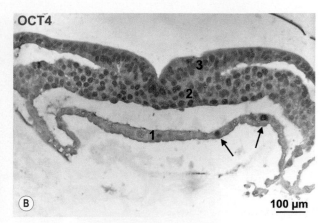

Fig. 4-1: Positioning of primordial germ cells in the endoderm. **A:** Embryonic disc of pig embryo at Day 14 of development. Note the primitive streak (1). The line 'B' indicates plane of section for Fig. 4-1B. **B:** Transverse section of the embryonic disc stained for Oct4. Note the individual Oct4 stained nuclei in the endoderm (1) identifying the primordial germ cells (arrows). 2: Mesoderm; 3: Ectoderm;.

Fig. 4-2: Migration of the primordial germ cells (red) from the yolk sac (1) along the yolk sac stalk (2) into the mesentery (4) of the primitive gut (3) and into the gonadal ridge (5) located medial to the mesonephros (6). 7: Allantois; 8: Urachus (allantois stalk). Courtesy Sinowatz and Rüsse (2007).

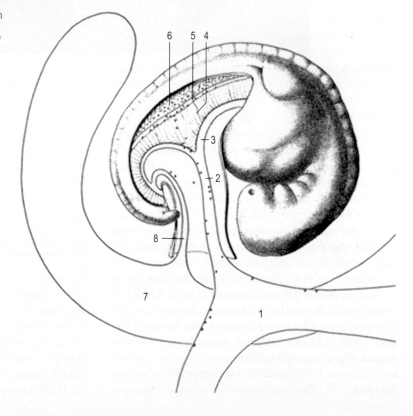

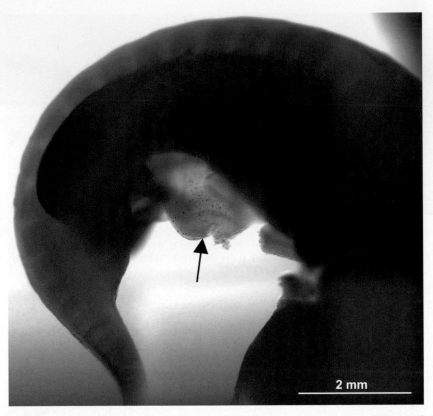

Fig. 4-3: Porcine embryo at Day 21 of development stained for OCT4. Note the primordial germ cells (small dark dots) in the stalk of the yolk sac (arrow) where they are returning to the embryo proper.

or passively, the primordial germ cells are brought along the caudal aspect of the yolk sac and the allantois into the primitive mesentery and then into the still undifferentiated, but developing, gonad. During their relocation, the primordial germ cells can be recognized by their relatively large size and by the use of special staining techniques such as those for alkaline phosphatase activity or the transcription factor OCT4 which is involved in maintaining cellular pluripotency (Figs 4-3, 4-4).

During and after their migration, the primordial germ cells proliferate by mitoses. The female (XX) and male (XY) primordial germ cells become engaged in sex-specific differentiation of the gonads and become surrounded by somatic cells (see Chapter 15). They are now referred to as **oogonia** and **spermatogonia**, respectively. These cells undergo further proliferation before they enter gametogenesis and, thus, meiosis.

THE CHROMOSOMES, MITOSIS AND MEIOSIS

The traits of a new individual are determined by specific **genes** identified as nucleotide sequences on the deoxyribonucleic acid (**DNA**). It is important to keep in mind that it is not the gene sequences themselves, but the balanced and controlled **expression** of genes controlled by epigenetic regulation that is crucial for the behaviour of the cells and, thus, for the development of the conceptus. Together with

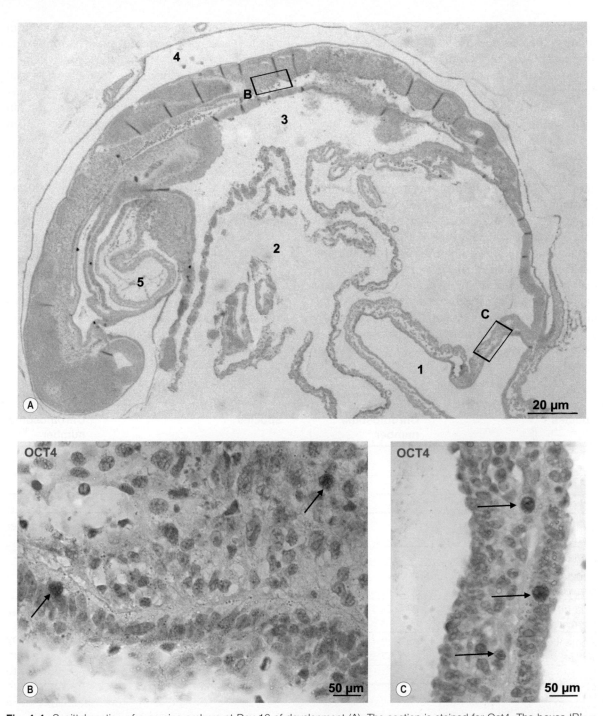

Fig. 4-4: Sagittal section of a porcine embryo at Day 16 of development (A). The section is stained for Oct4. The boxes 'B' and 'C' are enlarged. **B:** The nucleus of two primordial germ cells (arrows) located in the region of the developing gonadal ridge. **C:** The nuclei of three primordial germ cells (arrows) in the wall of the allantois (1). 2: Yolk sac; 3: Primitive gut; 4: Amniotic cavity; 5: Heart. Modified from Vejlsted et al. (2006). Reprinted with permission of John Wiley & Sons, Inc.

numerous proteins, DNA makes up the **chromosomes**. The chromosomes of an individual are inherited from the mother and the father. In humans, where the genes have been extensively mapped through the Human Genome Project (HUGO), it is estimated that there are about 25 000 genes on the 46 chromosomes. The number of functional genes in the domestic animals is probably similar.

In somatic cells, chromosomes appear as **homologous** pairs to form the **diploid** chromosome complement. The diploid chromosome number is designated 2n as it includes a maternal and a paternal copy of each chromosome. The diploid chromosome numbers in the domestic animals are listed in Table 4-1. One pair of chromosomes comprises the sex chromosomes, while the others are referred to as autosomes. If the sex chromosome pair is XX, the individual is genetically a female; if XY, genetically a male. One chromosome of each pair is inherited from the mother through the oocyte and the other from the father through the spermatozoon. Thus, in order to result in a normal diploid chromosome complement at fertilization, the gametes must contain only one chromosome from each pair, referred to as the **haploid** chromosome complement and designated 1n. Gametes, then, contain only half the number of chromosomes present in somatic cells.

Divisions of somatic cells occur through **mitosis** which transfers a copy of the full chromosome complement to each of the daughter cells. During gametogenesis, however, the special mechanisms of **meiosis** are responsible for producing the haploid chromosome complement in the germ cells.

Mitosis

Mitosis is the process whereby a cell divides its chromosome complement evenly between its daughter cells; **karyokinesis** describes the complete process, including mitosis, through which the nucleus of a

Table 4.1: Chromosome numbers in various animal species (Rüsse and Sinowatz, 1998)

Species	Chromosome number	Species	Chromosome number
Dog (*Canis familiaris*)	78	Sheep (*Ovis ammon aries*)	54
Wolf (*Canis lupus*)	78	Gorilla (*Gorilla gorilla*)	48
Hen (*Gallus gallus*)	78	Man (*Homo sapiens*)	46
Camel (*Camelus bactrianus*)	74	Rabbit (*Oryctolagus cuniculus*)	44
Lama (*Lama glama*)	74	Rat (*Rattus rattus*)	42
Reindeer (*Rangifer tarandus*)	70	Rhesus monkey (*Macca rhesus mulatta*)	42
Wild horse (*Equus przewalskii przewalskii*)	66	Mouse (*Mus musculus*)	40
Domestic horse (*Equus caballus*)	64	Pig (*Sus scrofa domesticus*)	38
Donkey (*Equus asinus*)	62	Cat (*Felis catus domesticus*)	38
Domestic cattle (*Bos primigenius taurus*)	60	European wild boar (*Sus scrofa*)	36
Bison (*Bison bison*)	60	Pigeon (*Columba livia*)	16
Goat (*Capra hircus*)	60		

cell gives rise to a nucleus in each of its daughter cells. Normally, karyokinesis is accompanied by **cytokinesis**, the division of the cytoplasm (including organelles and inclusions) between the daughter cells. Thus, karyokinesis and cytokinesis in combination give rise to two daughter cells that in principle are genetically identical to the parent cell, each receiving the complete diploid chromosomal complement (Fig. 4-5). Mitosis is one phase of the somatic cell cycle, the other phase being **interphase**. Interphase is subdivided into a gap phase 1 (G1), a DNA-synthetic phase (S) and a gap phase 2 (G2). During the S-phase, each chromosome replicates its DNA to produce two **chromatids**. As already mentioned, the diploid chromosome complement is referred to as 2n. Before the S-phase, each chromosome consists of a single DNA strand, and so each gene is present in two copies (2c), one of maternal and one of paternal origin. After the S-phase, because each chromosome now consists of two chromatids, each gene will be present in four copies (4c) although the chromosome number is maintained at 2n. During the G1-, S- and G2-phases the chromosomes are extremely long, spread through the nucleus in particular domains, and cannot be recognized with the light microscope.

Mitosis can be subdivided into pro-, meta-, ana- and telo- phases. When the cell moves from G2 of the interphase into the **prophase** of mitosis, the chromosomes coil, contract, condense and thicken (Fig. 4-5 B). They become visible with the light microscope and each can be seen to consist of two chromatids, joined at a narrow region known as the **centromere**. Also during the prophase, the **centriole pair** duplicates in the cytoplasm adjacent to the nucleus and the resultant two pairs become arranged at opposite poles of the nucleus. As the cell moves from pro- towards **metaphase** (a stage often referred to as pro-metaphase), microtubules starts to form from the two pairs of centrioles and the nuclear envelope begins to dismantle (Fig. 4-5 C). Some of the microtubules from each centriole pair then attach to structures on the chromatids, the **kinetochors**, that are found in the centromere of each chromosome. This establishes the **mitotic spindle** with a centriole pair at each pole. Other microtu-

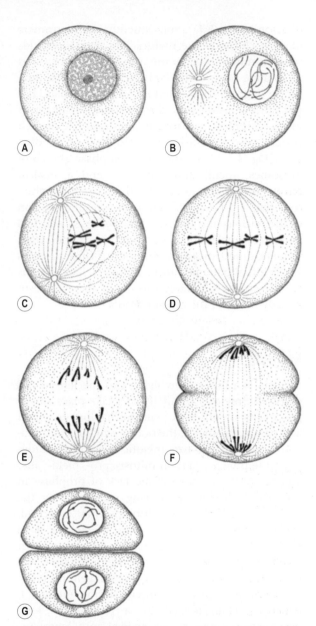

Fig. 4-5: Phases of mitosis: **A**: G2 of interphase; **B**: Prophase; **C**: Pro-metaphase; **D**: Metaphase; **E**: Anaphase; **F**: Telophase; **G**: Daughter cells in G1 of interphase. Courtesy Sinowatz and Rüsse (2007).

bules pass continuously from one centriole pair to the other without attaching to the chromosomes. As the spindle forms, the chromosomes line up in its equatorial plane, defining the metaphase of the cell division (Fig. 4-5 D). Subsequently, the centromere of each chromosome divides, the two chromatids separate and, pulled by the microtubules, they start to migrate towards the spindle poles during **anaphase** (Fig. 4-5 E). By this stage, each chromatid has transformed into a new chromosome. Arrangement of the chromosomes into two groups, one at each spindle pole, establishes the **telophase** of the division (Fig. 4-5 F). Further into telophase, the chromosomes uncoil and lengthen, and a nuclear envelope re-forms in each of the nascent daughter cells (Fig. 4-5 G). This event completes the division of the nucleus and its DNA (karyokinesis) into two daughter nuclei that contain the same DNA sequences and the same number of chromosomes as the initial parental nucleus (2n, 2c). Karyokinesis is followed by cytokinesis to divide the cytoplasm equally between the daughter cells.

Meiosis

Meiosis is a process involving two specialized cell divisions (meiosis I and II) that take place in the germ cells in order to generate haploid maternal and paternal gametes, the oocyte and the spermatozoon. Each of the two meiotic divisions includes the same phases as are in mitosis: pro-, meta-, ana- and telophase except for the lack of prophase in meiosis II. Besides producing gametes with the haploid complement of chromosomes, a second, and equally important, function of meiosis is to allow for **genetic recombination**; the process that ensures that the genome of the next generation will be a unique combination of parental genomes. The most complex processes occur during meiosis I, which is characterized by a particularly long prophase that can be subdivided into leptotene, zygotene, pachytene and diplotene stages, and diakinesis. It is beyond the scope of this text to address each of these substages beyond saying that they take their names from the morphological appearance of the chromosomes. As soon as the germ cell has initiated meiosis I the maternal one is referred to as a **primary oocyte** while the paternal equivalent is a **primary spermatocyte**. In the female, meiosis is ini-

tiated during fetal life, then becomes arrested at the **diplotene stage** of meiosis I until after puberty, and is only resumed shortly before ovulation. This prolonged duration of the diplotene stage is also known as the dictyate stage. In the male, on the other hand, meiosis is not initiated until after puberty but it then becomes a continuous process.

Crossover and genetic recombination

As in mitosis, maternal and paternal germ cells (oogonia and spermatogonia) undergo an S-phase before initiating meiosis. This forms two chromatids in each chromosome (2n, 4c) as in mitosis. This is the status of the germ cell when it enters the leptotene stage of the prophase of meiosis I (Fig. 4-6). In contrast to mitosis, however, the homologous chromosomes align in pairs during the prophase of meiosis I. Each chromosome pair therefore consists of four chromatids (4c) and is therefore referred to as a **tetrad**.

In the tetrad, each maternal chromatid becomes bound to its paternal counterpart over its full length by the **synaptonemal complex**. The chromatids match perfectly, point for point, in the female; so they do in the male, except for the XY-combination where the smaller Y-chromosome does not match the X-chromosome. This chromosome pairing allows for interchange of chromatid segments through a **crossover** process. The chromatids twist, or crossover, at certain points (the **chiasmata**) to form an X-like structure. Later during the prophase, the synaptonemal complex is gradually broken down, the DNA breaks in the chiasmata, and the free ends of the counterparts join up, thereby exchanging segments of DNA between maternal and paternal chromatids. This chromatin exchange, together with the random segregation of maternal and paternal chromosomes during meiosis II (see later), provide the molecular background for the genetic recombination that is characteristic of sexual reproduction.

During diakinesis, the homologous chromosomes are gradually released from each other. With the transition from diakinesis to metaphase of meiosis I, the nuclear envelope disappears and

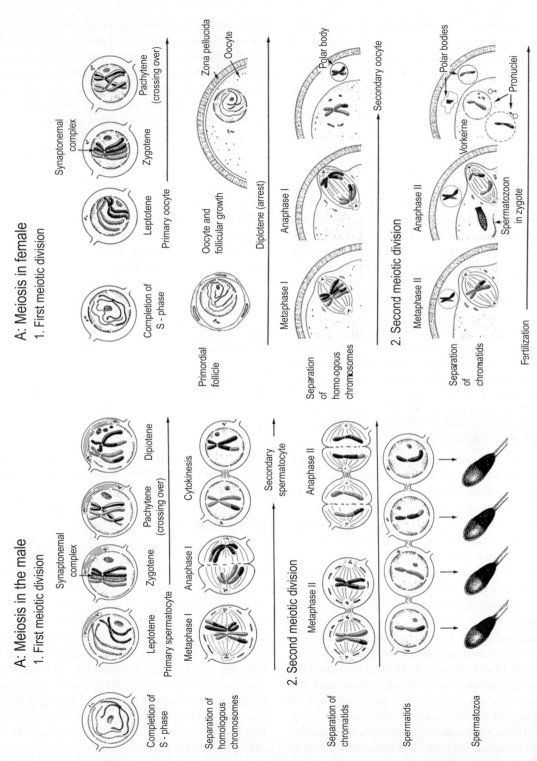

Fig. 4-6: Phases of meiosis in the male (**A**) and female (**B**). Courtesy Sinowatz and Rüsse (2007).

A: Meiosis in female
1. First meiotic division

Completion of S - phase · Leptotene · Zygotene · Pachytene (crossing over)

Synaptonemal complex

Primary oocyte

Primordial follicle · Oocyte and follicular growth · Diplotene (arrest)

Zona pellucida · Oocyte

Separation of homologous chromosomes

Metaphase I · Anaphase I

Polar body

Secondary oocyte

2. Second meiotic division

Separation of chromatids

Metaphase II · Anaphase II

Spermatozoon in zygote

Vorkerne · Pronuclei · Polar bodies

Fertilization

A: Meiosis in the male
1. First meiotic division

Completion of S - phase · Leptotene · Zygotene · Pachytene (crossing over) · Diplotene

Synaptonemal complex

Primary spermatocyte

Separation of homologous chromosomes

Metaphase I · Anaphase I · Cytokinesis

Secondary spermatocyte

2. Second meiotic division

Separation of chromatids

Metaphase II · Anaphase II

Spermatids

Spermatozoa

meiotic spindles are formed. In the male germ cell, the poles of the meiotic spindle are constituted by centriole pairs as during mitosis. However, in at least the large domestic species and in contrast to those of mice, the oocyte lacks centrioles and the spindle poles are made up by unknown material ultrastructurally recognizable as small clusters of vesicles. The microtubules of the spindle attach to each homologous chromosome in a tetrad in meiosis I instead of to the chromatids as they do in mitosis. During the metaphase of meiosis I the chromosomes align in the equatorial plane but, during anaphase, it is the homologous chromosomes, not their chromatids, that are pulled apart to become grouped at the poles of the spindle during telophase. Thus, in contrast to mitosis, meiosis I separates homologous chromosomes rather than chromatids. Upon completion of meiosis I, the germ cell is haploid, containing only one chromosome (1n) from each chromosome pair. It must be underlined, however, that the DNA content of the germ cell at this stage is still 2c because each chromosome consists of two chromatids.

Spermatocytes, spermatids, oocytes and polar bodies

At the end of telophase of meiosis I, the primary spermatocyte divides into two secondary spermatocytes by cytokinesis (Fig. 4-6). In the oocyte, however, the spindle is located at the periphery of the large spherical cell, and telophase is associated with a very uneven cytokinesis resulting in one of the two daughter cells being much larger than the other. The larger daughter cell is now referred to as a secondary oocyte while the small daughter cell, which is almost devoid of organelles, is the first polar body.

Immediately after completion of meiosis I, secondary oocytes and secondary spermatocytes initiate meiosis II without an interphase. Consequently, there is no S-phase, no DNA replication, and the chromosomes remain with the same amount of DNA (2c). The chromosomes also remain contracted, ready to progress directly through meta-, ana- and telophase of meiosis II without needing to go through a prophase. By telophase of meiosis II, the two chromatids of each chromosome have separated, and so each gamete receives only a single chromosome from each homologous pair (1n) containing a single DNA strand (1c). The secondary spermatocyte divides into two spermatids. The oocyte, on the other hand, again divides unequally giving rise to a large daughter cell, the precursor of the zygote and embryo, and a small second polar body. Moreover, in the oocyte, meiosis II becomes arrested in metaphase, the stage (M II) at which the oocyte is ovulated. Exceptions to this rule are found in the dog and the fox where the oocyte is ovulated in the prophase of meiosis I. In the large domestic species at least, the first and second polar bodies degenerate without dividing.

CYTODIFFERENTIATION OF THE GAMETES

While meiosis equips the gametes with the haploid chromosome number and allows for genetic recombination, there is a parallel need to construct the specialized cellular architecture that characterizes the two gametes. This cytodifferentiation forms oocytes from oogonia through oogenesis and spermatozoa from spermatogonia through spermatogenesis.

Oogenesis

Development of primordial follicles

After arriving and proliferating in the developing female gonad, the primordial germ cells become surrounded by follicular cells – flat somatic cells derived from the surface epithelium of the developing ovary (Fig. 4-7). This turns the primordial germ cells into oogonia that continue to proliferate, but without completing cytokinesis, leaving them attached to each other by narrow cytoplasmic bridges. The resultant clusters of oogonia derived from individual primordial germ cells can be identified in the embryo at stages of development that vary with species (Table 4-2).

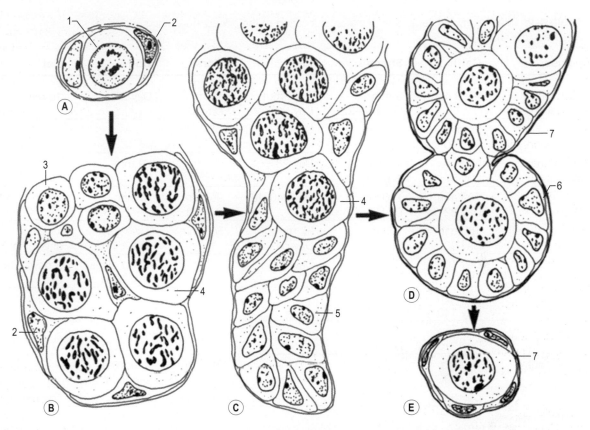

Fig. 4-7: The development of the primordial follicle. **A**: Primordial germ cell (1) surrounded by pre-follicle cells (2). **B**: Cluster of oogonia (3) and oocytes (4) associated with pre-follicle cells. **C**: Multiplication of pre-follicle cells (5). **D**: Development of the pre-follicle cells into follicle cells (6) surrounded by a basal lamina (7) and associated with individual oocytes. **E**: The final isolated primordial follicle. Courtesy Sinowatz and Rüsse (2007).

Most oogonia continue their mitotic proliferation but some differentiate into much larger **primary oocytes**. The latter immediately enter the S-phase of the cell cycle and then the prophase of meiosis I. Oogonia proliferate rapidly and in some species (notably the cow and human) are counted in millions (Table 4-3). However, this proliferation is followed by apoptosis which leads to most oogonia and primary oocytes being lost with only a small population near the surface of the developing ovary surviving. All surviving primary oocytes have entered the prophase of meiosis I when they become **arrested at the diplotene stage**, still with an intact nucleus. Covered by flat follicular cells, these oocytes form **primordial follicles** (Figs 4-8, 4-9, 4-10). The follicular cells rest on a basement membrane that separates them from the surrounding stromal cells. The primordial follicles constitute the pool of quiescent follicles from which the female will recruit follicles for growth and ovulation for the rest of her reproductive life. The numbers of primordial germ cells, oogonia and oocytes in various animal species and man are listed in Table 4-3.

Follicular and oocyte growth

Follicular growth occurs when follicles are recruited from the primordial pool and develop into

Table 4-2: Chronology of events during the differentiation of the gonad in various species (Rüsse and Sinowatz, 1998)

Species	Cattle	Sheep	Pig	Horse	Dog	Cat
[1]PGCs in the gonadal ridge	9–10 mm	8 mm Days 30–32	9–10 mm Day 20	12 mm Day 21	Day 28	10 mm
Differentiation of male gonad	25 mm Day 40	20 mm Day 31	Day 26	–	–	–
Development of oogonia	55 mm Day 57	46 mm Day 43	Day 28	–	29 mm	–
Onset of meiosis	125 mm Day 82	110 mm Day 55	Days 40–48	96 mm Day 73	At birth	Days 40–50
First primordial follicles	160 mm Day 90	150 mm Day 66	97 mm Day 64	305 mm	3 weeks after birth	11 days after birth
Last mitoses of oogonia	Day 160	Day 82	Day 100	–	15–17 days after birth	8 days after birth
First primary follicles	325 mm Day 140	255 mm Day 95	–	–	–	–
First secondary follicles	650 mm Day 210	320 mm Day 103	–	–	2 months after birth	–
First tertiary follicles	740 mm Day 230	500 mm Day 150	–	At birth	6 months after birth	–
Birth	Day 280	Day 150	Day 115	Day 336	Day 62	Day 63

[1]Primordial germ cells.

primary, secondary and tertiary follicles. It should be emphasized that the vast majority of follicles that enter a growth phase fail to complete it; most degenerate through a process referred to as **atresia** with only a minority completing their growth to the point of **ovulation**. At least in the large domestic species follicular growth is initiated during fetal life (Table 4-2). However, none of the oocytes enclosed in the follicles (except, perhaps, for some in atretic follicles) resume meiosis until puberty is reached.

Upon activation of the primordial follicle, the follicular cells start to proliferate and form a cuboidal monolayer around the oocyte to establish the **primary follicle** (Figs 4-8, 4-9, 4-10). The follicular cells are now referred to as **granulosa cells**. With this activation, a phase of **oocyte growth** is initiated in which the oocyte of the domestic species grows

from less than 30 μm to more than 120 μm in diameter. During this growth, the oocyte undergoes many morphological changes including the development of **cortical granules** (see below) in the cytoplasm. Furthermore, it becomes competent to both resume meiosis and sustain embryonic development after fertilization.

Granulosa cells proliferate to form several layers around the oocyte in what becomes known as the **secondary follicle** (Figs 4-8, 4-9, 4-10). The oocyte and the surrounding granulosa cells synthesize certain glycoproteins that are deposited between itself and the surrounding granulosa cells as the **zona pellucida**. This structure is traversed by numerous projections from the innermost granulosa cells which thereby maintain contact with the oocyte through gap junctions. The stromal cells surrounding the granulosa cells differentiate into an inner

Table 4-3: Numbers of oogonia and oocytes at various ages in different species (Rüsse and Sinowatz, 2000)

Species	Numbers of oogonia and/or oocytes
Cattle	Day 50: 16 000 Day 110: 2 700 000
Sheep	At birth: 54 000–1 000 000
Goat	6 months after birth: 24 000 3 years after birth: 12 000
Pig	Day 110: 491 000 10 days after birth: 60 000–509 000 9 months after birth: 50 000 2–10 years after birth: 16 000
Dog	At birth: 700 000 5 years after birth: 35 000 10 years after birth: 500
Man	Day 60: 600 000 Day 150: 6 800 000 At birth: 400 000–500 000 7 years after birth: 13 000

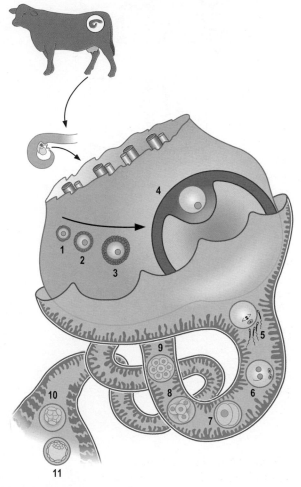

Fig. 4-8: Follicular development in the bovine ovary from the primordial (1) through the primary (2) and secondary (3) to the tertiary follicle (4). In the oviduct, the mature oocyte at the metaphase II (5), the fertilized zygote (6) presenting two pronuclei, the 2- (7), 4- (8), and 8-cell stage (9) are seen, and in tip of the uterine horn, the morula (10) and the blastocyst (11) are shown.

theca interna, a layer of steroid-producing cells, and the outer **theca externa**, made up of concentric layers of cells that have supportive functions. The steroidogenic cells of the theca interna and the granulosa cells are, together, responsible for the synthesis of estradiol in the follicle through a 'two-cell' system; the cells of the theca interna produce androgens that are transported to the granulosa cells where they are aromatized into oestrogens.

As development continues, fluid-filled spaces appear between the granulosa cells and coalesce into a single cavity, the **antrum,** characterizing the **tertiary follicle** (Figs 4-8, 4-9, 4-10). Such follicles are also referred to as antral follicles. In parallel with the expansion of the antrum, the oocyte becomes located in a protrusion of granulosa cells, **the cumulus oophorus**, extending into the antrum. The granulosa cells of the cumulus oophorus are referred to as **cumulus cells**. As the follicle develops, so does the oocyte until it achieves its characteristic structure. The process of ovulation is triggered by the preovulatory LH surge, but some evidence suggests that even before this stimulus the oocyte undergoes changes in the developing antral follicle that build up its competence to be fertilized and to support initial embryonic development. This process may be referred to as **oocyte capacitation**.

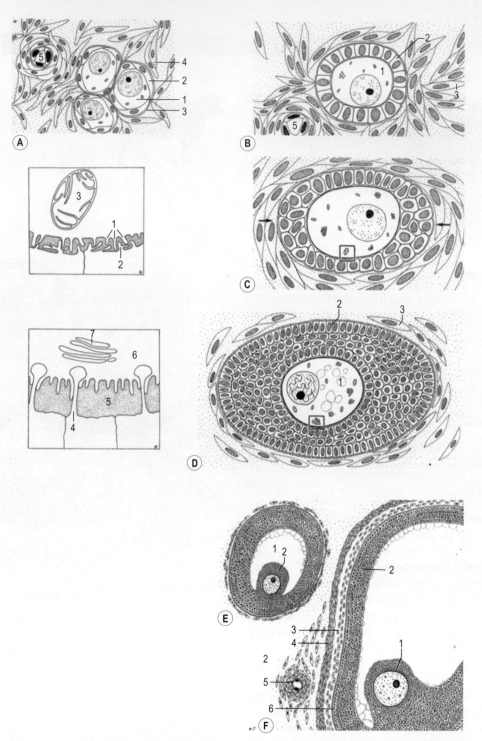

Fig. 4-9: Follicular development in cattle. **A:** Primordial follicle. The oocyte (1) is surrounded by flat follicular cells (2) resting on a basement membrane (3). 4: Stromal cell; 5: Arteriole. **B:** Primary follicle. The oocyte (1) is surrounded by cuboidal granulosa cells (2). **C:** Early secondary follicle in which polarization of the granulosa cell compartment has become evident (arrows). The insert shows a detail from the oocyte-granulosa cell interface with oocyte microvilli (1), granulosa cell projections (2). 3: Oocyte mitochondrion. **D:** Secondary follicle. The oocyte (1) is surrounded by a multilayered granulosa cell compartment (2), and the stromal cells have initiated the formation of the theca layers (3). The insert shows a detail from the oocyte-granulosa cell interface with granulosa cells projections (4) penetrating the developing zona pellucida (5). The granulosa cell projections form gap junctional contact with the oocyte (6). 7: Oocyte Golgi complex. **E:** Small tertiary follicle presenting the antrum (1) and the oocyte located in the cumulus oophorus (2). **F:** Large tertiary follicle presenting the oocyte in the cumulus oophorus (1) and the granulosa cell layer (2) surrounding the antrum. Theca interna (3) and externa (4) have differentiated and are separated from the granulosa cells by the basement membrane (6). Courtesy Sinowatz and Rüsse (2007).

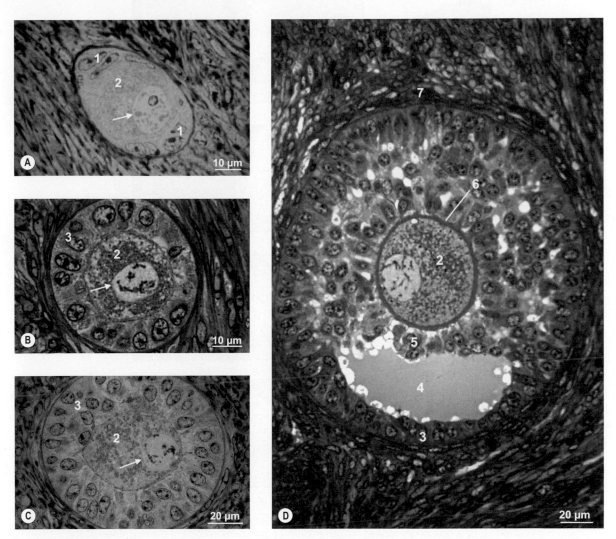

Fig. 4-10: Follicular development in cattle. **A:** Primordial follicle presenting flat follicular cells (1), and the oocyte (2) with its nucleus (arrow). **B:** Primary follicle presenting cuboidal granulosa cells (3). 2: Oocyte; Arrow: Oocyte nucleus. **C:** Secondary follicle presenting a multilayered granulosa cell layer (3). 2: Oocyte; Arrow: Oocyte nucleus. **D:** Tertiary follicle presenting the granulosa cell layer (3) and cumulus cells (5) enclosing the oocyte (2). The theca cell layers (7) have started to form. 2: Oocyte; 4: Antrum; 6: Zona pellucida.

Follicular and oocyte maturation

The tertiary follicle continues its development and, if selected for ovulation, enters a final phase of **follicular and oocyte maturation** stimulated by the preovulatory LH surge. The period from the onset of the LH surge to ovulation is species-specific and varies from less than 12 h to more than 40 h. During the preovulatory maturation of the follicle, steroid synthesis switches from oestradiol to progesterone production and the wall of the follicle prepares for rupturing to release the oocyte. The preovulatory maturation of the oocyte has nuclear as well as cytoplasmic components (Figs 4-11, 4-12). **Nuclear**

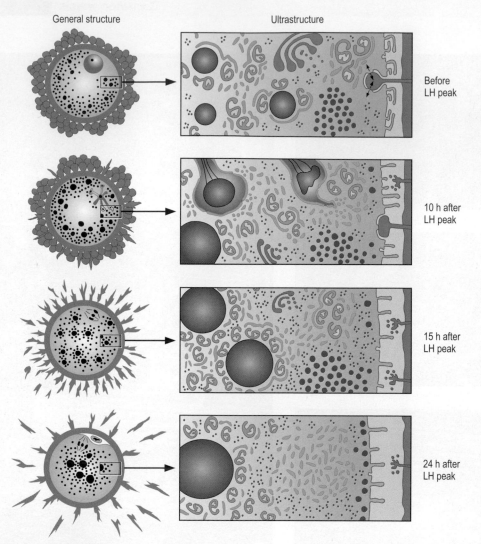

Fig. 4-11: Final oocyte maturation after the peak of the LH surge in cattle. *Before the LH peak*, the oocyte is in the diplotene stage and is characterized by a peripherally located nucleus (red) and a peripheral location of the organelles. At the ultrastructural level, the oocyte presents well developed smooth endoplasmic reticulum (SER; green), associated with lipid droplets (large black spheres) and mitochondria (blue), Golgi complexes (red), and clusters of cortical granules (small black spheres). The oocyte communicates through gap junctions with projections from the cumulus cells (arrows). *At about 10 h after the LH peak*, the oocyte has resumed meiosis and the nuclear envelope is dissolved into SER causing the nucleus, i.e. the germinal vesicle, to break down, and microtubules (black lines) appear adjacent to the condensing chromosomes (black in red nucleus). The perivitelline space between the oocyte and the zona pellucida develops, and in the oocyte the mitochondria tend to arrange around the lipid droplets and the Golgi complexes have decreased in size. The gap junctions between the oocyte and the cumulus cell projections are partially lost. *At about 15 h after the LH peak*, the oocyte has reached metaphase of the first meiotic division (metaphase I). The number and size of the lipid droplets have increased, mitochondria have assembled around the droplets, and these conglomerates have attained a more even distribution throughout the cytoplasm. Numerous ribosomes (black dots) have appeared, especially around the chromosomes, and the size of the Golgi complexes has decreased further. The gap junctions between the oocyte and the cumulus cell projections have been broken down. *At about 24 h after the LH peak*, the oocyte has reached the metaphase of the second meiotic division (metaphase II) and the first polar body has been abstricted. The bulk of the cortical granules are distributed at solitary positions along the plasma membrane. The lipid droplets and mitochondria have attained a more central location in the cytoplasm leaving a rather organelle-free peripheral zone in which the most prominent features are large clusters of SER. Golgi complexes are practically absent. Ovulation occurs around 24 h after the peak of the LH surge.

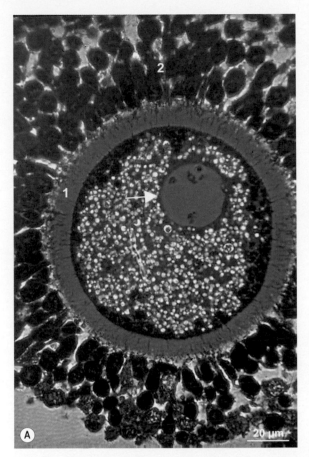
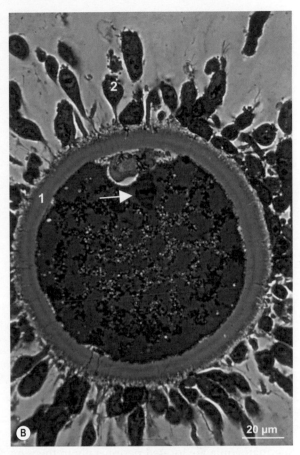

Fig. 4-12: Sections of bovine oocytes. **A:** Bovine oocyte at the diplotene stage. Arrow: Nucleus. 1: Zona pellucida; 2: Cumulus cells. **B:** Bovine oocyte at the metaphase of the second meiotic division (metaphase II). Arrow: Metaphase II plate with first polar body adjacent to it; 1: Zona pellucida; 2: Cumulus cells.

oocyte maturation refers to the process of meiosis which is resumed from the diplotene stage of meiosis I and continues to the metaphase of meiosis II when (except in the dog and fox) the oocyte is ovulated. The nucleus of the primary oocyte is often referred to as the **germinal vesicle**, and resumption of meiosis is morphologically evidenced by the breakdown of this structure (Fig. 4-11). **Cytoplasmic oocyte maturation** involves the restructuring and modulation of many of the organelles of the oocyte. It is particularly conspicuous in cattle where the cortical granules (which, before the LH-surge, are found in large clusters) migrate to

solitary positions adjacent to the plasma membrane in preparation for exocytosis at fertilization (Fig. 4-11).

Spermatogenesis

Development of spermatogonia and seminiferous tubules

After arriving and proliferating in the male developing gonad, the primordial germ cells become localized in solid cords of **primitive sustentacular cells**, the progenitors of the **Sertoli cells**, developed from the surface epithelium of the gonad. Shortly before puberty the cell cords acquire a lumen and develop into the **seminiferous tubules** of the testis. In parallel, the sustentacular cells gradually assume the characteristics of Sertoli cells and the primordial germ cells develop into spermatogonia (Figs 4-13, 4-14).

Spermatogenesis includes all the events by which the spermatogonia are transformed into spermatozoa. This process can be subdivided into **spermacytogenesis** (the development of spermatocytes from spermatogonia), **meiosis** (the two meiotic divisions of the spermatocytes), and **spermiogenesis** (the cellular re-structuring of the spermatids to spermatozoa without any cell divisions). Meiosis has already been described so the emphasis here will be on spermacytogenesis and spermiogenesis. There is a close cellular relationship between the spermatogenic cells and the Sertoli cells during spermatogenesis; Sertoli cells are required for both physical support and paracrine regulation of spermatogenesis, and also form the blood-testis barrier by sealing off the seminiferous tubules with tight junctions.

Spermacytogenesis

Spermatogonia are located peripherally in the seminiferous tubules adjacent to the basal lamina and outside (i.e. on the blood side) of the blood–testis barrier. Three types can be identified: **Type A, intermediate,** and **type B spermatogonia**. Type A_1 spermatogonia are the stem cells for spermatogenesis. Thus, the first mitoses in a type A_1 spermatogonium will result in a new type A_1 stem cell and a second-generation type A_2 spermatogonium with the ability to progress through spermatogenesis (Fig. 4-15). This ensures a perpetual population of stem cells for spermatogenesis. The type A_2 spermatogonium will, at least in ruminants, give rise to another subsequent generation of type A_3 spermatogonia, which finally divide into intermediate spermatogonia sharing morphological characteristics with both type A and type B spermatogonia. The intermediate spermatogonia give rise to type B spermatogonia of

which there are two generations, at least in ruminants.

Meiosis

The last mitotic division of type B spermatogonia results in the formation of **primary spermatocytes**. These cells enter meiosis I, with its characteristically prolonged prophase. In contrast to the oocyte, the spermatocyte is not arrested at the diplotene stage in the prophase. The spermatocytes re-locate through the blood-testis barrier to the luminal compartment of the seminiferous tubules. This is brought about by a zipper-like mechanism involving tight junctions; junctions are formed behind (basal to) the spermatocytes before the junctions ahead of them (on their luminal side) are dissolved to let the cells through. Completion of meiosis I results in the formation of two **secondary spermatocytes** that each divide into two **spermatids** through meiosis II. Throughout this series of divisions, from the second generation type A spermatogonia to the spermatids, cytokinesis is incomplete, leaving all cells within a generation still connected through thin cytoplasmic bridges.

Spermiogenesis

Spermatids are transformed into spermatozoa by spermiogenesis, which comprises four phases: the Golgi, cap, acrosome, and maturation phases. During the **Golgi phase**, the Golgi complex produces acrosomal granules which fuse to form a single large acrosomal granule that becomes localized adjacent to the nucleus (Fig. 4-16). The centriole pair of the spermatid re-locate to the opposite pole of the nucleus where the proximal centriole becomes attached to the nucleus. At the same time an axoneme, consisting of two central microtubules surrounded by nine doublets, develops from the distal centriole.

During the **cap phase**, the acrosomal granule flattens and covers a larger portion of the spermatid nucleus. During the **acrosomal phase**, the chromatin in the nucleus condenses as histones are

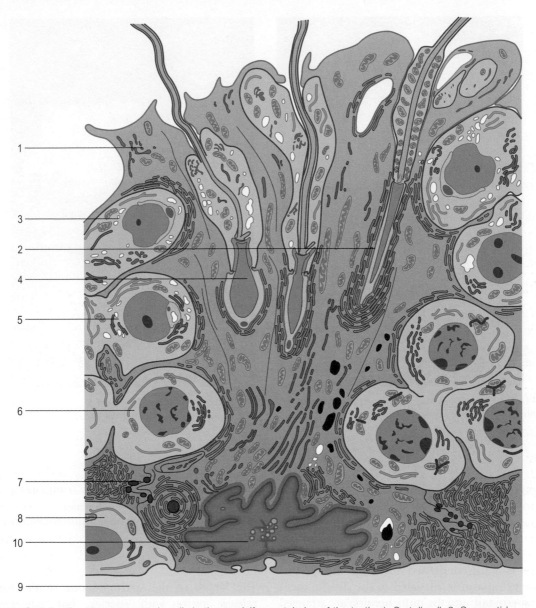

Fig. 4-13: Sertoli cell and spermatogenic cells in the seminiferous tubules of the testis. 1: Sertoli cell; 2: Spermatid – maturation phase; 3: Spermatid – cap phase; 4: Spermatid – acrosomal phase; 5: Spermatid – Golgi phase; 6: Primary spermatocytes connected by cytoplasmic bridges; 7: Blood-testis barrier; 8: Spermatogonium; 9: Basal lamina; 10: Sertoli cell nucleus. Modified from Liebich (2004).

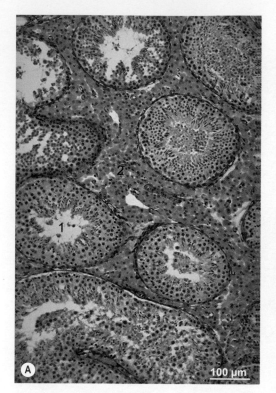 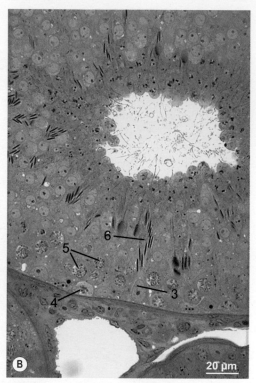

Fig. 4-14: Sections of the testis of a boar (A) and a ram (B). **A:** Seminiferous tubules (1) of the boar testis with Leydig cells (2) between them. **B:** Seminiferous tubule of the ram with Sertoli cells (3), spermatogonia (4), spermatocytes (5) and spermatids (6).

exchanged with protamines. The acrosomal granule is restructured into the **acrosome**, which contains enzymes of importance for the spermatozoon's penetration of the investments of the oocyte at fertilization. Eventually, the acrosome covers about two-thirds of the condensed nucleus of the spermatid, the cytoplasm is allocated to the development of the sperm tail, and the mitochondria are arranged around the growing axoneme. As these changes proceed, the spermatid rotates so that the acrosome faces the basal lamina of the seminiferous tubule and the developing tail faces the lumen.

During the **maturation phase**, the species-specific architecture of the sperm head and tail is developed. The major portion of the cytoplasm, including most of the organelles, is abstricted as the residual body (which is phagocytosed by the Sertoli cell) and the

spermatids are disconnected from each other. Finally, the spermatozoa are released from the Sertoli cells into the lumen of the seminiferous tubules.

Spermatozoa

The length of the **spermatozoon** at the time of release varies with species, but ranges from approximately 60 μm in the boar to 75 μm in the bull. At the light microscopical level, the spermatozoa appear to consist of two structures: the head and the tail. However, with the electron microscope, the tail can be subdivided into a neck, middle piece, principal piece, and end piece (Figs. 4-17).

The **head** of the spermatozoon contains the nucleus, which determines the shape of the head.

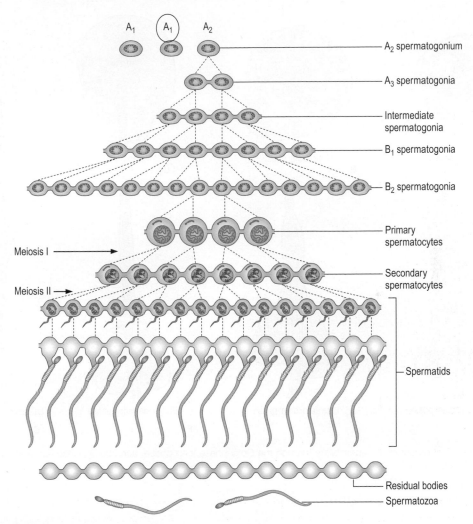

A₁ A₁ A₂

A₂ spermatogonium

A₃ spermatogonia

Intermediate spermatogonia

B₁ spermatogonia

B₂ spermatogonia

Primary spermatocytes

Meiosis I

Secondary spermatocytes

Meiosis II

Spermatids

Residual bodies

Spermatozoa

Fig. 4-15: Spermatogenesis in the bull. The encircled A₁ stem spermatogonium divides into an A₂ spermatogonium, which enters differentiation into spermatozoa, and an A₁ spermatogonium, which ensures the continuous supply of spermatogenic stem cells in the seminiferous tubules.

The anterior portion of the nucleus is covered by the **acrosome** delineated by an outer and inner acrosomal membrane. The acrosome contains hydrolytic enzymes that are released during fertilization as a result of the acrosome reaction (see Chapter 5). The posterior region of the acrosome is narrow, and this region of the sperm head is referred to as the **equatorial region**, which continues posteriorly into the **postacrosomal region**. The nucleus of the spermatozoon has a cytoskeletal coat known as the **perinuclear theca** which contains oocyte activating factors.

The **neck** is short and is connected to the head by a basal plate. It contains a **proximal centriole** and a **distal centriole** which continues into the axoneme of the tail. The centrioles are surrounded by nine peripheral **coarse fibres**, which are continued in the coarse fibres of the tail.

The **middle piece** of the tail has the characteristic structure of a flagellum, containing a central

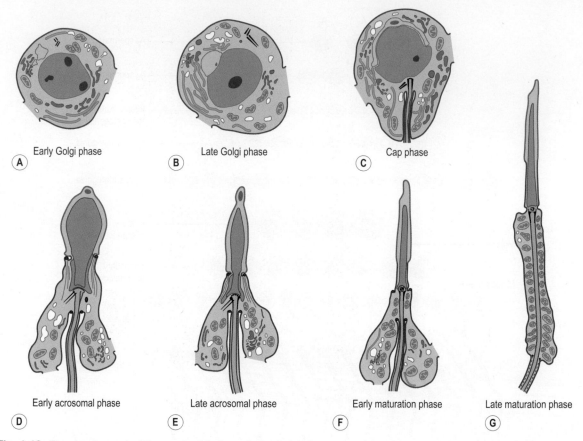

A   Early Golgi phase

B   Late Golgi phase

C   Cap phase

D   Early acrosomal phase

E   Late acrosomal phase

F   Early maturation phase

G   Late maturation phase

Fig. 4-16: The development of the spermatids through the Golgi-phase, cap phase, acrosomal phase and maturation phase. Modified from Liebich (2004).

axonema consisting of two central microtubules and nine peripheral doublets. The axoneme is surrounded by the nine coarse fibres, which, in turn, are surrounded by a helix of elongated mitochondria. In ruminants, the mitochondrial helix includes about 40 turns. A ring-shaped thickening of the plasma membrane of the middle piece, the **annulus**, marks the boundary between the middle piece and the principal piece of the tail.

The **principal piece** of the tail is the longest portion. It contains the axoneme surrounded by the nine coarse fibres. The mitochondrial helix is no longer present, and the coarse fibres are instead sur-rounded by semicircular ribs of structural proteins that have fused with two of the coarse fibres to form the **fibrous sheath**.

The transition between the principal piece and the **end piece** of the tail is marked by the end of the fibrous sheath. Proximally, the end piece still contains the axoneme, but distally the peripheral microtubule doublets are reduced into singlets which terminate at various levels.

The spermatozoa are transported by peristaltic contractions of the seminiferous tubules and subsequent ducts and, in the epididymal duct, they acquire motility and fertilizing capabilities.

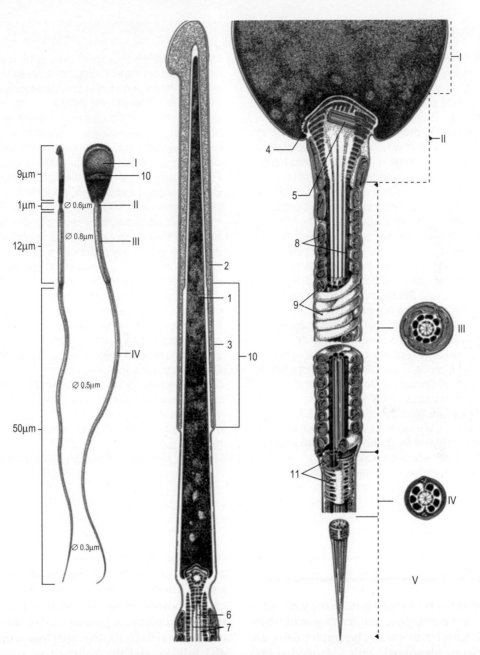

Fig. 4-17: The structure of the bull spermatozoon. The head (I) is connected to the middle piece (III) by the neck (II). The middle piece is continued in the principal piece (IV) and the end piece (V). The head presents a nucleus (1) with tightly packed chromatin, and the anterior portion of the nucleus is covered by the acrosome (2) with inner and outer acrosomal membranes located inside the plasma membrane (3). A basal plate (4) connects the head to the neck, which contains a proximal centriole (5) and a distal centriole extending into the axoneme located centrally in the middle piece and the principal piece of the tail consisting of two central (6) and 9 peripheral doublets (7) of microtubules. The middle piece presents 9 coarse fibres (8) surrounded by a mitochondrial helix (9). In the end piece, the axoneme is gradually lost. 10: Equatorial segment of the head; 11: Fibrous sheath. Courtesy Sinowatz and Rüsse (2007).

Box 4-1 Molecular regulation of germ line development

As for the three principal germ layers, specification of the germ line occurs during the process of gastrulation. At least in mice, specification is initiated by local signals originating outside the embryo proper. These include the **Bone Morphogenetic Proteins (BMP) 4 and 8b** acting through the Smad pathway. Responding epiblast cells then initiate expression of *fragilis/Ifitm3* and from this population of specified epiblast cells, germ line-restricted precursor cells are recruited. A key transcriptional regulator during this process is **Blimp1/Prdm1**. Functions related to Blimp1 include repression of the incipient somatic programs within the gastrulating epiblast cells, a hallmark being down-regulation of Hox gene expression. Other genes related to germ line specification include *Stella* and *c-kit*, the latter serving as a receptor for the stem cell factor/kit ligand being expressed in cells lining the path of germ cell transport to the developing gonad. Coupled to repression of somatic cell fate, germ line precursors maintain expression of pluripotency-associated genes including *Oct4*, *Sox2* and *Nanog* and show substantial epigenetic modifications. The latter include global DNA demethylation as the germ cells populate the genital ridge followed by de novo methylation and acquisition of sex-specific imprints during subsequent gametogenesis (see Chapter 2, Fig. 2-3).

In the female embryo, germ cells enter meiosis early during ovarian development. Molecular markers expressed during this developmental period include **Stra8** and **SCP3**, the latter a synaptonemal complex protein involved in pairing of homologue chromosomes. Apparently, entry into meiosis triggers loss of pluripotency in the germ cells. Oocytes guide early gonadal development. Folliculogenesis is initiated through expression of the transcription factor **Figα**, a factor specific for female germ cells, and essential for production of zona pellucida proteins for example. Further follicular development relies on a wealth of both endocrine and locally produced factors. In contrast to the situation in the female embryo, the presence of germ cells is apparently not necessary for testis development. Instead, differentiation of the gonad is controlled by the Sertoli cell lineage being induced by expression of the Y-linked **Sry gene** (Sex-determining region of the Y chromosome) in the somatic cells of the genital ridge. **Sox9**, **Fgf9**, and **Dax1** are among the genes expressed after initial Sry expression. On arrival in the genital ridge, male germ cells are prevented from entering meiosis. Instead they enter a state of mitotic arrest when they have reached a species-specific appropriate number.

SUMMARY

Primordial germ cells migrate from the wall of the yolk sac to the developing indifferent gonad where they proliferate by mitoses. The primordial germ cells associate with somatic cells and develop into **oogonia** and **spermatogonia**. Subsequently, they initiate **gametogenesis** which includes meiosis and cytodifferentiation of the gametes. **Meiosis** provides the gametes with the **haploid** chromosome number (half of the **diploid**) and with **recombination**, while **cytodifferentiation** results in cellular re-

structuring into the characteristic forms of the two gametes, the **oocyte** and the **spermatozoon**. In the female, the oogonia form **primary oocytes** that enter meiosis I but become arrested at the diplotene stage of prophase. A primary oocyte surrounded by its somatic cells (follicular cells) makes up a **primordial follicle**, and this follicle type constitutes the resting pool of follicles from which follicles are recruited for growth through the **primary**, **secondary** and **tertiary** stages. The primary oocyte does not resume meiosis and progress through its **nuclear maturation** to the metaphase of meiosis II until after puberty, shortly before ovulation. In parallel, the oocyte completes a **cytoplasmic maturation**. In the male, the spermatogonia are associated with somatic cells in solid cell cords that are the progenitors of the **seminiferous tubules**. **Spermatogenesis** begins after puberty and includes spermacytogenesis, meiosis and spermiogenesis. **Spermacytogenesis** includes several mitotic divisions of spermatogonia that divide into **primary spermatocytes**. By the two divisions of **meiosis**, primary spermatocytes produce haploid **secondary spermatocytes** and then **spermatids**. **Spermiogenesis** is the process of re-structuring spermatids into **spermatozoa**.

FURTHER READING

Berndston, W.E. and Desjardins, C. (1974): The cycle of the seminiferous epithelium in the bovine testis. Am. J. Anat. 140:167–179.

Brennan, J. and Capel, B. (2004): One tissue, two fates: molecular genetic events that underlie testis versus ovary development. Nature Rev. Gen. 5:509–521.

Dieleman, S.J., Kruip, T.A.M., Fontijne, P., de Jong, W.H.R. and van dr Weyden, G.C. (1983): Changes in oestradiol, progesterone, and testosterone concentrations in follicular fluid and in the micromorphology of preovulatory bovine follicles relative to the peak of luteinizing hormone. J. Endocr. 97:31–42.

Grøndahl, C., Hyttel, P., Grøndahl, M.L., Eriksen, T., Godtfredsen, P. and Greve, T. (1995): Structural aspects of equine oocyte maturation in vivo. Mol. Reprod. Dev. 42:94–105.

Heuser, C.H. and Streeter, G.L. (1927): Early stages in the development of pig embryos, from the period of initial cleavage to the time of the appearance of limb buds. Contr. Embryol. Carneg. Inst. 20:1–19.

Hyttel, P., Farstad, W., Mondain-Monval, M., Bakke Lajord, K. and Smith, A.J. (1990): Structural aspects of oocyte maturation in the blue fox. Anat. Embryol. 181:325–331.

Hyttel, P., Fair, T., Callesen, H. and Greve, T. (1997): Oocyte growth, capacitation and final maturation in cattle. Theriogenology 47:23–32.

Liebich, H.-G. (2004): Funktionelle Histologie der Haussaugtiere. Schatter, Stuttgart, Germany.

Moor, R.M. and Warnes, G.M. (1979): Regulation of meiosis in mammalian oocytes. Br. Med. Bull. 35:99–103.

Rüsse, I. and Sinowatz, F. (1998): Lehrbuch der Embryologie der Haustiere. 2nd edn. Parey Buchverlag, Berlin.

Sutovsky, P., Manandhar, G., Wu, A. and Oko, R. (2003): Interactions of sperm perinuclear theca with the oocyte: implications for oocyte activation, anti-polysperm defense, and assisted reproduction. Microsc. Res. Tech. 61:362–378.

Vejlsted, M., Offenberg, H., Thorup, F. and Maddox-Hyttel P. (2006): Confinement and clearance of OCT4 in the porcine embryo at stereomicroscopically defined stages around gastrulation. Mol. Reprod. Dev. 73:709–718.

Wrobel, K.-H. and Süss, F. (1998): Identification and temporospatial distribution of bovine primordial germ cells prior to gonadal sexual differentiation. Anat. Embryol. 197:451–467.

CHAPTER 5

Fred Sinowatz

Fertilization

Sexual reproduction occurs through **fertilization**, during which two haploid gametes fuse to produce a genetically unique individual. Fertilization, the process by which the spermatozoon and the egg unite, occurs in the **ampullary region** of the **oviduct** (see Chapter 3). The **mammalian egg complex**, which is ovulated and enters the oviduct via the infundibulum, consists of three components: (1) the **oocyte**, arrested at metaphase of meiosis II in most domestic mammals (with the exception of dogs, where the final maturation to metaphase II occurs in the oviduct), (2) the **zona pellucida**, an **extracellular matrix** surrounding the oocyte, consisting of glyco-proteins that are synthesized by both the oocyte and the surrounding cumulus cells in domestic animals, and (3) the **cumulus cells**, consisting of several layers of cells from the cumulus oophorus embedded in an extracellular matrix, composed mainly of hyaluronic acid. It has become common to consider the zona pellucida and the oocyte as one, leading the ovulated egg complex to be described as the **cumulus-oocyte complex (COC)** particularly in the context of biotechnological procedures (Fig. 5-1).

SPERM TRANSPORT IN THE FEMALE GENITAL TRACT

The duration of **copulation** varies among different domestic animals (see Chapter 3). It takes less than a minute for ruminants to copulate, somewhat longer in horses, several minutes in pigs, and in dogs five to 30 minutes may be necessary. In several mammalian species (cows, sheep, rabbit, dog, cat and primates) the semen is deposited into the cranial vagina. In others (pigs, horses and camelids) the semen is either ejaculated directly into the cervix (pig) or, via the processus urethralis, into both the cervix and uterus.

In **ruminants**, the ejaculate is small in volume (in general only 3 to 4 ml) but contains an enormous concentration of spermatozoa. It was assumed for a long time that, after being deposited in the uterus by artificial insemination, most spermatozoa ascend towards the oviducts. However, recent studies have clearly demonstrated that a high proportion of these spermatozoa are lost by retrograde transport; over 60% of spermatozoa deposited in the uterus are lost to the exterior within 12 hours after artificial insemination. This loss may be much higher if spermatozoa are deposited into the cervix and this can result in fertility being compromised.

In the **boar**, the volume of the ejaculate is large (200 to 400 ml) with a comparatively low concentration of spermatozoa. Due to its large volume, most of the ejaculate flows from the cervix into the uterus. The boar ejaculates a series of seminal fractions with different characteristics. The first fraction contains few spermatozoa and consists mainly of secretions from the accessory sex glands. The second fraction is rich in spermatozoa. Most of the final fraction originates from the bulbourethral glands, forming a coagulum that reduces retrograde sperm loss.

The **stallion** ejaculates in a series of 'jets', of which the first usually contains the fraction rich in spermatozoa. The seminal plasma of the later jets is highly viscous and, as in the pig, may serve to mini-mize retrograde sperm loss from the female's genital tract.

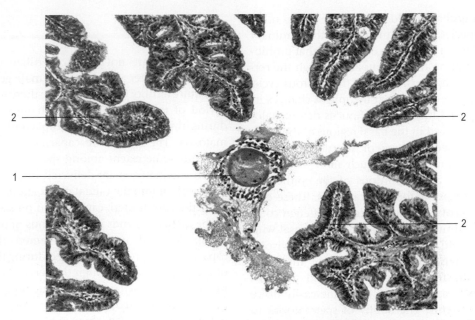

Fig. 5-1: Cumulus-oocyte-complex (1) in the ampulla of the sheep oviduct, where fertilization occurs. 2: Mucosal folds of the oviduct. Courtesy Sinowatz and Rüsse (2007).

In the **dog**, the first of the three fractions of the ejaculate originates from the prostate, the only accessory sex gland in this species. The volume of this clear and acellular so-called presperm fraction ranges from 0.5 to 5 ml, depending on the breed. The second fraction, opalescent in colour, is rich in spermatozoa. Its volume varies between 1 and 4 ml and it contains between 300 million and two billion spermatozoa. The last fraction is also contributed by the prostate. Its volume may vary over a broad range, from 1 to even 80 ml, depending on the breed. Ejaculated in surges, this last fraction of pro-static fluid may force the sperm-rich fraction crani-ally into the uterus. In the cat the ejaculate volume is small (0.2 to 0.3 ml) and it is unclear whether it comprises multiple fractions.

Retrograde loss of spermatozoa from the female genital tract depends on several factors. The more important are volume and physical nature of the ejaculate and the site of its deposition within the female genital tract. As already mentioned, in some species, like the pig, proteins from the seminal plasma form a conspicuous vaginal plug that pre-vents spermatozoa from being lost to the exterior.

In some laboratory rodents the solid vaginal plug that is formed after copulation can be seen from outside and is used to determine the time of mating (see Chapter 20).

Transport of spermatozoa to the ampulla of the oviduct is primarily the result of elevated tone and motility of the tunica muscularis of the female genital tract. It can be divided into two phases, a **rapid** and a **sustained transport phase**. Within a few minutes after mating, spermatozoa have already reached the oviduct. Although male gametes are close to the oocyte after a very short period, these spermatozoa are not viable and do not play a role in fertilization; it is the sustained phase of sperm transport that is important for successful fertiliza-tion. In the sustained phase, spermatozoa are trans-ported to the oviducts from presumed reservoirs in the uterotubal junction or the cervix over an extended time period, delivering them in a more uniform manner.

A **major barrier** for spermatozoal transport is the **cervix uteri** that can also serve as a reservoir of spermatozoa in several species. In ruminants, and to a lesser degree in the mare, the cervix possesses a convoluted system of folds and grooves. As in other domestic species, the epithelium of the ruminant cervix produces a highly viscous mucus that prohibits the penetration of spermatozoa through the cervical canal during most times of the oestrous cycle. It is only during oestrus that the mucus changes its viscosity, when a low viscosity mucus rich in sialomucins is produced in the basal regions of the cervical crypts. A second type of mucus, containing mainly sulphomucins and much more viscous, is secreted by the apical portions of the epithelium covering the tips of the cervical folds. These two different types of secretion create two different compartments within the cervical canal, one basal with low viscosity and one more central with high viscosity. The low viscosity environment in the basal regions of the folds offers a 'privileged pathway' through which spermatozoa can quite easily move towards the uterus. The ability of spermatozoa to use this privileged pathway depends on their ability to swim through the crypts of the cervix; non-motile spermatozoa cannot progress and are eliminated. Consequently, the cervix acts as a filter for removing non-viable spermatozoa.

CAPACITATION

Spermatozoa are not able to fertilize the oocyte immediately after arrival in the female genital tract; to acquire fertility they must reside there for a certain period of time (Fig. 5-2). The changes that occur during this period constitute **capacitation** of spermatozoa. The site where capacitation takes place varies to some extent among species. In species in which spermatozoa are delivered into the mid-cervix (sow), or into the caudal cervix and immediately enter the corpus uteri, capacitation probably begins in the uterus and ends in the isthmus of the oviduct. In species with intravaginal semen deposition, capacitation is probably initiated during the passage of the spermatozoa through the cervix. Not all spermatozoa are capacitated at the same time and, as the process usually extends over several hours, individual spermatozoa can show a different degree of capacitation depending on their location within the female genital tract.

Capacitation encompasses a number of complex processes. It has been clearly shown that the **plasma**

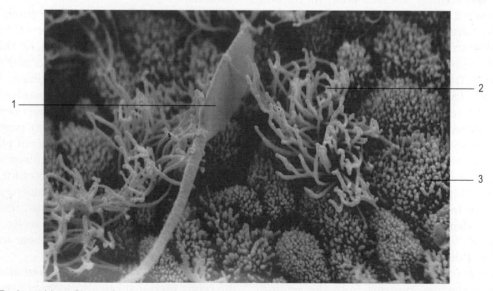

Fig. 5-2: Bovine oviduct. Spermatozoa can be temporarily bound to the epithelium of the isthmus in the oviduct by binding mechanisms mediated by sugars (for instance fucose). 1: spermatozoon; 2: kinocilia; 3 microvilli. Courtesy Sinowatz and Rüsse (2007).

membrane of the spermatozoon (particularly of the head) undergoes marked changes during capacitation. Important processes during capacitation are: removal of the glycoprotein coat and seminal plasma proteins (adsorbed during epididymal storage and ejaculation) from the spermatozoal surface; the functional coupling of the signal-transducing pathways that regulate the initiation of the acrosome reaction by the zona pellucida glycoproteins; alterations in the flagellar motility that are necessary to penetrate the zona pellucida; and, finally, development of the capacity to fuse with the plasma membrane of the oocyte. These processes are accompanied by changes in metabolism, the biophysical properties of the plasma membrane, and protein phosphorylation, together with elevation of intracellular calcium levels and pH, and hyperpolarization of membrane potential.

Capacitation can be reversed by returning already capacitated spermatozoa to seminal plasma. Once decapacitated in this way, they require additional capacitation before they can regain their fertility.

Much of our understanding of the capacitation process has been gained from studies in vitro. Several factors cause capacitation in vitro. First, cholesterol efflux from the sperm membrane is mediated by sterol-binding proteins and initiates many aspects of capacitation. The reorganization of the sperm membrane after cholesterol depletion is considered an early step in capacitation. Second, several sperm plasma membrane proteins are tyrosine phosphorylated through a cAMP-dependent mechanism. Spermatozoa express a bicarbonate-sensitive, soluble form of adenyl cyclase that may control these phosphorylation events. Third, elevation of the intracellular pH and bicarbonate levels may lead to a stimulation of cAMP production. By activating cyclic nucleotide-gated channels in the plasma membrane of the sperm flagellum, spermatozoa could switch to the hyperactivated motility pattern that is characteristic of capacitated spermatozoa.

In vivo, synergistic actions of multiple factors are likely to mediate capacitation. It has been shown that sterol-binding proteins, such as high-density lipoproteins, are present in the oviductal fluid and can accelerate cholesterol efflux from spermatozoa.

Additionally, progesterone, derived from the follicular fluid and from secretion by the cumulus cells surrounding the ovulated oocyte, may be involved in the regulation of some aspects of the process.

INTERACTIONS BETWEEN SPERMATOZOA AND THE ZONA PELLUCIDA

The **zona pellucida** (ZP) is an extracellular matrix surrounding the oocyte and the early embryo that exerts several important functions during fertilization and early embryonic development. In most mammalian species it is composed of three glycoproteins (ZPA, equivalent to mouse ZP2; ZPB, equivalent to mouse ZP1; ZPC equivalent to mouse ZP3), products of the gene families *ZPA*, *ZPB* and *ZPC* that have been found to be highly homologous within mammalian species. Most data on the structure and function of the ZP have been obtained from studies in the mouse. New data from pigs and other domestic animals, however, indicate that findings in the mouse model are not always applicable to other species. For example, whereas ZP3 is the primary sperm receptor in the mouse, it is ZPA and ZPC that possess receptor activity in the pig. Also contrary to the mouse (in which the growing oocyte is the only source of zona glycoproteins), these proteins are expressed in both the oocyte and granulosa cells in a stage-specific pattern in domestic animals.

The ZP is involved in several critical stages of fertilization: the adhesion and binding of capacitated spermatozoa to the ZP; the subsequent induction of the acrosome reaction and penetration of the ZP; and the fertilization-induced modifications of the ZP that prevent polyspermy.

Adhesion of spermatozoa to zona pellucida

The first contact between the spermatozoon and the ZP, **adhesion**, is a loose, non-specific association between the gametes and appears to be a disconcertingly random affair (Fig. 5-3). It is followed by a

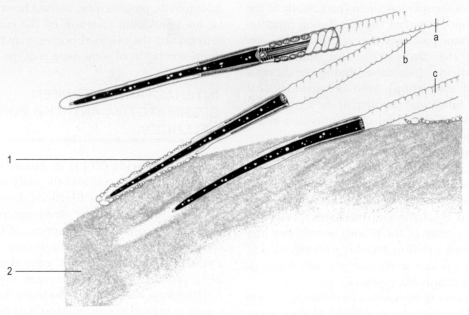

Fig. 5-3: Acrosome reaction. Once bound to the zona pellucida, the spermatozoa undergo the acrosome reaction, during which hydrolyzing enzymes are released from the acrosome of the sperm head. It begins when the plasma membrane of the spermatozoon forms multiple fusion sites with the outer acrosomal membrane resulting in the formation of many small vesicles. (a) Spermatozoon with intact acrosome. (b) Vesiculation of the plasma membrane and outer acrosomal membrane; (c) Penetration of the zona pellucida by the spermatozoon. 1: Fusion of the plasma membrane and the outer acrosomal membrane of the spermatozoon; 2: Zona pellucida. Courtesy Sinowatz and Rüsse (2007).

relatively **firm binding**, which is species-specific and mediated by complementary receptors on the ZP (sperm receptor) and on the sperm surface. In the mouse initial sperm-zona adhesion is mediated by ZP3, a constituent glycoprotein of the ZP that binds to receptors on the anterior head of acrosome-intact sperm. This adhesion to the ZP is probably based on protein-carbohydrate recognition processes, through the association of O-linked α-galactosyl residues from ZP3 with a cognate receptor on the sperm. Secondary binding is then mediated by ZP2. Other authors, however, consider that sperm-zona binding is a purely protein-based event.

In species other than the mouse, various carbohydrates of zona proteins have been suggested to be involved in sperm binding. Inhibition assays of sperm–ZP binding revealed a role for D-mannose on human and rat ZP. Pre-treatment of human sper-matozoa with D-mannose inhibited sperm penetration through the ZP. In the rat α-methyl mannoside and D-mannose turned out to be the most potent inhibitors. L-Fucose and fucoidin were shown to be involved in sperm-ZP recognition in guinea-pig, hamster, rat and human oocytes.

Acrosome reaction

Once bound, sperm undergo the **acrosome reaction** (Fig. 5-3) as a result of which hydrolytic enzymes are released from the acrosome of the sperm head. This permits the spermatozoon to penetrate the ZP matrix by a combination of enzymatic digestion of the ZP glycoproteins and vigorous propulsion by the tail of the spermatozoon. The acrosome reaction, induced by the ZP glycoproteins, consists of an orderly fusion of the plasma membrane of the sper-

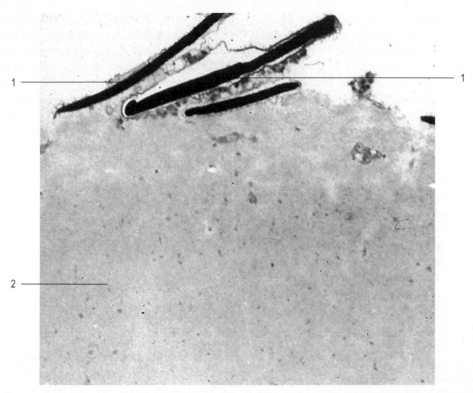

Fig. 5-4: Bovine spermatozoa undergoing the acrosome reaction on the surface of the zona pellucida. 1: Spermatozoa showing vesiculation of the plasma membrane and outer acrosomal membrane. 2: Zona pellucida, composed of glycoproteins (ZPA, ZPB, ZPC).

matozoon and the outer acrosomal membrane. It begins when the **plasma membrane forms multiple fusion sites with the outer acrosomal membrane** resulting in the formation of many small vesicles (**vesiculation**). After vesiculation has occurred, the enzymatic content of the acrosome is dispersed and the sperm nucleus remains covered by only the inner acrosomal membrane (Fig. 5-4). **Acrosin** and **hyaluronidase** are enzymes released during the acrosomal reaction. Acrosin hydrolyzes ZP proteins and also enhances the ability of the spermatozoa to bind to these proteins. During the process of ZP penetration, acrosome-reacted spermatozoa are temporarily bound and released by the ZP glycoproteins via secondary binding mechanisms involving proacrosin. The sperm are also pushed forward by

the vigorously beating tail towards the perivitelline space. Proacrosin is the inactive form of the enzyme acrosin and has a strong affinity for the ZP. Thus, proacrosin aids in binding to the zona as the acrosomal reaction proceeds. As proacrosin is converted to acrosin, the spermatozoon penetrates by using the enzyme to digest a small hole in the zona and passing through it.

ADHESION AND FUSION OF THE SPERMATOZOON AND OOCYTE

After penetration of the ZP, sperm **adhere** to and **fuse** with the plasma membrane of the oocyte. The membrane oocyte fuses with the membrane of the

equatorial segment of the spermatozoon (see Chapter 4), and the fertilizing spermatozoon, including its tail, is engulfed by the oocyte. Strictly, this process should be referred to as **syngamy**. The membrane fusion of the male and female gametes involves sperm fertilin-α (also known as disintegrin 1 or ADAM1), fertilin-β (ADAM2) and cyritestin (ADAM3) as well as CRISP1 (cystein-rich secretory protein 1). Integrins found on the plasma membrane of the oocyte are receptors for sperm ADAMs. The adhesion-mediating proteins on both gametes are thought to function as multimeric complexes at the plasma membranes. After adhesion, the sperm plasma membrane fuses with the plasma membrane of the oocyte. The molecular basis of this intercellular fusion process is not fully understood; the tetraspanin CD9, an integrin-associated protein, is implicated in certain types of membrane fusion, but it is not known if it plays a significant role in gamete fusion.

OOCYTE ACTIVATION

Immediately after entry of the spermatozoon, the oocyte undergoes **oocyte activation**, which establishes a block to polyspermic fertilization, resumption of meiosis, and initiation of embryonic development. In all animals investigated, activation involves an **increase in the cytosolic calcium ion concentration** to approximately 1 mM. Depending on the species, this increase in cytosolic calcium concentration occurs within several seconds to a few minutes after gamete membrane fusion, and often occurs as a 'wave' that travels across the oocyte. In mammals, a low-frequency oscillation in cytosolic calcium concentration persists for several hours preceding entry into the first embryonic cell division. Besides the induction of the block to polyspermic fertilization, the increase in cytosolic calcium concentration terminates meiotic arrest so that the reduction division can be completed (see Chapter 4). Later, oocyte activation responses include the recruitment of maternal mRNAs for translation, and changes in protein synthesis (see Chapter 6).

The use of intracytoplasmic sperm injection (ICSI; see Chapter 21) to fertilize oocytes has shown that extra-cellular sperm-egg contact is not necessary to activate eggs. Interestingly, neither is it simply the act of injection, nor the introduction of calcium from the medium, that induce egg activation. Constituents of the sperm nucleus, presumably its perinuclear theca, have been associated with oocyte-activating activities. Among the candidates for this property of the sperm are oscillin (a glucosamine-6-phosphate isomerase) and a truncated form of the tyrosine kinase c-Kit.

Block to polyspermic fertilization

The **block to polyspermic fertilization** is established through the exocytosis of a set of secretory granules, the **cortical granules**, from the oocyte (Fig. 5-5). This is referred to as the **cortical reaction** (see Chapter 4). The content of the cortical granules includes proteases, acid phosphatases, peroxidase, mucopolysaccharides and plasminogen activator. As a result of the release of cortical granules, the oocyte membrane and ZP become modified. Consequently, any further penetration of spermatozoa into the oocyte is prevented and the so-called zona-block to polyspermy is established.

Resumption of meiosis and pronucleus formation

As another consequence of oocyte activation, **meiosis is resumed** and the second meiotic division is completed. The daughter cell that receives hardly any cytoplasm is called the **second polar body** (see Chapter 4). The other daughter cell is the definitive oocyte, now referred to as the zygote. Its haploid chromosome set becomes surrounded by layers of smooth endoplasmic reticulum that contribute to the formation of a nuclear envelope, and a vesicular nucleus known as the **female** or **maternal pronucleus** is formed (Fig. 5-6). The sperm nucleus undergoes marked changes within the oocyte's cytoplasm. It becomes swollen ('decondensed'), surrounded by

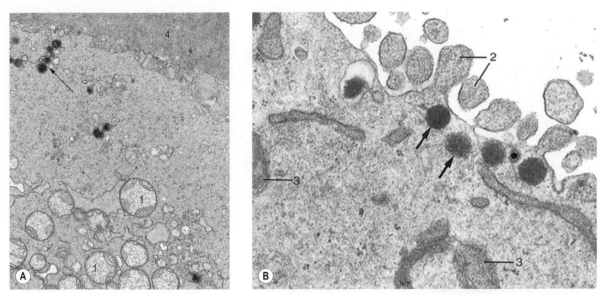

Fig. 5-5: The block to polyspermic fertilization is established through exocytosis of the cortical granules (cortical reaction). (A) shows an immature bovine oocyte with few and small cortical granules (arrow), (B) the exocytosis of peripherally located cortical granules of a mature oocyte. 1: Mitochondria of an immature oocyte; 2: Microvilli; 3: Mitochondrion of a mature oocyte; 4: Zona pellucida.

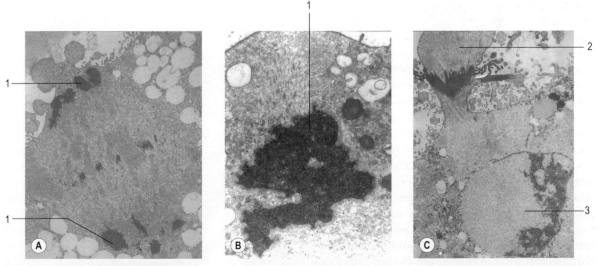

Fig. 5-6: Formation of the female pronucleus. As a consequence of oocyte activation, the second meiotic division is completed (A). One of the daughter cells (2 in Fig. 5-7 C) receives hardly any cytoplasm and is called second polar body. The other daughter cell (B) is the definitive oocyte. Its haploid chromosome set becomes surrounded by profiles of endoplasmic reticulum and a vesicular nucleus (3). The female pronucleus is formed.1: Haploid chromosome set; 2: Polar body; 3: Female pronucleus.

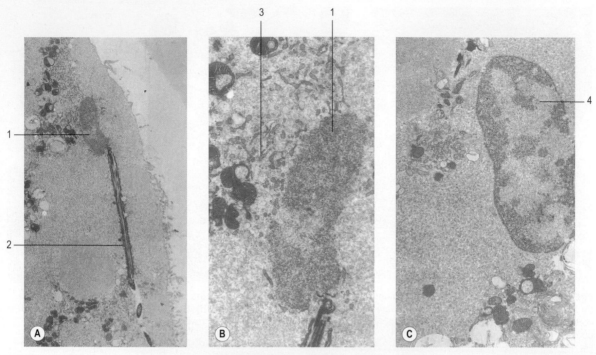

Fig. 5-7: Formation of the male pronucleus. The spermatozoon is taken up into the oocyte by a phagocytotic process (A). The sperm nucleus then becomes surrounded by layers of smooth endoplasmic reticulum (B) contributing to the formation of a nuclear envelope. A vesicular (decondensed) paternal pronucleus (C) is formed. 1: Decondensing sperm nucleus; 2: Degenerating sperm tail; 3: Endoplasmic reticulum; 4: Male pronucleus.

smooth endoplasmic reticulum contributing to a nuclear envelope, and forms the **male** or **paternal pronucleus** (Fig. 5-7). The decondensation of the sperm nucleus requires the reduction of the many disulphide cross-links. The primary reducing agent is glutathione from the oocyte cytoplasm. Furthermore, the protamines, by which the sperm DNA is packed, is exchanged with histones from the oocyte. The tail of the spermatozoon detaches and degenerates. Male and female pronuclei approach each other, helped by the cytoskeleton of the zygote (Figs 5-8, 5-9). Eventually, they come into close contact and lose their nuclear envelopes, which apparently dissolve into smooth endoplasmic reticulum. Upon dismantling of the nuclear envelopes, the male and female haploid genomes become united in the centre of the zygote. This mixing is referred to as **karyogamy** or **synkaryosis.** It should be noted that, in contrast to what occurs at fertiliza-

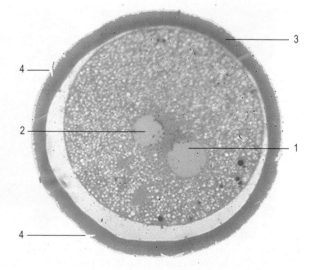

Fig. 5-8: Male (1) and female (2) pronucleus of a bovine oocyte. 3: Zona pellucida; 4: Spermatozoa penetrating the zona pellucida.

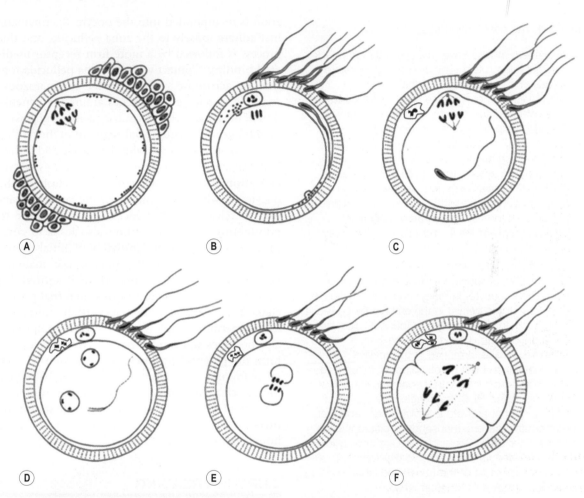

Fig. 5-9: Overview of mammalian fertilization (modified from Rüsse and Sinowatz, 1998). **A:** Anaphase of the first meiotic division in the follicle; **B:** Penetration of the spermatozoon into the perivitelline space; metaphase of the second meiotic division and activation of the oocyte results in release of cortical granules; **C:** First sperm is taken up into the oocyte by a phagocytotic process; anaphase of the second meiotic division; **D:** Formation of the male and female pronuclei, the tail of the spermatozoon degenerates; **E:** Karyogamy; **F:** First mitotic division of the zygote. Courtesy Sinowatz and Rüsse (2007).

tion in some lower orders, the pronuclei in mammals do not actually fuse. During the migration of the pronuclei, the S-phase of the first post-fertilization cell cycle is completed and, at the dissolution of the nuclear envelopes of the pronuclei, the chromatin condenses to form the **prophase of the first mitotic division**. The subsequent cleavage is normally completed within 24 hours after ovulation. If the oocyte is not fertilized within this period of time, it loses its developmental potential.

Box 5-1 The contribution of spermatozoa

Mature spermatozoa have little cytoplasm and lack any detectable protein synthesis. It had therefore been assumed for a long time that sperm contribute little other than the paternal genes to an embryo whereas the oocyte, with its abundant RNAs and proteins, exclusively directs the embryo's early development. Surprisingly, recent studies have shown that defects in sperm can disrupt embryo development even if the genes carried by the male germ cells are perfectly normal. It is now becoming clear that, besides the haploid set of chromosomes, **sperm also deliver a complex cargo of RNA and proteins** that may be crucial for an embryo's early development.

Contrary to earlier opinions, the entire spermatozoon, including the midpiece and tail, is taken into the oocyte. In many mammals, midpiece and tail structures persist in the embryo for several cell divisions. In most mammals (but not mice) the spermatozoon also delivers the centrioles, a prerequisite for the formation of the spindle apparatus and the first mitotic division. It has also been discovered recently that spermatozoa deliver a molecule called **PLC** that triggers the waves of calcium ions that activate a fertilized egg, and that sperm contain several thousands of different kinds of messenger RNA. Some of them are coding for proteins needed for early embryo development, but the function of most of the transferred RNA molecules remains to be established.

zoon is incorporated into the oocyte. Spermatozoa first **adhere** loosely to the zona pellucida, and this process is followed by a more **firm receptor-mediated binding**. Contact with the zona pellucida triggers the **acrosome reaction** in the spermatozoon, resulting in release of enzymes aiding the penetration of the zona pellucida. Subsequently, the plasma membrane of the **equatorial segment** of the fertilizing spermatozoon **fuses** with the oocyte and is then internalized into it. Gamete fusion induces **oocyte activation** including the **cortical reaction** in the oocyte, by which the content of the **cortical granules** is released and induces the **zona-block to polyspermy**. Oocyte activation also leads to **completion of meiosis II** and initiation of initial embryonic development. In the oocyte, the maternal haploid chromosome compartment is surrounded by a nuclear envelope forming the **maternal pronucleus**, and, after a decondensation of the chromatin in the sperm, its haploid chromosome component also becomes surrounded by a nuclear envelope to form the **paternal pronucleus**. The pronuclei then move towards each other in the centre of the zygote, their nuclear envelopes dissolve, and the chromatin condenses to enter prophase of the **first mitotic division**. First cleavage is normally seen within 24 hours after ovulation.

FURTHER READING

Brewis, I.A. and Moore, H.D. (1997): Molecular mechanisms of gamete recognition and fusion at fertilization. Hum. Reprod. 12:156–165.

Dean, J. (2005): Molecular biology of sperm-egg interactions. Andrologia 37:198–199.

Dunbar, B.S. and Avery, S. (1994): The mammalian zona pellucida: its biochemistry, immunochemistry, molecular biology, and developmental expression. Reprod. Fertil. Dev. 6:331–347.

Evans, J.P. and Florman, H.M. (2002): The state of the unions: the cell biology of fertilization. Nat. Cell. Biol. 4:57–63.

Farstad, W., Hyttel, P., Grøndahl, C., Mondain-Monval, M. and Smith, A.J. (1993): Fertilization and early embryonic development in the blue fox (*Alopex lagopus*). Mol. Reprod. Dev. 36:331–337.

Guraya, S.S. (2000): Cellular and molecular biology of capacitation and acrosome reaction in spermatozoa. Int. Rev. Cytol. 199:1–64.

SUMMARY

Spermatozoa are deposited in the female genital tract at **copulation** or **artificial insemination**. They are transported to the site of fertilization in the ampullary region of the oviduct in successive **rapid** and **sustained transport phases**, of which the latter results in fertilization. During transport, the spermatozoa undergo **capacitation** and achieve fertilizing capability. Fertilization is a stepwise process that includes a first series of interactions between the spermatozoa and the zona pellucida, and a second series of events whereby the fertilizing spermato-

Hyttel, P., Greve, T. and Callesen, H. (1988a): Ultrastructure of in-vivo fertilization in superovulated cattle. J. Reprod. Fert. 82:1–13.

Hyttel, P., Xu, K.P. and Greve, T. (1988b): Scanning electron microscopy of in vitro fertilization in cattle. Anat. Embryol. 178:41–46.

Kölle, S., Sinowatz, F., Boie, G., Totzauer, I., Amselgruber, W. and Plendl, J. (1996): Localization of the mRNA encoding the zona protein ZP3 alpha in the porcine ovary, oocyte and embryo by non-radioactive in situ hybridization. Histochem. J. 28:441–447.

Kölle, S., Sinowatz, F., Boie, G. and Palma, G. (1998): Differential expression of ZPC in the bovine ovary, oocyte, and embryo. Mol. Reprod. Dev. 49:435–443.

Kölle, S., Dubois, C.S., Caillaud, M., Lahuec, C., Sinowatz, F. and Goudet, G. (2007) : Equine zona protein synthesis and ZP structure during folliculogenesis, oocyte maturation, and embryogenesis. Mol. Reprod. Dev. 74:851–859.

Laurincik, J., Hyttel, P., Rath, D. and Pivko, J. (1994a): Ovulation, fertilization and pronucleus development in superovulated gilts. Theriogenology 41:447–452.

Laurincik, J., Kopecny, V. and Hyttel, P. (1994b): Pronucleus development and DNA synthesis in bovine zygotes in vivo. Theriogenology 42:1285–1293.

Laurincik, J., Hyttel, P. and Kopecny, V. (1995): DNA synthesis and pronucleus development in pig zygotes obtained in vivo: An autoradiographic and ultrastructural study. Mol. Reprod. Dev. 40:325–332.

Lyng, R. and Shur, B.D. (2007): Sperm-egg binding requires a multiplicity of receptor-ligand interactions: new insights into the nature of gamete receptors derived from reproductive tract secretions. Soc. Reprod. Fertil. Suppl. 65:335–351

Moore, H.D. (2001): Molecular biology of fertilization. J. Reprod. Fertil. Suppl. 57: 105–110.

Rüsse, I. and Sinowatz, F. (1998): Lehrbuch der Embryologie der Haustiere, 2nd edn. Parey Buchverlag, Berlin.

Sinowatz, F. and Wrobel, K.H. (1981): Development of the bovine acrosome. An ultrastructural and cytochemical study. Cell Tissue Res. 219(3):511–524.

Sinowatz, F., Gabius, H.J. and Amselgruber, W. (1988): Surface sugar binding components of bovine spermatozoa as evidence by fluorescent neoglycoproteins. Histochemistry 88:395–399.

Sinowatz, F., Volgmayr, J.K., Gabius, H.J. and Friess, A.E. (1989): Cytochemical analysis of mammalian sperm membranes. Prog. Histochem. Cytochem. 19:1–74.

Sinowatz, F., Amselgruber, W., Topfer-Petersen, E., Totzauer, I., Calvete, J. and Plendl J. (1995): Immunocytochemical characterization of porcine zona pellucida during follicular development. Anat. Embryol. 191:41–46.

Sinowatz, F., Plendl, J. and Kölle, S. (1998): Protein-carbohydrate interactions during fertilization. Acta Anat. (Basel) 161:196–205.

Sinowatz, F., Topfer-Petersen, E., Koelle, S. and Palma, G. (2001a): Functional morphology of the zona pellucida. Anat. Histol. Embryol. 30:257–263.

Sinowatz, F., Koelle, S. and Topfer-Petersen, E. (2001b): Biosynthesis and expression of zona pellucida glycoproteins in mammals. Cells Tissues Organs 168:24–35.

Sinowatz, F., Wessa, E., Neumueller, C. and Palma, G.: (2003): On the species specificity of sperm binding and sperm penetration of the zona pellucida. Reprod. Domest. Anim. 38:141–146.

Wassarman, P.M. (1995): Towards molecular mechanisms for gamete adhesion and fusion during mammalian fertilization. Curr. Opin. Cell Biol. 7:658–664.

Wassarman, P.M. and E.S. Litscher (1995): Sperm–egg recognition mechanisms in mammals. Curr. Top. Dev. Biol. 30:1–19.

CHAPTER 6

Embryo cleavage and blastulation

Morten Vejlsted

Upon fertilization, meiosis is completed and cell cyclicity returns to the mitotic pattern. The unique **embryonic genome** has been established through the mixing of the maternal and paternal chromosomes by dissolution of the two pronuclei. This equips the zygote with the full genetic make-up for building the embryo. The cytoplasm of the zygote, inherited from the oocyte, contains the complete molecular and structural composition necessary to initiate the first cleavages and, later, activate the embryonic genome for de novo embryonic transcription. Hence, the initial phase of development is driven by information stored in the oocyte and passed on to the zygote and the early embryo.

CLEAVAGES AND GENOME ACTIVATION

In the zygote, an S-phase is completed during the first post-fertilization cell cycle. Thus, when the zygote cleaves to the 2-cell embryo at the first mitosis, each of the two cells, referred to as **blastomeres**, obtains its full copy of the embryonic genome (Figs. 2-1, 6-1). The embryo is still surrounded by the **zona pellucida** and remains so for some days. A number of mitotic divisions follow. During this phase of development, the mitotic divisions are special in that they occur almost **without cellular growth**; the cells become smaller and smaller as the original cytoplasm of the zygote is divided into smaller and smaller portions. These cell divisions are referred to as **cleavages**. The blastomeres may be of unequal sizes because of asynchrony in cleavage. This asynchrony becomes apparent from the outset; even between the 2- and the 4-cell stages, it results in temporary 3-cell embryos. At least in the mouse, the point of sperm entry may position the plane of the first cleavage division. Furthermore, the 2-cell-stage blastomere inheriting the sperm entry site tends to divide earlier than the other and is more likely to give rise to cells that become positioned internally in the growing ball of cells.

Cleavages begin during the transport of the embryo through the **oviduct** but, at a species-specific stage of development, the embryo enters the **uterus** (Table 6-1). The mare is very unusual with regard to passage through the oviduct; only embryos are allowed to enter the uterus while unfertilized oocytes, by an unknown mechanism, are retained in the oviduct.

During the growth of the oocyte, transcripts and proteins are stored in this specialized cell for later use (Fig. 6-2). At the end of the growth phase transcription diminishes. However, by then the oocyte is more or less loaded with the transcripts and proteins required for driving initial embryonic development and these govern at least the first cleavage. The transcripts and proteins are gradually degraded after fertilization and, at a certain stage of development, activity of the embryonic genome is required. The embryonic genome is activated gradually; transcription is very limited initially but increases later, at species-specific stages, in two phases – those of **minor** and **major activation of the embryonic genome** (Table 6-2).

After a few cell divisions, the embryo takes the shape of a small ball of cells referred to as a **morula** after the Latin name for mulberry.

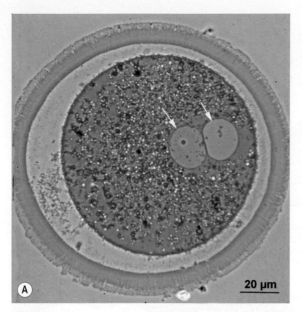 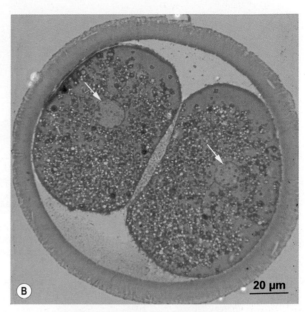

Fig. 6-1: Sections of a bovine zygote (A) with two pronuclei (arrows) and of a 2-cell embryo (B) with nuclei (arrows)

Table 6-1: Times of passage of the embryo from the oviduct into the uterus, and of blastocyst formation, in different species

Species	Passage into the uterus		Time of blastocyst formation (days after ovulation)
	Days after ovulation	Stage of development	
Pig	2	4–8 cell	5–6
Cattle	3–3 ½	8–16 cell	7–8
Sheep	3	8–16 cell	6–7
Horse	5–6	Morula	6
Dog	8	Blastocyst	8

COMPACTION

Individual cells of the morula all look identical to start with, their spherical shapes giving the morula its typical mulberry-like appearance. Later, however, the outer cells differentiate into an epithelium, attach firmly to each other, and give the embryo a smoother surface. This process is referred to as com-paction (Fig. 6-3). The outer cells constitute the **trophectoderm** or trophoblast. In the present book, the term trophectoderm will be used before placentation and the term trophoblast when these cells become engaged in placental formation. The firm attachment between neighbouring cells of the trophectoderm results from specialized intercellular junctions including tight junctions and

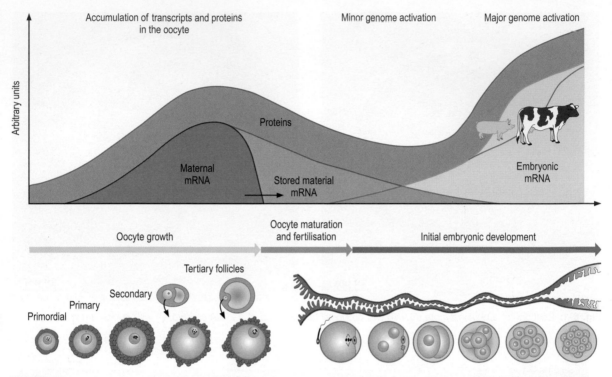

Fig. 6-2: Maternal versus embryonic control of initial embryonic development. During the oocyte growth phase in the follicles, transcripts and proteins are accumulated in the oocyte. With development, these components are gradually used and degraded. In parallel, the embryonic genome undergoes first a minor and later a major activation. The latter occurs at the 4-cell stage in pig and the 8-cell stage in cattle.

Table 6-2: Timing of the minor and major activation of the embryonic genome in different species

Species	Minor genome activation	Major genome activation
Mouse	G2 of first cell cycle (zygote)	Second cell cycle (2-cell embryo)
Pig	Unknown	Third cell cycle (4-cell embryo)
Cattle	First cell cycle (zygote)	Fourth cell cycle (8-cell embryo)
Dog	Unknown	Fourth cell cycle (8-cell embryo)
Horse	Unknown	Fourth to fifth cell cycle (8–16-cell embryo)
Sheep	Unknown	Fourth to fifth cell cycle (8–16-cell embryo)

desmosomes. Hence, a typical epithelium with apical and basolateral cell compartments is formed. There are some species differences in the timing of compaction: in the pig it occurs very early in development, around the 8-cell stage, whereas in cattle it happens later, around the 16- to 32-cell stage.

At the molecular level, differentiation of outer blastomeres, at least in the mouse, appears to rely on down-regulation of the transcription factor Oct4, followed by an up-regulation of other transcription factors such as Cdx2 and Eomesodermin (Fig. 6-4). The inner cells, meanwhile, retain expression of Oct4.

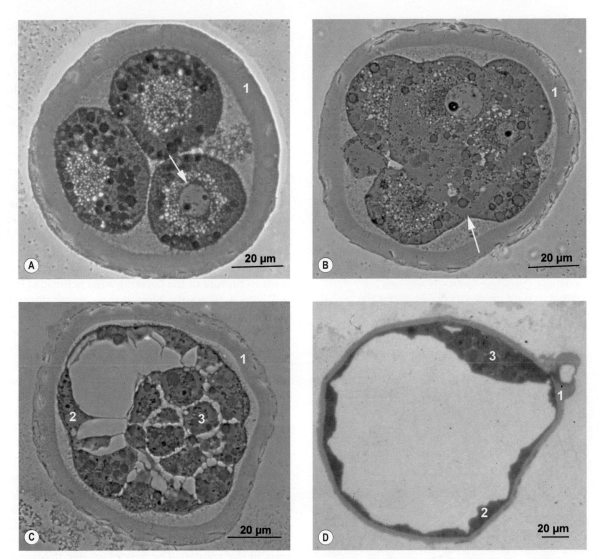

Fig. 6-3: Sections of pig embryos. A: 4-cell embryo presenting three blastomeres and one nucleus (arrow) in the section. 1: Zona pellucida. B: Morula in the process of compaction. Note the close connections (arrow) between the outer cells. 1: Zona pellucida. C: Blastocyst. 1: Zona pellucida; 2: Trophectoderm; 3: ICM. D: Expanded blastocyst. 1: Zona pellucida; 2: Trophectoderm; 3: ICM.

BLASTULATION

Compaction of the morula is a prerequisite for subsequent blastulation – the formation of a central fluid-filled cavity, the **blastocyst cavity**, within the early embryo. Blastulation transforms the embryo into a **blastocyst**, usually within the uterine lumen during the first week of development (Fig. 6-5).

Blastulation is brought about mainly by the trophectoderm and its control of fluid transport into the blastocyst cavity. Eventually, the inner blastomeres become positioned at one pole of the embryo forming the **inner cell mass (ICM)**.

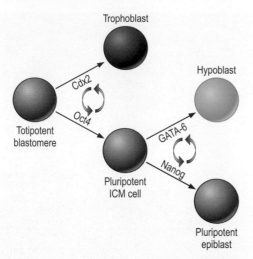

Fig. 6-4: The sequential action of the transcription factors Oct4, Nanog, Cdx2, and GATA-6 during initial cell differentiation in the mouse embryo. At compaction two cell lineages are derived from the totipotent blastomeres: the pluripotent inner cell mass (ICM) and the trophectoderm. The epiblast later differentiates into hypoblast and epiblast.

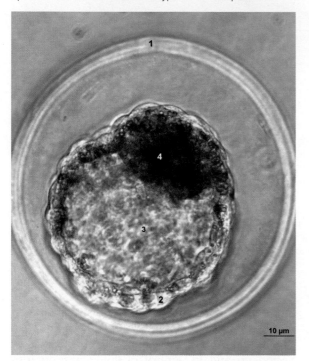

Fig. 6-5: Pig blastocyst at Day 6 of development as seen through the stereo microscope. 1: Zona pellucida; 2: Trophectoderm; 3: Blastocyst cavity; 4: Inner cell mass (ICM).

Descendants of the ICM will form the embryo proper; cells of the trophectoderm will give rise to the embryonic part of the placenta (see Chapter 9). The ratio of cells in the ICM to those in the troph-ectoderm is around 1:3. The portion of the trophectoderm covering the ICM is referred to as the **polar trophectoderm** whereas the rest is known as the **mural trophectoderm** (Fig. 6-6).

With the osmotic pressure inside the blastocyst cavity rising, the blastocyst gradually expands. Upon flushing of a blastocyst from the uterus (for embryo transfer for example), it is common to see the blastocyst collapse and re-expand several times. Whether this is an in vitro artefact or a normal physiological phenomenon also occurring in the uterus is unknown. Eventually, expansion of the blastocyst leads to rupture of the covering zona pellucida (Fig. 6-7) which allows the blastocyst to escape through the opening. In some species, this process, which is known as **hatching**, is aided by proteolytic enzymes released from the endometrium acting upon the glycoproteins forming the zona pellucida. In the horse, a 'compensatory' capsule forms between the trophectoderm and the overlying zona pellucida before the zona is shed. The capsule plays an important role in the maintenance of early pregnancy (see Chapter 9).

Around the time of hatching, the ICM differentiates into two cell populations: those facing the blastocyst cavity become flattened and delaminate, forming an inner cell sheet referred to as the **hypoblast** (Fig. 6-8); the remaining cells form the multi-layered **epiblast**. Small intercellular cavitations may arise in the epiblast. The hypoblast, like the trophectoderm, is epithelial in character. Gradually, it forms a complete inner lining beneath not only the epiblast, but also the trophectoderm. In the horse, the hypoblast first forms separate 'colonies' before coalescing into an internal closed compartment. In either case, a cavity, referred to as the **primitive yolk sac**, is formed. At the molecular level, the expression of the transcription factor Nanog is essential for the cells forming the epiblast at least in mice (Fig. 6-4) while the transcription factor GATA-6 is a key regulator of hypoblast formation. The epiblast will later form the embryo proper whereas the hypoblast will

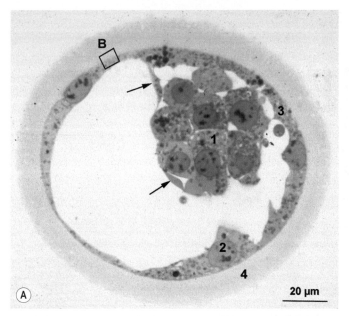
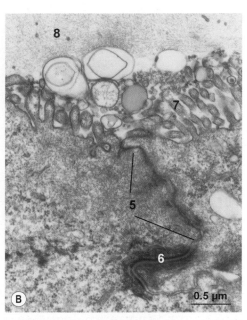

Fig. 6-6: Bovine blastocyst at Day 6 of development. The box (B) is seen at the ultrastructural level in 'B'. A: Light microscopical section. Note that flat hypoblast cells (arrows) have started to form from the ICM. 1: ICM; 2: Mural trophectoderm; 3: Polar trophectoderm; 4: Zona pellucida. B: Transmission electron micrograph of two adjacent trophectoderm cells. 5: Tight junction; 6: Desmosome; 7: Microvilli; 8: Zona pellucida.

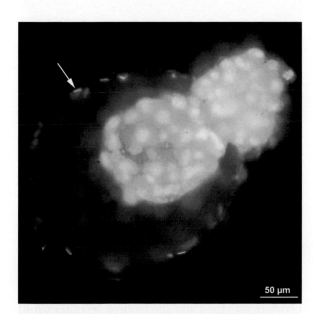

Fig. 6-7: Hatching of the pig blastocyst. The nuclei are stained with the fluorescent dye Hoechst 33342 and supernumerary spermatozoa are seen embedded in the zona pellucida (arrow). (Photo: Wouter Hazeleger.)

form the inner epithelium of the yolk sac which, depending on the species, may become engaged in placentation (see Chapter 9). However, at least in the mouse and rabbit, the hypoblast has also been shown to play a significant role in regulating the survival, proliferation and differentiation of the overlying epiblast. This regulation is, in part, mediated through formation of a basement membrane between the hypoblast and epiblast.

In the domestic species, the polar trophectoderm covering the epiblast (known as Rauber's layer) gradually disintegrates and is lost, exposing the epiblast to the uterine environment. However, before the shedding of Rauber's layer, tight junctions are formed between the outermost epiblast cells to seal the embryo despite the loss of the polar trophectoderm. After the loss of Rauber's layer, the epiblast is clearly discernable as a lucent structure, circular at first but becoming oval. Together with its underlying hypoblast this structure is known as the **embryonic disc** (Figs 6-9, 6-10).

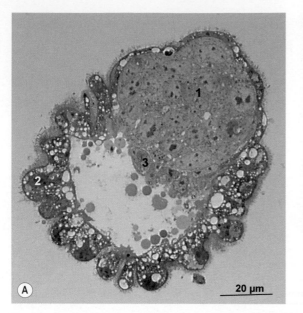
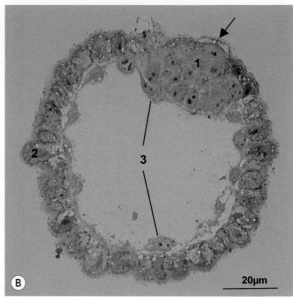

Fig. 6-8: Bovine blastocysts at Days 10 (A) and 12 (B) of development. 1: Epiblast; 2: Trophectoderm; 3: Hypoblast. Note that Rauber's layer is in the process of degenerating in B (arrow).

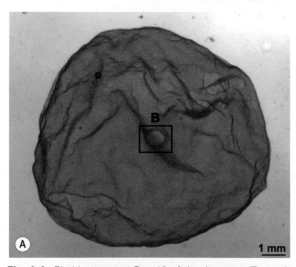
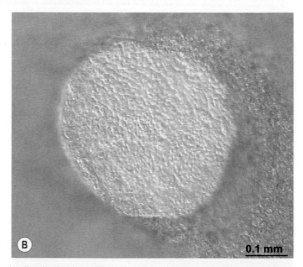

Fig. 6-9: Pig blastocyst at Day 10 of development. The embryonic disc in the box (B) is seen at a higher magnification in B.

BLASTOCYST ELONGATION

During the formation of the embryonic disc, the blastocyst is still expanding. Once the disc is formed, the trophectoderm with its underlying hypoblast becomes reshaped and the embryo becomes **ovoid** (Fig. 6-10). In the ruminants and pig, the process of elongation continues, and the embryo becomes first **tubular** and later **filamentous** (Fig. 6-11). The total

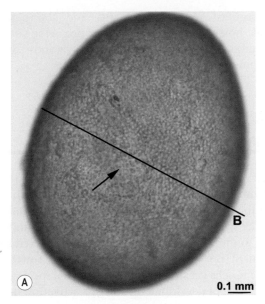

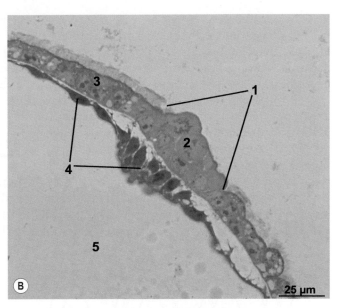

Fig. 6-10: The embryonic disc in a bovine embryo. A: Ovoid embryo at Day 14 of development faintly presenting the embryonic disc (arrow). The line (B) indicates the section displayed in B. B: Section through the embryonic disc (1). 2: Epiblast; 3: Trophectoderm presenting microvilli; 4: Hypoblast; 5: Primitive yolk sac.

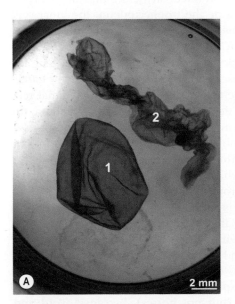

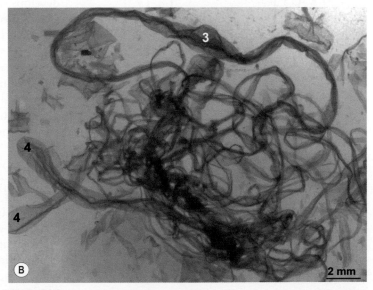

Fig. 6-11: Elongation of the pig embryo. A: A spherical (1) and a tubular (2) embryo at Day 11 of development. The tubular embryo is a bit folded. B: Intermingled filamentous embryos at Day 13 of development. Note the embryonic disc (3) and the dilated ends of the embryo (4).

mass of the embryo does not increase at the same rate as its length and so the embryo becomes thread-like and tremendously long. This phenomenon is particularly pronounced in the pig where the embryo develops from a sphere, about 1 cm in diameter, on Day 10 of development to a filamentous structure about one metre long on Day 13. Elongation is particularly dramatic on Days 12 and 13 (30–45 mm per hour!). This increase cannot be explained by mitoses alone; it involves restructuring of cells' cytoskeletons and shape as well. In ruminants, embryo elongation is less pronounced; in cattle the length increases by up to 35 cm between Days 12 and 21 (Fig. 6-12).

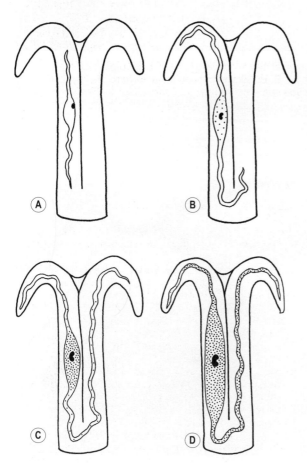

Fig. 6-12: Elongation of bovine embryos around Days 16 (A), 18 (B), 22 (C), and 27 (D) of development. Courtesy Sinowatz and Rüsse (2007).

In contrast to the ruminants and the pig, in the horse the embryo does not elongate but stays spherical during this period of development.

SUMMARY

In the zygote, meiosis is completed and the unique **embryonic genome** is assembled. Having completed the S-phase of the first post-fertilization cell cycle, the zygote enters the **mitotic cell cycle** and cleaves to the 2-cell stage. This cleavage, and several subsequent ones, occur **without cellular growth** and so the cells get smaller and smaller. At a species-specific stage of development, a **major activation of the embryonic genome** occurs. After a certain number of cleavages, the embryo enters the uterus from the oviduct and its cells form a mulberry-like cell cluster referred to as a **morula**. During the process of **compaction**, the outer cells of the morula adhere to each other and develop into the **trophectoderm**. A fluid-filled cavity, the **blastocyst cavity**, develops inside the trophectoderm, the inner cells gather at one pole of the embryo to form the **inner cell mass (ICM)**, and the embryo becomes a **blastocyst**. At a species-specific stage of development, the blastocyst escapes from the zona pellucida by **hatching**. Around the time of hatching, the internal cells of the ICM delaminate and form an epithelium, the **hypoblast**, inside the blastocyst. The cavity enclosed by the hypoblast may be referred to as the **primitive yolk sac**. The external cells of the ICM form the **epiblast**, which will later give rise to the embryo itself. The trophectoderm covering the epiblast, Rauber's layer, is subsequently lost, and the epiblast is exposed to the uterine environment and becomes confluent with the trophectoderm. At this stage, the epiblast and the hypoblast have established the **embryonic disc**. After hatching, the blastocyst retains its spherical shape at first but, in pigs and ruminants (but not horses), becomes **ovoid** and, with further elongation, successively **tubular** and **filamentous**.

Box 6-1 Molecular regulation of blastulation

Around the morula stage, the blastomeres have lost totipotency and two distinct cell lineages become apparent: inner cells, forming the ICM, and outer cells forming the trophectoderm. Formation of ICM and trophectoderm constitutes the first differentiation process during embryonic development. At the molecular level, however, recent findings in mice have shown that the molecular background for this differentiation is laid down as early as at the 4-cell stage. As mentioned in Chapter 2, cell differentiation and embryonic development are epigenetically controlled since all cells (with a few exceptions, e.g. the lymphocyte lineage) descended from the zygote share the same DNA sequences. Histone modification is one such epigenetic control mechanism. In the mouse, depending on the spatial arrangement of individual 4-cell blastomeres and the order in which they are generated, some blastomeres apparently end up with more methylation of arginine residues at histone H3 than do others. The more methylated blastomeres tend to form inner cells and, consequently, the ICM; the less methylated ones tend to form outer cells and thence trophectoderm.

At the morphological level, differentiation of ICM and trophectoderm is first evidenced by cell surface changes that increase adhesion between blastomeres. This is mediated through the expression of the calcium-dependent trans-membrane cell adhesion molecule, **ovomorulin**, also known as **E-cadherin**. When E-cadherin-mediated adhesion occurs, all blastomeres have a surface covered with microvilli facing the outside of the embryo and a smoother surface facing the centre. Subsequently to the E-cadherin-dependent adhesions, tight junctions develop between the outer cells, clearly defining apical and basolateral plasma membrane domains. Thus, outer cells become polarized and epithelial. Later, Na^+,K^+ pumps are established basolaterally in the trophectoderm to drive formation of the blastocyst cavity during blastulation.

FURTHER READING

Betteridge, K.J. (2007): Equine embryology: An inventory of unanswered questions. Theriogenology 68S, S9–S21.

Betteridge, K.J. and Fléchon, J.–E. (1988): The anatomy and physiology of pre-attachment bovine embryos. Theriogenology 29:155–187.

Degrelle, A.A., Campion, E., Cabau, C., Piumi, F., Reinaud, P., Richard, C., Renard, J.–P. and Hue, I. (2005): Molecular evidence for a critical period in mural trophoblast development in bovine blastocysts. Dev. Biol. 288:448–460.

Denker, H.–W., Eng, L.A., Mootz, U. and Hammer, C.E. (1978): Studies on the early development and implantation in the cat. I. Cleavage and blastocyst formation. Anatomischer Anzeiger 144:457–468.

Heuser, C.H. and Streeter, G.L. (1927): Early stages in the development of pig embryos, from the period of initial cleavage to the time of the appearance of limb-buds. Contributions to Embryology, 20, Carnegie Institution of Washington, Publication number 109:1–19.

Holst, P.A. and Phemister, R.D. (1971): The prenatal development of the dog: preimplantation events. Biol. Reprod. 5:194–206.

Hunter, R.H.F. (1974): Chronological and cytological details of fertilization and early embryonic development in the domestic pig, Sus scrofa. Anat. Rec. 178:169–186.

Maddox-Hyttel, P, Bjerregaard, B. and Laurincik, J. (2005): Meiosis and embryo technology: renaissance of the nucleolus. Reprod. Fertil. Dev. 17:3–14.

Patten, B.M. (1948): Embryology of the pig, 3rd edn. Blakiston, New York.

Reynaud, K., Fontbonne, A., Marseloo, N., Viaris de Lesegno, C., Saint-Dizier, M. and Chastant-Maillard, S. (2006): In vivo canine oocyte maturation, fertilization and early embryogenesis: a review. Theriogenology 66:1685–1693.

Rüsse, I. and Sinowatz, F. (1998): Lehrbuch der Embryologie der Haustiere, 2nd edn. Parey Buchverlag, Berlin.

Schier, A.F. (2007): The maternal-zygotic transition: death and birth of RNAs. Science 316:406–407.

Sharp, D.C. (2000): The early fetal life of the equine conceptus. Anim. Reprod. Sci. 60–61:679–689.

Stroband, H.W.J. and van der Lende, T. (1990): Embryonic and uterine development during early pregnancy in pigs. J. Reprod. Fert. Suppl. 40:261–277.

Vejlsted, M., Du, Y., Vajta, G. and Maddox-Hyttel P. (2006): Post-hatching development of the porcine and bovine embryo – defining criteria for expected development in vivo and in vitro. Theriogenology 65:153–165.

Watson, A.J. (1998): Trophectoderm differentiation in the bovine embryo: characterization of a polarized epithelium. J. Reprod. Fert. 114:327–339.

Watson, A.J. and Barcroft, L. (2001): Regulation of blastocyst formation. Frontiers in Bioscience 6:D708–730.

CHAPTER 7

Morten Vejlsted

Gastrulation, body folding and coelom formation

As was described in the previous chapter, blastulation results in the formation of the ICM, trophectoderm, epiblast, and hypoblast. The hypoblast and trophectoderm are extra-embryonic cell lineages that will participate in fetal membrane formation (see Chapter 9) whereas derivatives of the epiblast will found all of the embryonic cell lineages. Initially, this occurs through formation of three somatic germ layers from the epiblast: **ectoderm**, **mesoderm** and **endoderm**. A prominent derivative of the endoderm is the primitive gut, the formation of which lends its name to the entire process of germ layer formation – **gastrulation**, from the Greek term gastrula meaning small stomach. Besides the three germ layers, gastrulation also establishes the **germ line**, in the form of the **primordial germ cells**. Only the initial establishment of the germ line is covered in this chapter; further development of the primordial germ cells within the genital ridges is described in Chapters 4 and 15.

While gastrulation proceeds, the embryonic disc gradually becomes covered by extra-embryonic membranes to form the **amniotic cavity**. In domestic species, amnion formation results from an 'upfolding' of the trophectoderm with its underlying extra-embryonic mesoderm, as will be described first, followed by focus on the events occurring in the disc itself.

DEVELOPMENT OF THE AMNION

During the early phases of gastrulation, the trophectoderm is lined by a thin layer of extra-embryonic mesoderm (see below), the two layers together constituting the **chorion**. During gastrulation, the chorion forms folds – **chorioamniotic folds** – that surround the embryonic disc (Fig. 7-1). Gradually, the folds extend upwards to meet and fuse above the embryonic disc thereby enclosing the disc in a sealed **amniotic cavity**. The term **amnion** is generally used collectively for the cavity and its wall. The inner epithelium of the amnion originates from the trophectoderm and so, at the embryonic disc, it is continuous with the epiblast and later the embryonic surface ectoderm (see below). The outside covering of the amnion is composed of extra-embryonic mesoderm. Later, the amnion will become surrounded by yet another cavity, the **allantois** (see below and Chapter 9).

The site where the chorioamniotic folds meet and fuse is known as the **mesamnion** (Fig. 7-2). In the horse and carnivores, the mesamnion disappears leaving no connection between the amnion and chorion. As a result, foals, pups and kittens are born covered by an intact amnion which can be suffocating if not removed by the mother or an attendant. In contrast, in the pig and ruminants, the mesamnion persists; as a result, the amnion gets torn during parturition and offspring are generally born without covering membranes.

EARLY PHASES OF GASTRULATION

The onset of gastrulation has traditionally been linked to the morphological appearance of the **primitive streak**, an elongated accumulation of cells at the caudal pole of the future embryo proper. This structure is formed by epiblast cells accumulating

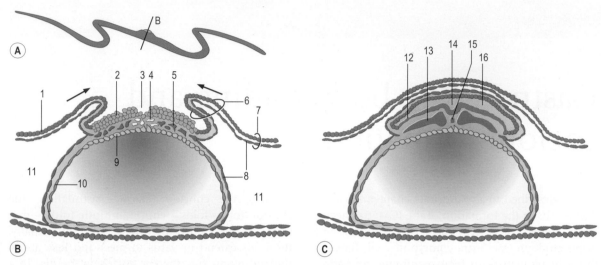

Fig. 7-1: Formation of the amnion from chorioamniotic folds in the pig at Days 13 to 15 of development. 1: Trophectoderm; 2: Epiblast; 3: Primitive streak; 4: Mes-endodermal precursor cells; 5: Intra-embryonic mesoderm; 6: Chorioamniotic fold; 7: Chorion; 8: Extra-embryonic mesoderm; 9: Endoderm; 10: Hypoblast; 11: Coelom; 12: Surface ectoderm; 13: Mesoderm; 14: Neural groove; 15: Notochord; 16: Amniotic cavity.

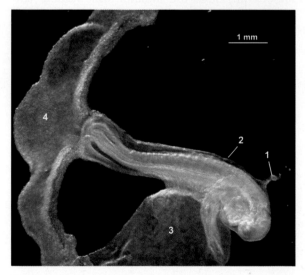

Fig. 7-2: A sheep embryo at Day 17 of development. When embryos are flushed from the uterus, the chorion is usually pinched off, leaving the mesamnion looking like an antenna on the amnion. 1: Mesamnion; 2: Amnion; 3: Yolk sac; 4: Allantois.

posteriorly and gradually establishing a **crescent-shaped thickening** of the embryonic disc – the earliest morphological sign of the onset of gastrulation yet identified, at least in pigs and cattle (Figs 7-3, 7-4). The caudal crescentic thickening appears around Days 10 to 11 of gestation in the pig and around Days 14 to 15 in cattle. When the crescent-shaped thickening is established, ingression of epiblast cells to the space between the epiblast and hypoblast is initiated (Fig. 7-5). In laboratory animals, these early morphological signs of gastrulation in the epiblast are preceded by morphological and molecular changes in the hypoblast underlying the anterior pole of the epiblast (see Box 7-1 on molecular regulation).

The epiblast cells constituting the posterior crescent soon gather in the embryonic disc midline to form the primitive streak (Fig. 7-3). In the streak, cells start to involute from the epiblast through its basement membrane to establish **mes-endodermal precursors**, i.e. cells capable of forming either

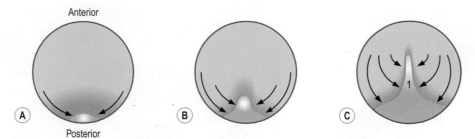

Fig. 7-3: Accumulation of epiblast cells in the posterior portion of the embryonic disc results in the formation of the primitive streak (1).

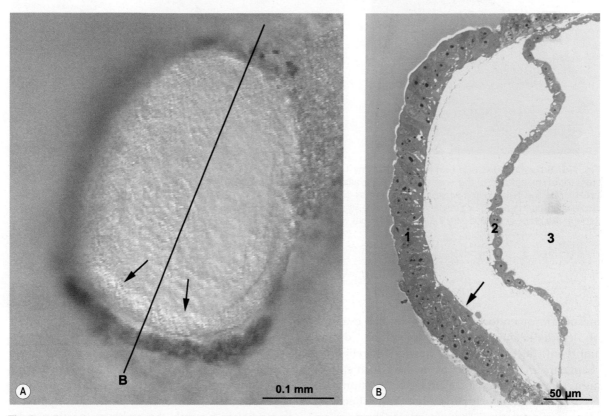

Fig. 7-4: Embryonic disc of a pig embryo at Day 10 of development showing the gathering of epiblast cells forming a posterior crescent. **A:** The embryonic disc with the posterior crescent (arrows). The line (B) indicates the plane of section shown in 'B'. **B:** Median section through the embryonic disc presenting a posterior thickening (arrow) of the epiblast (1). 2: Hypoblast; 3: Primitive yolk sac.

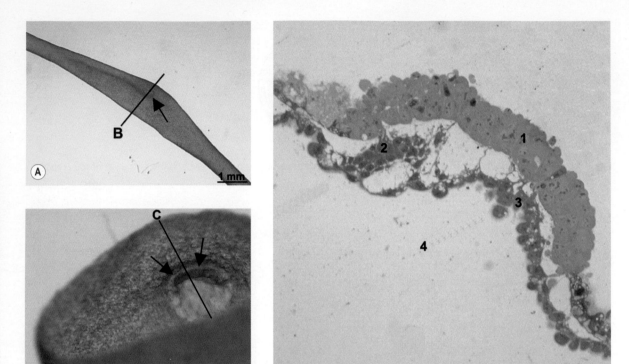

Fig. 7-5: Embryonic disc of a bovine embryo at Day 14 of development showing the ingression of cells from the caudal crescent of the epiblast to the space between epiblast and hypoblast. **A:** Tubular embryo presenting the embryonic disc (arrow). The line (B) indicates where the embryo was cut in order to produce the image in B. **B:** Internal view of the embryonic disc displaying the posterior crescent (arrows). The line (C) indicates the plane of section shown in C. **C:** Median section through the embryonic disc with the epiblast (1) from which cells ingress (2). 3: Hypoblast; 4: Primitive yolk sac.

mesoderm or **endoderm**. This is the first example of **epithelio-mesenchymal transition** during embryonic development, the process whereby cells change their characteristics from those of an epithelium (having strong intercellular connections) to become more loosely organized and, therefore, capable of migration. The term **mesenchyme** refers to loosely organized embryonic tissue regardless of germ layer origin. Interestingly, just as the initiation of gastrulation is marked by this epithelio-mesenchymal transition, so the cessation of this phase of development is marked by a suppression of this process.

INITIAL FORMATION OF THE MESODERM AND ENDODERM

The mes-endodermal precursor cells give rise to **endoderm** and **mesoderm**. The endoderm-forming cells integrate into, and displace, the hypoblast immediately beneath the epiblast, forming endoderm (Fig. 7-6). Other cells remain positioned under the epiblast and trophectoderm forming intra- and extra-embryonic mesoderm, respectively. The endoderm enlarges to form the upper lining of the **primitive yolk sac** under the epiblast and, at the margin of the embryonic disc, is continuous with the hypo-

The development of the **intra-embryonic meso-derm** parallels that of the endoderm. It arises from a portion of the presumptive mes-endodermal cells that ingressed through the primitive streak but now remain in the space between the epiblast and the hypoblast. Formation of mesoderm is not limited to the area of the embryonic disc, however; meso-dermal cells migrate far beyond the disc as the **extra-embryonic mesoderm** (Figs 7-6, 7-7). Intra- and extra-embryonic mesoderm each split into two sheets: one associating with the epiblast and tro-phectoderm to form the **somatic** or **parietal meso-derm**, the other associating with the endoderm and hypoblast as the **visceral** or **splanchnic mesoderm** (Figs 7-6, 7-7). Together, the trophectoderm and the extra-embryonic somatic mesoderm will form the outer layers of the embryonic part of the pla-centa, the **chorion** (see Chapter 9). The cavity forming between the somatic and visceral meso-derm is referred to as the **coelom**. Initially, the coelom is only located outside the embryonic disc and is therefore referred to as the **extra-embryonic coelom** or **exocoelom**. Soon, however, the split between the somatic and visceral mesoderm also involves intra-embryonic mesoderm portions, establishing an **intra-embryonic coelom** which, with the cranio-caudal and lateral foldings of the embryo, will later give rise to the body cavities (Fig. 7-8). When this happens, the somatic mesoderm gives rise to the parietal portions of the **peritoneum** and **pleura**, whereas the visceral mesoderm gives rise to the visceral portions of these serous membranes.

The intra-embryonic mesoderm is established in a posterior to anterior direction, in part progressing in parallel with the growing primitive streak. After involution, cells spread both laterally, forming the extra-embryonic mesoderm, and cranially, forming intra-embryonic mesoderm. Soon, the rate of growth of the entire embryonic disc overtakes that of the primitive streak, and the disc is lengthened into an initially oval, later pear-shaped, structure (Fig. 7-9). From extending well over half the length of the embryonic disc, the primitive streak gradually becomes more and more posteriorly located as a result of this differential growth.

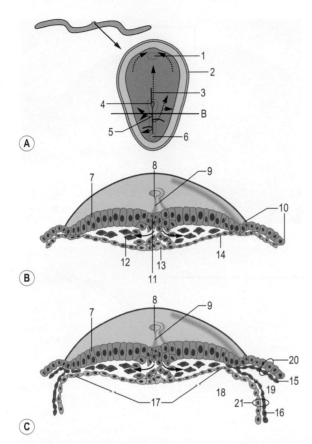

Fig. 7-6: Two different phases in the ingression (arrows) of cells through the primitive streak and node. **A:** The embryonic disc seen from above. The line (B) indicates the section presented in the oblique view in 'B'. 1: Buccopharyngeal membrane; 2: Cut edge of trophectoderm and hypoblast; 3: Mesoderm cells forming the notochord; 4; Primitive node; 5: Primitive streak; 6: Cloacal membrane. **B:** Oblique section through the primitive streak. 7: Epiblast; 8: Primitive node; 9: Primitive streak; 10: Trophectoderm; 11: Mes-endoderm cells (orange); 12: Mesoderm cells (red); 13: Endoderm cells (yellow); 14: Hypoblast cells (green). **C:** Oblique section some hours later. 15: Somatic mesoderm; 16: Visceral mesoderm; 17: Transition between endoderm and hypoblast; 18: Primitive yolk sac; 19: Coelom; 20: Chorion; 21: Yolk sac wall.

blast (Figs 7-6, 7-7). The endodermally lined portion of the primitive yolk sac will later become enclosed within the embryo proper and develop into the **primitive gut,** whereas the hypoblast-lined portion of the cavity will be displaced extra-embryonically to form the **definitive yolk sac** (Fig. 7-8).

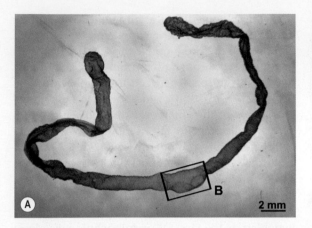

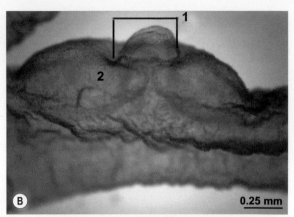

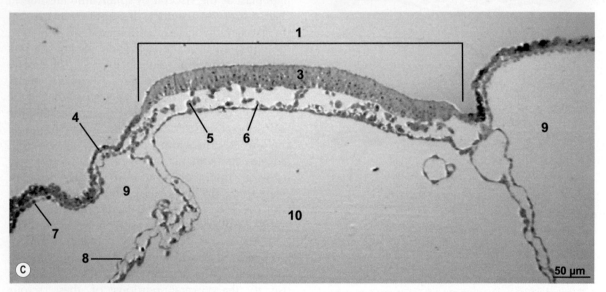

Fig. 7-7: Gastrulation in a sheep embryo at Day 13 of development. **A:** Tubular sheep embryo. The box (B) is enlarged in 'B'. **B:** The embryonic disc (1) surrounded by chorioamniotic folds (2). **C:** Longitudinal section through B. 1: Embryonic disc; 3: Epiblast; 4: Trophectoderm; 5: Mesoderm; 6: Endoderm; 7: Somatic mesoderm; 8: Visceral mesoderm; 9: Coelom; 10: Primitive yolk sac.

Along with the relative posterior withdrawal of the primitive streak, a midline structure, the **notochord,** is laid down – a pivotal step in the establishment of the anterior-posterior embryonic axis (Figs 7-1, 7-6). The notochord is formed by epiblast cells ingressing through the **primitive node**, a specialized population of epiblast cells located at the anterior end of the primitive streak. The first cells that ingress through the primitive node form the **prechordal**
plate, a mesodermal structure located just anterior to the tip of the notochord.

During the process of gastrulation, involution of cells forming the mesoderm and endoderm occurs through different organizer regions within the primitive streak. In the mouse, three such organizer regions have been identified: an early-gastrula organizer, contributing mainly to formation of extra-embryonic mesoderm; a mid-gastrula

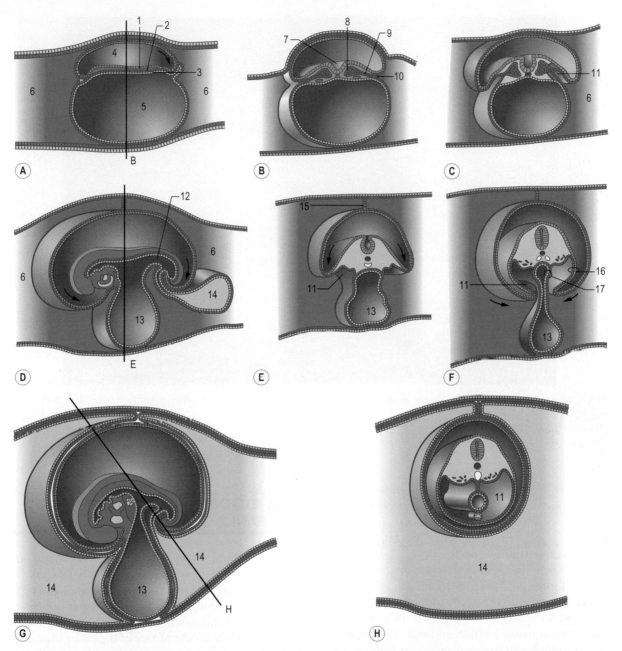

Fig. 7-8: Formation of the coelomic cavities. **A, D, and G:** Median sections of embryos at different stages of the cranio-caudal folding. Arrows indicate the direction of folding. **B, C, E, F, and H:** Cross sections of embryos at different stages of lateral folding. Arrows indicate the direction of folding. The section plane B is indicated in A, the section plane E is indicated in D, and the section plane H is indicated in G. 1: Ectoderm; 2: Mesoderm; 3: Endoderm; 4: Amniotic cavity; 5: Primitive yolk sac; 6: Extra-embryonic coelom; 7: Neural groove; 8: Paraxial mesoderm; 9: Intermediate mesoderm; 10: Lateral plate mesoderm; 11: Intra-embryonic coelom; 12: Hindgut; 13: Yolk sac; 14: Allantois; 15: Mesamnion; 16: Somatopleura; 17: Splanchnopleura. Modified from Sadler (2004).

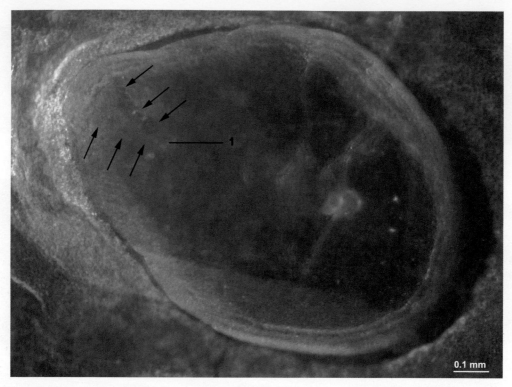

Fig. 7-9: Pear-shaped embryonic disc in a pig embryo at Day 12 of development. The primitive streak (arrows) and node (1) are faintly visible.

organizer, contributing mainly to endoderm and intra-embryonic mesoderm formation; and a late-gastrula organizer region giving rise to the prechordal plate and notochord. The late organizer region is the primitive node.

Anteriorly, the notochord is delimited by the **prechordal plate**, and anterior to this the epiblast is so tightly adherent to the newly formed endoderm that there is no space for intervening mesoderm (Fig. 7-6). This apposed epiblast and endoderm develops into the **buccopharyngeal membrane** which for a time seals the future opening between the oral cavity and the pharynx (see Chapter 14). Posteriorly, the notochord is delimited by a similar structure, the **cloacal membrane**, which for a time seals the common openings of the gut, urinary organs, and reproductive tract into the cloaca (see Chapter 14).

THE ECTODERM AND ITS EARLY DERIVATIVES

The notochord's signalling molecules, including Sonic hedgehog (Shh), induce the overlying epiblast to differentiate into neuroectoderm (see Chapter 8). Hence, for a while, both the primitive streak (posteriorly) and the nascent neural ectoderm (anteriorly) are visible on the surface of the embryonic disc (Fig. 7-10).

Neuroectoderm

In the embryonic disc region anterior to the primitive node, epiblast cells are induced to differentiate into **neuroectoderm**, in part by the recently established notochord. This is first recognized by the formation of the **neural plate** (Fig. 7-10). Soon, the lateral edges of the neural plate become elevated, forming the **neural folds** that enclose a midline depression known as the **neural groove**. The neural folds gradually fuse over the neural groove to complete the **neural tube**. Fusion is initiated in the future embryonic cervical region and proceeds from there in both anterior and posterior directions like a double zipper. Hence, the neural tube initially opens into the amniotic cavity anteriorly and posteriorly through the anterior and posterior **neuropores** (Fig. 7-11). These pores eventually close, the anterior one first and then the posterior. This process represents the foundation of the first embryonic organ system, the **central nervous system** (see Chapters 8 and 10).

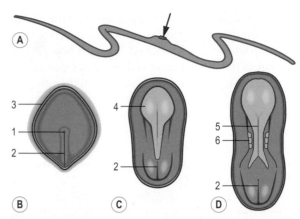

Fig. 7-10: The embryonic disc seen from above displaying the gradual development (B through D) of the neuroectoderm in relation to the relative withdrawal of the primitive streak. 1: Primitive node; 2: Primitive streak; 3: Cut edge of trophectoderm and hypoblast; 4: Neural plate; 5: Neural groove; 6: Somite.

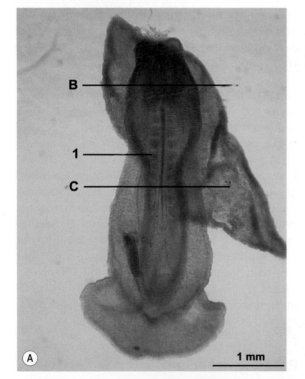

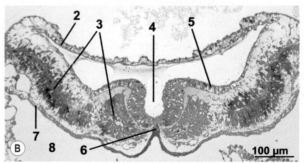

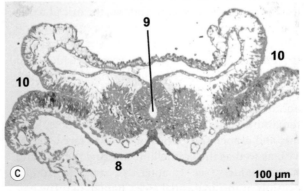

Fig. 7-11: Formation of the neural groove and tube in a bovine embryo at Day 21 of development. The chorion has been pinched off during collection of the embryo and so the extra-embryonic coelom is not delineated. **A:** The section planes (B, C) indicate the location of the cross sections in 'B' and 'C'. 1: Somite; 2: Inner epithelium of amniotic wall; 3: Mesoderm; 4: Rostral neuropore; 5: Surface ectoderm; 6: Notochord; 7: Endoderm; 8: Primitive yolk sac; 9: Neural tube; 10: Extra-embryonic coelom.

Along with the elevation and fusion of the neural folds, certain cells at the lateral border or crest of the neural folds become detached. This cell population, known as the **neural crest cells,** will not participate in formation of the neural tube; instead they migrate widely and participate in the formation of many other tissues, such as the integument (melanocytes), other parts of the nervous system (including neurons for the central, sympathetic and enteric nervous system) and large parts of the craniofacial mesenchymal derivatives (see Chapter 8).

The mechanism whereby the neural crest cells detach from the neural folds is comparable with that occurring during ingression of epiblast cells in the primitive streak and node – a second example of **epithelio-mesenchymal transition**. As mentioned above, the term **mesenchyme** refers to loosely organized embryonic tissue regardless of germ layer origin. Thus, both neuroectoderm (through the neural crest cells) and mesoderm may give rise to mesenchyme.

Surface ectoderm

After having allocated cells for endoderm, mesoderm, the germ line and neuroectoderm, most of the remaining more laterally located epiblast will differentiate into surface ectoderm. Once the anterior and posterior neuropores have closed, two bilateral thickenings of the surface ectoderm, the **otic placode** and the **lens placode**, are established in the embryonic cephalic ectoderm (Fig. 7-12). The otic placode invaginates to form the **otic vesicle**, which will develop into the inner ear for hearing and balance (see Chapter 11), while the lens placode invaginates and forms the **lens** of the eye (see Chapter 11). The remaining surface ectoderm gives rise to the **epidermis** and **associated glands of the skin** (see Chapter 17), as well as the epithelium covering the oral and nasal cavities (see Chapter 14) and the caudal portion of the anal canal (see Chapter 14). The epithelium covering the oral cavity gives rise to the **enamel** of the teeth (see Chapter 14) and also part of the **pituitary gland**, the adenohypophysis (see Chapter 10).

THE MESODERM AND ITS EARLY DERIVATIVES

Formation of the notochord provides an embryonic midline axis as a template for the axial skeleton. Initially, cells of the mesoderm form a thin sheet of loosely woven mesenchyme on either side of the notochord. Soon, however, starting in the occipital region of the embryo, the mesoderm closest to the notochord (the **paraxial mesoderm**) proliferates and forms pairs of segmental thickened structures known as **somitomeres**. In the head region, the somitomeres, together with lateral plate mesoderm and neural crest cells differentiate further into connective tissue, bone, and cartilage. In the body region they form **somites** from which dermis, skeletal muscle and vertebrae develop (Figs 7-8, 7-10, 7-11). In large animal species, somites are formed at a rate of, on average, about six pairs a day. The number of somites formed during this phase of development therefore forms a basis for estimating embryonic age.

More laterally, the mesoderm remains thin and is therefore referred to as the **lateral plate mesoderm**. The lateral plate mesoderm is continuous with the extra-embryonic mesoderm. As described above, formation of the extra-embryonic coelom divides this part of the mesoderm into **somatic** and **visceral mesoderm** (Fig. 7-8). With the continued development of the coelom, an intra-embryonic coelom similarly divides the lateral plate mesoderm. Within the embryo, the somatic mesoderm associates with the surface ectoderm to constitute the **somatopleura** while the **visceral mesoderm** associates with the endoderm to form the **splanchnopleura** (Fig. 7-8). Between the paraxial and lateral plate mesoderm, the **intermediate mesoderm** is established.

Paraxial mesoderm

As a general rule, development proceeds in an anterior to posterior direction (one exception to this was the development of the primitive streak). Accordingly, formation of somites progresses from the

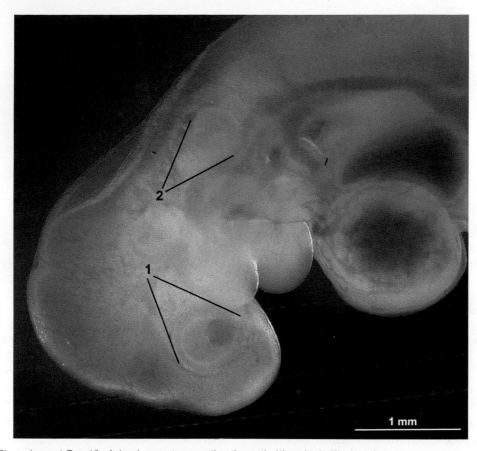

Fig. 7-12: Pig embryo at Day 18 of development presenting the optic (1) and otic (2) placodes.

occipital region posteriorly. In the head region, the somitomeres, together with a similar segmentation of the neural plate, form **neuromeres** (see Chapters 9, 10). From the occipital region and posteriorly, the somitomeres gradually organize into **somites**. Each somite subsequently differentiates into three components (Fig. 7-13). The ventro-medial part of the somite associates with the notochord establishing the **sclerotome** which patterns formation of the vertebral column (see Chapter 16). The dorso-lateral part of each somite forms regionalized precursors of both dermal and muscle tissue, the **dermamyotome**. From this structure, dorso-medially and ventromedially located cell populations forms the **myotome** and a dorso-laterally located group becomes the **dermatome**. The myotome of each

somite contributes to muscles of the back and limbs (see Chapter 16), while the dermatome disperses and forms the dermis and subcutis of the skin (see Chapter 17).

Later, each myotome and dermatome will receive its own segmental nerve component (see Chapter 10). Clinically speaking, it is important to appreciate that this innervation from the segment of origin is retained throughout life.

Intermediate mesoderm

The intermediate mesoderm, which connects paraxial and lateral plate mesoderm, differentiates into structures of both the urinary system and the gonads, together referred to as the **urogenital system** (see

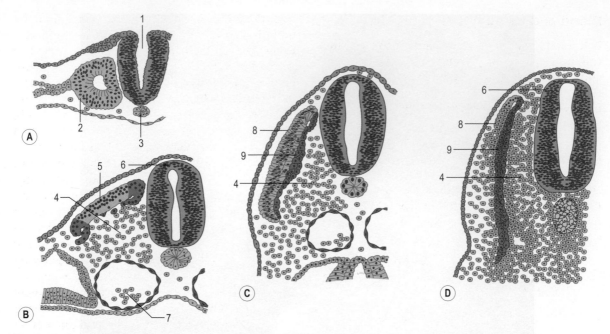

Fig. 7-13: Cross sections of embryos showing the gradual (A, B, C through D) differentiation of the somites. 1: Neural groove; 2: Somite; 3: Notochord; 4: Sclerotome; 5: Dermamyotome; 6: Neural tube; 7: Dorsal aorta; 8: Dermatome; 9: Myotome. Modified from Sadler (2004).

Chapter 15). Analogously to processes described for the paraxial mesoderm, the intermediate mesoderm in the cervical and cranial thoracic regions forms segmental cell clusters known as **nephrotomeres**. However, more caudally an unsegmented mass of tissue is formed. This is the **nephrogenic cord** forming a temporary kidney, the mesonephros, on the medial aspect of which the gonads start to form at a relatively early stage of development in order to receive the **primordial germ cells**. The primordial germ cells initially escape from the epiblast during formation of the somatic germ layers, but later return to populate the developing gonad (see Chapters 4 and 15).

Lateral plate mesoderm and body folding

During a series of anterior-posterior and lateral foldings, the subdivision of the coelom into intra- and extra-embryonic cavities becomes progressively better defined and the embryonic body gradually assumes the shape of a closed tube enclosing another tube, the **primitive gut** (Fig. 7-8). The somatopleura will form the lateral and ventral body wall of which the somatic mesoderm will provide the inner lining (giving rise to the **peritoneum** and **pleura**) and the ectoderm the outer lining (the **epidermis)**. The splanchnopleura will form the wall of the primitive gut and its derivatives in which the endoderm will provide the inner lining (the **lamina epithelialis of the tunica mucosa**). The visceral mesoderm will provide **all other components of the gut** and its derivatives. Soon, the intra-embryonic coelom will be divided into the peritoneal, pleural and pericardial cavities. Thus the serous membranes lining the *parietal* surfaces of each of these cavities are derived from the somatic mesoderm, whereas the serous membranes lining the *visceral* surfaces (and hence covering the organs) are derived from the visceral mesoderm.

Blood and blood vessel formation

Both blood and blood vessels appear to arise from common mesoderm precursor cells, the **haemangioblasts**. These differentiate into **haematopoietic stem cells** (forming blood cells) and **angioblasts** that form endothelial cells which coalesce to form blood vessels (see Chapter 12).

The first sign of blood and blood vessel formation is seen in the visceral mesoderm of the splanchnopleura covering the extra-embryonic yolk sac. However, this appears to be only a transient phenomenon; later, haematopoiesis moves first to the liver and spleen and then to the bone marrow (see Chapter 12).

THE ENDODERM AND ITS EARLY DERIVATIVES

The inner epithelial lining of the gastrointestinal tract and its derivatives is the main component derived from the endoderm (Fig. 7-8). Initially, the epithelium of the roof of the primitive yolk sac is formed by the endoderm, which is continuous with, and displaces, the hypoblast. With the anterior-posterior and lateral foldings of the embryo, the endoderm-enclosed portion of the primitive yolk sac is enclosed within the embryo forming the **primitive gut**, whereas the hypoblast-enclosed portion becomes localized outside the embryo to form the **definitive yolk sac**. The term yolk sac may be confusing, as the cavity may seem to share very little similarity with the yolk sac of the fowl. As will be described in Chapter 9, the yolk sac plays only a transient role in the pig and ruminants. However, in both the horse and carnivores it is essential during at least the initial establishment of the placenta. Thus, the yolk sac of domestic animals is somewhat analogous to the structure in the fowl, in that it has a nutritive function during embryonic development.

The primitive gut comprises cranial (foregut), middle (midgut) and caudal (hindgut) parts. The midgut communicates with the yolk sac through the **vitelline duct** (Fig. 7-8). This duct is wide initially but, as development proceeds, becomes long and narrow and is eventually incorporated into the **umbilical cord** (see Chapter 9). The endoderm forms the epithelium of the gastro-pulmonary system and the parenchyma of its derivatives. Endoderm of the **foregut** gives rise to the pharynx and its derivatives, including the middle ear, the parenchyma of the thyroid gland, the parathyroid glands, the liver and the pancreas, and the reticulated stroma of the tonsils and thymus, as well as the oesophagus, stomach, liver and pancreas (see Chapter 14). At its anterior end, the foregut is temporarily closed by an ectodermal-endodermal membrane, the **buccopharyngeal membrane**. At a certain stage of development, this membrane ruptures and open communication between the amniotic cavity and the primitive gut is established. The **midgut** gives rise to most of the small and the large intestine down to the transverse colon whereas the **hindgut** gives rise to the transverse and descending colon as well as the rectum and part of the anal canal. At its caudal end, the hindgut temporarily dilates to form the **cloaca**, a cavity transiently common to both the developing gastrointestinal and urogenital systems (see Chapters 14 and 15). The cloaca is separated from the amniotic cavity by the **cloacal membrane**, composed of closely apposed ectoderm and endoderm, like the buccopharyngeal membrane. After separation of the gastrointestinal and urinary systems, the cloacal membrane breaks down, opening the two systems into the amniotic cavity via the **anus** and **urogenital sinus** respectively.

Formation of the allantois

During the second or third week of development, depending on the species, the **allantois** is formed as an outgrowth from the hindgut into the extra-embryonic coelom (Fig. 7-8). In ruminants and the pig, the allantois assumes a T-shaped appearance with the top bar of the T being located as a transverse cavity just caudal to the embryo proper and the stem of the T connected with the hindgut (Fig. 7-2). Like the vitelline duct, the **allantoic duct**, connecting the allantoic cavity and the hindgut, becomes incorporated into the umbilical cord as a consequence of embryonic foldings. Since the allantois is diverticulum of the hindgut, its wall is composed of an inner epithelial lining of endodermal origin and an outer layer derived from the visceral mesoderm. As the allantois enlarges, the visceral mesodermal part of its wall fuses with the somatic mesoderm of the chorion and, finally, more or less covers the amnion. The fusion of the allantoic and chorionic walls forms the embryonic part of the **allantochorionic placenta** found in the domestic animals (Fig. 7-8; see Chapter 9). The intra-embryonic proximal portion of the allantoic duct, extending from the hindgut to the umbilicus, is referred to as the **urachus** and gives rise to the urinary bladder (see Chapter 15). Through initial gestation, the allantoic cavity serves as a repository of the wastes excreted through the embryo's developing urinary system.

THE PRIMORDIAL GERM CELLS

During formation of the mesoderm and endoderm, a certain population of epiblast cells is set aside for formation of the future germ line. These **primordial germ cells** are not well described in the domestic animals but, at least in pigs and cattle, they seem to become recognizable for the first time in the posterior rim of the embryonic disc during gastrulation. As the somatic germ layers form, the primordial germ cells are displaced from the embryonic disc area to the wall of the definitive yolk sac and, to some degree, of the allantois (see Chapter 4). How this comes about is not known, but probably involves passive carriage with the endoderm. The primordial germ cells multiply in the yolk sac wall and then, by active or passive means, relocate into the area of the genital ridges as the ridges develop from the intermediate mesoderm (see Chapter 4). The relocation pathway, in the pig at least, passes through the visceral mesoderm connecting the stalks of both the yolk sac and the allantois to the hindgut. On arrival in the genital ridge, the primordial germ cells continue to multiply for a while (the time varying with species) until they either initiate meiosis (female embryo) or enter mitotic arrest until puberty (male embryo; see Chapter 4).

SUMMARY

During the **gastrulation**, the epiblast forms the **primitive streak** through which cells involute to form the **endoderm** and **mesoderm** and the **primordial germ cells**. The remaining epiblast gives rise to the ectoderm.

The first organ to form in the developing embryo is the central nervous system, derived from the **ectoderm**. During **neurulation**, neuroectoderm is formed and establishes the neural tube that eventually differentiates into brain vesicles and spinal cord. Before closure of the neural tube a population of **neural crest cells** is detached. This specialized cell population participates in the formation of many tissues including components of the central, enteric and peripheral nervous systems. After differentiation of the neuroectoderm, the remaining part of the ectodermal germ layer forms **surface ectoderm** giving rise to the epidermis including hair, horn, claws, hooves and subcutaneous glands.

The **endoderm** gives rise to the gastrointestinal tract, respiratory tract, parts of the urinary system, parts of the middle ear, the parenchyma of the thyroid gland, the parathyroid glands, the liver and the pancreas, and the reticular stroma of the tonsils and thymus.

The **mesoderm** is partitioned into **paraxial, intermediate** and **lateral plate mesoderm**. In the cranial region, the paraxial mesoderm forms paired **somitomeres** that will later participate in head formation. More caudally, the somitomeres form **somites**. Each somite gives rise to a **sclerotome**, a **myotome** and a **dermatome**. The sclerotome forms the basis of the axial skeleton (the vertebral column). From the myotome comes the body wall, limb and epaxial musculature. The dermatome gives rise to the dermis and subcutis of the skin. The urogenital system is derived from the intermediary mesoderm. Essential to the genital system are the primordial germ cells; formed early during gastrulation, these cells are allocated to the yolk sac and allantois during germ layer formation, and are finally incorporated into the genital ridges derived from the intermediate mesoderm. The lateral plate mesoderm splits into somatic and visceral sheets thereby forming the intra-embryonic coelom. The **somatic mesoderm** associates with the trophectoderm, forming the **chorion,** and with the surface ectoderm to form the **somatopleura.** Likewise, the **visceral mesoderm** associates with the endoderm forming the **splanchnopleura.**

The somatopleura gives rise to the parietal serous membranes of the body cavities including the peritoneum, pleura and pericardium, whereas the splanchnopleura gives rise to the serous membranes covering internal organs. Blood and blood vessels, the cortical portion of the adrenals and the spleen are also mesodermal derivatives.

Box 7-1 Molecular regulation: establishment of the body axes

The dorso-ventral embryonic axis is established during blastulation when the ICM becomes positioned at one pole of the blastocyst with its external cells facing the overlying trophectoderm and its internal cells facing the blastocyst cavity (see Chapter 6). With differentiation, the internal ICM cells delaminate and form the hypoblast while the epiblast is provided a dorso-ventral axis with its dorsal cells facing the trophectoderm, i.e. Rauber's layer. The anterior-posterior (future cranial-caudal) embryonic axis is apparently not established until gastrulation. In laboratory species, an anterior-posterior axis is first evident when the anterior embryonic pole becomes marked by an area of hypoblast cells expressing a range of factors with neural-inducing properties. These include transcription factors such as Otx2 and Hesx1, and signalling molecules such as Dickkopf 1 (Dkk1) and Cerberus-like 1 (Cer-l). This area of the hypoblast is known as the **anterior visceral endoderm** (AVE) in the mouse, and as the **anterior marginal crest** (AMC) in the rabbit. At least in these species, the AVE or AMC hypoblast induces the overlying epiblast to start differentiating in a neural direction, thereby establishing the future embryonic head region. Interestingly, this occurs even before formation of the primitive streak at the posterior pole of the embryonic disc. Later, signalling

molecules from the primitive node and the notochord, including Chordin, Noggin and Follistatin, are important for further neural differentiation. In pigs and cattle, formation of the **caudal crescent-shaped epiblast thickening** preceding formation of the primitive streak, is so far the first sign of the future embryonic anterior-posterior axis.

The final embryonic axis to be established is the left-right axis. In the mouse, left-right sidedness has been shown to be mainly regulated by the cells in the primitive node that secrete fibroblast growth factor 8 (FGF-8), initiating a cascade of expression of other growth factors. Beating cilia on the ventral side of node cells establish an FGF-8 gradient that results in more FGF-8 being supplied to the left side of the primitive streak than to the right. The pattern of the cascade of gene expression initiated by FGF-8 selectively defines the left side of the embryo. The signalling molecule **Sonic hedgehog (Shh)** is expressed in the notochord and may serve as a midline barrier, repressing expression of left-side genes in the right side of the embryonic disc. Cilia on node cells aberrantly beating towards the right may be involved in the condition known as **situs inversus,** in which all the body organs develop mirrored to their normal position.

FURTHER READING

Barends, P.M.G., Stroband, H.W.J., Taverne, N., te Kronnie, G., Leën, M.P.J.M. and Blommers, P.C.J. (1989): Integrity of the preimplantation pig blastocyst during expansion and loss of polar trophectoderm (Rauber cells) and the morphology of the embryoblast as an indicator for developmental stage. J. Reprod. Fert. 87:715–726.

Degrelle, A.A., Campion, E., Cabau, C., Piumi, F., Reinaud, P., Richard, C., Renard, J.–P. and Hue, I. (2005): Molecular evidence for a critical period in mural trophoblast development in bovine blastocysts. Dev. Biol. 288:448–460.

Fléchon, J.-E., Degrouard, J. and Fléchon, B. (2004): Gastrulation events in the prestreak pig embryo: ultrastructure and cell markers. Genesis 38:13–25.

Gilbert, S.F. (2006): Developmental Biology, 8th edn. Sinauer Associates, Inc., Publishers, Sunderland, Massachusetts.

Maddox-Hyttel, P., Alexopoulos, N.I., Vajta, G., Lewis, I., Rogers, P., Cann, L., Callesen, H., Tveden-Nyborg, P. and Trounson, A. (2003): Immunohistochemical and ultrastructural characterization of the initial post-hatching development of bovine embryos. Reproduction 125:607–623.

Ohta S., Suzuki K., Tachibana K., Tanaka H. and Yamada G. (2007). Cessation of gastrulation is mediated by supression of epithelial-mesenchymal transition at the ventral ectodermal ridge. Development 134:4315–4324.

Robb, L. and Tam, P.P.L. (2004): Gastrula organiser and embryonic patterning in the mouse. Semin. Cell Dev. Biol. 15:543–554.

Sadler, T.W. (2006): Langman's Medical Embryology. 10th edition, Lippincott Williams and Wilkins, Baltimore, Maryland, USA.

Stern, C.D. (2004). Gastrulation. From cells to embryo. Ed. Cold Spring Harbor Laboratory Press, Cold Spring Harbor, New York.

Vejlsted, M., Du, Y., Vajta, G. and Maddox-Hyttel, P. (2006): Post-hatching development of the porcine and bovine embryo – defining criteria for expected development in vivo and in vitro. Theriogenology 65:153–165.

CHAPTER 8

Neurulation

Fred Sinowatz

Neurulation is a fundamental event of embryogenêsis. It leads to the formation of the **neural tube**, the precursor of the **central nervous system** including the brain and spinal cord. This organ system is the first to initiate its development; functionally, however, it is overtaken by the development of the vascular system, which is the first organ system to gain function.

FORMATION OF THE NEURAL TUBE: PRIMARY AND SECONDARY NEURULATION

During neurulation, which is conventionally divided into primary and secondary phases, the epiblast is induced to form **neural ectoderm** (Fig. 8-1). The first morphological sign of **primary neurulation** is a dorsal thickening in the anterior ectoderm concomitant with regression of the primitive streak. This elliptical region of specialized thickened ectoderm is referred to as the **neural plate**. Subsequently, the neural plate undergoes a **shaping** which converts it into a more elongated key-hole-shaped structure with broad anterior and narrow posterior regions. The main driving force of neural plate shaping seems to come from convergent extensions that cause a net medially directed movement of cells with intercalation in the midline. This leads to lengthening and narrowing of the neural plate. Neural plate shaping is followed by the development of two lateral elevations, the **neural folds**, on either side of a depressed midregion referred to as the **neural groove**. In pigs and cattle the neural folds become clear during the third week of development.

Development of the anterior neural folds seems to be highly dependent on the underlying mesenchyme which proliferates and expands markedly, with a notable increase in its extracellular spaces, as the elevation of the folds begins. In the spinal part of the neural tube, expansion of the paraxial neural fold elevation is not accompanied by elevation of mesenchyme.

The neural folds continue to elevate, appose in the midline, and, eventually, fuse to create the **neural tube** which becomes covered by the surface ectoderm that will develop into the future epidermis. This process is facilitated by the cytoskeleton (microfilaments and microtubuli) of neural plate cells, and by extrinsic forces from underlying paraxial and notochordal tissues. This **primary neurulation** creates the **brain** and most of the **spinal cord**.

In the tail bud, the neural tube is formed by **secondary neurulation**. This is a different mechanism, without neural folding, in which the spinal cord initially forms as a solid mass of epithelial cells, and a central lumen develops secondarily by **cavitation**. The transition from primary to secondary neurulation occurs at the future upper sacral level.

Bending of the neural plate and apposition of neural folds

The bending of the neural plate, which is observed during primary neurulation, occurs at three principal sites: the **median hinge point (MHP)**, overlying the notochord, and the **paired dorsolateral hinge points (DLHP)** at the points of attachment of the surface ectoderm to the outside of each neural fold.

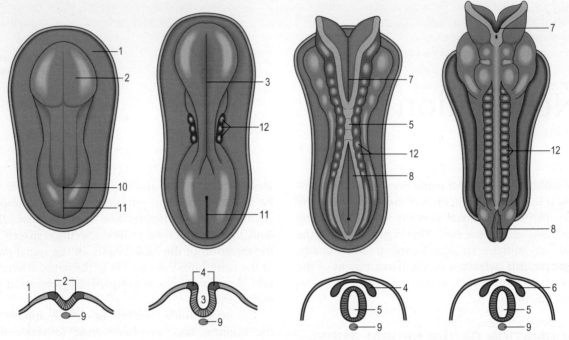

Fig. 8-1: Development of the neural tube and the neural crest. The lateral edges of the neural plate are elevated and become the neural folds. The depressed midregion of the neural plate is called the neural groove. The neural folds continue to rise, appose in the midline and fuse to create the neural tube, which becomes covered by future epidermal ectoderm. As the neural folds rise and fuse, cells at the lateral border of the neuroectoderm (neural crest cells) begin to dissociate from their neighbours, undergo an epithelio-mesenchymal transition, and leave the neuroectoderm. 1: Surface ectoderm; 2: Neural plate; 3: Neural groove; 4: Neural crest; 5: Neural tube; 6: Spinal ganglion; 7: Anterior neuropore; 8: Posterior neuropore; 9: Notochord; 10: Primitive node; 11: Primitive streak; 12: Somites.

The MHP is induced by signals from the notochord and is the sole site of bending in the upper spinal neural plate.

Gradually, the neural folds approach each other in the midline, where they eventually fuse. The actin microfilaments of the neuroepithelial cells play a significant role in anterior neurulation. This has become apparent from mouse mutant data and from studies using cytochalasin (a drug that disassembles actin microfilaments) which, in several species, have shown that neural tube closure, especially in the anterior part, is highly dependent on the actin cytoskeleton. Spinal neurulation, on the other hand, is more resistant to the disruption of actin microfilaments.

Cellular protrusions extend from apical cells of the neural folds as they approach one another in the dorsal midline and interdigitate as the folds come into contact. This allows a first cell-cell recognition and provides an initial adhesion pending later establishment of permanent cell contacts.

Fusion of neural folds

Fusion begins in the cervical region and proceeds anteriorly and posteriorly from there. This fusion is mediated by cell-surface glycoconjugates. As a result of these processes, the **neural tube** is formed and separated from the overlying ectodermal sheet. Until fusion is complete, the anterior and posterior ends of the neural tube communicate with the amniotic cavity via two openings, the **anterior** and **posterior neuropores**. Closure of the anterior neuropore occurs in the bovine embryo at approximately Day 24 (18 to 20 somite stage), whereas the posterior neuropore closes two days later (25 somite stage). Neurulation is then complete. The central nervous system is represented at this time by a closed tubular structure with a narrow posterior portion, the anlage of the **spinal cord**, and a much broader cephalic portion, the primordium of the **encephalon**. During neurulation, the neuroepithelium is entirely proliferative; cells do not begin to exit the cell cycle and start neuronal differentiation until after the neural tube closure is complete.

Apoptosis during neurulation

During neurulation, cell proliferation is also accompanied by some degree of **apoptosis** in the neuroepithelium. The rate of apoptosis appears to be finely tuned and it seems to be equally detrimental if the intensity of apoptosis is increased or decreased. Excessive apoptosis disturbs anterior neurulation by leaving too few normally functioning cells for morphogenesis, but there are also data indicating that reduced cell death from too little apoptosis can lead to neural tube closure defects.

Apoptosis at the tips of the neural folds may serve a special function. After opposing neural folds have made contact and adhered to each other, midline epithelial remodelling by apoptosis breaks the continuity between the neuroepithelium and surface ectoderm. Inhibition of apoptosis produces spinal neural tube defects, probably by preventing this dorsal midline remodelling.

NEURAL CREST

Formation of neural crest

As the neural folds elevate, cells of the lateral border or crest of the neuroepithelium, the **neural crest**, undergo an **epithelio-mesenchymal transition** as they leave the neuroectoderm by active migration into the underlying mesoderm (Fig. 8-1). Induction of neural crest cells requires interactions between neural and overlying surface ectoderm. Neural crest cells are specified as the result of an inductive instruction by the surface ectoderm. The instruction is possibly mediated by a gradient of bone morphogenetic protein 4 (BMP4), BMP7, and Wnt. Bone morphogenetic proteins secreted by surface ectoderm initiate this process. Thus stimulated, neural crest cells express slug, a transcription factor of the zinc finger family that characterizes cells that break away from an embryonic cell layer to migrate as mesenchymal cells.

Neural crest cell migration and neurulation are temporally and spatially related in the anterior parts of the neural tube, but in the midbrain and hindbrain, neural crest cells begin to detach from the apices of the neural folds and start to migrate well in advance of neural tube closure. In contrast, in the spinal cord region, migration of neural crest cells does not begin until several hours after spinal neural tube closure is complete.

Migration of neural crest cells

The pathway by which the neural crest cells leave the neural tube depends on the region. Migrating crest cells give rise to a heterogeneous array of cells and tissues. Neural crest cells that leave the anterior parts of the neural folds, before closure of the neural tube in this region, contribute to the craniofacial skeleton and other mesenchymal derivatives, but can also differentiate into several other cell types including neurons of the cranial ganglia, Schwann cells and melanocytes Table 8-1.

Neural crest cells break free from the neural plate or neural tube by changing their shape and other properties from those of typical neuroepithelial cells to those of **mesenchymal cells**. In the head region, incipient neural crest cells send out processes that penetrate the basal lamina underlying the neural epithelium. After the basal lamina is further degraded, the neural crest cells, by this time mesenchymal in appearance, pass through the remnants of the basal lamina and migrate into the surrounding mesenchyme.

Table 8-1: Major derivatives of the cranial and circumpharyngeal neural crest

Sensory nervous system	Ganglia of trigeminal nerve (V), facial nerve (VII), glossopharyngeal nerve (superior ganglion), vagus nerve (jugular ganglion)
Autonomic nervous system	Parasympathetic ganglia: ciliary, ethmoidal, sphenopalatine, submandibular, visceral Satellite cells of sensory ganglia, Schwann cells of peripheral nerves, leptomeninges of prosencephalon and part of mesencephalon
Endocrine cells	Carotid body, parafollicular cells of thyroid
Pigment cells	Melanocytes
Mesectodermal cells	Cranial vault (squamosum and part of os frontale), nasal and orbital bones, part of the otic capsule, palate, maxilla, visceral cartilage, part of external ear cartilage
Connective tissue	Dermis and adipocytes of the skin, cornea of the eye, odontoblasts, stroma of glands (thyroid, parathyroid, thymus, salivary, lachrymal), outflow tract of heart, cardiac semilunar valves, walls of aorta and aortic-arch derived arteries
Muscle	Ciliary muscle; dermal smooth muscles, vascular smooth muscle

A significant change accompanying the epithelial-mesenchymal transition of the neural crest cells is their **loss of cell adhesiveness** due to loss of adhesion molecules (CAMs) characteristic of the neural tube (e.g. N-CAM, and N-cadherin).

After leaving the neuroepithelium, the neural crest cells encounter an environment relatively poor in cells but rich in extracellular-matrix molecules. In this specialized environment, neural crest cells migrate along several well-defined pathways to extents that are influenced by both intrinsic properties of the cells and the environment they encounter.

Migration is supported by components of the extracellular matrix: molecules found in the basal lamina, such as fibronectin, laminin and type IV collagen. Attachment to, and migration over, these substrate molecules is mediated by integrins (a family of attachment molecules) on the migrating cells. Balancing the process, other molecules of the extracellular matrix, such as chondroitin sulphate proteoglycans, inhibit the migration of neural crest cells.

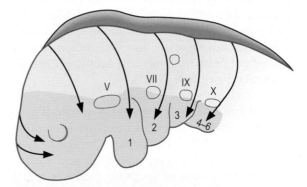

Fig. 8-2: Migratory paths of neural crest cells in the head region (modified after Sadler, 2006). Cells leaving the neural crest migrate and form structures in the face and neck. 1–6: Pharyngeal arches; V, VII, IX and X: Epibranchial placodes. Reproduced with permission from Lippincott Williams & Wilkins.

Anterior neural crest

Neural crest cells in the developing head (Fig. 8-2) and trunk follow different migration pathways. The **anterior neural crest** is a **major component of the developing cephalic end of the embryo**. Comparative anatomical and developmental research suggests that the anterior neural crest is the major morphological substrate for the evolution of the vertebrate head. Leaving the nascent neurotube well before fusion of the neural folds, the anterior neural crest cells migrate in diffuse streams throughout the anterior mesenchyme to reach their final destinations in the developing head, their paths controlled by local differences in the extracellular matrix.

The origins of the neural crest in the anterior rhombencephalon significantly influence their ultimate destination within the pharyngeal arches (see Chapter 14), and the expression of certain gene products. Neural crest cells from **rhombomeres 1** and **2** migrate into the **first pharyngeal arch** and form the bulk of its mesenchyme. Neural crest cells of **rhombomere 4** migrate into the **second arch**, and those of **rhombomeres 6** and **7** into the **third arch**. A close correlation can be demonstrated between migration pattern of the rhombomeric neural crest cells and the expression of products of the *HoxB* gene complex (see Chapter 14). Products of the *HoxB 2*, *HoxB-3*, and *HoxB-4* genes are expressed in a regular sequence in both the neural tube and the neural-crest-derived mesenchyme of the second, third, and fourth pharyngeal arches, but not in rhombomere 2 nor in the first pharyngeal arch mesenchyme. After the pharyngeal arches have become populated with neural crest cells, the ectoderm overlying the arches also expresses a similar pattern of *HoxB* gene products. These interactions between the neural crest cells and the surface ectoderm of the pharyngeal arches may influence how the ectoderm of the arches differentiates.

It was assumed for a long time that, in contrast to trunk neural crest cells, cells from the anterior neural crest are pre-programmed, having already been imprinted with distinct morphogenetic instructions before they left the neural tube. However, recent experiments have shown that environmental factors play a decisive role in determining the fate of the anterior neural crest cells: many of the regional influences on their differentiation are now recognized to result from interactions encountered during migration.

Anterior neural crest cells differentiate into a wide variety of cell and tissue types (Table 8-2; see

Table 8-2: Major derivatives of the trunk neural crest

Sensory nervous system	Spinal ganglia
Autonomic nervous system	Ganglia of the sympathetic chain, coeliac and mesenteric ganglia, visceral and pelvic plexuses, Schwann cells of peripheral nerves Satellite cells of sensory ganglia, enteric glial cells
Endocrine cells	Adrenal medulla, neurosecretory cells of heart and lung
Pigment cells	Melanocytes
Mesectodermal cells	None
Connective tissue	None
Muscle	None

Chapters 14 and 16) including connective tissue and skeletal tissues of the head.

Circumpharyngeal neural crest

The **circumpharyngeal neural crest** arises in the posterior rhombencephalic region, and in the lower part of the pharynx. Cells from this region migrate towards the gut (parasympathetic vagal neural crest cells, originating from the levels of somites 1 to 7) and the heart (cardiac neural crest cells, originating from the anterior rhombenecephalon to the level of somite 5), where they significantly contribute to the cardiac outflow tract (see Chapter 12). **Vagal neural crest cells** migrate into the developing gut as precursors of the parasympathetic neurons of the digestive tract. They migrate posteriorly until, together with neural crest cells from the sacral region, they populate the entire length of the gut. These cells form **the submucosal** and **myenteric plexuses**.

The **cardiac neural crest cells** contribute massively to the **truncoconal folds** that separate the outflow tract of the heart into aortic and pulmonary segments, to the leaflets of the **semilunar valves** at the base of the outflow tract, and to the walls of the proximal **coronary arteries** near their attachment to the ascending aorta (see Chapter 12). They may also modify the signals leading to the normal differentiation of myocardial cells. The cardiac neural crest cells can also differentiate into **Schwann cells** of the cranial nerves.

A significant fraction of the cardiac neural crest population becomes associated with other organs, including the thymus, parathyroid, and thyroid glands. Several severe abnormalities of these organs result from deficiencies of the cardiac neural crest. One such is the DiGeorge syndrome, caused by a deletion on chromosome 22 in humans. This syndrome is characterized by hypoplasia and reduced function of the thymus, thyroid, and parathyroid glands, as well as cardiovascular defects, such as persistent truncus arteriosus and abnormalities of the aortic arches.

Circumpharyngeal neural crest cells also migrate ventrally to the pharynx. There, they accompany the somite-derived myoblasts that are migrating anteriorly to form the intrinsic muscles of the tongue and the hypopharyngeal muscles, and also contribute to the connective tissue of these muscles. A disturbance in this region of cardiac neural crest cells can result in cardiac septal defects (aorticopulmonary septum), as well as glandular and craniofacial malformations.

Trunk neural crest

The **trunk neural crest** extends from the sixth somite to the most posterior somites. Within the trunk, three main migratory pathways of neural crest cells can be discerned. One is a **dorsolateral pathway** between the ectoderm and the somites. The cells that take this pathway disperse beneath the ectoderm and ultimately enter it as pigment cells (**melanocytes**). In the **second ventromedial pathway**, neural crest cells initially move into the space between the somites and the neural tube in the anterior half of the embryo. The pathway continues just under the ventromedial surface of the somites, leading the migrating cells to the dorsal aorta. Cells that use this branch belong to the

sympathoadrenal lineage and contribute to the **sympathetic nervous system** and to the **adrenal medulla**. A **third ventrolateral pathway** goes into the anterior halves of the somites. Cells that follow this pathway form the segmentally arranged **sensory** or **spinal ganglia**.

The **sympathoadrenal lineage** is derived from committed sympathoadrenal progenitor cells that have already passed a number of restriction points so that they can no longer form sensory neurons, glia, or melanocytes. These progenitor cells give rise to four types of cellular progeny: (1) **adrenal chromaffin cells**, (2) **small, intensely fluorescent cells found in the sympathetic ganglia**, (3) **adrenergic sympathetic neurons**, and (4) a **small population of cholinergic sympathetic neurons**.

Somewhat further down this cellular lineage, a bipotential progenitor cell that can give rise to either adrenal chromaffin cells or sympathetic neurons is found. The bipotential progenitor cells already possess some neuronal traits, but final differentiation depends on their environment. In the presence of fibroblast growth factor (FGF) and nerve growth factor (NGF) in early sympathetic ganglia, these precursors differentiate into definitive sympathetic neurons. If, on the other hand, precursor cells in the developing adrenal medulla encounter glucocorticoids secreted by adrenal cortical cells, they lose their neuronal properties and differentiate into adrenal chromaffin cells. This choice, however, is not absolute; chromaffin cells can be stimulated after birth to transdifferentiate into neurons if they are exposed to NGF in vitro.

The entire length of the gut is populated by neural-crest-derived parasympathetic neurons and associated cells, the enteric glia. These arise from neural crest cells at the cervical (vagal) and sacral levels which, under the influence of glial-derived neurotrophic factor (GDNF), migrate extensively along the developing gut. Sacral neural crest cells colonize the hindgut, but even there they form only a minority of the enteric neurons; the majority are derived from vagal neural crest cells. Within the gut the neural crest cells form the **enteric nervous system** which, in many respects, acts like an independent component of the nervous system. The number of enteric neurons nearly matches the number of neurons in the spinal cord, and most of them are not directly connected to the brain or spinal cord. This independence explains how the bowel can maintain reflex activity in the absence of input from the central nervous system.

Neural crest cells are not committed to form gut-associated nervous tissue before leaving the spinal cord. Experimentally, if vagal neural crest is replaced by the neural crest of the trunk (which normally does not give rise to gut-associated derivatives) the gut is colonized by the transplanted trunk-level neural crest cells. Evidence that the pathways of migration affect differentiation is seen in the neuro-transmitters produced by these transplanted crest cells. Hence, the parasympathetic neurons, differentiated from ectopically transplanted trunk neural crest cells, produce serotonin, not catecholamines, in the gut. Had they differentiated in their normal sites in the trunk, these neurons would have produced catecholamines and not serotonin.

Despite the strong influence of the environment of the gut on the differentiation of neural crest cells, the cells retain a surprising degree of developmental flexibility. If crest-derived cells already in the gut of avian embryos are re-transplanted into the trunk region of younger embryos, they seem to lose the memory of their former association with the gut. They enter the pathways common to all trunk crest cells (with the exception of pigment cell pathways) and differentiate accordingly.

Most neural crest precursors of gut-associated parasympathetic neurons express the basic helix-loop-helix transcription factor, Mash 1, which is also expressed in the precursors of sympathetic, but not of sensory, neurons. Expression of Mash 1, which appears to maintain the competence of the postmigratory cells in the gut to differentiate into neurons, is stimulated by the growth factors BMP2 and BMP4. Other environmental factors are required for complete commitment of these cells to form autonomic neurons.

Compared to the anterior neural crest, the trunk neural crest has a relatively limited range of differentiation options. The derivatives of the trunk neural crest are summarized in Table 8-2.

Phylogenetic origin of the neural crest

Phylogenetically, the neural crest is a typical vertebrate feature. Its derivatives are often regarded as being homologous with the epidermal and visceral nerve plexus found in non-vertebrates. Therefore, it is assumed that the neural crest arose as a result of the centralization of the nervous system seen in vertebrates.

During evolution, vertebrates also developed special sense organs and locomotor structures. To protect and support these evolutionarily 'new' acquisitions, skeletal structures also developed. Therefore, it can be assumed that the neural crest of vertebrates evolved as a result of changes of the nervous system and in the need to protect structures for the special sense organs and muscles. With this in mind, it should not be surprising that neural crest cells have two basic developmental fates: they form the **ganglionic elements and supporting structures of the peripheral nervous system** and they can differentiate into **mesenchyme (ectomesenchyme)**. Depending on the level from which neural crest cells start to migrate, developmental fates differ: anterior neural crest, formed anterior to somite 7, can form neurons and ectomesenchyme. Trunk neural crest, posterior to somite 7, forms neural structures and somites but, under physiological conditions, no ectomesenchyme.

SUMMARY

During **primary neurulation**, the **neural plate** is formed in the anterior portion of the epiblast. Subsequently, **neural folds** define the **neural groove** and **neural tube**. The posterior portion of the neural tube is formed by **secondary neurulation** where a solid neural cord develops a lumen secondarily. The anterior and posterior ends of the neural tube communicate with the amniotic cavity via the **anterior** and **posterior neuropores** that close later.

As the neural folds elevate, cells of the lateral border or crest of the neuroepithelium, the **neural crest**, undergo an **epithelio-mesenchymal**

transition as they leave the neuroectoderm to enter the underlying mesoderm by active migration. The neural crest is now regarded as a pluripotent stem cell population that makes vital contributions to a wide array of both neural and non-neural organ systems. Neural crest cells migrate to peripheral locations throughout the body. They differentiate into many cell types, such as neurons, glial cells of the peripheral nervous system, melanocytes, and adrenal medullary cells. **Cranial and circumpharyngeal neural crest cells** also differentiate into cartilage, bone, dentin, dermal fibroblasts, smooth muscle cells, stroma of pharyngeal glands and several structures of the heart and great vessels. Neural **crest cells in the trunk** take three main paths for their migration: a **dorsolateral pathway** for melanocytes, a **ventral pathway** for cells of the sympatho-adrenal lineage, and a **ventrolateral pathway** running through the anterior halves of the somites for cells forming sensory ganglia. In contrast to cranial and circumpharyngeal neural crest cells, neural crest cells in the trunk cannot differentiate into skeletal elements.

Box 8-1 Formation of the neural crest and migration of neural crest cells

The formation of the neural crest is induced by interactions of the neural plate with paraxial mesoderm or non-neural ectoderm. Several signalling pathways converge at the border between neural and non-neural ectoderm where the neural crest is established. Among the molecules identified in this process are members of the **BMP**, **Wnt**, **FGF** and **Notch** signalling pathway families. The concerted action of these signals and their downstream targets will define the identity of the neural crest. Although the neural crest is a vertebrate innovation, comparative genomic results suggest that its migratory properties evolved by utilizing programs that are already present in the common vertebrate-invertebrate ancestor. Various mechanisms control neural crest cell migration in different regions of the body. In the trunk, cell-cell interactions predominate and the mesodermal somites control the rostro-caudal patterning of neural crest cells. The notochord prevents neural crest cells from crossing the midline. In the hindbrain, the segmental migration of neural crest cells is influenced both by information inherent to the rhombomeres and environmental signals from neighbouring tissues, such as the otic vesicle. There is clearly an intimate relationship between migrating neural crest cells, the neural tube from which they emerge, and tissues through which they move. The developmental program that determines neural crest cell fate is both fixed and plastic: fixed in that a cohort of neural crest cells carries information that directs the axial pattern and species-specific morphology of the head and face; plastic because, as individual cells, neural crest cells are responsive to signals from each other as well as from non-neural-crest tissues in the environment.

FURTHER READING

Anderson, D.J. (1997): Cellular and molecular biology of neural crest cell lineage determination. Trends Genet. 13:276–280.

Barrallo-Gimeno, A. and Nieto, M.A. (2006): Evolution of the neural crest. Adv. Exp. Med. Biol. 589:235–244.

Basch, M.L. and Bronner-Fraser, M. (2006): Neural crest inducing signals. Adv. Exp. Med. Biol. 589:24–31.

Bronner-Fraser, M. (1995): Patterning of the vertebrate neural crest. Perspect. Dev. Neurobiol. 3:53–62.

Dupin, E. Creuzet. S. and Le Douarin, N.M. (2006): The contribution of the neural crest to the vertebrate body. Adv. Exp. Med. Biol. 589:96–119.

Farlie, P.G., McKeown S.J., Newgreen, D.F. (2004): The neural crest: basic biology and clinical relationships in the craniofacial and enteric nervous systems. Birth Defects Res. C. Embryo Today 72:173–189.

Kee, Y., Hwang, B.J., Sternberg, P.W. and Bronner-Fraser, M. (2007): Evolutionary conservation of cell migration genes: from nematode neurons to vertebrate neural crest. Genes Dev. 21: 391–396.

Maschoff, K.L. and Baldwin, H.S. (2000): Molecular determinants of neural crest migration. Am. J. Med. Genet. 97:280–288.

Noden, D.M. and Schneider, R.A. (2006): Neural crest cells and the community of plan for craniofacial development: historical debates and current perspectives. Adv. Exp. Med. Biol. 589:1–23.

Patterson, P.H. (1990): Control of cell fate in a vertebrate neurogenic cell lineage. Cell 62:1035–1038.

Sandell, L.L. and Trainor, P.A. (2006): Neural crest cell plasticity. Size matters. Adv. Exp. Med. Biol. 589:78–95.

Trainor, P.A. and Krumlauf, R. (2001): Hox genes, neural crest cells and branchial arch patterning. Curr. Opin. Cell Biol. 13:698–705.

CHAPTER 9

Morten Vejlsted

Comparative placentation

Upon entering the uterine cavity, the embryo is initially nourished by secretions from the uterine glands. Collectively, these products are known as **histotrophe** or 'uterine milk'. However, with development this arrangement rapidly becomes inadequate. To counteract the insufficiency, a close relationship has to be established between extra-embryonic tissues, which are vascularized from the embryo proper, and the maternal circulatory system. This allows the embryo to import blood-borne maternal nutrients, the **haemotrophe**, and to export its own waste products. Together, histotrophe and haemotrophe are referred to as **embryotrophe**. To accomplish exchange between the mother and her embryo a temporary organ, the **placenta**, is formed by contributions of both extra-embryonic and maternal tissues. As will be explained below, formation of the placenta (**placentation**) necessitates close synchrony between the state of uterine receptivity and the stage of embryonic development.

In rodents and primates, the newly hatched blastocyst attaches to the endometrial epithelium and, due to the invasive nature of the trophectoderm in these species, the embryo actually penetrates the epithelium and invades the endometrial connective tissue in which it becomes completely embedded. This process, whereby the embryo leaves the uterine lumen, is known as **implantation**. In domestic animals, however, the embryo remains **attached** to the internal endometrial surface throughout gestation and, except in carnivores, placentation is non-invasive.

PERI-IMPLANTATION CONCEPTUS DEVELOPMENT

In most domestic species, the embryo reaches the uterine cavity prior to blastulation (see Chapter 6). At the end of blastulation, the embryo consists of a sphere of **trophectoderm** surrounding the **inner cell mass** and the **blastocyst cavity** (Fig. 9-1). When engaged in placental formation, the trophectoderm is referred to as trophoblast. As is true of most of the extra-embryonic tissues, the trophoblast is essential during intra-uterine life but it is expelled at parturition as part of the afterbirth.

At about the time of hatching from the zona pellucida, the inner cell mass differentiates into the **epiblast** and **hypoblast** (Fig. 9-1). The hypoblast gradually forms an inner lining of the epiblast and trophectoderm. When complete, the enclosed cavity may be referred to as the **primitive yolk sac**, analogous to the yolk sac found in avian embryos. The process of gastrulation results in establishment of the three germ layers: endoderm, mesoderm and ectoderm (see Chapter 7). During this process, the **endoderm** gradually displaces the hypoblast beneath the epiblast. Meanwhile the **extra-embryonic mesoderm** is split into somatic (or parietal) and visceral (or splanchnic) sheets lining the **extra-embryonic coelom**. The extra-embryonic somatic mesoderm associates with the overlying trophectoderm to give rise to the **chorion,** whereas the visceral mesoderm together with the hypoblast and endoderm forms the **splanchnopleura**. Eventually,

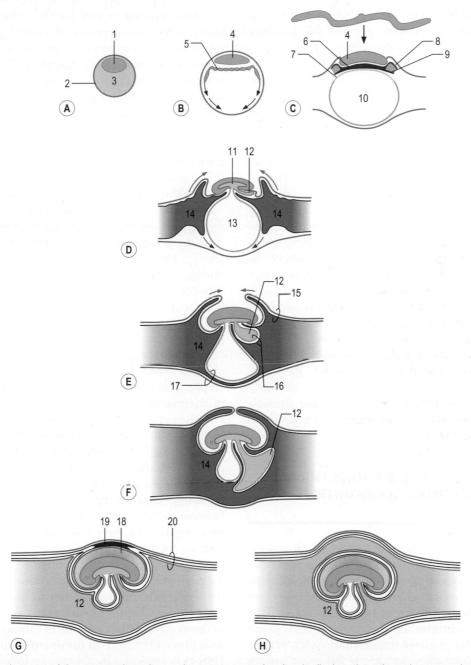

Fig. 9-1: Development of the extra-embryonic membranes presented as longitudinal sections through progressively older embryos (A to F). 1: Inner cell mass; 2: Trophectoderm; 3: Blastocyst cavity; 4: Epiblast; 5: Hypoblast; 6: Intra-embryonic mesoderm; 7: Endoderm; 8: Somatic extra-embryonic mesoderm; 9: Visceral extra-embryonic mesoderm; 10: Primitive yolk sac; 11: Primitive gut; 12: Allantois; 13: Definitive yolk sac; 14: Extra-embryonic coelom; 15: Chorion; 16: Splanchnopleura; 17: Fusion between yolk sac wall and chorion allowing for formation of choriovitelline placenta; 18: Amniotic cavity; 19: Mesamnion; 20: Chorioallantois allowing for formation of chorioallantoic placenta. **G:** In cattle and pigs, the chorion and the dorsal portion of the amniotic wall remain fused in the mesamnion. **H:** In horse and dog, the allantois surrounds the amnion completely.

the body foldings of the embryo proper result in the formation of the **primitive gut** and the **definitive yolk sac** from the primitive yolk sac (see Chapter 7). The definitive yolk sac wall fuses with the chorion in some species to establish a **choriovitelline placenta**.

The **allantois** develops as an evagination from the hindgut (Fig. 9-1). The evagination occurs after formation of the definitive yolk sac and, due to its origin from the hindgut, its wall is made up of endoderm on the inside with a covering of visceral mesoderm on the outside, the two layers together forming the splanchnopleura. The visceral mesoderm of the yolk sac is the area where blood and blood vessel formation is first seen, and this development is later followed by vascularization of the visceral mesoderm associated with the allantois (see Chapter 12). In contrast, the somatic mesoderm, including that of the chorion, remains avascular initially. As the embryo grows, the allantois gradually expands into the extra-embryonic coelom, eventually occupying most of this cavity. Where the allantoic wall and the chorion meet, they fuse, forming the **chorioallantois** which gradually becomes vascularized from vessels in the allantoic visceral mesoderm and gives rise to the **chorioallantoic placenta**.

CHANGES IN THE ENDOMETRIUM AND MATERNAL RECOGNITION OF PREGNANCY

During the period when the embryo is still moving freely in the uterine cavity, the uterus prepares for placentation. **Oestrogens** and **progesterone** are the principal hormones produced within the ovary (see Chapter 3). High levels of oestrogens are secreted into the bloodstream during prooestrus and oestrus (the follicular phase of the oestrous cycle); progesterone predominates during the following periods of metoestrus and dioestrus (the luteal phase) when the early embryo moves from the oviduct into the uterus. It is these cyclic phases of hormone production in the ovary that stimulate marked changes in the **endometrium**, the lining of the uterus.

During prooestrus and oestrus, rising oestrogen levels induce proliferation of uterine glands and simultaneous engorgement of the stroma with blood (as a result of hyperaemia and congestion) and extracellular fluid (oedema). The external genitalia, notably the vulva, become oedematous, which can help the diagnosis of oestrus. During metoestrus, the endometrial oedema decreases and some of the congested blood vessels break down. This phenomenon, referred to as metorrhagia, may lead to the presence of blood in the vulvar discharge; a sign, in the cow, that oestrus has passed.

Proliferation of the endometrial glands continues during metoestrus, and during the following dioestrus the glands reach a stage of maximal secretory activity. Hence, uterine gland secretion is greatest during the first 11 days of dioestrus, providing histotrophe for potential embryos. If pregnancy does not occur, endometrial involution follows, reflecting the regression of the corpus luteum or corpora lutea.

Luteolysis must be prevented if pregnancy is to continue. The maintenance of the corpus luteum or corpora lutea is based upon **maternal recognition of pregnancy**, a series of events depending upon synchronous development of the embryo on the one hand and of a receptive endometrium on the other. By signalling its presence in the uterus, the embryo prevents luteolysis while apposing, and then adhering to, the endometrium. The effectiveness of the signalling depends upon the degree of contact between the trophoblast and endometrium, ensured by elongation of the conceptus in ruminants and pigs but by intrauterine migration in horses.

In ruminants, the corpus luteum produces oxytocin as well as progesterone. Oxytocin stimulates the endometrium to synthesize **prostaglandins** (PGF2α; see Chapter 3) which have been identified as the main cause of luteolysis in ruminants (as well as in pigs and horses). In **ruminants**, **interferon-tau (IFN-t)** is produced by the trophectoderm, inhibiting formation of endometrial oxytocin receptors. Thus, in the presence of an embryo, oxytocin cannot stimulate synthesis of PGF2α and luteolysis is prevented. In addition, IFN-t stimulates production of histotrophe from the endometrial glands.

Pigs employ another strategy to interrupt the luteolytic pathway. Although oxytocin is also produced by the corpora lutea in the pig, and promotes synthesis of endometrial PGF2α, pig embryos prevent luteolysis differently. **Oestradiol** is produced from their trophectoderm around Days 11 to 12 of development causing PGF2α to be secreted into the uterine lumen instead of into the maternal blood stream. In the lumen, PGF2α is quickly degraded. In addition to changing the secretion of PGF2α from endocrine (into the maternal circulation) to exocrine (into the uterine lumen), oestradiol is also believed to stimulate myometrial contraction facilitating distribution of embryos within the very long uterine horns. It has been shown that at least four embryos must be present in order to prevent luteolysis in the pig.

Yet another strategy for maintenance of early pregnancy is seen in the **mare**. Here, direct cell-to-cell contact between the trophoblast and endometrium is prevented until about Day 21 by the capsule (see below) and is slow to be established even after that. It is the capsule that enables the spherical horse conceptus to **migrate** over the entire endometrial surface between 12 to 14 times per day during Days 6 to 17 of pregnancy in order to prevent luteolysis. This migration has been shown to be essential for pregnancy maintenance but the nature and roles of signals exchanged with the mare in the process are still not fully identified or understood. Considering that the mare 'recognizes' a difference between embryos and unfertilized oocytes even in the oviduct ('allowing' only embryos to pass into the uterus), it may be inappropriate to apply the term 'recognition of pregnancy' to horses in the sense used in ruminants and pigs. Perhaps more likely is the concept that a continuum of dialogue, rather than specific signals at 'critical' junctures, is essential to pregnancy maintenance in the mare.

In **carnivores**, too, a signal for maternal recognition of pregnancy has not been identified. The canine met- and dioestrous periods are long. Under normal conditions these phases of the oestrous cycle may last 20 to 30 days and, in many cases, the nonpregnant bitch develops a syndrome referred to as pseudopregnancy in which the corpora lutea maintain their progesterone production for even longer periods. In most cases this condition reverses by itself but it may sometimes require treatment. Due to the long lifespan of the corpus luteum, early embryonic signals for recognition of pregnancy may be less important or even unnecessary in dogs. Hence, rising levels of the luteotrophic pituitary hormone, prolactin, appears to be responsible for maintenance of the corpora lutea later in canine pregnancy.

CLASSIFICATION OF PLACENTA

There are enormous differences among species with respect to how placentation is initiated and, accordingly, how its final architecture develops. Many different classification schemes for the placenta, based on a variety of criteria, have been proposed over the years. One scheme is based on nature of the extraembryonic tissue that contributes to the placenta, leading to placentae being classified as either choriovitelline or chorioallantoic. In the **choriovitelline placenta**, the yolk sac wall combines locally with the chorion to form an area for exchange (Fig. 9-1). In domestic animals a functional choriovitelline placenta is seen only in carnivores and horses. The **chorioallantoic placenta**, which is the primary functional placenta in all domestic species, is established by fusion between the allantoic wall and chorion establishing the chorioallantois. In pigs and ruminants, the yolk sac involutes 3 to 4 weeks after conception and never forms a functional placenta.

Another classification scheme is based on the structure of the chorioallantoic surface and its interaction with the endometrium. Areas where the chorioallantois interacts with the endometrium and engages in placental formation are referred to as **chorion frondosum**. In contrast, areas where the chorioallantois is free, not engaged in placental formation, and therefore has a smooth surface, are known as **chorion laeve**. In **pigs** and **horses**, chorion frondosum is diffusely distributed over the entire chorioallantoic surface and so the placenta is categorized as being **diffuse.** The porcine chorioallantoic surface area is increased by foldings, revealed as primary **plicae** and secondary **rugae**, and is thus referred to as being **folded**. In the horse, because **chorionic villi** are gathered in numerous specialized 'microzones', known as **microcotyledons**, and extending into crypts of the endometrium, the equine placenta is also referred to as being **villous**.

In **ruminants**, chorion frondosum is organized as arborizing chorionic villi assembled into larger macroscopically visible tufts called **cotyledons**. Hence, the ruminant placenta is known as **cotyledonary** or **multiplex** and **villous**. The cotyledons combine with endometrial prominences known as **caruncles**, forming **placentomes** in which the chorioallantoic villi of the cotyledon extend into crypts of the caruncle. A chorion laeve is present between the cotyledons.

In **carnivores**, the chorion frondosum is organized into a broad belt extending around the longitudinal axis of the embryo where it forms lamellae. This type of placenta is consequently referred to as being **zonary** and **lamellar**.

A third classification scheme is based on the number of tissue layers separating the fetal and maternal circulations, thereby forming the placental barrier (Fig. 9-2). There are always three fetal extraembryonic layers in the chorioallantoic placenta:

the **endothelium** lining the allantoic blood vessels; **chorioallantoic mesenchyme**, originating from the fused somatic (chorionic) and visceral (allantoic) mesoderm; and the **chorionic epithelium**, i.e. the trophoblast. However, the numbers of layers retained in the maternal portion of the placenta varies with species. Before placentation, the endometrium presents three layers that could contribute to the placental barrier: the **endometrial epithelium**, **connective tissue**, and **vascular endothelium**.

In domestic animals, the number of maternal layers in the placental barrier results in two main placental classes: the **epitheliochorial** and the **endotheliochorial placentae**. The former is seen in the pig, horse and ruminants. Here, the chorionic and endometrial epithelia are apposed, and there is no loss of maternal tissue. The epitheliochorial placenta in ruminants is modified as particular trophoblast cells cross into, and fuse with, some of the endometrial epithelial cells. Hence, the placenta is referred to as **synepitheliochorial**. In carnivores, on the other hand, the placenta is endotheliochorial, because endometrial epithelium and connective tissue are lost during placentation, leaving the trophoblast in direct contact with maternal vascular

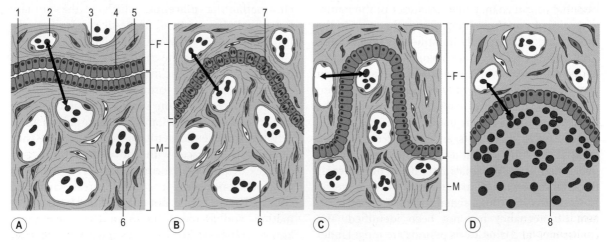

Fig. 9-2: The placental barrier. **A:** The epitheliochorial placenta in the sow. **B:** The synepitheliochorial placenta of the cow. **C:** The endotheliochorial placenta of the dog. **D:** The haemochorial placenta of the mouse. F: Fetal components of the placenta; M: Maternal components of the placenta; 1: Endometrial epithelium; 2: Fetal vessels; 3: Fetal endothelium; 4: Trophoblast; 5: Mesenchyme; 6: Maternal vessels; 7: Binucleate cell; 8: Red blood cells. The placental barrier is indicated by the double arrow.

endothelium. In rodents and humans, the reduction of the maternal placental barrier is complete, leaving the trophoblast in direct contact with the blood in a **haemochorial placenta**. The number of tissue layers separating the fetal and maternal circulations has important implications for the transfer of immunoglobulins and other maternal proteins to the fetus and, therefore, for the development of the immune system in utero (see Chapter 13).

In carnivores, the endotheliochorial placenta results in a tight adherence between the fetal and maternal components of the placenta. As a result, a portion of the endometrium is shed when the fetal membranes and the placenta are expelled as the afterbirth. The shed portion of the endometrium is referred to as the **decidua**, and this type of placenta as **deciduate**. The placenta in rodents and humans is also deciduate. In contrast, the placenta in ruminants, pigs and horses is **adeciduate**.

SPECIES DIFFERENCES

Pig

The pig embryo enters the uterus at the 4-cell stage, approximately 2 days after ovulation. The hatched blastocyst undergoes a phase of extreme elongation during Days 10 to 14 of development coincident with spacing of embryos within the long uterine horns. Oestradiol secreted by the trophoblast brings about maternal recognition of pregnancy around Days 11 to 12 and implantation is initiated around Days 13 to 14 along the mesometrial side of the uterus.

A yolk sac is transiently present, but involutes around Day 20 without forming a functional choriovitelline placenta. Thus, the placenta is formed by the chorioallantois and is **diffuse, folded, epitheliochorial** and **adeciduate**. The placental exchange area is increased by foldings in the form of primary (macroscopic) **plicae** and secondary (microscopic) **rugae** (Figs 9-3, 9-4). At the extremities of the fetal membranes, the allantois does not extend to the end of the chorion which forms necrotic tips. The diffuse placenta covers the entire endometrial surface

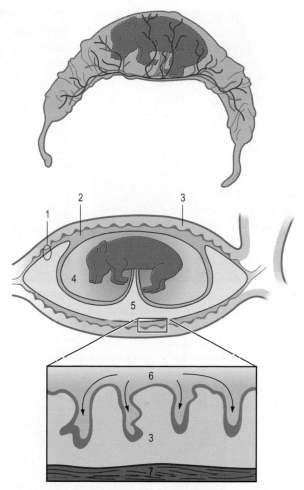

Fig. 9-3: The diffuse placenta in the sow. 1: Chorioallantois; 2: Mesamnion; 3: Endometrium; 4: Amnion; 5: Allantois; 6: Chorioallantoic plicae with secondary rugae; 7: Myometrium.

including the openings of the endometrial glands. Therefore, to allow for the glandular secretions of histotrophe to escape, the chorioallantois forms rosette-like cavities, **areolae,** over the openings of the glands (Fig. 9-5).

Formation of the amnion is followed by a persistent **mesamnion** (see Chapter 7). Thus, piglets are, in general, born without being covered in fetal membranes. The allantois begins to form about Day 15 and, due to involution of the yolk sac, occupies the entire extra-embryonic coelom except for the area of the mesamnion.

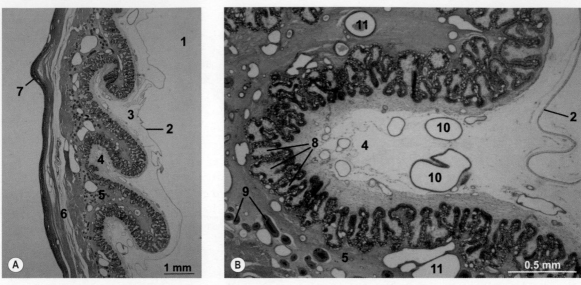

Fig. 9-4: Sow placenta at low (A) and high magnification (B). 1: Allantois; 2: Endodermal epithelium of allantois; 3: Mesenchyme; 4: Chorioallantoic plica; 5: Endometrium; 6: Myometrium; 7: Perimetrium; 8: Chorioallantoic rugae; 9: Uterine glands; 10: Fetal vessels; 11: Maternal vessels.

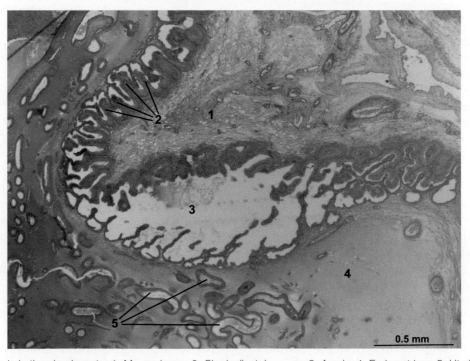

Fig. 9-5: Areola in the pig placenta. 1: Mesenchyme; 2: Chorioallantoic rugae; 3: Areola; 4: Endometrium; 5: Uterine glands.

Ruminants

In general, the ruminant embryo enters the uterus at the 8- to 16-cell stage, 3 to 4 days after ovulation. The blastocyst rapidly elongates after hatching from the zona pellucida. In cattle, the conceptus extends equally into both horns around Day 22 (see Chapter 6). More embryos seem to locate to the right horn, reflecting the facts that ovulation is more common from the right ovary and that embryo migration is not as pronounced as in the pig and horse. Maternal recognition of pregnancy occurs around Day 12 to 13 (sheep) and 16 to 17 (cattle), as a result of IFN-t secretion by the trophoblast, and is followed by implantation beginning at Days 15 to 20 (sheep) and 16 to 18 (cattle).

A yolk sac is present only transiently, degenerating shortly after implantation has begun. Thus, a chorioallantoic placenta is formed and is **cotyledonary** or **multiplex**, **villous**, **synepitheliochorial**, and **adeciduate**.

Placentation occurs by chorioallantoic villi developing opposite the prominent endometrial **caruncles** and forming the button-like **cotyledons**, corresponding to the shape of the caruncle. The caruncle and cotyledon together form a **placentome** (Figs 9-6, 9-7). In cows, 75 to 120 caruncles are present; in sheep around 80 to 100.

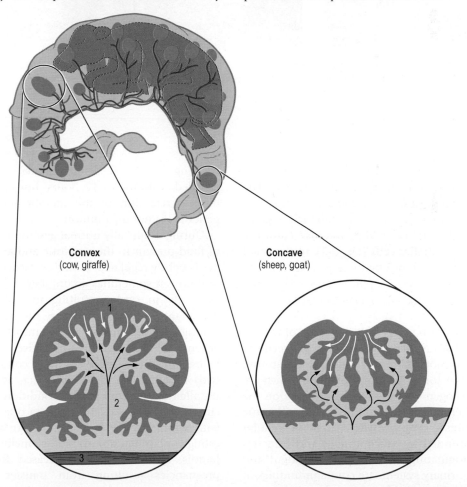

Convex
(cow, giraffe)

Concave
(sheep, goat)

Fig. 9-6: The cotyledonary placenta of the ruminants. 1: Chorioallantois (cotyledon) forming villi; 2: Caruncle with crypts enclosing the villi; 3: Myometrium.

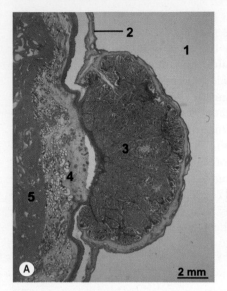
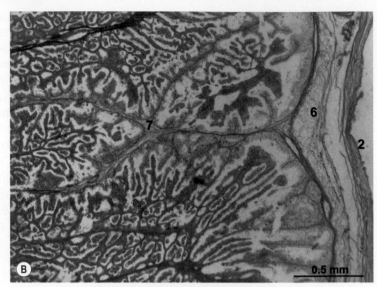

Fig. 9-7: Cow placentome at low (A) and high magnification (B). 1: Allantois; 2: Endodermal epithelium of allantois; 3: Placentome; 4: Endometrium; 5: Myometrium; 6: Mesenchyme; 7: Branching villus from chorioallantois.

In cattle, the placentomes are convex, in sheep they are concave, and in goats they are flat. The trophoblast covering the cotyledons gives rise to a unique population of hormone-producing **giant binucleate cells** that cross into, and **fuse with, the endometrial epithelial cells** (Fig. 9-2). In the small ruminants this fusion phenomenon, giving rise to the synepitheliochorial placenta, is even more pronounced resulting in a **syncytium** replacing the maternal epithelium.

The caruncles do not possess openings of uterine glands and, because the chorion laeve between the cotyledons is not attached to the endometrium, areolae do not form. **Amniotic plaques**, which are stratified glycogen-rich epithelial elevations on the inner epithelium of the amnion, and **allantoic calculi**, whitish or brownish masses of cellular debris surrounded by mucoproteins and minerals probably originating from the fetal hindgut and developing urinary system, are common findings in cattle and sheep. As in the pig, a **mesamnion** persists and so the calf is born without membranes covering it. The fetal membranes are normally expelled within 6 to 12 hours, but retained afterbirth – retention of the membranes for longer periods – is not uncommon.

During a clinically normal gestation, the amount of fluid present in the amniotic and allantoic cavities is tightly regulated. However, excessive amounts of fluid can sometimes accumulate in either cavity, especially in cattle, resulting in hydramnion or hydrallantois. Thus, whereas the normal fluid volumes in the amnion and allantois in cattle are around 15 and 10 litres, respectively, in cases of hydrallantois (the more common condition of the two) a total of 100 to 200 litres may accumulate in the allantois. Reasons for this condition include vascular disturbances in the placenta often associated with twinning and embryonic malformations. Interestingly, placental abnormalities, including hydrallantois, are seen at an increased frequency in pregnancies resulting from transfer of cloned embryos produced by somatic cell nuclear transfer (see Chapter 21).

Horse

The equine embryo enters the uterus approximately 6 days after ovulation, at the morula or blastocyst stage. Only embryos enter the uterine cavity; unfertilized oocytes are retained in the uterine tubes for reasons that are not yet fully clarified. Hatching from the zona pellucida occurs around Days 7 to 8 of development. However, even before hatching the blastocyst becomes surrounded by a tough elastic glycoprotein **capsule**, produced in large part by the trophectoderm, inside the zona pellucida. In contrast to other species, the conceptus, due to the presence of the capsule, remains spherical during gastrulation until around Day 21 when the capsule is lost. The capsule allows the spherical embryo to traverse the entire uterine lumen during Days 6 to 17, providing the signal(s) essential for pregnancy maintenance. This extended mobility is terminated by **fixation** – an increased uterine tone fixing the embryo at the base of one of the uterine horns. It is at the time of fixation that the equine conceptus has to become properly positioned (orientated) in the uterus, with the embryo proper facing the antimesometrial wall, or 'downward' as seen by transrectal ultrasonography. However, placentation is not initiated before about Day 40.

In the horse, the yolk sac is a prominent structure forming a first **choriovitelline placenta** providing the basis for fetal-maternal exchange until around Day 42 when it gradually involutes, and a **chorioallantoic placenta** takes over the function for the rest of pregnancy. The involuted yolk sac persists to term and, partly due to this, the umbilical cord is long in the horse, measuring 50 to 100 cm at birth.

Initiation of placentation is preceded by formation of the **chorionic girdle** at the junction between the developing chorioallantois and the yolk sac at about Day 34 (Figs 9-8, 9-9). This structure consists of a thickened band of trophoblast cells that invade the endometrium, traverse the placental barrier and form **endometrial cups** in the endometrium. These

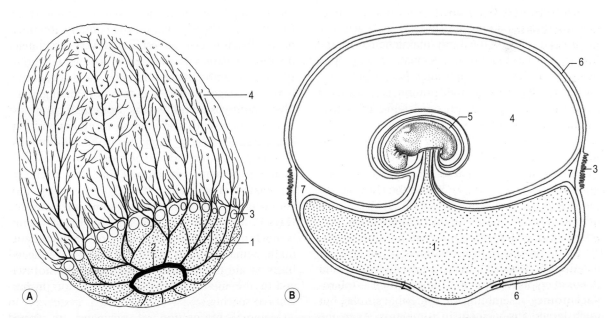

Fig. 9-8: Horse embryo during the presence of the chorionic girdle. **A:** View of the vascular ramifications. **B:** Section through the embryo. 1: Yolk sac; 2: Sinus terminalis; 3: Chorionic girdle; 4: Allantois; 5: Amnion; 6: Mesoderm with vessels; 7: Extra-embryonic coelom. Courtesy Sinowatz and Rüsse (2007).

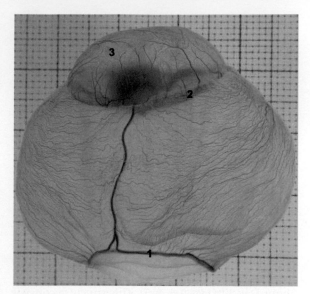

Fig. 9-9: Horse embryo at Day 25 of gestation, before formation of the chorionic girdle. 1: Sinus terminalis; 2: Site of future girdle formation; 3: Chorioallantois covering the allantoic cavity. Photo: Keith Betteridge.

cell clusters produce the hormone **equine chorionic gonadotropin (eCG)**, formerly known as pregnant mare's serum gonadotropin (PMSG). eCG acts as a luteotropin stimulating both maintenance of the primary corpus luteum and formation of supplementary (accessory) corpora lutea (see Chapter 3).

The development of the amnion is completed around Day 21. There is **no persistence of a mesamnion.** Therefore, foals may be born covered by the amnion, potentially risking suffocation if this membrane is not quickly removed. From Day 21 to Day 40, the allantois expands into the extra-embryonic coelom (Figs 9-8, 9-9). Where the chorioallantois forms, it gradually develops diffusely distributed tufts of chorioallantoic villi, **microcotyledons**, projecting into endometrial indentations, the **crypts**. The entire process of placentation may not be completed until Day 120. Fetal microcotyledons and maternal crypts together may be described as **microplacentomes**, resembling the somewhat similar, but much larger, arrangement in ruminants. As in the pig, there is no loss of maternal endometrium at birth in the horse. Hence, the horse placenta is

diffuse, **villous**, **epitheliochorial**, and **adeciduate**. Numerous **areolae** are scattered between the microcotyledons, facilitating uptake of histotrophe (Figs 9-10, 9-11).

When a mare conceives **twins**, there is a reduction in the endometrial area available to each embryo for placentation. This poses a problem, and the expansion of one twin's placenta is often restricted by growth of the other's, potentially resulting in death of one or both twins. Therefore, an early diagnosis of pregnancy is often sought in order to be able to remove one of the twins by **embryo reduction** (manual rupture transrectally).

As in ruminants, **allantoic calculi** are commonly found floating in the allantoic cavity. In the horse they are particularly big and are referred to as **hippomanes**. **Amniotic plaques** or pustules are also quite commonly observed in the amnion.

Carnivores

It is difficult to time the events of gestation precisely in the bitch both because mating may take place before ovulation, and because sperm remain viable for a long time in the female genital tract (see Chapter 3). In the queen, on the contrary, the time of fertilization can be estimated very accurately because ovulation is induced by coitus. For both species, the embryos seem to enter the uterus at the blastocyst stage, around 6–8 days post-mating. Carnivore embryos do not emerge from their coverings in the same way that expanding ruminant and pig blastocysts so clearly 'hatch' from the still-obvious zona pellucida. Instead, the **blastocyst** of the cat, for example, **remains enveloped in an extremely attenuated membrane**, strongly resembling the equine embryonic capsule, until sometime between Days 12 and 15 after coitus. Whether this covering is much-modified zona pellucida, or a replacement for it, remains to be established. The covering is likely to aid the extensive migration of blastocysts within the uterine horns that allows for proper embryo spacing.

Maternal recognition of pregnancy in these species is probably not required for preventing regression of the corpora lutea. Placentation is initiated around Days 17 to 18 of development in the bitch and Days 12 to 14 in the queen.

The yolk sac initially forms a broad **choriovitelline placenta**. Later, the central areas of the choriovitelline placenta degenerate leaving a transient choriovitelline placenta in the periphery of the initial structure. The **chorioallantoic placenta**, however, soon provides the major basis for fetal-maternal exchange. Due to the belt-shaped appearance of the chorion frondosum, the chorioallantoic placenta in carnivores is referred to as being **zonary** (Fig. 9-12). In the chorion frondosum, the trophoblast gives rise to two different cell populations: basally located **cytotrophoblast cells** and superficially located **syncytiotrophoblast cells**, which are formed by fusion of many trophoblast cells. The syncytiotrophoblast is highly invasive and destroys both apposing endometrial epithelium and underlying connective tissue. This brings the trophoblast into close contact with the maternal endothelium, making the carnivore placenta **endotheliochorial** (Fig. 9-2). Furthermore, since maternal tissue is lost at parturition, the placenta is classified as **deciduate**. As in the pig, the surface area of the chorion frondosum is increased by straight foldings referred to as **lamellae**. These structures may, depending on the species of carnivore, be more or less branched and twisted, resulting in the formation of a **labyrinth**. The placental zone is organized into an interior **lamellar zone** with chorioallantoic lamellae, an intermediate **junctional zone** containing the terminal parts of the lamellae, maternal vessels, cell debris, and glandular secretions, and an exterior **glandular zone** containing the dilated upper parts of the uterine glands (Fig. 9-13). In summary, the carnivore placenta is **zonary**, **lamellar** or **labyrinthine**, **endotheliochorial** and **deciduate**.

In the margins of the placental zone, some of the maternal endothelium degenerates. In the dog and mink, the resulting local bleeding and haematoma formation is compartmentalized into so-called **marginal haematomas**. In the cat, haematomas are more irregularly positioned. In both species, the blood contained in the haematomas is thought to serve as a source of iron for the embryo. Due to differences in haemoglobin breakdown, the

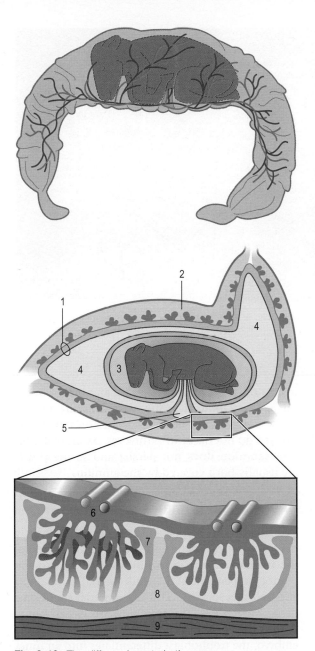

Fig. 9-10: The diffuse placenta in the mare.
1: Chorioallantois; 2: Endometrium; 3: Amnion; 4: Allantois; 5: Yolk sac; 6: Chorioallantoic microcotyledons with villi; 7: Endometrial cups; 8: Endometrium with crypts enclosing the villi. 9: Myometrium.

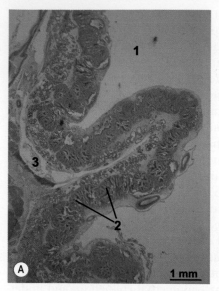

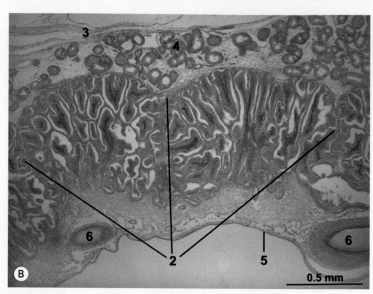

Fig. 9-11: Mare placenta at low (A) and high magnification (B). 1: Allantois; 2: Microcotyledons; 3: Endometrium; 4: Uterine glands; 5: Endodermal epithelium of allantois; 6: Fetal vessels.

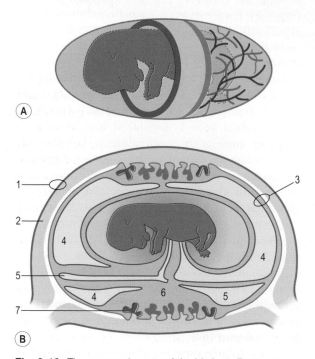

Fig. 9-12: The zonary placenta of the bitch. 1: Perimetrium; 2: Endometrium and myometrium; 3: Chorioallantois; 4: Allantois; 5: Yolk sac; 6: Chorioallantois forming lamellae in the placental zone; 7: Marginal haematoma.

haematomas are green in the dog and brown in the cat. Areas peripheral to the placental zone, known as the paraplacenta, are considered non-functional. Areolae do not occur in carnivores. As in the horse, a **mesamnion does not persist** and so the young are usually born covered by the amnion.

Rodents and primates

The rodent and primate placentae will be briefly described for comparative reasons. In these species, the **trophectoderm** is highly **invasive** and so the blastocyst penetrates the endometrial epithelium and becomes located in the endometrial connective tissue. Hence, the term **implantation** is well suited in these species. Along with the development of the embryo, the trophoblast differentiates into an inner **cytotrophoblast** and an outer **syncytiotrophoblast**. The allantois never develops and there is therefore no chorioallantois to give rise to a placenta. However, the migrating visceral mesoderm results in ample vascularization of the placenta, which takes the shape of a disc, making the placenta **discoid** (Fig. 9-14). It is from the resemblance of

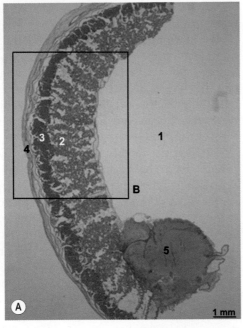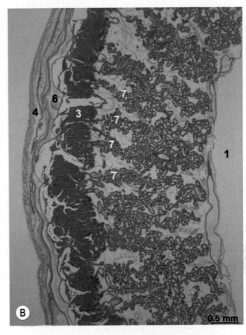

Fig. 9-13: Mink placenta. **A:** The boxed area in A is enlarged in 'B'. 1: Allantois; 2: Lamellar zone; 3: Junctional zone; 4: Endometrium; 5: Marginal haematoma; 6: Glandular zone; 7: Individual lamellae of the lamellar zone.

this spongy disc to a cake (placenta = flat cake in Latin) that we take the term 'placenta'.

In the disc, the trophoblast forms villi with a core of cytotrophoblast and an outer layer of syncytiotrophoblast. Later, the core is invaded by mesoderm carrying blood vessels. Due to the invasive nature of the syncytiotrophoblast, the maternal connective tissue and endothelium are removed and the trophoblast-covered fetal villi are directly surrounded by maternal blood contained in intervillous spaces. Hence, the placenta is **haemochorial** (Fig. 9-2). At birth, the discoid placenta and decidua are expelled as the afterbirth. Thus, the rodent and primate placentae are **discoid**, **villous**, **haemochorial**, and **deciduate**.

ECTOPIC PREGNANCY

Pregnancies occurring elsewhere than in the uterine cavity are termed **ectopic**. This rare, but life-threatening, condition occurs mainly in the **oviducts** or in the **abdomen**. Oviductal pregnancies may account for more than 95% of all ectopic pregnancies in humans; in contrast, this type does not occur in domestic animals. One may speculate whether this is due to species-specific oviduct environments not being conducive to further embryonic development, or to interruptions of the pathways leading to maternal recognition of pregnancy. The abdominal type of ectopic pregnancy may occur either as a result of a zygote entering the abdominal cavity and attaching to the mesentery or abdominal viscera (primary abdominal form) or, more commonly, by rupture of the oviduct or uterus followed by expulsion of the embryo/fetus (secondary abdominal form). In most cases, the embryo/fetus becomes calcified and is often found by chance. However, in both sheep and cats, live offspring resulting from the secondary form have been recovered at caesarean section, showing that full-term development is in fact possible outside the uterine cavity.

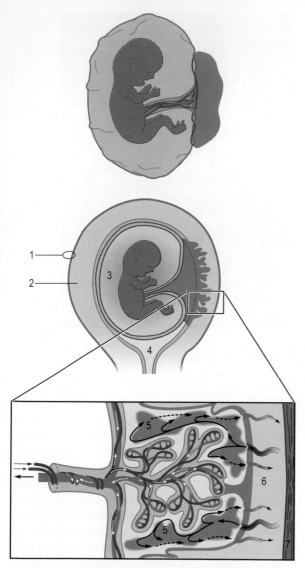

Fig. 9-14: The discoid primate placenta. 1: Perimetrium; 2: Endometrium and myometrium; 3: Amnion; 4: Uterine cavity; 5: Intervillous space with maternal blood; 6: Endometrium; 7: Myometrium.

SUMMARY

Upon entering the uterus, the embryo is initially nourished by **histotrophe** from the uterine glands. Placentation establishes the basis for an uptake of blood-borne nutrients, the **haemotrophe**. An

important pre-implantation event is the **maternal recognition of pregnancy** mediated through signals produced from the embryo. Around the time of implantation, the embryo develops multiple membranes and cavities. The outer covering of the embryo consists of the trophectoderm with an internal lining of the somatic extra-embryonic mesoderm, together making up the **chorion**. Folding of the chorion results in formation of the **amnion** enveloping the embryo proper. The hypoblast, covered with the visceral extra-embryonic mesoderm on the outside, encloses a cavity referred to as the **primitive yolk sac**. The **extra-embryonic coelom** is found between the somatic and visceral extra-embryonic mesoderm. The endoderm is inserted into the embryonic portion of the hypoblast sac and, with the anterior-posterior and lateral foldings of the embryo, the endoderm-lined portion of the primitive yolk sac becomes internalized into the embryo proper, forming the **primitive gut,** whereas the hypoblast-lined portion forms the **definitive yolk sac**. Finally, the **allantois** develops as an endoderm-lined outgrowth from the hindgut and comes to occupy most of the extra-embryonic coelom. With time, the allantois more or less surrounds the amnion. However, in cattle and pigs, a mesamnion, where the amnion and the chorion are attached, persists.

A temporary **choriovitelline placenta** is formed by interaction of the fused yolk sac and chorion with the endometrium in the horse and dog. The permanent **chorioallantoic placenta** is formed by interaction between the fused allantois and chorion and the endometrium. The placenta is classified according to its gross anatomical appearance (diffuse, multiplex, zonary or discoid), its surface-enlarging characteristics (villi, folds, lamellae/labyrinth), and the thickness of the placental barrier (epitheliochorial, synepitheliochorial, endotheliochorial, or haemochorial). In the **pig**, the placenta is **diffuse, folded, epitheliochorial** and **adeciduate**. In **ruminants**, the placenta is **cotyledonary** or **multiplex**, **villous**, **synepitheliochorial**, and **adeciduate**. In the **horse**, the placenta is **diffuse, villous, epitheliochorial**, and **adeciduate**. In **carnivores**, the placenta is **zonary**; **lamellar** or **labyrinthine**, endotheliochorial and **deciduate**. In **rodents and primates**, the placenta is **discoid, villous, haemochorial**, and **deciduate**.

FURTHER READING

Allen, W.R. (2005): Maternal recognition and maintenance of pregnancy in the mare. Anim. Reprod. 2:209–223.

Allen, W.R. and Stewart F. (2001): Equine placentation. Reprod. Fert. Dev. 13:623–634.

Cencic, A., Guillomot, M., Koren, S. and La Bonnardière, C. (2003): Trophoblastic interferons: Do they modulate uterine cellular markers at the time of conceptus attachment in the pig? Placenta 24:862–869.

Concannon, P., Tsutsui, T. and Shille, V. (2001): Embryo development, hormonal requirements and maternal responses during canine pregnancy. J. Reprod. Fert. Suppl. 57:169–179.

Corpa, J.M. (2006): Ectopic pregnancy in animals and humans. Reproduction 131:631–640.

Dantzer V. (1984): Scanning electron microscopy of exposed surfaces of the porcine placenta. Acta Anat. 118:96–106.

Dantzer V. (1985): Electron microscopy of the initial stages of placentation in the pig. Anat. Embryol. 172:281–293.

Dantzer, V. and Leiser, R. (1994): Initial vascularisation in the pig placenta: I. Demonstration of nonglandular areas by histology and corrosion casts. Anat. Rec. 238:177–190.

Dantzer, V. and Winther, H. (2001): Histological and immunohistochemical events during placentation in the pig. Reproduction Suppl. 58:209–222.

Denker, H.-W. (2000): Structural dynamics and function of early embryonic coats. Cells Tissues Organs 166:180–207.

Denker, H.-W., Eng, L.A. and Hammer, C.E. (1978): Studies on the early development and implantation in the cat. II. Implantation: Proteinases. Anat. Embryol. 154:39–54.

Lee, K.Y. and DeMayo, F.J. (2004): Animal models of implantation. Reproduction 128:679–695.

Leiser, R. and Dantzer V. (1988): Structural and functional aspects of porcine placental microvasculature. Anat. Embryol. 177:409–419.

Leiser, R. and Dantzer, V. (1994): Initial vascularisation in the pig placenta: II. Demonstration of gland and areola-gland subunits by histology and corrosion casts. Anat. Rec. 238:326–334.

Leiser, R., Krebs, C., Ebert, B. and Dantzer, V. (1997): Placental vascular corrosion cast studies: a comparison between ruminants and humans. Microsc. Res. Tech. 38:76–87.

Rüsse, I. and Sinowatz, F. (1998): Lehrbuch der Embryologie der haustiere, 2nd edn. Parey Buchverlag, Berlin.

Spencer, T.E., Johnson, G.A., Bazer, F.W. and Burghardt, R.C. (2004). Implantation mechanisms: insights from the sheep. Reproduction 128:657–668.

Swanson, W.F., Roth, T.I. and Wildt D.E. (1994): In vivo embryogenesis, embryo migration, and embryonic mortality in the domestic cat. Biol. Reprod. 51: 452–464.

CHAPTER 10

Development of the central and peripheral nervous system

Fred Sinowatz

The **central nervous system (CNS)** develops from the ectoderm once the latter has become specified into **surface ectoderm** and **neuroectoderm**. Some of the early features of nervous system development have already been addressed in relation to neurulation (see Chapter 8) and will be briefly recapitulated here in discussing the development of the CNS more specifically. The **peripheral nervous system (PNS)** develops in association with the CNS as the communication system between the CNS and the rest of the body.

NEURAL PLATE

The development of the **neural plate**, a thickening of the ectoderm that represents the primordium of the nervous system, is induced by the notochord (see Chapter 8) a major axial signalling centre of the trunk of the early embryo. Subsequently, the neural plate folds and forms the **neural tube**. Some of the molecular mechanisms underlying these processes have been clarified recently in mice. The notochord, which is in close proximity to the midline neural plate during this stage, releases sonic hedgehog (Shh). Much of the surface ectoderm of an embryo during gastrulation produces Bone Morphogenetic Protein-4 (BMP4). This signalling protein prevents the dorsal ectoderm from forming neural tissue. Under the influence of Hepatic Nuclear Factor-3beta (HNF-3beta), cells of the developing notochord secrete noggin and chordin. These two molecules are potent neural inducers that block the inhibitory influence of BMP4 and thus allow the ectoderm dorsal to the notochord to form neural tissue.

NEURAL TUBE

The neural tube is a prominent structure that dominates the anterior (future cephalic) end of the embryo. In the following we will see how the early neural tube develops into the major morphological and functional components of the mature nervous system (Fig. 10-1). Before neurogenesis, the neural plate and the neural tube are composed of a single layer of **neuroepithelial cells (neuroepithelium)**. Neuroepithelial cells are highly polarized along their apical-basal axis. This is reflected, for example, in the organization of their plasma membranes: certain transmembrane proteins such as prominin-1 (CD133) are found selectively in the apical plasma membrane.

Shortly after induction, the epithelium of the neural plate and early neural tube organizes into a **pseudostratified epithelium** in which the nuclei appear to be located in several separate layers because they are at different heights within the elongated neuroepithelial cells. The nuclei shift extensively within the cytoplasm as the cell cycle progresses (Fig. 10-2). DNA synthesis (the S-phase) occurs in nuclei located near the external limiting membrane (the basal lamina surrounding the neural tube). As these nuclei prepare to go into mitosis, they migrate within the cytoplasm towards the lumen of the neural tube where mitosis is completed. The **orientation of the mitotic spindle** during this division is important for the fate of the daughter cells. If the cleavage plane is perpendicular to the apical (inner) surface of the neural tube, the two daughter cells slowly migrate towards the periphery of the neural tube, where they prepare for

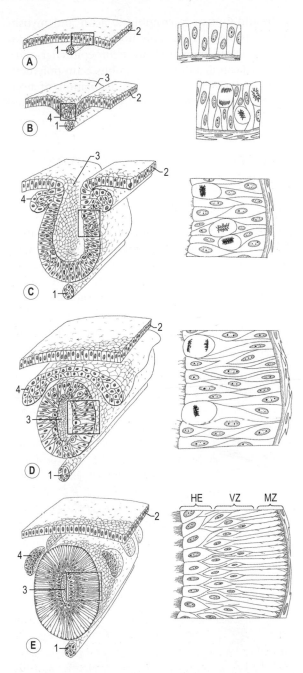

Fig. 10-1: Formation of the neural tube and the neural crests. The boxed areas in A–C are enlarged to the right (modified after Rüsse and Sinowatz, 1998). **A:** 1: Notochord; 2: Surface ectoderm: **B:** 1: Notochord; 2: Surface ectoderm; 3: Neural groove; 4: Neural plate. **C:** 1: Notochord; 2: Epithelium of the neural groove; numerous mitoses occur in the neural epithelium; 3: Neural groove; 4: Neural crest; **D:** 1: Notochord; 2: Surface ectoderm; 3: Neural tube; 4: Neural crest, which at this stage is still a continuous sheet of cells. **E:** 1: Notochord; 2: Surface ectoderm; 3: Neural tube; 4 Neural crests, which are segmented into groups of cells giving rise to different cell types. E: Ependymal cells; VZ; Ventricular zone; MZ: Marginal zone. Courtesy Sinowatz and Rüsse (2007).

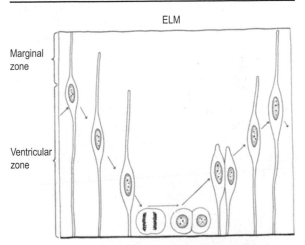

Fig. 10-2: Interkinetic nuclear migration within the neural tube. Within the pseudostratified epithelium of the neural tube, nuclei that synthesize DNA (S-phase) are located near the external limiting membrane (ELM) but then move toward the inner margin of the neural tube, where mitosis occurs. Courtesy Sinowatz and Rüsse (2007).

very slowly and remains a proliferative **progenitor cell** that is still capable of mitosis. The daughter cell that is **closer to the basal surface** (external limiting membrane) inherits a high concentration of the Notch receptor on its surface and can now be called a **neuroblast**. The neuroblasts are the precursor cells of neurons and begin to produce cell processes that ultimately become axons and dendrites.

Interkinetic nuclear migration in the neuroepithelium is accompanied by a change in nuclear morphology: the nucleus adopts an elongated shape along the apical-basal axis when migration begins and rounds up when migration stops. This is consistent with the idea that the nucleus is pulled by some

another round of DNA synthesis. If, on the other hand, the cleavage plane runs parallel to the inner surface of the neural tube, the two daughter cells have completely different fates. The **daughter cell that is closer to the inner surface** migrates away cytoskeletal machinery. Early work on interkinetic nuclear migration indicated the involvement of microtubules, an idea that is supported by the observation that nuclear positioning is a microtubule-dependent process in many cell types. Recent studies of the *lissencephaly 1* (*LIS1*) gene also support this idea. Mutations in the human *LIS1* gene are responsible for the type I form of lissencephaly (smooth brain), a severe genetically caused malformation of the brain. The LIS1 protein forms a complex with cytoplasmic dynein and dynactin which binds to microtubules and disturbs microtubule dynamics. Mice with reduced *LIS1* expression show defects in the interkinetic nuclear migration in neuroepithelial cells and abnormal neuronal migration.

In addition to microtubules, actin and myosin filaments are also probably involved in the interkinetic nuclear migration in neuroepithelial cells. Cytochalasin B, a drug that inhibits actin polymerization, blocks the process, and ablation of non-muscle myosin heavy chain II-B results in disordered nuclear migration in the cells.

CELL LINEAGES OF THE CENTRAL NERVOUS SYSTEM

During development, **neural stem cells** give rise to all the neurons of the mammalian CNS (Figs 10-3, 10-4, 10-5) and also the two types of macroglial

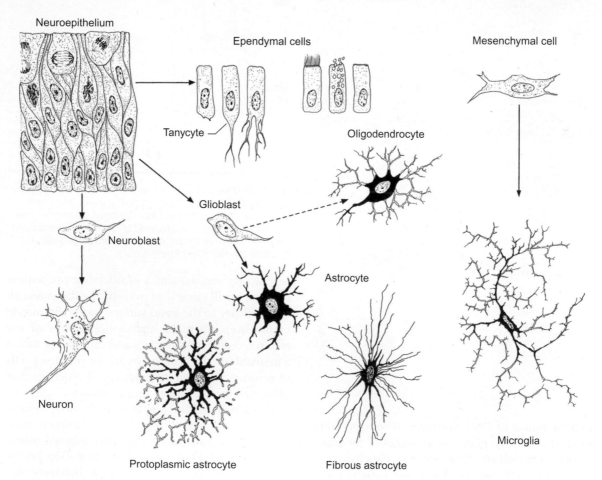

Fig. 10-3: Cell lineages in the developing central nervous system. Courtesy Sinowatz and Rüsse (2007).

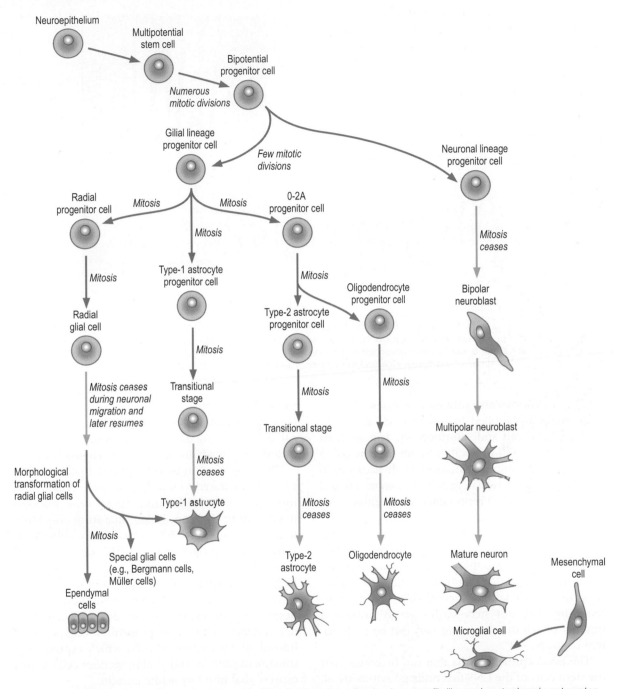

Fig. 10-4: Origins of neurons and various types of glial cells. Neurons, oligodendrocytes, fibrillar and protoplasmic astrocytes, and ependymal cells orginate from neuroepithelial cells. Microglia (Hortega glia) develop from mesenchyme cells.

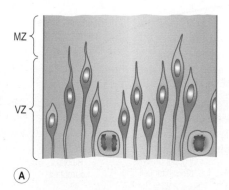

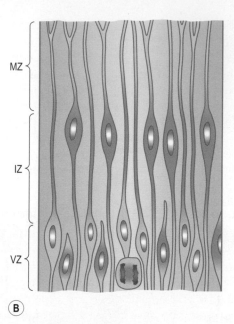

Fig. 10-5: A: During its early development, the epithelium of the neural tube consists of the ventricular zone (VZ), where neural epithelial cells undergo mitoses, and the marginal zone (MZ), which contains elongated processes of the cells. B: Section through the neural tube at a slightly more advanced stage than A. Neuroepithelial cells, which have left the mitotic cycle, migrate away from the lumen of the neural tube and form an intermediate cell layer (IZ: intermediate zone).

cell, the **astrocytes** and **oligodendrocytes**. Usually, two criteria are applied to define a cell as a stem cell: self-renewal and pluripotency (or at least multipotency). Self-renewal indicates that the cell is capable of an unlimited number of divisions each resulting in either two stem cells or a stem cell and a committed cell. Pluripotency or multipotency implies that the cell can give rise to numerous types of differentiated cells – all cell types of the mammalian body in the case of pluripotency (see Chapter 2). However, this concept has to be somewhat modified when applied to the CNS: 'stem cells' in this context are neural cells that are self-renewing, but not necessarily for an unlimited number of cell divisions, and they can be multipotent or unipotent.

The neuroepithelial cells that can be considered the stem cells of the CNS first undergo symmetrical, proliferative divisions, each generating two daughter stem cells. These divisions are followed by numerous asymmetrical, self-renewing divisions, each of which results in a daughter stem cell and a more differentiated cell such as a progenitor cell. Neural progenitor cells typically undergo symmetrical, differentiating divisions that generate two postmitotic cells ready for terminal differentiation.

The origins of most cells found in the mature CNS can be traced to multipotent stem cells within the early neuroepithelium. These cells undergo many mitotic divisions before maturing into **bipotent progenitor cells**, which give rise to either **neuronal** or **glial progenitor cells**. This developmental bifurcation is accompanied by a significant change in gene expression. For example, multipotent stem cells express an intermediate filament protein called nestin. Nestin expression is down-regulated as descendants of bipotent progenitor cells separate into neuronal progenitor cells, which express neurofilament protein, and glial progenitor cells, which express glial fibrillary acidic protein.

The **neuronal progenitor cells** give rise to a series of neuroblasts. The earliest **bipolar neuroblasts** possess two slender cytoplasmic processes that contact both the external limiting membrane and the central luminal border of the neural tube. By retracting the inner process, a bipolar neuroblast loses contact with the inner luminal border and becomes a **unipolar neuroblast**. The unipolar neuroblasts accumulate a large amount of rough endoplasmic reticulum (Nissl substance) in their cytoplasm and then begin to send out several cytoplasmic processes. At this point, they are known as **multipolar neuroblasts** with the principal developmental activities of sending out axonal and dendritic processes and making connections with other neurons or end organs.

The other major lineage stemming from the bipotential progenitor cells is that of the **glial progenitor cells**. Glial progenitor cells continue to undergo mitosis, and their progeny split into several lines. One, the **O-2A progenitor cell**, is a precursor to two important lines of glial cells that ultimately form the **oligodendrocytes** and **type-2 astrocytes**, the latter distinguished by its antigenic phenotype from **type-1 astrocytes** derived from another glial lineage. Anatomically, the astrocytes can be divided into protoplasmic astrocytes, found in the grey matter, and fibrous astrocytes found in the white matter. The origin of **oligodendrocytes** has long been a matter for debate, but studies have shown that they probably arise from progenitor cells located in the ventral ventricular zone alongside the floor plate. From there, they spread throughout the brain and spinal cord and ultimately form the myelin coverings around axons in the white matter of the CNS. The formation of oligodendrocyte precursors depends on sonic hedgehog (Shh), produced by cells in the notochord, as an inductive signal.

A third glial lineage has a more complex history. **Radial progenitor cells** give rise to **radial glial cells**, which act as guide wires in the brain for the migration of young neurons. When the neurons are migrating along the radial glial cells of the fetus during midpregnancy, they inhibit the proliferation of the radial glial cells. After neuronal cell migration, the radial glial cells, now free from the inhibitory influence of the neurons, re-enter the mitotic cycle and produce progeny that can transform into a number of cell types: some can seemingly cross lineage lines and differentiate into type-1 astrocytes;

others differentiate into various specialized glial cell types; yet others even into ependymal cells and neurons.

Another type of glial cell of the CNS does not originate from the neuroepithelium. These **microglial cells**, which act as motile macrophages after damage to the CNS, are mesoderm-derived cells that enter the CNS along with vascular tissue and are therefore not found in the developing CNS until it is penetrated by blood vessels.

Whether neural stem cells and their derivative progenitor cells proliferate (by symmetrical divisions) or differentiate (through asymmetrical division) is closely linked to their epithelial characteristics, especially their apical–basal polarity and cell-cycle length. Generally, the period of neuron production precedes that of gliogenesis. The time at which the precursor of a neuron undergoes its last division is called its birthday. Neurogenic cells in the ventral part of the spinal cord and the hindbrain are usually the first to stop dividing, with dorsal and intermediate neurons following. Cortical neurons in the cerebrum and cerebellum are the last population to be formed; they continue to proliferate until the third to fourth month after birth in the dog and the third year of life in humans. In precocial species, including cattle and horses, most cortical neurons are already formed by the time of birth.

HISTOLOGICAL DIFFERENTIATION OF THE CENTRAL NERVOUS SYSTEM

Nerve cells

Neuroblasts arise by division of **neuroepithelial cells** and, once formed, they lose their ability to divide (Fig. 10-4). Initially, neuroblasts develop two processes and extend from the the lumen of the neural tube to the external limiting membrane. When they start to migrate into the intermediate layer, the central process is retracted and the neuroblasts appear temporarily unipolar. During further differentiation, several small cytoplasmic processes extend from their cell body. One of these processes elongates rapidly, forming the primitive **axon**, while arborization of the others gives rise to the primitive **dendrites**. These cells can be now called **multipolar neuroblasts** that eventually become mature **multipolar neurons**. Axons of neurons in the basal plate, which leave the marginal zone on the latero-ventral aspect of the cord, form the efferent **ventral root** of the spinal cord. Axons of neurons in the alar plate penetrate into the marginal zone of the cord where they ascend to higher or lower levels to form **association neurons**.

Glial cells

The other major cell lineage originating from bipotent progenitor cells is that of the **glial progenitor cells (glioblasts)**, which are formed by neuroepithelial cells after the production of neuroblasts ceases, and their progeny split into several lines. One of them, the **0–2A progenitor cell**, is the precursor of two glial cell types that ultimately differentiate into **type-2 astrocytes** and **oligodendrocytes**. It has been recently shown that oligodendrocytes are derived from progenitor cells located in the ventral ventricular zone. From there they migrate throughout the spinal cord and brain and form the myelin sheath around neuronal processes. The formation of oligodendrocytes depends on the signalling molecule sonic hedgehog (Shh) produced by cells of the notochord. In contrast to the Schwann cells of the peripheral nervous system, each of which can only wrap itself around one axon, the flat processes of a single oligodendroglial cell in the central nervous system can myelinate several nerve fibres. Myelin sheaths begin to form in the spinal cord during the late fetal period. In general, fibre tracts become myelinated at about the time they become functional (Table 10-1).

Not all glial cells of the spinal cord originate from the neuroepithelium. **Microglial** cells, which appear in the second half of fetal development, are highly phagocytotic cells derived from the mesoderm.

When neuroepithelial cells cease to produce neuroblasts, they differentiate into the **ependymal epithelial cells** lining the central canal of the spinal cord. With the generation of neurons, the neuroepithelium is transformed into an epithelium with several cell layers. With the switch to neurogenesis, neuroepithelial cells down-regulate certain epithelial features (notably their expression of tight-junction proteins) at the same time that astroglial hallmarks appear. In essence, after the onset of neurogenesis, neuroepithelial cells give rise to a distinct, but related, cell type: the **radial glial cells** which exhibit residual neuroepithelial as well as astroglial properties.

Radial glial cells represent more fate-restricted progenitors than neuroepithelial cells and gradually replace them. As a consequence, many of the neurons in the central nervous system are derived from radial glial cells. The neuroepithelial properties that are maintained by radial glial cells include the expression of neuroepithelial markers (such as the intermediate-filament protein nestin) and the maintenance of an apical surface and important features of apical–basal polarity (such as an apical localization of centrosomes and prominin-1). Like neuroepithelial cells, radial glial cells show interkinetic nuclear migration, with their nuclei undergoing mitosis at the apical surface of the ventricular zone and migrating basally for completion of the S-phase of the cell cycle. However, in contrast to neuroepithelial cells, radial glial cells show several properties of astroglia, such as the expression of astrocyte-specific glutamate transporter (GLAST), Ca^{2+}-binding protein S100β, and glial fibrillary acidic protein.

In contrast to early neuroepithelial cells, most radial glial cells have a limited developmental potential; usually they generate only a single cell type, either astrocytes, or oligodendrocytes, or (most commonly) neurons.

DEVELOPMENT OF THE SPINAL CORD

With the beginning of cellular differentiation in the neural tube, the neuroepithelium thickens and appears layered (Fig. 10-6). The layer closest to the lumen of the neural tube is called the **ventricular** or **neuroepithelial layer**; it remains epithelial and still shows mitotic activity. However, with further

Table 10-1: Beginning of formation of the myelin sheath in the central and peripheral nervous systems.

Species	Tissue	Stage of gestation
Cat	N. vestibularis	Day 53 p.c.
	N. cochlearis	Day 57 p.c.
	N. opticus	Day 1–2 p.n.
Pig	Spinal cord	Week 8 p.c. (cervical)
		Week 9 p.c. (lumbar)
Sheep	N. oculomotorius	Day 63 p.c.
	N. trochlearis	
	N. vestibularis	
	N. hypoglossus	
	N. trigeminus (sens.)	Day 66 p.c.
	N. glossopharyngeus	
	N. vagus	
	N. accessorius	
	N. opticus	Day 78 p.c.
	N. trigeminus (mot.)	Day 60 p.c.
	N. facialis	Day 78 p.c.
	N. trochlearis	
	N. abducens	
	N. vestibularis	Day 80 p.c.
	Spinal cord	Day 60 p.c.
	Medulla oblongata	
	Mesencephalon	
	Cerebellum	Day 80 p.c.
	Telencephalon	Day 100 p.c.
Cattle	Medulla oblongata	Week 21 p.c.
	Spinal cord	Week 16 p.c.
	N. abducens	Week 20 p.c.
	N. intermediofacialis (mot.)	
	N. cochlearis	
	N. glossopharyngeus	
	N. vagus	
	N. hypoglossus	
	N. trigeminus	Week 21 p.c.
	N. vestibulocochlearis	Week 16 p.c.
	N. accessorius	
	N. opticus	Week 24 p.c.

p.n. = post natum; p.c. = post coitum

development, the proliferating cell population in the neuroepithelial layer becomes largely exhausted and the remaining cells differentiate to become the **ependyma** of the **central canal** and the **ventricular system** of the brain.

The ventricular zone is surrounded by the **intermediate** or **mantle layer** (Figs 10-1, 10-5) which contains the cell bodies of postmitotic neuroblasts and presumptive glial cells. As the spinal cord matures, the intermediate layer becomes the **grey**

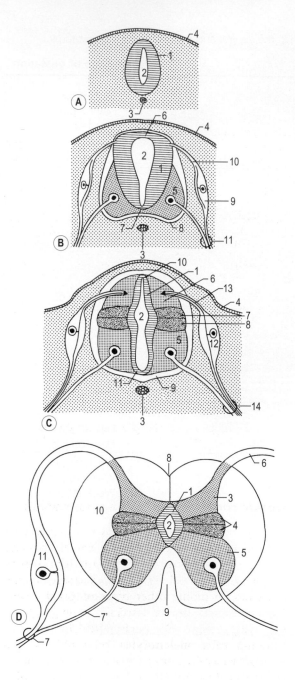

Fig. 10-6: Four successive stages in the development of the spinal cord. A and B: 1: Neuroepithelium; 2: Central canal; 3: Notochord; 4: Surface ectoderm; 5: Basal plate; 6: Roof plate; 7: Floor plate; 8: Marginal zone; 9: Spinal ganglion; 10: Dorsal (sensory) horn; 11: Spinal nerve. C: 1: Neuroepithelium; 2: Central canal; 3: Notochord; 4: Surface ectoderm; 5: Basal plate; 6: Alar plate; 7 and 8: Intermediate horn; 9: Marginal zone; 10: Roof plate; 11: Floor plate; 12: Spinal ganglion; 13: Dorsal root; 14: Spinal nerve; D: 1: Ependyma; 2: Central canal; 3: Dorsal (sensory) horn; 4: Intermediate horn; 5: Ventral (motor) horn; 6: Dorsal (sensory) root; 7: Spinal nerve. 7': Ventral (motor) root; 8: Septum dorsale; 9: Median fissure; 10: White matter; 11: Spinal ganglion. Courtesy Sinowatz and Rüsse (2007).

neural cell bodies and later forms the **white matter** of the spinal cord.

Continous addition of neuroblasts to the intermediate layer thickens the neural tube ventrally and dorsally on each side (Figs 10-6, 10-8). The ventral thickenings are referred to as the **basal plates**. They contain motor neurons (general somatic efferent nerve fibers) and autonomic neurons (visceral efferent nerve fibres; Table 10-2). The dorsal thickenings, the **alar plates**, form the sensory area with neurons receiving their input from the skin, joints and muscles (general somatic afferent nerve fibres), from the pharynx (special visceral afferent nerve fibres) and from the viscera and heart (general visceral afferent nerve fibres). A small longitudinal groove, the sulcus limitans, marks the boundary between these two areas (Fig. 10-6). The left and right alar plates are connected dorsally over the **central canal** by the thin **roof plate**, the two basal plates are connected by the **floor plate** ventral to the central canal. The roof and floor plates do not contain neuroblasts, their nerve fibres serving primarily to connect one side to the other.

The mature spinal cord is organized similarly to the embryonic pattern except that the basal and alar plates become subdivided into somatic and visceral components. Transformation of the embryonic into the mature spinal cord (Fig. 10-9) results from proliferation, asymmetrical cell movement of immature neurons in the intermediate layer, and the development of neuronal processes. In the process, the intermediate layer becomes shaped like a butterfly,

matter, where the cell bodies of the neurons are located. (Fig. 10-7)

As the neuroblasts continue to develop axons and dendrites, a peripheral **marginal layer** (marginal zone) is formed. It contains neural processes but not

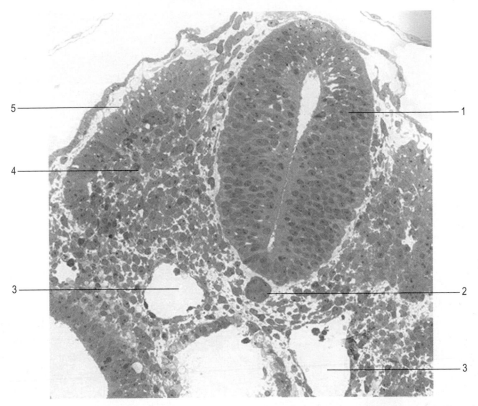

Fig. 10-7: Porcine embryo, Day 16, transverse section. 1: Primordium of the spinal cord; 2: Notochord; 3: Dorsal aorta; 4: Myotome; 5: Dermatome.

with prominent dorsal and ventral grey horns arranged around the central canal. In addition to the ventral efferent and the dorsal afferent horns, a small lateral projection of grey matter can be observed between the dorsal and ventral columns at spinal levels thoracic 1 (T1) to lumbar 2 (L2). This is the lateral horn; it contains cell bodies of sympathetic autonomic (visceral efferent) neurons.

The marginal layer develops into the white matter of the spinal cord, named because of its whitish appearance that results from the dominance of **myelinated axons**. This outer layer contains tracts of ascending and descending axons that are grouped together in bundles (**funiculi**). The dorsal, lateral and ventral funiculi are separated by the efferent spinal nerve roots emerging from the cord and afferent roots entering the cord (Fig. 10-9).

Dorsal root ganglia and spinal nerves

As more fully described in Chapter 8, **neural crest cells** migrate from the edge of the neural folds and give rise to sensory or **spinal ganglia (dorsal root ganglia)** of the spinal nerves, as well as several other cell types, including **other types of ganglia cells** (sensory ganglia, general visceral efferent ganglia of the sympathetic and parasympathetic system), **Schwann cells, melanocytes, odontoblasts**, and **mesenchyme** of the pharyngeal arches. Neuroblasts of the spinal ganglia develop two processes, which soon unite in a T-shaped fashion (**pseudo-unipolar neurons**). Both processes of spinal ganglion cells have the structural characteristics of axons, but the peripheral process can be functionally classified as a dendrite in that conduction within it is toward the

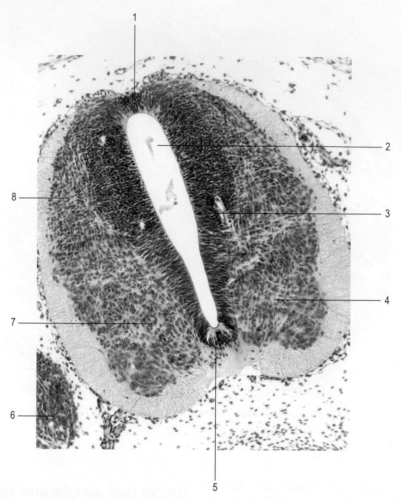

Fig. 10-8: Cat embryo, 17 mm CRL. 1: Roof plate; 2: Central canal; 3 Ependymal zone; 4: Marginal zone; 5: Floor plate; 6 Spinal ganglion; 7: Basal plate; 8: Alar plate.

cell body. The centrally growing processes enter the dorsal portion of the neural tube and constitute the afferent **dorsal root** of the spinal cord. In the spinal cord, they either form synapses with afferent dorsal horn interneurons or ascend through the marginal layers to one of the higher brain centres. The peripherally growing processes join the fibres of the ventral root to form the trunk of the **spinal nerve** through which they eventually terminate in sensory receptors. The common trunk of the spinal nerve almost immediately splits into a **dorsal** and a **ventral ramus**. The dorsal rami of the spinal nerves

innervate dorsal axial musculature, vertebral joints and the skin of the back. Ventral primary rami innervate the limbs and the ventral body wall and form the two major nerve plexuses, the **brachial** and **lumbosacral plexuses**.

Positional changes of the spinal cord: ascensus medullae spinalis

Intitially, the spinal cord runs the entire length of the embryo with spinal nerves passing through the intervertebral foramina at the levels of their origin.

Table 10-2: Origin of structures in the central nervous system

	Dorsal roof plate	Alar plate	Basal plate
Spinal cord	Obliterated	Most tracts and the dorsal grey columns	Ventral grey and intermediate columns
Metencephalon and Myelencephalon	Rostral and caudal vela, tela chorioidea	Afferent nuclei of cranial nerves V, VII, VIII, IX and X; cerebellum; pons	Efferent nuclei of cranial nerves V, VI, VII, IX, X, XI and XII
Mesencephalon	No derivatives	Corpora quadrigemina, tectum, substantia nigra, red nucleus, etc.	Efferent nuclei of cranial nerves III and IV
Diencephalon	Pineal gland, tela choroidea of roof of ventricle III	Epithalamus, metathalamus, thalamus, hypothalamus, retina	
Telencephalon	Corpus callosum (dorsal plate fibres grow into the roof plate)	Cerebral cortex, basal ganglia	

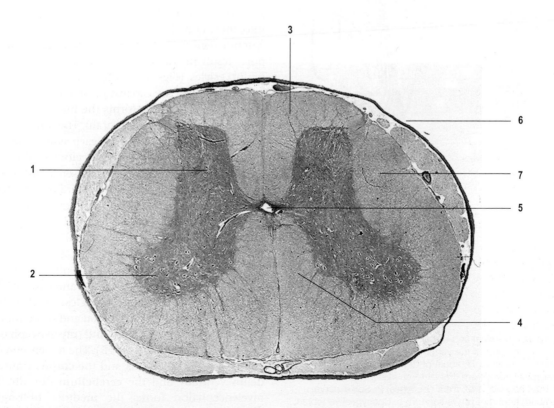

Fig. 10-9: Adult dog, cross-section through the spinal cord. 1: Dorsal (sensory) horn; 2: Ventral (motor) horn; 3: Funiculus dorsalis; 4: Funiculus ventralis; 5: Central canal; 6: Dura mater; 7: Funiculus lateralis.

Later, however, the vertebral column and the dura grow more rapidly than the spinal cord, leaving the posterior end of the cord terminating at a gradually higher level in the vertebral column (Fig. 10-10). This phenomenon is called **ascensus medullae**

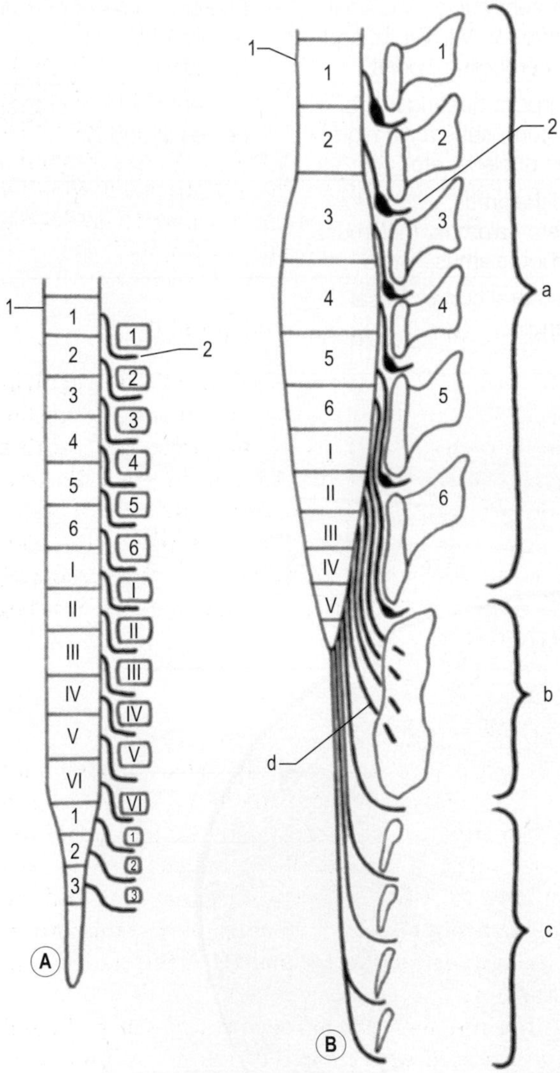

Fig. 10-10: Terminal end of the bovine spinal cord in relation to the end of the vertebral column at two stages (A: 3 months gestation, B: adult) of development. 1: Segments of the spinal cord, from cranial to caudal: 1–6: Pars lumbalis; I–VI: Pars sacralis; 1–3: Pars coccygea; 2: Spinal nerve; a: lumbar vertebrae; b: Os sacrum; c: Coccygeal vertebrae; d: Cauda equina. Courtesy Sinowatz and Rüsse (2007).

spinalis. The disproportionate growth also forces the spinal nerves to run obliquely from the spinal cord to their corresponding vertebral foramina.

In adult animals the spinal cord terminates at the level L2 to L3, depending on the species. The surrounding dural sac and the subarachnoidal space extend more posteriorly, usually to sacral 2 (S2). From the posterior end of the spinal cord, a threadlike glial and ependymal extension, the **filum terminale**, runs posteriorly and attaches to the periosteum of the first coccygeal vertebrae. Bundles of nerve fibres running posteriorly within the vertebral column collectively form the **cauda equina**. To collect cerebrospinal fluid during a lumbar puncture, the needle has to be inserted at the lower lumbar levels to avoid hitting the lower end of the spinal cord.

DEVELOPMENT OF THE BRAIN

The anterior two-thirds of the neural tube develop into the brain. Fusion of the neural folds in the anterior region, and closure of the anterior neuropore, result in the formation of the three primary brain vesicles (Figs 10-11, 10-12) from which the brain develops. An expansion at the most rostral end of the neural tube forms the first brain vesicle, the **prosencephalon** or forebrain. The **optic vesicles** grow out as evaginations from each side of the prosencephalon. The two enlarged regions of the brain posterior to these become the **mesencephalon** and **rhombencephalon** (second and third primary brain vesicles). The prosencephalon partly divides into two vesicles, the **telencephalon** and **diencephalon** (Figs 10-13, 10-14). The lateral walls of the telencephalon soon become domed, presaging the future **cerebral hemispheres**. The diencephalon remains undivided, located in the midline and connected to the laterally expanding optic vesicles. The rhombencephalon also divides into rostral and posterior portions: the **metencephalon** and **myelencephalon**, respectively (Figs 10-14, 10-15). The metencephalon will give rise to the **pons** and the **corpus trapezoideum** ventrally and the **cerebellum** dorsally. The myelencephalon forms the **medulla oblongata**, which is the most posterior part of the brain stem

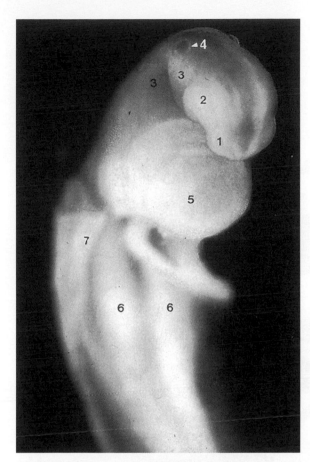

Fig. 10-11: Sheep embryo with three brain vesicles. 1: Prosencephalon; 2: Mesencephalon; 3: Rhombencephalon; 4: Otic placode; 5: Heart; 6: Mesonephros; 7: Body wall.

and connects it with the spinal cord (Figs. 10-14, 10-16).

The brain flexures

Differential growth of the five secondary brain vesicles (telencephalon, diencephalon, mesencephalon, metencephalon and myelencephalon) gives rise to flexures (Fig. 10-12). As head folding occurs, the mesencephalon bends ventrally to produce the midbrain flexure (**cephalic flexure**). A second more gradual ventral bend between the hindbrain and the spinal cord is termed the **cervical flexure**. In the rhombencephalon a slight dorsal bending, the

pontine flexure, occurs. The pontine flexure is located in the future pontine region and causes a thinning of the roof of the hindbrain.

At first, the developing brain shows the same basic structure as the spinal cord, but the flexures produce considerable variations in the outline of transverse sections at different levels of the brain and in the relative positions of white and grey matter. The sulcus limitans extends anteriorly only to the junction of the mesencephalon and diencephalon. Alar and basal plates, which are separated by the sulcus limitans, are therefore only recognizable posterior to this junction. In the diencephalon and telencephalon, however, the alar plates become accentuated and the basal plates regress.

Rhombencephalon (hindbrain)

The rhombencephalon consists of the **myelencephalon**, the most posterior brain vesicle, and the **metencephalon**, which extends from the pontine flexure to the rhombencephalic isthmus. Posteriorly, the cervical flexure demarcates the myelencephalon from the developing spinal cord. Later, this junction is defined as the level of the roots of the first cervical spinal nerve, roughly at the foramen magnum.

Myelencephalon

The myelencephalon resembles the spinal cord both developmentally and structurally and develops into the **medulla oblongata** – the posterior part of the brain stem. The medulla oblongata serves as a conduit for tracts between the spinal cord and the higher regions of the brain and also contains important centres for the regulation of respiration and heartbeat.

The fundamental arrangement of alar and basal plates, which are separated by the sulcus limitans as seen in the spinal cord, is retained almost unchanged, but the lateral walls are everted. This causes a pronounced expansion of the roof plate, closing the central canal dorsally, and a widening of the canal to the **fourth ventricle**. The roof plate of the myelencephalon is reduced to a single layer of

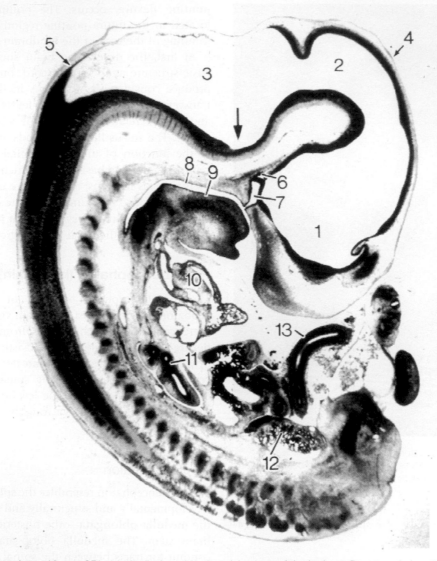

Fig. 10-12: Cat embryo, 10 mm CRL, longitudinal section, 3-vesicle stage of the brain. 1: Prosencephalon; 2: Mesencephalon; 3: Rhombencephalon with pontine flexure (arrow); 4: Cephalic flexure; 5: Cervical flexure; 6: Primordium of neurohypophysis; 7: Rathke's pouch, primordium of adenhypophysis; 8: Primary oral cavity; 9: Tongue; 10: Heart; 11: Lung; 12: Mesonephros; 13: Intestine.

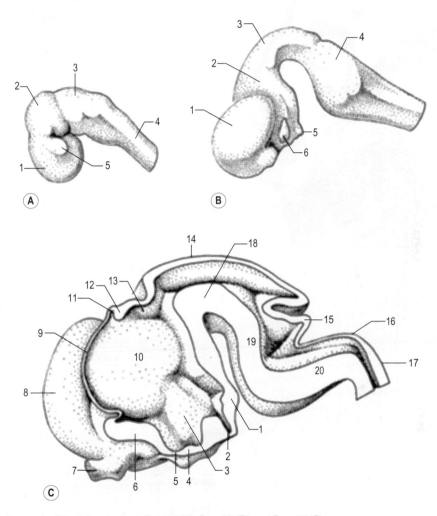

Fig. 10-13: Development of the feline brain at Day 18 (A), Day 22 (B) and Day 25 (C).
A: 1: Prosencephalon; 2: Mesencephalon: 3: Rhombencephalon; 4: Spinal cord; 5: Optic vesicle.
B: 1: Telencephalon; 2: Diencephalon; 3: Mesencephalon; 4: Rhombencephalon; 5: Infundibulum; 6: Stalk of the optic vesicle.
C: 1: Primordium of corpus mammilare; 2: Infundibulum; 3: Hypothalamus; 4: Chiasma opticum; 5: Lamina terminalis; 6: Commissural plate; 7: Bulbus olfactorius; 8: Cerebral hemisphere; 9: Roof of the IIIrd ventricle; 10: Thalamus; 11: Primordium of epiphysis; 12: Commissura caudalis; 13: Metathalamus; 14: Corpora quadrigemina; 15: Cerebellum; 16: Lamina tectoria; 17: Cervical flexure; 18: Crus cerebri; 19: Pons; 20: Medulla oblongata. Courtesy Sinowatz and Rüsse (2007).

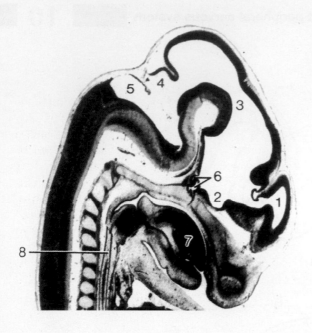

Fig. 10-14: Feline embryo, 17 mm CRL, 5-vesicle stage of brain development, longitudinal section, from Rüsse and Sinowatz, 1998. 1: Telencephalon; 2: Diencephalon; 3: Mesencephalon; 4: Metencephalon; 5: Myelencephalon; 6: Hypophysis; 7: Tongue; 8: Oesophagus. Courtesy Sinowatz and Rüsse (2007).

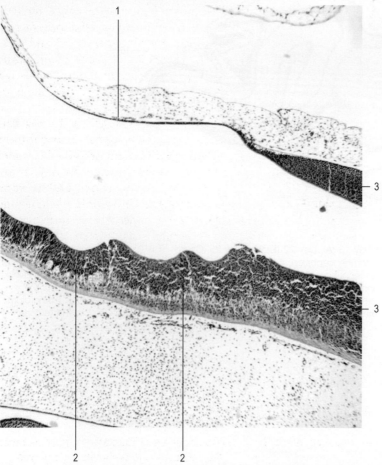

Fig. 10-15: Pig embryo, Day 21.5, longitudinal section through the metencephalon and myelencephalon. 1: Roof plate of the IVth ventricle; 2: Neuromeres of the rhombencephalon; 3: Myelencephalon. Courtesy Sinowatz and Rüsse (2007).

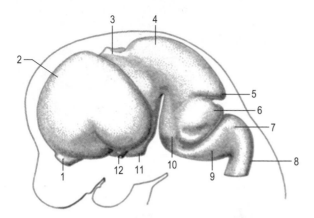

Fig. 10-16: Development of the feline brain at day 33.
1: Bulbus olfactorius: 2: Cerebral hemisphere;
3: Epithalamus; 4: Primordium of corpora quadrigemina;
5: Colliculus caudalis; 6: Cerebellum; 7: Lamina tectoria;
8: Cervical flexure; 9: Medulla oblongata; 10: Pons; 11: Crus
cerebri; 12: N. opticus. Courtesy Sinowatz and Rüsse
(2007).

ependymal cells that is covered by mesenchymal cells forming the pia mater. Active proliferation of the vascular mesenchyme produces a number of sac-like invaginations into the underlying fourth ventricle. They form a **choroid plexus**, which produces the **cerebrospinal fluid**.

As a result, instead of being arranged dorsoventrally, the alar and basal plates come to lie in the floor of the hindbrain like the pages of an open book so that the efferent areas of the basal plates become situated medially to the afferent areas of the alar plates. The cavity of this part of the myelen-

cephalon (posterior part of the future fourth ventricles) becomes rhomboid shaped.

The basal plates, as in the spinal cord, contain the **nuclei** (aggregations of neuron cell bodies) of efferent nerves. On each side, these nuclei are arranged into three groups (Table 10-3). The first is the medial **general somatic efferent group**, represented by neurons of the hypoglossal (XII) and accessory (XI) nerves, a cephalic continuation of the ventral horn of the spinal cord. This general somatic efferent group expands rostrally into the mesencephalon and is also called the general somatic efferent motor column. The second group is the intermediate **special visceral efferent group**, represented by neurons that innervate muscles derived from the pharyngeal (branchial) arches (the glossopharyngeal (IX), vagus (X) and accessory (XI) nerves innervating the musculature of the third and fourth pharyngeal arches). The third, lateral **general visceral efferent group**, is represented by neurons of the vagus (X) and glossopharyngeal (IX) nerves. The axons of the vagus neurons supply the thoracic and abdominal viscera and the heart while the axons of the glossopharyngeal neurons supply the parotid gland.

Neuroblasts of the alar plates in the myelencephalon migrate into the marginal zone and form isolated areas of grey matter, the **gracile nuclei** medially and the **cuneate nuclei** laterally. These nuclei are associated with the corresponding tracts ascending from the spinal cord within the funiculus dorsalis. Another group of neuroblasts from the alar plates migrates ventrally and forms the **olivary**

Table 10-3: Functional regions in the brain and spinal cord

Alar plate (afferent or sensory)	General somatic afferent	Input from the skin, joints, and muscles
	Special visceral afferent	Input from taste buds and pharynx
	General visceral afferent	Input from the viscera and heart
Basal plate (Efferent motor or autonomic)	General visceral efferent	Autonomic links from the intermediate horn to the viscera
	Special visceral efferent	Motor nerves to striated muscles of the branchial arches
	General somatic efferent	Motor nerves to the striated muscles other than those of the branchial arch nerves

nuclei. Yet other neuroblasts of the alar plates cluster into nuclei that are arranged in four columns at each side. From lateral to medial, these are: (1) **special somatic afferent**, receiving impulses from the inner ear; (2) **general somatic afferent**, receiving input from the surface of the head; (3) **special visceral afferent**, receiving input from the taste buds, and (4) **general visceral afferent**, receiving impulses from the viscera.

Metencephalon

The metencephalon represents the anterior portion of the rhombencephalon (Figs 10-17, 10-18). It develops into two main parts: the **pons**, a transverse structure demarcating the anterior end of the medulla oblongata, and the **cerebellum**, a phylogenetically newer and ontogenetically later developing structure, acting as a coordination centre for posture and movement. In mice it has been shown that the development of these structures depends on the expression of the gene *engrailed-1* in this area during early development.

The metencephalon, like the myelencephalon, is characterized by basal and alar plates, but with very different developmental fates. As in the anterior parts of the myelencephalon, the pontine flexure causes a divergence of the lateral walls and so the alar plates are, again, situated laterally to the basal plates instead of being arranged dorsoventrally.

Each basal plate of the metencephalon contains three groups of motor neurons: (1) the medial **general somatic efferent group**, which forms the nucleus of the abducens (VI) nerve; (2) the intermediate **special visceral efferent group**, which gives rise to the nuclei of the trigeminal (V) and facial (VII) nerves, innervating the musculature of the first and second pharyngeal arches; and (3) the lateral **general visceral efferent group** giving rise to the nucleus of the facial (VII) nerve, supplying the mandibular and sublingual glands. Some alar plate neurons migrate ventrally to form the **pontine nuclei**. Axons from neurons in the cerebral cortex terminate on pontine nuclei. Ventrally, the axons of these pontine neurons form a superficial band of nerve fibres known as the transverse fibres of the pons.

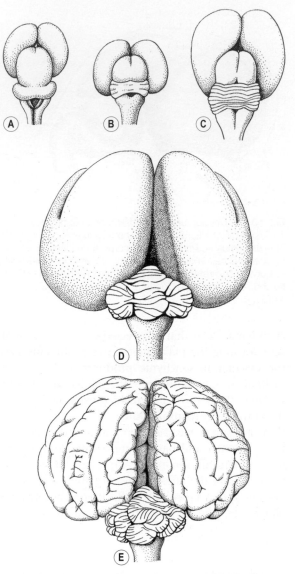

Fig. 10-17: Prenatal development of the bovine cerebrum and cerebellum. A: Day 60; B: Day 65; C: Day 80; D: Day 120; E: Day 180. Courtesy Sinowatz and Rüsse (2007).

The **cerebellum**, an alar plate derivative, is formed in the roof of the metencephalon and is structurally and functionally very complex (Fig. 10-17). It arose phylogenetically as a specialization of the vestibular system and acquired other important functions, (such as orchestration of general coordination, and involvement in auditory and

Fig. 10-18: Development of the bovine metencepahlon from Day 65 to Day 120 of gestation; median sections. **A:** Day 65. 1: Pons; 2: Medulla oblongata; 3: Vermis; 4: Fissura postculminata; 5: Fissura uvulonodularis; 6: Lobus flocculonodularis; 7: Choroid plexus of the IVth ventricle; 8: IVth ventricle. **B:** Day 80. 1: Pons; 2: Medulla oblongata; 3: Lobus rostralis; 4: Fissura postculminata; 5: Lobus caudalis; 6: Fissura postpyramidalis; 7: Fissura flocculonodularis; 8: Lobus flocculonodularis; 9: IVth ventricle; 10: Velum medullare rostrale; 11: Velum medullare caudale; 12: Choroid plexus. **C:** Day 120. 1: Pons; 2: Medulla oblongata; 3: Trigeminal ganglion; 3': Nucleus sensibilis pontinus n. trigemini; 3'': Nucleus tractus mesencephali; 3''': Nucleus tractus spinalis n. trigemini; 4: Velum medulare rostrale; 5: Velum medullare caudale; 6: Fissura postculminata; 7: Fissura postpyramidalis; 8: Pyramis, 9: Uvula; 10: Fissura uvulonodularis; 11: Lobus flocculonodularis. Courtesy Sinowatz and Rüsse (2007).

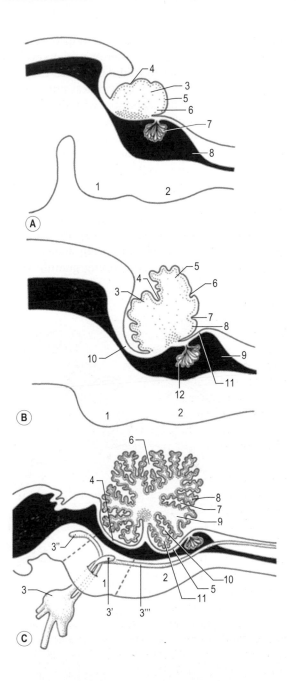

visual reflexes) later in evolution. Both the morphology of the cerebellum and the spatial arrangement of its neurons have been highly conserved during evolution. Developmental defects of the cerebellum cause abnormalities of locomotion and posture (see Chapter 19).

The primordia of the cerebellum are the **rhombic lips**, the dorsolateral regions of the alar plates of the metencephalon. In mice it has been shown that the rhombic lips extend between rhombomeres 1–8, but the cerebellum proper is only derived from the anterior rhombic lip (r1). The more posterior parts of the rhombic lips (r2–r8) give rise to migratory precursor cells that form a variety of ventrally located nuclei, including the olivary and pontine nuclei.

Viewed from above, the rhombic lips appear as V-shaped structures. Thus the rhombic lips are close together in their anterior region and further apart posteriorly, where they merge with the myelencephalon. Rostrally, the medial extensions of the rhombic lips are fused by an isthmus. As a result of a further deepening of the pontine flexure, the rhombic lips compress antero-posteriorly and form the cerebellar plate.

During the early fetal period, the developing cerebellum expands dorsally forming a dumb-bell structure with transverse fissure dividing it into a larger anterior and a smaller posterior portion. The medial part of the anterior region gives rise to the vermis, and the lateral areas develop into the **hemispheres** of the cerebellum. The anterior region grows considerably and later becomes the dominant component of the mature cerebellum. This enlargement is characterized by a marked folding of the surface, resulting in close, parallel, transverse folds – the **folia cerebelli**. The posterior portion evolves into the paired **flocculo-nodular lobes**. They are regarded as the phylogenetically oldest structures of the cerebellum and are associated with the development of the vestibular apparatus.

Initially, the cerebellar plate consists of neuroepithelial, intermediate, and marginal layers. During the early fetal period, cells from the neuroepithelium migrate through the intermediate and marginal layers to the surface of the cerebellum, where they are arranged into a second germinal layer, the **external granular layer** (Fig. 10-19). Cells of this layer are still able to divide mitotically and later give rise to various cell types, including **granule cells**,

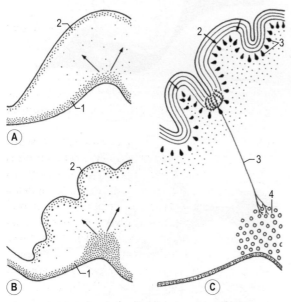

Fig. 10-19: Histological differentiation of the cerebellum (sagittal section). **A and B:** Neuroblasts migrate from the neuroepithelium (1) to the surface of the cerebellum and form an external granular layer (2). Cells of this layer retain their ability to divide and form a proliferative zone on the surface of the cerebellum. **C:** Later in development, the cells of the external granular layer give rise to various cell types which migrate inwards and pass the differentiating Purkinje cells (3). They give rise to the granule cells of the definitive cerebellar cortex. Basket and stellate cells are produced by proliferating cells in the cerebellar white matter. 4: Neurons of the nucleus dentatus. Courtesy Sinowatz and Rüsse (2007).

basket cells, and **stellate cells**. The granule cells are by far the largest population formed by the external granular layer.

The remaining cells of the neuroepithelial layer divide and form the **inner germinal layer**. Neuroblasts originating from the inner germinal layer migrate into the cerebellar hemisphere where they come to rest in three paired groups just above the ependyma of the fourth ventricle as precursors of the **cerebellar nuclei** (the nucleus dentatus, nucleus interpositus, and nucleus fastigii) which are responsible for relaying signals to and from the cerebellar cortex.

Cells from the inner germinal layer also migrate towards the external granular layer where they differentiate into **Purkinje cells**. The cell bodies of Purkinje cells become aligned in a single layer under the external granular layer. Each of these neurons develops a large, superficial dendritic arborization in a single plane transverse to the longitudinal axis of the folium. In bovine fetuses, the Purkinje cell layer is already well developed at Day 100 of gestation.

After their last mitotic division, the **external granule cells** become immature bipolar neurons, with their axons running in a plane parallel to the longitudinal axis of the folium. Concomitantly, the cell bodies of the external granule cells undergo a second and centrally oriented migration toward the interior of the future cerebellum. En route, these cells pass through the layer of precursors of the larger Purkinje cells and establish numerous synapses with them (Fig. 10-19). When they have passed the Purkinje cells they form a thick layer in the cerebellar cortex called the **granular layer**, which is thickest over the centre of each folium and thinner around the sulci between them. From each granule cell, a single axon runs superficially and bifurcates at the level of the Purkinje cell dendrites. These axons, called parallel fibres, traverse the folia cerebelli perpendicular to the plane of the Purkinje dendrite trees. Each Purkinje cell makes synaptic contact with several hundred thousand parallel fibres. The exact mechanisms controlling cell migration in the cerebellum are largely unknown, but it is established that a special type of glial cells (radial glial

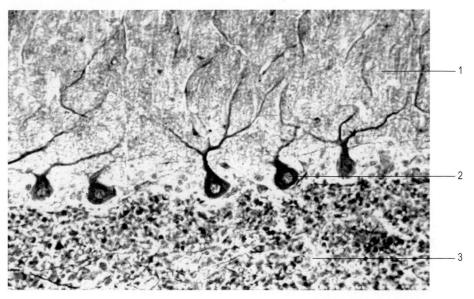

Fig. 10-20: Histological section through the differentiated cerebellar cortex of an adult dog. 1: Molecular layer; 2: Purkinje cell layer; 3: Granular layer.

cells) guide the radial migration of Purkinje cells. The inward migration of the external granule cells depletes the outer zone of the cerebellar cortex, which is then referred to as the **molecular layer**. Thus, in its final form the cerebellar cortex shows three clearly separated layers: an outer **molecular layer**, the **Purkinje cell layer** and an inner **granular layer** (Fig. 10-20).

How well the cerebellum is developed at birth is closely correlated with the age at which the animal is able to stand and walk. In carnivores, much of the differentiation of the cerebellar cortex occurs post-natally; kittens and puppies do not walk in a coordinated manner for about 3 weeks postnatally. At the time of birth, there is only some layering in the intermediate layer and some in the external germinal layer where cells are still actively dividing. The other layers are formed during the first two postnatal weeks, as the inward migration from the external germinal layer begins. The external germinal layer peaks in development at about 7 days and begins to be reduced in size by 14 days post-natally, as the definitive granule layer becomes established. Differentiation of the Purkinje cell layer in cats and dogs is completed in the vermis by the end of Day 30 after birth and in the rest of the cerebellum at about 10 weeks.

In calves and foals (precocial and able to stand and walk within an hour of birth) the cerebellum is much more differentiated and functional at birth. In the bovine fetus the external germinal layer appears around Day 57 of gestation and reaches its maximal thickness at around Day 183. Although the external germinal layer is still recognizable at birth in these species, the three definitive layers of a mature cerebellum are already apparent. The external germinal layer is gradually depleted of cells over the first several months post-natally and eventually disappears. During this time, the functional capacity of the cerebellum matures, evidenced by the appearance of 'learned' reflexes (e.g. postural reflexes) and better coordinated locomotion.

Mesencephalon (midbrain)

The mesencephalon (midbrain) remains structurally relatively simple and the fundamental relationships between the basal and alar plates are essentially preserved. The part of the midbrain dorsal to the aqueduct becomes the **tectum** and forms the **corpora quadrigemina**, derived from the alar plates. Ventral to the aqueduct the basal plates form the **tegmentum** which contains the efferent nuclei of the oculomotor (III; general somatic efferent and general visceral efferent) and trochlear (IV; general somatic efferent) nerves. Their axons supply most of the extrinsic muscles that move the eyeball. A relatively small special visceral efferent nucleus, the Edinger-Westphal nucleus, innervates the pupillary sphincter muscle of the eye through the oculomotor nerve (III). It is still not clear whether the **red nuclei** and the **substantia nigra** are derived from the basal plate, or by migration of neurons from the alar plate.

Neurons from the intermediate layer of both basal and alar plates contribute to the **formatio reticularis**, an aggregation of nerve cells concentrated in nuclei around the aqueduct that extends from the myelencephalon to the diencephalon and is concerned with the state of consciousness of the animal.

The marginal layer, associated with each basal plate, enlarges considerably and forms the **crus cerebri**. The crura (cerebral peduncles) serve as pathways for axons descending from the cerebral cortex to lower centres in the metencephalon and spinal cord. These fibres are corticonuclear and corticospinal (pyramidal), respectively.

Neuroblasts from the alar plates migrate into the tectum, the roof of the mesencephalon, and form two prominent longitudinal bulges separated by a shallow midline depression. These elevations become separated by a transverse groove that divides each of them into a **rostral** and a **caudal colliculus**. The caudal colliculi are relatively simple in structure and have auditory functions. The rostral colliculi show a more complex layered architecture and are an integral part of the visual system. In lower vertebrates, the rostral colliculi act as primary integrative centres of visual inputs. In mammals neurons of the rostral colliculi send their axons to appropriate motor nuclei via tectobulbar and tectospinal tracts. The rostral colliculi are involved in subconscious eye movements. In higher mammals, the function of the rostral colliculi also depends on input from the visual cortex. Cortical damage produces apparent total blindness. In birds the optic lobe, the equivalent of the rostral colliculi, provides all visual functions. Connections between the rostral and caudal colliculi coordinate visual and auditory reflexes.

Prosencephalon (forebrain)

The prosencephalon is the most anterior of the three primitive brain vesicles. The anterior part of the forebrain, the **telencephalon**, forms the **cerebral hemispheres** and the **olfactory bulbs**. The posterior part, the **diencephalon**, gives rise to the **epithalamus including the epiphysis**, **thalamus**, **metathalamus** and **hypothalamus** as well as the **neurohypophysis** and **optic cups**. The cavity developing within the diencephalon is the **third ventricle**; cavities in the telencephalon form the **lateral ventricles**. All forebrain structures (telencephalon and diencephalon) are regarded as highly **modified derivatives of the alar and roof plates** without significant representation by basal plates. This is supported by the fact that the sulcus limitans, which separates alar and basal plates in the more posterior brain vesicles, does not extend anteriorly beyond the mesencephalon. Interestingly, molecular studies in the mouse have shown that sonic hedgehog (Shh), the ventral midline marker, is expressed in the ventral parts of the diencephalon, implying that a basal plate may exist, at least in this species.

Patterning of the prosencephalic region

Distinct patterns of gene expression strongly influence the basic regional organisation of the prosencephalon. Six so-called **prosomeres** extend from the prosencephalic-mesencephalic junction to the anterior tip of the prosencephalon. Prosomeres 1–3 (p1–p3, the most posterior), become incorporated into the diencephalon with p2 and p3 contributing significantly to the thalamus. P4 to p6 contribute to both diencephalic and telencephalic structures. The basal area of p4 to p6 develops into the major regions that integrate autonomic nervous functions and control hormone release from the pituitary. The alar plates of these domains develop into structures that include the cerebral cortex, basal ganglia, and optic vesicles.

As development advances, the p2 to p3 combination folds sharply posteriorly on top of p4 to p6. In humans, it has been shown that an enormous outgrowth of the alar plate of p4 to p6 forms the telencephalic vesicles, which envelop the other prosomeres and later form the cerebral cortex.

Diencephalon

Development of the diencephalon is characterized by the appearance of three pairs of swellings on the medial aspect of the lateral wall of the diencephalon (Fig. 10-21). They form a dorsal **epithalamic**, an intermediate **thalamic**, and a ventral **hypothalamic primordium** on each side. The largest pair of masses is represented by the developing **thalamus**, which is separated by a groove, the hypothalamic sulcus, from the ventrally located **hypothalamus** (Fig. 10-22). The hypothalamic masses, originally paired, later fuse to form a single structure that becomes a master regulatory centre. It differentiates into a number of nuclear areas controlling many basic homeostatic functions such as sleep, body temperature, hunger, fluid and electrolyte balance, emotional behaviour, and activity of the pituitary. Paired subthalamic nuclei, the **mamillary bodies**, can be seen as distinct protuberances on the midventral surface of the hypothalamus.

The highly proliferative thalamic primordia gradually project into the lumen of the diencephalon. In domestic animals this expansion is often so great that the thalamic regions from both sides fuse in the midline, forming the **interthalamic adhesion**, or massa intermedia. The central region of the vertically expanded neural canal of the diencephalon consequently becomes obliterated resulting in a **ring-shaped third ventricle** (Fig. 10-22). Ventral to the adhesion, the third ventricle forms a vertical slit between the walls of the developing hypothalamus extending ventrally into the stalk of the neurohypophysis. Dorsal to the interthalamic adhesion, the third ventricle is covered by the roof plate (reduced to a single layer of ependymal cells)

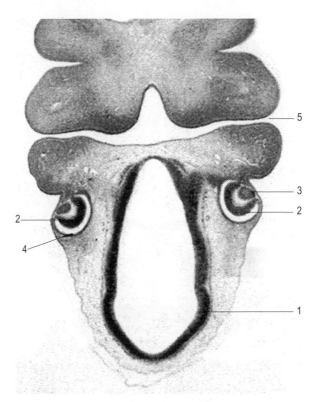

Fig. 10-21: Pig embryo, Day 21.5. 1: Diencephalon; 2: Retina; 3: Lens; 4: Pigment epithelium of the retina; 5: Stomodeum. Courtesy Sinowatz and Rüsse (2007).

covered by vascular mesenchyme. This combined layer forms the **choroid plexus** of the third ventricle and the lateral ventricles. In the thalamus, neural tracts from higher brain centres synapse with those of other regions of the brain and brainstem. Thus, the thalamus acts as an important centre for relaying sensory impulses (auditory, visual and tactile), along with signals from the basal ganglia and cerebellum, to the corresponding areas of the cerebral cortex.

On the dorsolateral aspect of the thalamic primordia, the **metathalamus** forms the lateral and medial geniculate bodies, structures that make connection with the rostral and caudal colliculi, respectively, to relay visual and auditory impulses.

Epiphysis (pineal gland). The most posterior portion of the roof plate of the diencephalon develops a small diverticulum. Within it, cellular

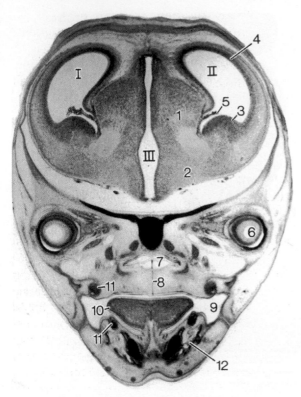

Fig. 10-22: Dog embryo, 35 mm CRL, coronal section. I and II: Lateral ventricles; III: Third ventricle. 1: Thalamus; 2: Hypothalamus; 3: Corpus striatum; 4: Cerebral hemispheres; 5: Choroid plexus; 6: Eye; 7: Cavum nasi; 8: Suture of the lateral palatine processes; 9: Cavum oris; 10: Tongue; 11: Dental cups; 12: Mandible. Courtesy Sinowatz and Rüsse (2007).

proliferation produces the **epiphysis** (including the **pineal gland**) as a cone-shaped structure. The cone remains attached to the roof of the diencephalon by the **habenulae**, two thin stalks of nerve fibres also containing some clusters of neurons (nuclei habenulares). The neuroepithelial cells differentiate into two types of cells, **pinealocytes** and **glial cells**. The pinealocytes develop cellular processes and release a hormone, melatonin, into the surrounding capillaries or into the cerebrospinal fluid of the third ventricle. The pineal gland is involved in the control of the circadian rhythm. In the absence of light, it produces melatonin which has antigonadotropic activity and inhibits the function of the pituitary-gonadal axis in some species, such as the mare, but

has an opposite effect in other species, such as the ewe (see Chapter 3). Production of melatonin by the pineal gland is under the influence of the supra-chiasmatic nucleus of the hypothalamus, which receives information from the retina about the daily pattern of light and darkness. Recent data in experimental animals suggest that it is mainly the supra-chiasmatic nucleus that controls the daily cycle; not the melatonin signal, as was once postulated.

Hypophysis (pituitary gland). The hypophysis develops from two quite separate parts: (1) an **ecto-dermal outpocketing** of the stomodeum immediatly in front of the buccopharnygeal membrane, known as **Rathke's pouch**, forming the **adenohypo-physis**, and (2) a **ventral downgrowth of the diencephalon, the infundibulum**, forming the **neurohypophysis**. When the stomodeum is first formed, the ectoderm of its dorsal aspect is close to the ventral neuroectoderm of the diencephalon (Fig. 10-23). At the site of apposition, the stomodeal ectoderm thickens and invaginates, forming **Rathke's (or the adenohypophyseal) pouch**. The distal end of this pouch grows towards the **infundibular primordium**, just dorsal and adjacent to Rathke's pouch. Once in intimate contact with the anterior edge of the forming infundibulum, the pouch flattens again while still attached to the stomodeal lining by an epithelial stalk. The connection is lost a few days later and the epithelium at the anterior edge of the pouch proliferates and begins to form cords and clumps of cells. Less proliferation is seen in the part of Rathke's pouch that is in contact with the developing neurohypophyis. The cellular proliferation at the rostral edge continues to a varying degree, depending on the species, and forms the adenohypophysis. The cells of the adenohypophysis surround those of the neurohypophysis to varying extents, very extensively in the pig.

Telencephalon

Development of the telencephalon is dominated by the tremendous expansion of the the **telecencephalic vesicles**, which will give rise to the two **cerebral hemispheres** that completely overgrow the anterior parts of the brain stem (Figs 10-17, 10-24).

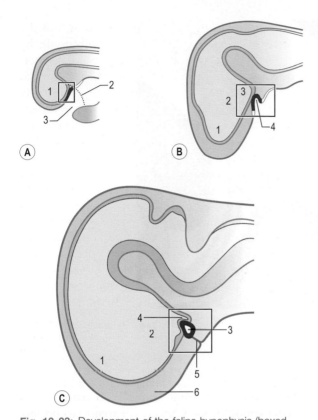

Fig. 10-23: Development of the feline hypophysis (boxed areas). A: 5 mm CRL. 1: Prosencephalon; 2: Buccopharyngeal membrane; 3: Stomodeum; B: 11 mm CRL. 1: Telencephalon; 2: Diencephalon; 3: Evagination of the infundibulum from the diencephalon: primordium of the neurohypophysis; 4: Rathke's pouch: primordium of the adenohypophysis. C: 14 mm CRL. 1: Telencephalon; 2: Diencephalon; 3: Adenohypophysis; 4: Neurohypophysis; 5: Craniopharyngeal canal; 6: Os sphenoidale.

The walls of the telencephalic vesicles surround the expanding **lateral ventricles**, which are outpocketings from the third ventricle, communicating with it via the **interventricular foramina**.

Although the cerebral hemispheres expand greatly during early pregnancy, their external surface remains smooth. Later, they undergo folding at several levels of organization and several major sulci and fissurae begin to appear. At the end of pregnancy, the surface of each hemisphere becomes folded and develops the species-specific **sulci** (grooves) and **gyri** (elevations) characteristic of the mature brain. The external pattern of sulci and gyri is produced by unequal growth of the cortex and its related white matter.

A multitude of internal cellular events determine how the telencephalon functions. Details are beyond the scope of this book and only general principles will be discussed here. Generally, the functional development of the telencephalon begins with an early regionalization followed by the generation and directed migration of neural precursors. The migration is radial and its pattern is established at very early stages of embryo development.

The **neuroblasts migrate from the ventricular layer**, where they are formed, **to the external surface** of the telencephalic vesicles. There are genetically predetermined loci in the ventricular layer of the neural tube that match particular areas on the surface of the hemispheres; neuroblasts originating at a given locus and developmental time will end up at defined points in the future cortex. This matching depends on special glial cells (radial glial cells) that extend from the ventricular layer of the neural tube to the corresponding area on the surface of the hemisphere; the migrating neuroblasts follow the glial processes to reach their specified destinations.

Besides the position within the neural tube, the time of migration strongly influences the placement of neurons in the cerebral cortex. In the mature cortex, the first neurons to organize on the surface will be found in the deepest layer. As more neurons leave the ventricular layer, they must migrate through layers of neurons already present. The last neurons to form are found in the most superficial layers of the cerebral cortex (**inside-out layering of the cerebral cortex**).

Once the neuronal cells have reached their final position, axonal processes (and, somewhat later, dendritic processes) grow out from them to specific target cells along tightly guided paths. The axons of the pyramidal cells, for instance, pass as long fibre bundles (the capsula interna) between the basal ganglia and run to the general somatic efferent cells of the spinal cord. On the ventral surface of the medulla oblongata, they are seen as the pyramids, which are the gross manifestation of the corticospinal tracts.

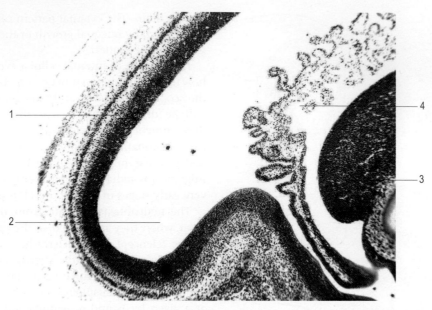

Fig. 10-24: Pig embryo, Day 21.5, sagittal section through the telencephalon. 1: Cerebral hemisphere; 2: Lateral ventricle; 3: Basal ganglia; 4: Choroid plexus.

Thus, the tangential position of a neuron in the cerebral cortex is determined by its origin in the ventricular layer and, in turn, the layer in which the cell is finally located is strongly influenced by the time at which it migrated. The genetically pre-determined neuronal migration pattern during the formation of the cerebral cortex probably contributes significantly to the development of **modular organized neuron columns** that comprise the functional and organizational unit of the cerebral cortex of the mature brain.

As the cerebral cortex develops, axons of its neurons synapse to other neurons in the following ways: (1) with neurons within the **same hemisphere**, (2) with neurons of the **other hemisphere**, and (3) with neurons of **other regions of the brain and spinal cord**. Neurons that synapse with neurons of the same hemisphere are called **association neurons**; their processes course between adjacent gyri (short association neurons) or more distant gyri (long association neurons). Neurons with axons that connect corresponding regions of the two hemispheres are classified as **commissural neurons**.

Those with axons that connect the cortex with deeper region of the CNS are referred to as **projection neurons**.

Based on its phylogenetic development, the cerebral cortex can be subdivided into the evolutionarily older **allocortex** and the newer **neocortex** (Fig. 10-25). The allocortex comprises the **archicortex** and the **palaeocortex**. The allocortex displays a wide variety of histological patterns in different regions, but is generally characterized by **three histological layers** (molecular, pyramidal or granular, and polymorphic layer). The neocortex, on the other hand, presents a more complex **five or six-layered histological structure**.

In carnivores, the major connections between the hemispheres are completed by the third postnatal week but full maturation is delayed until the sixth week or even later, when myelination of the major pathways has been completed. The general somatic efferent pathways and the pathways for proprioreception are the last to become myelinated. Gross anatomical and functional evidence for the postnatal maturation processes of the brain comes from a

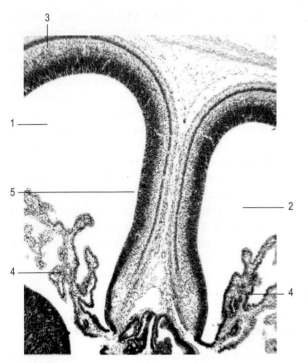

Fig. 10-25: Pig embryo, Day 21.5, coronal section through the telencephalon. 1: Right lateral ventricle; 2: Left lateral ventricle; 3: Neopallium; 4: Choroid plexus; 5 Archipallium.

rapid growth of the hemispheres, the increasing prominence of the gyri, and increasingly complex motor behaviour of the animal during the first six postnatal weeks. In the precocial species (ruminants and horses) the cortex has already reached functional maturity by the time of birth.

Archicortex (archipallium) (Fig. 10-25). The archicortex consists of the **genicular gyrus, supracallossal gyrus, parahippocampal gyrus**, as well as the **hippocampal gyrus** and **dentate gyrus**, which are collectively called the **hippocampal formation**. The primordium of the hippocampal formation appears early in development in the dorsomedial wall of the telecephalon, where a restricted area of the ventricular wall bulges into the ventricular lumen. The hippocampal formation then comes to lie external to the choroid fissure. Further development is delayed and the migrating phase of the neuroblasts does not start until late in the

embryonic period. During the fetal period, when the neocortex and the big commissure, the corpus callosum, develop, the hippocampal formation retreats posteriorly along the dorsomedial wall of the hemispheres. Only small remnants, the indusium griseum and the longitudinal striae, remain along the hippocampal sulcus. The hippocampus is displaced into the temporal lobe where it forms an eminence that projects dorsally into the inferior horn of the lateral ventricle. The efferent system of the hippocampus is the fornix, which curves over the thalamus to reach the mamillary bodies ventrally.

Palaeocortex (palaeopalleum). The palaeocortex is located on the medial and basal aspects of the hemispheres. It comprises the **olfactory bulbs, olfactory tracts, olfactory tubercle**, and **piriform lobe**. Outgrowths from rostral regions of the telencephalon form the olfactory bulbs. They receive axons from neurons in the olfactory mucosa which, with mitral cells of the olfactory bulb, form complicated synapses called olfactory glomeruli. The axons of the bulb neurons form the olfactory tract and synapse with neurons of the olfactory cortex of the cerebral hemisphere.

Neocortex (neopallium). The neocortex makes up most of the **cerebral cortex**. It is distinguished from the allocortex by having more nerve cells in six histological layers. During its formation, cells from the ventricular layer migrate superficially to form an intermediate layer and later an additional subventricular layer and the cortical plate. The cortical plate is established by migration of neuroblasts formed in the ventricular layer. Layers 2–6 of the mature neocortex are derived from the cortical plate. Although the layering of the cortex is completed during fetal development, the cerebral cortex does not become functional and morphologically mature until later. This is especially evident in carnivores, but is also true of ungulates and horses. Postnatal functional maturation involves the arrival of afferent fibres, myelination of important fibre tracts in the CNS and the completion of necessary intracortical synaptic connections.

Commissures. As the cerebral cortex develops, neuronal processes synapse with neurons within the same hemisphere, between the left and right hemispheres (commissures), and also between the hemisphere and other regions of the CNS. The first commissural fibres are found in the **anterior commissure** which consists of axons connecting the olfactory bulb and related brain areas of one hemisphere to those of the opposite side. The second commissure to develop is the **fornix** or **hippocampal commissure**. Its axons arise in the hippocampus and converge on the lamina terminalis. The fibres continue from there, forming an arching system outside the choroid fissure that runs to the mamillary body and the hypothalamus. The most important commissure in adult life is the **corpus callosum**, which connects the non-olfactory areas of the cortex of the right and left cerebral hemispheres and is essential for the coordination of activities between the two. Initially, axons of the corpus callosum form a small fibre bundle in the lamina terminalis. In association with the continous expansion of the neopallium, it extends both anteriorly and posteriorly, arching over the thin roof of the diencephalon. In ungulates, the corpus callosum is well developed at birth but in carnivores its development continues well into the first year of life. In addition to these three major commissures that originate in the lamina terminalis, there are other commissural fibre bundles. Two of them, the **posterior** and **habenular commissures** cross just below and rostral to the stalk of the pineal gland between the right and left hemispheres.

Basal nuclei. In addition to populating the cerebral cortex, neurons originating from the intermediate layer of the diencephalic and telencephalic vesicles form aggregations of cell bodies known as the basal ganglia. The base of each telencephalic vesicle thickens and forms a medial and lateral eminence. The smaller **medial eminence**, which is derived from the diencephalic vesicle, is involved in the fomation of the **amygdaloid body**. The **globus pallidus** has its origin from an adjacent area of the diencephalon. The larger **lateral eminence** is derived from the telencephalic vesicle and is concerned with the formation of the **caudate nucleus** and the **putamen**. The caudate nucleus, putamen and other basal nuclei collectively form the **corpus striatum**. The basal nuclei develop first

near the interventricular foramina but become elongated and C-shaped as the cerebral hemispheres grow posteriorly. The caudate nucleus in particular bulges into the rostral horn and central part of the lateral ventricle. It also courses into the temporal lobe and eventually lies on the roof of the inferior horn of the lateral ventricle. With the histodifferentiation of the cerebral cortex, many nerve fibres converge in the area of the **corpus striatum**, which becomes subdivided by the **internal capsule** into two major components: the **lentiform nucleus** ventrolaterally, consisting of the putamen and pallidum, and **claustrum**; and the **caudate nucleus** dorsomedially. These structures, which are components of the complex aggregation of nuclei also referred to as the basal ganglia, are involved in the unconscious control of muscle tone and complex body movements.

Ventricular system of the brain

In contrast to the narrow central canal of the spinal cord, the lumen of the neural tube expands in the developing brain region. As certain parts of the brain take shape, the lumen of the neural tube expands into well-defined ventricles, connected by thinner channels. Ventricles and channels are lined by the **ependymal epithelium**, derived from the neuroepithelial layer, and filled with clear cerebrospinal fluid.

Within each telencephalic vesicle a **lateral ventricle** develops (Figs 10-22, 10-24, 10-25). The central cavity of the telencephalon and of the diencephalon forms the **third ventricle**, which surrounds the interthalamic adhesion. The third ventricle is connected to each lateral ventricle through the **interventricular foramina**. Posteriorly, the third ventricle is connected via the narrow **mesencephalic aqueduct** to the **fourth ventricle**. The **tela choroidea**, from which the **choroid plexus** is suspended into the ventricular lumen, form from regions along the roof of the diencephalon, in the medial wall of each lateral vesicle, and in the roof of the third and fourth ventricle, which are composed of ependymal cells and vascular pia mater.

The primary function of the plexus is the production of **cerebrospinal fluid**, formed by filtration of blood plasma, active transport of certain plasma components and secretory activity of the ependymal cells. As it is formed, the cerebrospinal fluid flows from the lateral ventricles into the third and, ultimately, the fourth ventricle. Much of the fluid escapes through two or three small holes in the roof of the fourth ventricle (two **lateral apertures**, the **foramina Magendii**, and one **dorsal aperture**, the **foramen Luschkae**) and enters the subarachnoid space between the pia mater and the arachnoidea. This allows cerebrospinal fluid produced by the plexus to pass out of the lumen of the CNS and circulate within the meninges from where it is absorbed by veins.

Meninges

In the embryonic and early fetal period, two layers of mesenchyme surround the brain and spinal cord. These coverings develop into an outer **ectomeninx**, derived from the axial mesoderm, and a thinner **endomeninx**, considered to be a derivative of the neural crest cells. The ectomeninx forms the tough **dura mater**, composed of collagen and elastic fibres. The endomeninx later subdivides into a thin **pia mater**, which is closely apposed to the neural tissue, and a middle **arachnoidea**, a delicate non-vascular layer.

The dura mater and the arachnoidea are separated by a very thin, fluid-filled **subdural space**. In contrast to the dura mater of the spinal cord, the dura mater of the brain is composed of two distinct fibrous layers: the outer layer fuses with the periosteum of the developing bones of the cranium; the inner layer forms a large fold, the **falx cerebri**, which separates the cerebral hemispheres. Because the outer layer of the dura mater is fused with the periosteum of the cranial bones, **no epidural space is found in the cranium**. In the spinal cord, the space between the dura mater and the wall of the developing vertebral canal, the **epidural space**, contains fluid, loose connective tissue, blood vessels and adipose tissue, which gives support for the spinal cord and the roots of the spinal nerves.

PERIPHERAL NERVOUS SYSTEM

Classification of peripheral nerves

The peripheral nervous system (**PNS**), which develops from various sources, consists of the **cranial**, **spinal**, and **visceral nerves** and the **cranial** (Fig. 10-26), **spinal**, and **autonomic ganglia**. It comprises **efferent** (motor) nerve fibres that conduct impulses away from the CNS and **afferent** (sensory) fibres that conduct impulses towards the CNS. Nerves usually contain both kinds of fibres.

Efferent as well as afferent nerves of the PNS can also be classified as being **somatic** or **visceral** (Table 10-2). This subdivision is based on whether a peripheral nerve terminates in tissues derived from the splanchopleura (i.e. visceral tissue), or somatopleura (i.e. body wall tissue). Somatic afferent and general somatic efferent neurons innervate voluntary muscles and related connective tissue and structures in which epithelia derived from ectoderm are present (skin, mouth, and sense organs). The **general somatic efferent neurons** give rise to **general somatic efferent fibres** concerned with voluntary muscles derived from the somatopleura. The **somatic afferent neurons** can give rise to **special somatic afferent fibres** concerned with vision, hearing, and balance (only in the brain region), and **general somatic afferent fibres** concerned with the remaining somatic afferent impulses. The **visceral efferent neurons** control the movement of voluntary muscles derived from the pharyngeal arches, involuntary muscles and glands in the pulmonary and digestive tracts, and the cardiovascular system. **Visceral efferent neurons** give rise to **special visceral efferent fibres** concerned with the pharyngeal arch muscles (only in the brain region), and **general visceral efferent fibres** concerned with remaining functions. The visceral afferent neurons project from the same tissues as well as from the taste buds and olfactory mucosa. Again, the **visceral afferent neurons** can give rise to **special visceral afferent fibres** concerned with taste buds and olfactory mucosa (only in the brain region), and **general visceral afferent fibres** concerned with the remaining functions.

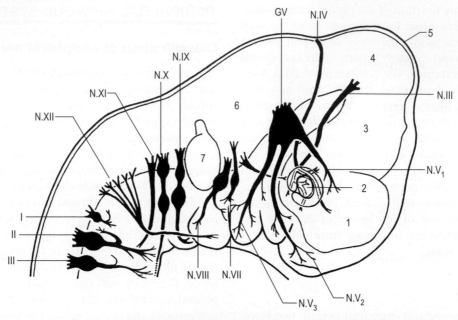

Fig. 10-26: Cranial nerves and their ganglia in a pig embryo of 12 mm CRL. 1: Telencephalon; 2: Optic cup with lens; 3: Diencephalon; 4: Mesencephalon; 5: Skin; 6: Rhombencephalon; 7: Otic vesicle. N. III: N. oculomotorius; N. IV: N. trochlearis; NV₁: N. ophthalmicus of the N. trigeminus; NV₂: N. maxillaris of the N. trigeminus; NV₃: N. mandibularis of the N. trigeminus; GV: Ganglion trigeminale; N. VII: N. facialis with ganglion geniculi; N. VIII: N. vestibulocochlearis; N. IX: N. glossopharyngeus with ganglion proximale and ganglion distale; N. X: N. vagus with ganglion proximale with ganglion distale; N. XI: N. accessorius; N. XII: N. hypoglossus. I–III: Cervical spinal ganglia. Courtesy Sinowatz and Rüsse (2007).

General somatic efferent and afferent system

Voluntary muscles in the body are derived from the paraxial mesoderm. The neurons that innervate these muscles are located in the **ventral horn** of the grey substance of the spinal cord or within discrete efferent (motor) nuclei in the brain stem. Their axons, which are referred to as carrying **general somatic efferent fibres**, project directly to the target muscles.

Somatic afferent neurons transmit information about physical and chemical stimuli impinging on an animal. The **general somatic afferent fibres** convey information of two types: **exteroreceptive fibres** convey information from different receptors in the skin, while the **proprioreceptive fibres** carry information from the muscle spindles of voluntary muscles and associated connective tissue (fascia and tendons) or ligaments and joint capsules. The latter provide the necessary information for the control of posture and movement.

In the head, somatic afferent fibres also include nerves associated with specialized receptors of the optic, vestibular and auditory systems, and such fibres are referred to as being **special somatic afferent fibres**.

In the trunk, the somata of both the afferent somatic and visceral (see later) neurons are located in **spinal ganglia** (Figs 10-27, 10-28) associated with the dorsal root of the spinal nerves. Afferent **cranial ganglia** are less regular in their location (Fig. 10-26). Most cranial ganglia are derived from thickenings of the lateral surface ectoderm referred

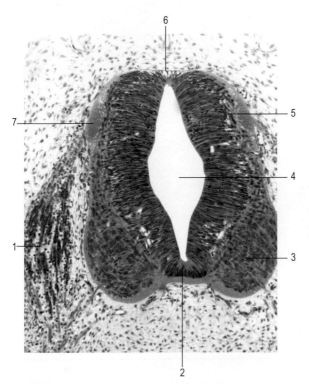

Fig. 10-27: Pig embryo, Day 21.5, cross section through the spinal cord. 1: Spinal ganglion; 2: Floor plate; 3: Basal plate; 4: Central canal; 5: Alar plate; 6: Roof plate; 7: Marginal zone. Courtesy Sinowatz and Rüsse (2007).

to as **neurogenic placodes**; the rest originate from neural crest cells. For example, the vestibular and cochlear ganglia are formed exclusively from cells that separate from the medioventral wall of the otic placode.

Neurons in the afferent ganglia are **initially bipolar**, with a peripheral and central process emerging from opposite sides of the soma. As the cells mature, these two projections approach and form a single convoluted stem that divides into a T-shape, making the cells **pseudo-unipolar neurons**. The centrally running process from neurons in the spinal ganglia enters the spinal cord via the dorsal root of a spinal nerve. Most of these axons synapse with neurons in the dorsal horn. The cell body of each afferent neuron is closely surrounded by glial cells, the **satellite cells**, which are also derived from the neural crest.

Spinal nerves

General somatic efferent (motor) nerve fibres appear in the developing spinal cord at the end of the third to fourth week of gestation, depending on the species. Axons grow out from nerve cells of the basal plate and assemble in bundles, the **ventral roots**. Nerve fibres originating from spinal ganglia, on the other hand, connect to form **dorsal roots** (Fig. 10-27). The central processes of the neurons in the dorsal root ganglia grow towards the dorsal horns of the spinal cord and establish synapses with sensory interneurons located in the area. Distal processes join the general somatic efferent ventral nerve root and form a **spinal nerve**. This common trunk of the spinal nerve splits almost immediately into a **dorsal** and **ventral ramus**. The dorsal rami of the spinal nerves innervate dorsal axial musculature, vertebral joints, and the skin of the back. Ventral rami innervate the limbs and ventral body wall and form the major nerve plexuses.

The major nerve plexuses (**cervical**, **brachial** and **lumbosacral plexuses**) are formed by secondary rami of the ventral rami, joined by connecting loops of nerve fibres. The developing plexuses supply the muscles and skin of the limbs. As the limbs develop, the nerves from the corresponding spinal cord segments grow into the mesenchyme, elongate, and form neuromuscular synapses with the developing muscle fibres. The dorsal divisions of these plexuses supply the extensor muscles and the extensor surface of the limbs; the ventral division supply the flexor muscles and flexor surfaces. The skin of the developing limbs is also innervated by segmental nerves fibres.

Origin of cranial nerves and their composition

Although they are arranged according to the same fundamental plan as the spinal nerves, the cranial nerves have lost the regular segmental arrangement and have become highly specialized. By convention, roman numerals are used to designate the cranial nerves, with cranial nerve I being the most rostral and cranial nerve XII the most caudal. The

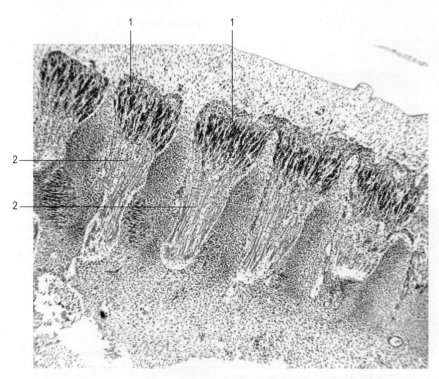

Fig. 10-28: Pig embryo, Day 21.5, sagittal section. 1: Spinal ganglion; 2: Spinal nerve. Courtesy Sinowatz and Rüsse (2007).

nomenclature of cranial nerves also uses the region or structure that they innervate; cranial nerve I, for example, is also called the olfactory nerve.

One of the major differences between cranial and spinal nerves is the tendency of many cranial nerves to be either afferent or efferent rather than mixed. Cranial nerves can be classified into three categories according to their embryonic origin and their future: (1) nerves with **special sensory function** (special somatic afferent or special visceral afferent fibres), (2) mixed nerves that innervate **pharyngeal arch derivatives** (special visceral efferent and afferent fibres), and (3) nerves with **exclusively general somatic efferent fibres.**

Cranial nerves I (olfactory) and **II (optic)** are often regarded more as extensions of brain tracts than as true nerves. Together with **cranial nerve VIII (vestibulocochlear)** they constitute the cranial nerves with special afferent functions. The facial nerve (VII) might also be considered a member of this group due to its special visceral afferent fibres

concerned with taste, but because the major task of this nerve relates to its branchial origin, it is classified according to that function. **Cranial nerves III (oculomotor), IV (trochlear), VI (abducent),** and **XII (hypoglossal)** are general somatic efferent nerves. **Cranial nerves V (trigeminal), VII (facial), IX (glossopharyngeal), X (vagus),** and **XI (accessory)** are classified as mixed nerves with both special visceral efferent and afferent components and each nerve supplies derivatives of a different pharyngeal arch. At the end of the first month of development, nuclei of all 12 cranial nerves are established. All of them, except the olfactory (I) and optic nerves (II), arise from the brain stem and only the oculomotor nerve (III) arises outside the region of the rhombencephalon.

In the rhombencephalon, proliferation centres in the neuroepithelium establish eight distinct segments, called **rhombomeres**. The establishment of this segmental pattern appears to be directed by mesoderm surrounding the neuroepithelium. The rhombomeres give rise to the efferent nuclei of cranial nerves IV, V, VI, VII, IX, X, XI and XII.

Whereas the efferent neurons of the cranial nerves are located within the brainstem, **sensory ganglia harbouring the afferent neurons are situated outside of the brain**. The sensory ganglia of cranial nerves originate from ectodermal placodes or neural crest cells. Ectodermal placodes include the **nasal, optic, otic** and four **epibranchial placodes**, represented by ectodermal thickenings dorsal to the pharyngeal arches (Table 10-4).

Cranial nerves with special sensory function

The group of special sensory nerves comprises the **olfactory (I)**, **optic (II)**, and **vestibulocochlear (VIII) nerves**.

The neurons of the **olfactory nerve (I)** develop from the nasal placode. Their unmyelinated axons are collected into a number (15 to 20) of smaller bundles around which the **cribriform plate** of the ethmoid bone is formed. These nerve fibres end in the **olfactory bulb**, where they form special synapses (olfactory glomeruli) with the mitral cells of the olfactory bulb.

The **optic nerve (II)** is formed by nerve fibres that are derived from ganglion cells of the primitive retina. Because the optic nerve develops from the evaginated wall of the diencephalon, it is usually considered as a fibre tract of the brain. The details of the development of the optic nerve are described in Chapter 11.

The **vestibulocochlear nerve (VIII)** comprises two kinds of sensory nerve fibres running in two bundles, the **vestibular** and the **cochlear nerves**. The vestibular nerve takes its origin from the bipolar neurons of the vestibular ganglion. The central processes of these cells terminate in the vestibular nuclei in the floor of the fourth ventricle. The cochlear nerve is formed by axons of the bipolar neurons of the spiral ganglion. Their dendrites innervate the organ of Corti (spiral organ), and their axons end in the ventral and dorsal cochlear nuclei in the medulla oblongata.

The nerves of the pharyngeal arches

The **cranial trigeminal (V)**, **facial (VII)**, **glossopharyngeal (IX)**, and **vagus (X)** nerves supply derivatives of the pharyngeal arches.

The **trigeminal nerve (V)** innervates the **first pharyngeal arch**. It is mainly general somatic afferent and is the principal afferent nerve of the head. Its large **trigeminal ganglion** is situated beside the rostral end of the pons and its neurons originate from the most anterior part of the neural crest. The centrally running processes from this ganglion form the large sensory root of the trigeminal nerve, which enters the lateral portion of the pons. The peripheral processes separate into three large divisions, the **ophthalmic, maxillary** and **mandibular** nerves. Their afferent fibres innervate the skin of the face as well as the mucosa of the mouth and nose. The efferent fibres of this cranial nerve arise from neurons in the most anterior part of the special visceral efferent column in the metencephalon and form the special visceral efferent nucleus of the trigeminal nerve, which lies at the midlevel of the pons. Its axons supply the muscles of mastication and other muscles that develop in the mandibular prominence of the first pharyngeal arch.

The **facial nerve (VII)** supplies derivatives of the **second pharyngeal arch**. The **special visceral efferent nuclei** are located in the special visceral efferent column in the caudal part of the pons. The efferent fibres of these neurons are distributed to the muscles of facial expression and to other muscles developing from the mesenchyme of the second arch. A small **general visceral efferent portion** (see later) of the facial nerve ends in the peripheral autonomic ganglia of the head. The geniculate ganglion provides the **special visceral afferent fibres** of the facial nerve. The peripheral processes pass to the greater superficial petrosal nerve and, via the chorda tympani, to the taste buds of the anterior two-thirds of the tongue. The central processes of the geniculate ganglion enter the pons.

The **glossopharyngeal nerve (IX)** innervates the **third pharyngeal arch**. It forms several rootlets which arise from the medulla oblongata, just caudal to the otic vesicle, the primordium of the inner ear.

Table 10-4: Cranial nerves

Cranial nerve	Origin	Distribution/Structures served	Functional role of components
Olfactory (I)	Olfactory placode, telencephalon	Olfactory region of the nose	Special visceral afferent (smell)
Optic (II)	Diencephalon	Retina of the eye	Special somatic afferent (vision)
Oculomotor (III)	Mesencephalon	Dorsal, ventral and medial rectus muscles, ventral oblique muscle, levator palpebrae muscle M. sphincter and dilator pupillae, m. ciliaris	General visceral efferent (parasympathetic, minor) General somatic efferent
Trochlear (IV)	Metencephalon	Superior oblique ocular muscle	General somatic efferent
Trigeminal (V)	Metencephalon	Derivatives of first branchial arch: Muscles of mastication	General somatic afferent Special visceral efferent
Abducens (VI)	Metencephalon	Lateral rectus, retractor bulbi muscles	General somatic efferent
Facialis (VII)	Metencephalic/ myelencephalic junction	Derivatives of second branchial arch: Muscles of facial expression, caudal belly of m. digastricus, m. stapedius Taste (rostral two-thirds of tongue) Mandibular and sublingual salivary glands; lacrymal glands Skin of auditory meatus	General visceral afferent Special visceral afferent (taste) Special visceral efferent General visceral efferent (parasympathetic)
Vestibulo-cochlear (VIII)	Metencephalic / myelencephalic junction	Inner ear	Special somatic afferent (hearing, balance)
Glossopharyngeal (IX)	Myelencephalon	Derivatives of third branchial arch: Stylopharyngeal muscle Taste (caudal third of tongue) Parotid, zygomatic glands in carnivores Carotid sinus, pharynx External ear	General visceral afferent Special visceral afferent (taste) Special visceral efferent General visceral efferent (parasympathetic)
Vagus (X)	Myelencephalon	Derivatives of fourth branchial arch: Constrictor muscles of pharynx Intrinsic muscles of larynx Caudal pharyngeal mucosa, mucosa of larynx Trachea, bronchi, heart, smooth muscles of digestive tract External auditory meatus	General visceral afferent Special visceral efferent General visceral efferent (parasympathetic)
Accessory (XI)	Myelencephalon, spinal cord	M. trapezius, M. sternocephalicus, M. brachiocephalicus	Special visceral efferent General somatic efferent
Hypoglossal (XII)	Myelencephalon	Tongue muscles	General somatic efferent

The **special visceral efferent fibres** arise from nuclei in the myelencephalon and innervate muscles of the third pharyngeal arch located in the region of the pharynx. The **general visceral efferent fibres** run to the otic ganglion. The postganglionic axons pass to the parotid gland and to the posterior lingual glands. **Special visceral afferent fibres** innervate the taste buds of the posterior part of the tongue.

The **vagus nerve (X)** results from the fusion of nerves of the **fourth to sixth pharyngeal arches**. Its large **general visceral efferent** and **general visceral afferent** components innervate the heart, the foregut and its derivatives, and a large part of the midgut. **Special visceral efferent fibres** originating from the fourth pharyngeal nerve (cranial laryngeal nerve) innervate the cricothyroid muscle, whereas analogous fibres from the sixth arch gives rise to the recurrent laryngeal nerve, which supplies the remaining intrinsic laryngeal muscles (see Chapter 12).

The cranial root of **the accessory nerve (IX)** is an extension of the vagus nerve. The spinal roots arise from the spinal cord (from the five or six most cranial cervical segments). The **special visceral efferent fibres** of the cranial root join the vagus nerve and supply the muscles of the soft palate and the intrinsic muscles of the larynx. The **general somatic efferent fibres** of the spinal roots innervate the sternocleidomastoideus and trapezius muscles.

The general somatic efferent cranial nerves

The **trochlear (IV)**, **abducens (VI)**, **hypoglossal (XII)**, and the greater part of the **oculomotor (III)** nerves can be considered to be homologous with the ventral roots of spinal nerves, i.e. being general somatic efferent. The corresponding neurons are located in general efferent (motor) nuclei of the brain stem. Their efferent axons supply the muscles derived from the preotic and occipital myotomes. The **oculomotor nerve (III)** supplies muscles of the eyeball that are derived from the first preotic myotomes (i.e. the dorsal, ventral, and medial recti, the ventral oblique, and medial portion of retractor muscles). The **trochlear nerve (IV)** is the only cranial nerve that leaves the brain stem dorsally and innervates the dorsal oblique muscle. The **abducens**

nerve (VI) arises from nuclei in the metencephalon. It supplies the lateral rectus and the lateral portion of the retractor muscle of the eye, both of which are derived from the most posterior of the three preotic myotomes.

Autonomic nervous system

The autonomic (involuntary) nervous system regulates many of the involuntary functions of the body (Fig. 10-29). It has a central regulatory role in the innervation of smooth muscle, cardiac muscle, exocrine, and several endocrine glands. Functionally, the efferent portion of the autonomic system nerves (the **general visceral efferent fibres**) can be divided into the **sympathetic nervous system**, originating from the **thoracolumbar region**, and the **parasympathetic nervous system**, originating from the **cranial** and **sacral regions**. While the axons of the general somatic efferent system project from cell bodies located within the CNS directly to their target muscles, the visceral efferent network involves at least two neurons: the cell body of the first, **preganglionic neuron**, is located in the CNS (in the lateral horn of the grey matter of the spinal cord or equivalent nuclei of the brain); the second, **postganglionic neuron**, is in a peripheral ganglion. All second neurons are derived from the neural crest and their axons are termed postganglionic axons. In the **parasympathetic system**, the first and second neurons utilize **acetylcholine** as the transmitter. In the sympathetic nervous system, on the other hand, the first and second neurons use different transmitters: preganglionic telodendria release acetylcholine whereas most **sympathetic second neurons release norepinephrine** at their distal terminals. The development of the second neurons proceeds in several steps. First, the migrating neural crest cells are committed to develop into an autonomic neuron. Second, biochemical markers and transmitters characteristic of a sympathetic or a parasympathetic neuron appear. These initial steps are followed by a maturation process that elevates these characteristics to adult levels.

The autonomic nervous system also includes the general visceral afferent neurons and interneurons

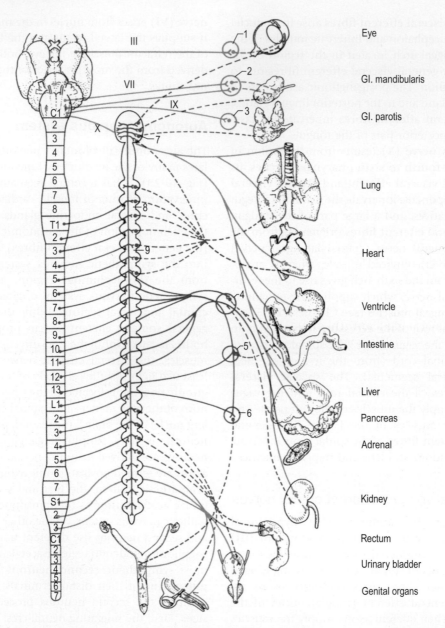

Fig. 10-29: Sympathetic (red) and parasympathetic (blue) nervous system. Continuous lines: preganglionic fibres; dotted lines: postganglionic fibres. III; N. oculomotorius; VII: N. facialis; IX: N. glossopharyngeus; X: N. vagus. I: Ganglion ciliare; 2: Ganglion mandibulare; 3: Ganglion oticum; 4: Ganglion coeliacum; 5: Ganglion mesentericum craniale; 6: Ganglion mesentericum caudale; 7: Ganglion cervicale craniale; 8: Ganglion cervicale medium; 9: Ganglion stellatum. Courtesy Sinowatz and Rüsse (2007).

in the brain and spinal cord. The peripheral component of the autonomic nervous system can be further subdivided into the **sympathetic, parasympathetic,** and **enteric system**.

Sympathetic nervous system

Towards the end of the embryonic period, cells originating in the neural crest of the thoracic regions migrate on each side of the spinal cord toward the region immediately dorsal to the aorta, where they form aggregations. Segmentally arranged **paravertebral (sympathetic) ganglia** develop from these aggregations, interconnected by longitudinal nerve fibres forming the **sympathetic trunk**. Although these ganglia are initially arranged segmentally, this arrangement is later partially lost by fusion of ganglia, especially in the cervical region: the first three cervical paravertebral ganglia fuse and form the **cranial cervical ganglion**. The **middle cervical ganglion** is formed by the aggregation of the fourth, fifth and sixth paravertebral ganglia, and the **caudal cervical ganglion** is derived by the fusion of the seventh and eight ganglia. The aggregation of the caudal cervical ganglia with the first two thoracic paravertebral ganglia gives rise to the **cervico-thoracic** or **stellate ganglion**.

Neural crest cells that migrate close to the branches of the aorta that supply the abdominal viscera form **preaortic ganglia**, such as the **coeliac ganglion** and the **cranial** and **caudal mesenteric ganglia**.

After the sympathetic trunks have formed, axons of sympathetic neurons, located in the lateral horn of the thoracolumbar segments of the spinal cord, pass via a ventral root of a spinal nerve and a white ramus communicans to a paravertebral ganglion. Since the visceral efferent column extends only from the first thoracic to the second or third lumbar segment of the spinal cord, white rami communicantes are found only at these levels.

The preganglionic fibres either synapse with neurons of the paravertebral ganglion or ascend or descend in the sympathetic trunk to synapse with neurons of paravertebral ganglia at other levels. Other preganglionic fibres bypass the paravertebral ganglia without synapsing and form the splanchnic nerves to the **preaortic ganglia**. Other fibres, the grey communicating rami, run from the sympathetic chain of ganglia to spinal nerves and from there to peripheral blood vessels, hair, and sweat glands. Grey communicating rami can be seen at all levels of the spinal cord.

The **postganglionic sympathetic fibres are relatively long** and typically release norepinephrine at their distal terminals

Parasympathetic nervous system

The preganglionic parasympathetic fibres arise from neurons in nuclei of the brain stem and from the sacral region of the spinal cord. Fibres from the cranial part of the parasympathetic nervous system travel via the **oculomotor (III), facial (VII), glossopharyngeal (IX),** and **vagus nerves (X)**. The postganglionic neurons are located in peripheral ganglia or plexuses near or within the organ being innervated (e.g. the pupil of the eye, salivary glands, or viscera).

Both the location and transmitters of the parasympathetic second neurons differ from those of the sympathetic neurons. The **second neurons of the parasympathetic component** of the autonomous nervous systems are located **in, or close to, the organ innervated and have short axons**. Most of them release **acetylcholine** at their synapses

The preganglionic neurons associated with the vagus nerve are derived from the ventricular layer of the neural tube in the medulla oblongata. They migrate into the intermediate layer of the neural tube and later form the parasympathetic nucleus of the vagus nerve.

Enteric nervous system

The wall of the gut has a large number of neurons (approximately 10^8 in large species). The neurons are often categorized as a special group. Since only several thousand fibres of the vagus nerve supply the gut, very few enteric neurons receive direct input from the CNS. Most of the neurons of the intestine project to one another. The enteric ganglia are also biochemically extremely heterogeneous: more than

the cerebral cortex is organized with the grey matter in layers outside the white matter. Based on its phylogenetic development, it can be subdivided into two different regions: the phylogenetically older **allocortex (archicortex and palaeocortex)** and the newer **neocortex**. The **allocortex** is the original part of the cerebral cortex and displays a wide variety of histological patterns in different regions, but is generally characterized by **three histological layers**: molecular, pyramidal or granular, and polymorphic layers. The **neocortex**, on the other hand, presents a more complex five- or **six-layered histological structure**.

In addition to populating the cerebral cortex, neurons originating from the intermediate layer of the diencephalic and telencephalic vesicles form aggregations of cell bodies known as the **basal ganglia**.

The **peripheral nervous system (PNS)**, which develops from various sources, consists of the **cranial**, **spinal**, and **visceral nerves** and the **cranial**, **spinal**, and **autonomic ganglia**. It comprises **efferent (motor) nerve fibres** that conduct impulses away from the CNS and **afferent (sensory) fibres** that conduct impulses towards the CNS. Spinal nerves contain both afferent and efferent fibres. The cranial nerves have lost their segmental patterns and have become highly specialized. Some are purely afferent, some are efferent, and still others are mixed, containing autonomic nerve fibres as well. The **autonomic nervous system** consists of two efferent components, the **sympathetic** and **parasympathetic nervous system**. Both components contain **preganglionic neurons**, derived from the CNS, and **postganglionic neurons**, of neural crest origin.

Box 10-1 Molecular regulation of the development of CNS and PNS

Molecular regulation of spinal cord development

As early as the neural plate stage, the presumptive spinal cord region expresses the homeobox-containing transcription factors **paired box gene 3 (Pax3)**, **Pax7**, **Msx1**, and **Msx2**. This expression pattern is modified by **Sonic hedgehog (Shh)**, a transcription factor originating from the notochord that is released even before the neural plate has folded to become the neural tube. This local Shh signalling stimulates the neural plate cells directly above the notochord to transform into the floor plate and basal plate whereupon the floor plate starts to express Shh.

Within the basal plate, efferent neurons (alpha-motor neurons and gamma-motor neurons) and interneurons become arranged in a well-defined dorso-ventral pattern. These different types of neurons are specified by a characteristic combination of homeodomain transcription factors, with a pattern of expression determined by the gradient of Shh emanating from the floor plate. As a result, a specific combination of transcription factors at each level of the developing spinal cord

determines each of the different types of neurons which, in turn, show their own molecular signature. For instance, general somatic efferent neurons are specified by the expression of *islet-1* that can be regarded as the earliest marker of developing motor neurons.

Shortly after the production of efferent neurons has ceased in the basal plate, a shift in regulatory factors stimulates the production of glial precursor cells from the ventral neuroepithelium.

The **Bone morphogenetic proteins 4** and **7 (BMP4** and **BMP7)**, expressed in the surface ectodermal cells at the lateral border of the neural plate, maintain and upregulate **Pax4** and **Pax7** in the dorsal half of the neural tube. These dorsalizing inductive effects cause the formation of roof and alar plates. After closure of the neural tube, the BMPs influence the formation of sensory interneurons in the alar plate of the later spinal cord.

Ventral to the central canal, neuronal processes cross from one side of the spinal cord to the other through the floor plate as commissural axons. These nerve fibres originate from neurons in the dorsal half of the neural tube. They are attracted to the floor plate by specific molecules, for example **netrin 1**.

Molecular regulation of mesencephalic and rhombencephalic development

Different brain regions respond to different signals and this helps specify regional differences. Furthermore, expression patterns of genes regulating the dorsoventral and anterior-posterior patterning of the brain overlap and interact at the borders of these regions.

The **mesencephalon** (midbrain) and **metencephalon** (hindbrain) are specified by the **isthmic organizer,** a signalling centre at the border between the mesencephalon and metencephalon. The principal signalling molecule is **FGF8** which is expressed in a narrow ring-shaped area at the anterior border of the first rhombomere. In cooperation with **Wnt1**, FGF8 induces the expression of engrailed genes *En-1* and *En-2*, two homeobox-containing genes, as well as *Pax2* and *Pax5*. The expression of these genes decreases with increasing distance from the FGF8-signalling centre. *En-1* regulates development throughout its expression domain, including the dorsal mesencephalon (tectum) and anterior rhombencephalon (cerebellum). *En-2* acts only in the development of the cerebellum.

The **mesencephalon** is highly patterned along its dorso-ventral axis. As in all other regions of the CNS, ventral patterning is controlled by **Shh**. Besides promoting neuronal development in the basal plate of the mesencephalon, Shh inhibits the ventral expression of molecules, such as **Pax7**, that are characteristic of the alar plates. Anteriorly, the mesencephalon becomes separated from the diencephalon through a distinct set of molecular interactions: the diencephalon is characterized by the expression of *Pax6*, whereas the mesencephalon is a domain of *En-1* expression. Mediated by the action of several negative regulators, Pax6 inhibits *En-1* expression, whereas **En-2** directly inhibits *Pax6* expression, leading to a sharp diencephalic-mesencephalic border.

The **rhombencephalon** consists of eight segments (rhombomeres) that show a variable expression of a cluster of **Hox genes**. Genes at the most 3'end of a cluster have more anterior boundaries and are also expressed earlier than those at the 5'end. These genes, which are expressed in overlapping spatio-temporal patterns, confer positional information along the antero-posterior axis of the hindbrain, determine the identity of the rhombomeres, and specify their derivatives. Many details of Hox-gene expression are still unclear, but **retinoic acid** may play a critical role because retinoic acid deficiency results in a small hindbrain.

The **cerebellum**, like the cerebrum, includes a nuclear structure and an overlying cortical structure. The initial molecular steps in cerebellar development depend on inductive signalling involving **FGF** and **Wnt** proteins produced at the mesencephalic/metencephalic boundary. Interlocking codes of transcription factors (mammalian homologues of LIM homeodomain-containing proteins, basic helix-loop-helix proteins, and three-amino-acid-loop-containing proteins) define precursors of the cerebellar nuclei, and both Purkinje cells and granule neurons of the cerebellar cortex.

Molecular regulation of prosencephalic development

Specification of the prosencephalon and mesencephalon is also regulated by genes containing a homeodomain. At the neural plate stage, *LIM1* is expressed in the prechordal plate, and *OTX2* in the neural plate. Both genes are important for designating the prosencephalic and mesencephalic areas. With the appearance of neural folds and pharyngeal arches, additional homeobox genes are expressed in patterns that specify the later prosencephalic and mesencephalic regions.

After the establishment of these boundaries, the **anterior neural ridge (ANR)** becomes an important organizing centre at the anterior junction between the neural plate and surface ectoderm. Cells of the ANR secrete **FGF8**, a key signalling molecule that induces subsequent gene expression important for further differentiation. FGF8-induced expression of **brain factor 1 (BF1)** then regulates the development of the cerebral hemispheres and regional specification within the prosencephalon,

Continued

including the basal telencephalon and retina. Dorsoventral and mediolateral patterning also occurs in the prosencephalic areas. Ventral patterning is controlled, as in all other parts of the central nervous system, by expression of **Shh** which is secreted by the prechordal plate and induces the expression of **Nkx2.1**, a homeodomain-containing gene product that regulates the development of the hypothalamus.

FURTHER READING

Abematsu, M., Kagawa, T., Fukuda, S., Inoue, T., Takebayashi, H., Komiya, S., and Taga, T. (2006): Basic fibroblast growth factor endows dorsal telencephalic neural progenitors with the ability to differentiate into oligodendrocytes but not gamma-aminobutyric acidergic neurons. J. Neurosci. Res. 83:731–743.

Aboitiz, F. (2001): The origin of isocortical development. Trends Neurosci. 24:202–203.

Agawala, S., Sanders, T.A. and Ragsdale, C.W. (2001): Sonic hedgehog control of size and shape in midbrain pattern formation. Science 291:2147–2150.

Andersen, B. and Rosenfeld, M.G. (1994): Pit-1 determines cell types during development of the anterior pituitary gland. A model for transcriptional regulation of cell phenotypes in mammalian organogenesis. J. Biol. Chem. 25:29335–29338

Armstrong, C.L. and Hawkes, R. (2000): Pattern formation in the cerebellar cortex. Biochem. Cell Biol. 78: 551–562.

Barlow, R.M. (1969): The foetal sheep: morphogenesis of the nervous system and histochemical aspects. J. Comp. Neurol. 135:249–262.

Briscoe, J. and Ericson, J. (2001): Specification of neuronal fates in the ventral neural tube. Curr. Opin. Neurobiol. 11:43–49.

Carpenter E.M. (2002): Hox genes and spinal cord development. Dev. Neurosci. 24:24–34.

Cecchi, C., Mallamaci, A. and Boncinelli, E. (2000): Otx and Emx homeobox genes in brain development. Int. J. Dev. Biol. 44:663–668.

Colello, R.J. and Pott, U. (1997): Signals that initiate myelination in the developing mammalian nervous system. Mol. Neurobiol. 15:83–100.

Fox, M.W. (1963): Gross structure and development of the canine brain. Am. J. Vet. Res. 24:1240–1247.

Gershon, M. (1997): Genes and lineages in the formation of the enteric nervous system. Curr. Opin. Neurobiol. 7:101–109.

Götz, M. and Huttner, W.B. (2005): The cell biology of neurogenesis. Nat. Rev. Mol. Cell Biol. 6:777–788.

Houston, M.L. (1968): The early brain development of the dog. J. Comp. Neurol. 134: 371–384.

Jastrebski, M. (1973): Zur Entwicklung der Markscheiden der Gehirnnerven im Markhirn des Rindes. Zbl. Vet. Med. C 2:221–228.

Kirk, G.R. and Breazile, J.E. (1972): Maturation of the corticospinal tract in the dog. Exp. Neurol. 35:394–397.

Lange, W. (1978): The myelinisation of the cerebellar cortex in the cat. Cell Tiss. Res. 188:509–520.

LeDouarin, N. and Smith, J. (1988): Development of the peripheral nervous system from the neural crest. Annu. Rev. Cell Biol. 4:375–381.

Louw, G.J. (1989): The development of sulci and gyri of the bovine cerebral hemispheres. Anat. Histol. Embryol. 18:246–264.

Lumsden, A., and Krumlauf, R. (1996): Patterning of the vertebrate neuraxis. Science 274:1109–1115.

Marquardt, T. and Pfaff, S.L. (2001): Cracking the transcriptional code for cell specification in the neural tube. Cell 106:1–4.

Noden, D.M. (1993): Spatial integration among cells forming the cranial peripheral nervous system. J. Neurobiol. 24:248–261.

Noden, D.M. and DeLahunta, A. (1985): Central nervous system and eye. In: Embryology of Domestic Animals, Developmental Mechanisms and Malformations. Williams and Wilkins, Baltimore, MD, p 92–119.

Patten, I. and Placzek, M. (2000): The role of sonic hedgehog in neural tube patterning. Cell Mol. Life Sci. 57:1695–1708.

Rakic, P. (1988): Specification of cerebral cortical areas. Science 241:170–176.

Rüsse, I. and Sinowatz, F. (1998): Lehrbuch der Embryologie der Haustiere, 2nd edn. Parey Buchverlag, Berlin.

Scully, M.C., and Rosenfeld, G. (2002): Pituitary development: regulatory codes in mammalian organogenesis. Science 295:2231–2235

Sinowatz, F. (1998): Nervensystem. In: Lehrbuch der Embryologie der Haustiere. Rüsse I. and Sinowatz, F., Verlag Paul Parey, Berlin und Hamburg, 2nd edn, p 247–286.

Tessier-Lavigne, M. and Goodman, C.S. (1996): The molecular biology of axon guidance. Science 274:1123–1133.

Wingate, R.J.T. (2001): The rhombic lip and early cerebellar development. Curr. Opin. Neurobiol. 11:82–88.

CHAPTER 11

Fred Sinowatz

Eye and ear

DEVELOPMENT OF THE EYE

The eye is an organ of remarkable complexity and apparently flawless design. Eyes develop from three sources: (1) the **neuroectoderm** of the forebrain, (2) the **surface ectoderm** of the head, and (3) head **mesenchyme** of neural crest origin between these layers. Ectodermal outgrowth from the brain gives rise to the **retina**, **iris** and **optic nerve**, the surface ectoderm forms the **lens**, and the surrounding mesenchyme forms the **vascular** and **fibrous coats** of the eye.

Optic cup and lens vesicle

The area of the neural plate that gives rise to the eyes is initially a single medial region, the **optic field**, near the anterior margin of the future prosencephalon. Interactions of the neuroectoderm of the optic field with underlying mesoderm lead to a separation of the single optic field into **lateral eye-forming regions**. At the end of the third week of gestation in most species, shallow grooves are formed on the sides of the forebrain. With closure of the neural tube, these grooves expand as outpockets of the prosencephalon – the **optic vesicles** (Figs 11-1, 11-2). The optic vesicles remain attached to the prosencephalon by the optic stalk. It has been shown in the mouse that the transcription factor Rx is expressed very early in the optic field. In its absence, the optic vesicles fail to form.

Each optic vesicle grows laterally until it comes into contact with the surface ectoderm, where it induces a circumscribed thickening of the ectoderm,

the **lens placode**. This placode subsequently invaginates and forms a **lens vesicle**, which loses its contact with the surface ectoderm. As the lens vesicles develop, the optic vesicles invaginate and become double-walled structures, the **optic cups** (Figs 11-1, 11-3). The inner and outer layers of the optic cups are at first separated by a lumen, the **intraretinal space**, but it soon disappears, and the two layers appose each other. The inner layer of the optic cup later develops into the **neural retina** with its three layers of neurons that function in visual perception. The outer layer of the optic cup becomes the **pigmented layer** of the retina (Figs 11-4, 11-5). The optic stalk connects the optic cup with the prosencephalon and, later, the diencephalon; the stalk serves to guide the growth of neuronal axons from the retinal ganglion layer back to the developing brain.

Retina

The retina develops from the optic cups. The outer, thinner, layer, characterized in most species by cells containing small pigment granules, becomes the **pigmented layer** of the retina. The inner layer of the optic cup thickens, and the epithelial cells begin a complicated process of differentiation into neurons and light receptor cells of the multilayered **neural retina** (Figs 11-6, 11-7). The outer lips of the optic cup undergo a quite different transformation. They give rise to the **iris** and **ciliary body**, which control the amounts of light that reach the retina and the curvature of the lens, respectively.

In the adult, the neural retina is a multilayered structure. The sensory pathway of the retina consists

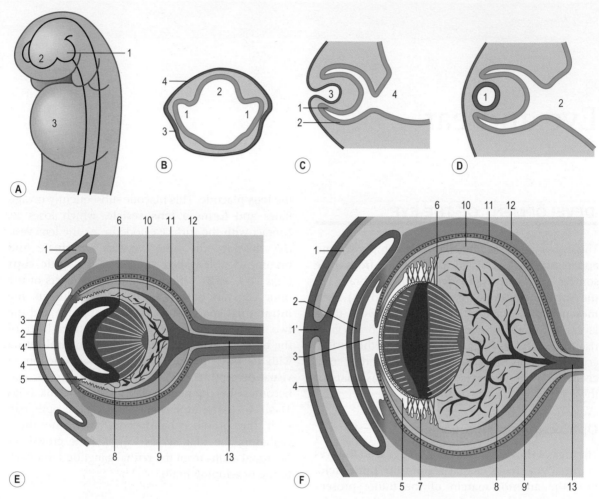

Fig. 11-1: Development of the eye. A: Evagination of the optic vesicles (1) from the prosencephalon (2); 3: Heart. B: Cross section through the optic vesicles (1) and the prosencephalon (2); 3: lens placode; 4: Ectoderm. As a result of the contact of the optic vesicles with the surface ectoderm, the ectoderm thickens and forms the lens placode. C: Longitudinal sections through the developing eye, showing the invagination of the lens placode (3). 1: Inner layer of the optic cup; 2: outer layer of the optic cup; 4: Diencephalon. D: The lens vesicle (1) loses contact with the surface ectoderm and lies in the mouth of the optic cup. 2: Diencephalon. E and F: Differentiation of the eye-ball. 1: Eyelid; 1': Suture of the fused eyelids; 2: Cornea; 3: Anterior chamber of the eye; 4: Iris; 4': Pupillary membrane; 5: Posterior chamber of the eye; 6: Lens; 7: Ciliary body with zonular fibres; 8: Vitreous body; 9: Hyaloid artery; 9': Central retinal artery; 10: Neural layer of the retina; 11: Pigment layer of the retina; 12: Choroid and sclera; 13: N. opticus. Courtesy Sinowatz and Rüsse (2007).

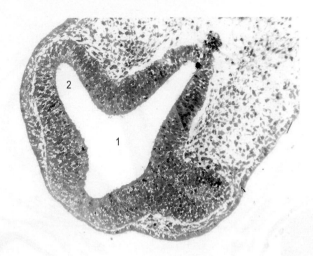

Fig. 11-2: Optic vesicles evaginating from the prosencephalon. Pig embryo of 6 mm CRL. 1: Prosencephalon; 2: Optic vesicle.

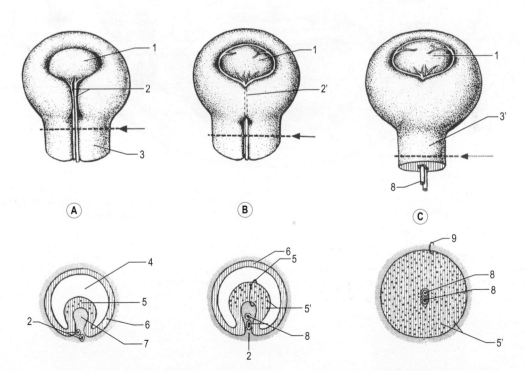

Fig. 11-3: Transformation of the optic stalk into the optic nerve. Upper series: Ventral view of the optic cup and optic stalk at progressive stages of development. Lower series: Cross sections of the optic stalk at different levels (A, B, C). 1: Lens; 2: Choroid fissure; 2': Closed choroid fissure; 3: Optic stalk; 3': N. opticus; 4: Lumen of optic vesicle; 5: Inner layer of the optic stalk; 5': Axons of the N. opticus; 6: Outer layer of the optic stalk; 7: Mesenchyme; 8: Central retinal artery and vein; 9: Pia and arachnoid layer of the nerve. Courtesy Sinowatz and Rüsse (2007).

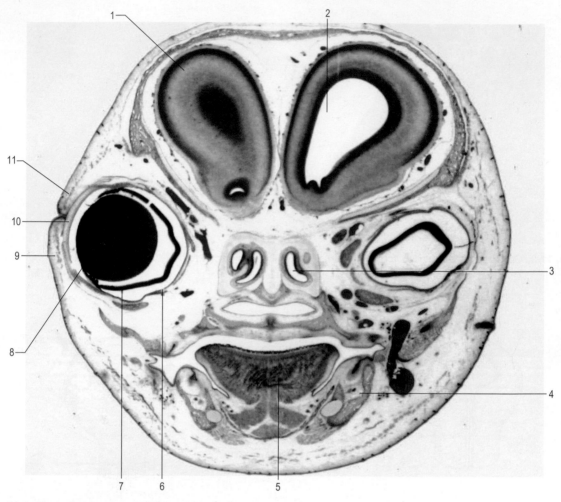

Fig. 11-4: Transverse section of a 45 mm feline fetus. 1: Telencephalon; 2: Lateral ventricle; 3: Nasal cavity; 4: Mandible; 5: Tongue; 6: Pigment epithelium of the retina; 7: Nervous layer of the retina; 8: Lens; 9: Lower eyelid; 10: Cornea; 11: Upper eyelid.

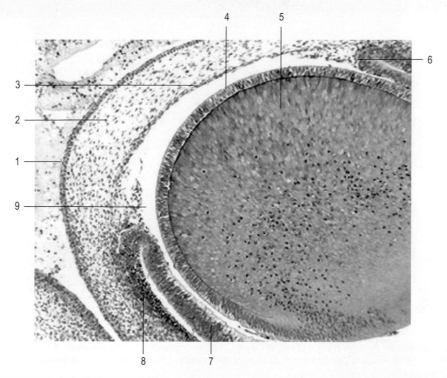

Fig. 11-5: Section through the anterior part of the eye of a 17 mm feline embryo. 1: Anterior corneal epithelium; 2: Corneal stroma; 3: Posterior corneal epithelium; 4: Anterior lens epithelium; 5: Lens fibres; 6: Margin of iris; 7: Neural (sensory) layer of the retina; 8: Pigment layer of the retina; 9: Anterior chamber.

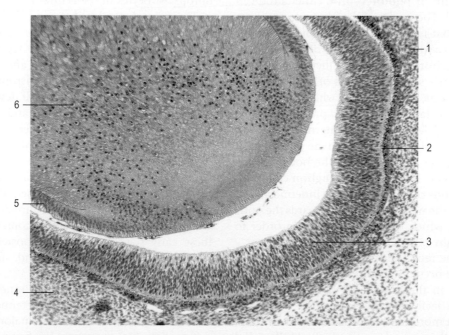

Fig. 11-6: Section through the posterior part of the eye of a 17 mm feline embryo. 1: Mesenchyme of the choroidea; 2: Pigment layer of the retina; 3. Neural layer of the retina; 4: Undifferentiated mesenchyme, which later forms the sclera; 5: Lens epithelium; 6: Lens fibres.

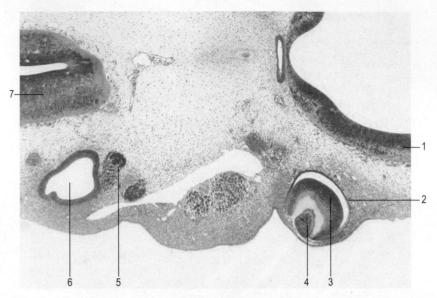

Fig. 11-7: Horizontal section through a pig embryo at Day 21. 1: Diencephalon; 2: Pigment layer of the retina; 3: Neural (sensory) layer of the retina; 4: Lens primordium; 5: Statoacoustic ganglion; 6: Otic vesicle; 7: Metencephalon. Courtesy Sinowatz and Rüsse (2007).

of a **chain of three neurons**. The first link in the chain is a **light- or photoreceptor**, either a rod cell or a cone cell. The nuclei of the photoreceptors are located in what is referred to as the **outer nuclear layer**. The rod and cone cells send processes towards the **outer plexiform layer**, where they synapse with processes of the second neurons of the chain, the **bipolar neurons**, the nuclei of which occupy the **inner nuclear layer**. The other process of each bipolar neuron leads into the **internal plexiform layer** and establishes synapses with the third neuron in the chain, the **ganglion cell**. The bodies of the ganglion cells are located in the **ganglion cell layer**. Their long axons course through the innermost layer of the retina, the **nerve fibre layer**, towards the optic disc through which they leave the eye in order to reach the brain as the optic nerve (II).

Even in the retina, many levels of integration of visual signals occur: **horizontal** and **amacrine cells** are involved in the horizontal distribution of the signals. This facilitates the integration of simple signals into a more complex visual pattern. Another important cell type in the retina is the **Müller glial cell**; these cells provide mechanical support and

nutrition to the retina, a role analogous to that of fibrous astrocytes in the central nervous system.

The normal development and differentiation of the neural retina depends upon its close contact and interaction with the pigmented layer, as well as interactions between the neural and the glial elements within the neural layers. Disruptions of these contacts result in abnormal retinal development. In ungulates, retinal differentiation and maturation is essentially completed at birth whereas in carnivores they continue for up to 5 weeks after birth.

In the originally single-layered columnar inner layer of the optic cup many mitoses occur, transforming the primordium of the neural retina into a thickened pseudostratified columnar epithelium. The **polarity of the retina** also becomes fixed during these early stages; the anterior-posterior axis first then the dorso-ventral axis and, finally, radial polarity.

As the number of cells in the inner layer of the early retina increases, the differentiation of the neurons begins. There are two major gradients of differentiation of the retina: the first proceeds more or less **vertically from the inner to the outer layers**;

the second is more **horizontal, from the centre towards the periphery**. Differentiation in the horizontal gradient starts with the appearance of ganglion cells. As the ganglion cell layer is established, premature differentiation of neighbouring neural precursor cells is prevented by expression of the *Notch* gene. The protein coded by *Notch* keeps these cells in an undifferentiated state that will be overcome later by differentiation signals from the neighbourhood of the neuroblasts. Differentiation of amacrine and horizontal cells completes the differentiation of the inner and outer nuclear layers of the retina. These neurons send out processes that contribute to the definition of the inner and outer plexiform layers. The last retinal cells to differentiate are the bipolar neurons and receptor cells – the rod and cone cells.

Optic axon guidance

At a later stage of retinal differentiation, axons from the ganglion cells grow along the innermost layer of the retina towards and into the optic stalk, following molecular cues. The **optic stalk** connects the retina with the diencephalon (Fig. 11-3). On its ventral surface the stalk has a groove, the **choroid fissure**, that contains the hyaloid vessels. The optic stalk also serves as a guide directing axons from the ganglion cells of the retina back into the developing brain.

Later, the choroid fissure closes and a narrow tunnel is formed inside the optic stalk. The number of outgrowing nerve fibres in the inner wall of the stalk increases continuously and eventually the inside and outside walls of the stalk fuse, transforming the optic stalk into the **optic nerve** carrying the **central artery of the retina**, a portion of the hyaloid artery. Myelinization of the optic nerve fibres is incomplete at birth and continues postnatally.

During the phase of axonal outgrowth from the retina, a precise **retinal map** is maintained in the organization of the optic nerve and passed on to the visual centres of the brain. The formation of a retino-optic map involves the establishment of an initial, very coarse map that subsequently undergoes large-scale remodelling to generate a refined map.

Attachment of the retina

The cleft between the inner and outer layer of the optic cup is never completely obliterated, even into adulthood, and so **no firm attachment between the pigment epithelium and the nervous epithelium** of the retina is established. The major factor keeping the two layers in contact is the maintenance of normal intraocular pressure, a major function of the aqueous humour and vitreous body.

Iris and ciliary body

Differentiation of the **iris** and **ciliary body** occurs at the lip of the optic cup, where the neural and pigment layers of the retina meet. The iris develops by the peripheral extensions of both layers of the optic cup so that they cover the edges of the lens vesicle. This brings the lens vesicle entirely inside the boundary of the optic cup (Fig. 11-1). Thus the iris consists of an **inner non-pigmented epithelial layer** and an **outer pigmented layer**, which are continuous with the neural and pigmented layers of the retina, respectively. The stroma of the iris is of neural crest origin and migrates into the iris separately. The muscles of the iris, the **sphincter pupillae** and **dilator pupillae** are, interestingly, of **neuroectodermal origin**; they result from a transformation of the anterior epithelial layers of the iris into smooth muscle cells. The levels and distribution of pigmentation in the iris determine eye colour. The bluish colour of the iris seen in most newborn animals is caused by the pigmentation of the outer pigmented layer of the iris. Pigment cells, however, also appear in the stroma of the iris; the greater the density of pigment cells in the stroma, the browner is the eye colour. Definitive pigmentation of the eye develops during the first months of postnatal life.

The **ciliary body**, containing the **ciliary muscle**, takes shape between the iris and the neural retina. The neural-crest-derived ectomesenchyme of this area proliferates unevenly and forms a series of ridges (**processus ciliaris**) that are covered by a two-layered epithelium (Fig. 11-1). The pigmented epithelium of the ciliary body is derived from the outer layer of the optic cup and is continuous with the retinal pigmented layer. The inner epithelial layer is continuous with the neural layer of the retina posteriorly and the epithelium of the iris anteriorly. This inner epithelium later becomes the source of aqueous humour. The ciliary body is connected to the lens by a set of radial elastic fibres (**zonular fibres**) forming the suspensory ligaments of the lens. Contraction of the ciliary muscle, which is derived from the ectomesenchyme within the ciliary body, diminishes the tension of the zonular fibres and results in a more spherical, relaxed shape of the lens, critical to the focusing of the lens.

Lens

When the optic vesicles contact the surface ectoderm, the ectoderm thickens to form the **lens placodes** (Fig. 11-1). These structures subsequently invaginate and form the **lens vesicles**, which break away from the surface ectoderm. Shortly after formation of the lens vesicles, cells of the posterior wall of the vesicles elongate to form **primary lens fibres** which fill the hollow lens vesicle cavity and thereby transform it into a solid lens (Fig. 11-5). Growth of the lens is not finished at this stage; new, **secondary lens fibres** are continuously added to the central core of the lens, extending almost pole to pole. On the posterior side of the lens, less differentiated cells that do not elongate move to the poles of the lens, proliferate and serve as a source for new lens fibres. The cells of the lens secrete a basal-membrane-like, elastic material rich in glycoproteins that covers the surface of the lens. This **lens capsule** contributes to the elastic properties of the lens, essential to its function. **Zonular fibres**, essentially collagenous fibres that are formed from mesenchymal cells situated between the ciliary body and the lens, attach to this capsule.

Differentiation of the lens is precisely controlled at several levels of organization. At the cellular level, cytodifferentiation transforms mitotically dividing anterior lens epithelial cells into **elongated postmitotic transparent lens fibres**. Most of the soluble protein (up to 90%) of the lens fibres consists of three crystalline proteins: α, β, and γ. This process is under control of the transcription factor Sox2 and other proteins paired with the oncogene *Maf*. During cell differentiation in the lens, all cell organelles gradually disappear, leaving lens fibres with an intact outer membrane, an inner cytoskeleton and transparent cytoplasm filled with crystalline proteins. The crystalline proteins appear in a characteristic sequence: first α-crystalline proteins, then, when the cells elongate, β-crystallins; then, and only in the terminally differentiated lens fibres, γ-crystallins

Formation of crystallin-containing lens fibres starts with the elongation of epithelial cells from the posterior pole of the lens vesicle. These **primary lens fibres** make up the lens nucleus. The remaining lens fibres originate from the elongation of the cuboidal cells of the anterior lens epithelium. They form concentric layers (**secondary lens fibres**) around the primary fibres of the lens nucleus. Consequently, the most peripheral lens fibres are the youngest and, as long as the lens grows, new secondary lens fibres move in from the equator to the outer cortex of the lens. The midline regions, where secondary lens fibres from opposite points on the equator meet, are called the **anterior** and **posterior lens sutures**.

The development of the lens is strongly influenced by the retina. Fibroblast growth factor secreted by the retina accumulates in the vitreous humour behind the lens and stimulates the formation of lens fibres. During its rapid growth, the lens also requires a rather extensive blood supply. This is established by a **vascular tunic that covers the lens**, supplied by blood vessels from two sources: the blood supply for the front of the lens comes from the vessels of the stroma of the iris; the posterior surface of the lens is invested by the **hyaloid artery**, a branch of the choroid vessels that passes through the optic fissure and crosses the vitreous chamber. Branches of the vessels from the stroma of the iris form a vascular membrane called the **pupillary membrane**, which extends across, and temporarily occludes, the pupil. Both the pupillary membrane and the hyaloid artery normally regress long before birth. The more proximal part of the hyaloid arterial systems persists as the central artery of the retina.

Vitreous body

The vitreous body arises from a **loose mesenchyme** that, by way of the choroid fissure, invades the cavity of the optic cup where it forms a loose fibrillar mesh. The interstitial spaces of this delicate network later fill with transparent **gelatinous substance**, forming the vitreous body. During much of embryonic development the hyaloid artery supplies the vitreous body. However, as development progresses, the vitreous part of the hyaloid artery, as well as its branches supplying the lens, regress, leaving a hyaloid canal in the vitreous body.

Choroid, sclera, and cornea

During early development of the eye, the optic cup is surrounded by a layer of **loose mesenchyme**, largely derived from the neural crest. Under the influence of the pigmented epithelium of the retina, the inner layer of these cells differentiates into the **highly vascularized pigmented layer of the choroid**. The outer cells form the white, densely collagenous **sclera** that provides mechanical support for the eye and attachment for the extraocular muscles that move the eyeball. The sclera is continuous with the cornea.

Formation of the cornea results from several sequential inductive events (Fig. 11-5) that transform the surface ectoderm and the underlying mesenchyme into a transparent structure that allows light to pass towards the retina. The cornea is formed by: (1) an **epithelial layer** derived from the surface ectoderm; (2) the **primary stroma**, originating from mesenchyme surrounding the optic cup; and (3) an epithelial layer, the **corneal endothelium**, that borders the anterior chamber. After the corneal endothelium has formed, its cells synthesize and secrete large amounts of hyaluronic acid into the primary stroma. The large water-binding capacity of hyaluronic acid causes the primary stroma to swell greatly, providing the proper environment for a wave of migration of cells of neural crest origin into the developing cornea.

Once the migrating mesenchymal cells have settled, they are transformed into fibroblasts, estab-

lishing the **secondary stroma**. The fibroblasts secrete protocollagen that assembles outside the cells into coarse collagen fibres. Secretions of the corneal epithelium and corneal endothelium provide the remaining layers of the cornea: **Bowman's membrane (lamina limitans anterior**; a thick basal lamina under the corneal epithelium) and the **Descemet's membrane (lamina limitans posterior**; basal lamina of the corneal endothelium), respectively. Bowman's membranes are especially well developed in humans and higher primates. The fully differentiated cornea comprises the following layers: (1) the **multilayered corneal epithelium**, (2) the **lamina limitans anterior**, (3) the **secondary stroma**, (4) the **lamina limitans posterior**, and (5) the **corneal endothelium**. During the final stages of development, the transparency of the cornea is greatly increased, allowing almost 100% transmission of light. This is accomplished by removing most of the water from the secondary stroma, initially by degradation of the water-binding hyaluronic acid within it. During a second phase, thyroxin from the maturing thyroid gland causes a further dehydration of the cornea. Thyroxin acts on the corneal endothelium to pump sodium ions from the secondary stroma into the anterior chamber of the eye. Water molecules follow the transport of sodium ions, thus, effectively completing the dehydration of the cornea. A rather late event of corneal development is a change in its radius of curvature, bringing light rays into focus on the retina.

The **anterior chamber** of the eye develops from a cleft-like space within the mesenchyme between the developing cornea and the lens. The **posterior chamber** of the eye arises from a space that forms in the mesenchyme posterior to the developing iris and anterior to the developing lens. When the pupillary membrane disappears, anterior and posterior chambers of the eye can communicate with each other through the pupil opening. The anterior and posterior chambers are filled with **aqueous humour**, which is secreted into the posterior chamber by the epithelial cells of the ciliary body. The aqueous humour passes through the pupil opening in the anterior chamber, where it is removed into the bloodstream via a trabecular meshwork of connective tissue fibres that bring it into very close proximity to capillaries. The meshwork is located at the junction of the cornea, iris and sclera – the iridocorneal angle. This angle is initially obstructed by a layer of epithelial cells that extends between the endothelium of the cornea and the anterior surface of the iris. As the mesenchyme in this area does not proliferate quickly enough to keep up with the growth of the eye, fluid-filled spaces develop, which later becomes the spaces of the meshwork. The epithelial sheet also becomes perforated by rarefaction. The morphogenetic events forming the meshwork of the filtration angle continue after birth.

Eyelids and lacrimal glands

Each eyelid is formed from a **fold of ectoderm** with a **mesenchymal core**. Once their formation starts, the eyelids grow rapidly towards each other over the developing cornea until they meet and **fuse with one another**. The temporary fusion involves only the epithelial layer of the eyelid, resulting in a persisting common epithelial lamina between them. Separation of the eyelids occurs before birth in humans (around the seventh month of gestation), horses, and ruminants, and after birth in carnivores (at about the eight and tenth days postnatally in pups and kittens, respectively). Before the eyelids reopen, eyelashes and small modified sebaceous glands lying along the margins of the lids (the **tarsal glands**) begin to differentiate from the common epithelial lamina. Each lash also has its own modified sweat gland. In dogs, no eyelashes develop in the lower eyelids.

The thin, transparent mucous membrane covering the inner surface of the eyelid continues over the anterior surface of the sclera and is called the **conjunctiva**. The space between the eyelids and the front of the eyeball is known as the **conjunctival sac**. In domestic animals, a fold of mesenchyme covered by conjunctiva develops into the **third eyelid**. Later, within the mesenchymal tissue, a cartilage forms that gives rigidity to the third eyelid.

Around the time when the eyelids fuse, the **lacrimal glands** develop from a number of solid buds from the surface ectoderm at the dorsolateral angles of the orbits. These buds branch and become canalized to form the ducts and alveoli of the glands. Soon after birth they produce a watery secretion that lubricates the outer surface of the cornea. The lacrimal glands do not function fully at birth in humans; newborn babies do not produce tears when crying during the first six weeks.

EAR

The ear is a complex organ consisting of three compartments, the **outer**, **middle**, and **inner ear**, each of different embryonic origin. The structures of the outer and middle ear are derived from the first and second pharyngeal arches and the intervening first pharyngeal cleft and pharyngeal pouch (see Chapter 14). The inner ear develops from a thickened ectodermal placode at the level of the hindbrain.

The external ear consists of the **auricle**, the **external auditory meatus**, and the **outer layers of the tympanic membrane**. The middle ear conducts sound waves from the external to the inner ear. This is achieved through a chain of **three middle ear ossicles**, which connect the inner side of the tympanic membrane to the oval window of the middle ear. The middle ear ossicles are located within the **tympanic, or middle ear, cavity**. Other components of the middle ear are the **auditory tube** (Eustachian tube), the **middle ear muscles**, and the **inner layer of the tympanic membrane**. The inner ear consists of the **membranous labyrinth** and the **vestibular** and **acoustic (spiral) ganglia** associated with the **vestibulocochlear nerve** (VIII). The inner ear contains the **vestibulocochlear organ**, the sensory apparatus involved in both hearing (through the cochlea) and balance (by means of the vestibular apparatus). The inner ear is surrounded by the cartilaginous otic capsule, which becomes the ossified petrous (and, postnatally, the tympanic bulla) region of the os temporale.

Development of the inner ear

The primordia of the inner ear are **otic placodes**, bilateral thickenings of the surface ectoderm immediately adjacent to the middle of the myelencephalon. Recent studies have shown that FGF19, produced by the paraxial mesoderm, induces the expression of *Wnt-8c* in the neuroepithelium of the rhombencephalon, which in turn stimulates the secretion of FGF3. Possibly under the influence of FGF3, the otic placodes invaginate to form the **otic pits**, which make contact with the wall of the myelencephalon. After a short time, the lips of the pit close, separating the **otic vesicle** from the surface ectoderm (Figs 11-8, 11-9). The cavity of the otic vesicles fills with a fluid called **endolymph**. Some cells that break away from the ventromedial wall of the otic epithelium later give rise to the sensory ganglia of the **vestibulocochlear nerve** (VIII).

Next, a series of outpocketings from the otic vesicle establish the primordia of the **endolymphatic, semicircular,** and **cochlear ducts** (Fig. 11-10). A finger-like evagination of the dorsomedial region of the otic vesicle gives rise to the **endolymphatic duct** which, upon dilation of its terminal end, forms the endolymphatic sac. FGF3, secreted by rhombomeres, appears to be necessary for this development. The otic vesicle itself soon begins to elongate and differentiates into two distinct parts: the **utricle** dorsally, and the **saccule** ventrally (Fig. 11-10). The two main parts of the inner ear are under the control of different genes: *Paired box gene 2 (Pax2)* for the auditory portion and *Nkx5* for the vestibular portion including the semicircular ducts. Knockout of *Pax2* specifically suppresses the development of the cochlea and spiral ganglion.

Two flat, disc-like diverticula grow from the utricular portion of the otic vesicle. One of these flat diverticula takes a vertical position, parallel to the median plane while the second is horizontal, at a right angle to the first. Division of the vertical diverticulum gives rise to the anterior and posterior semicircular structures. Subsequently, the central portions of these vanish due to apoptosis and the two tubes remaining are termed the **anterior** and **posterior semicircular ducts** that later become

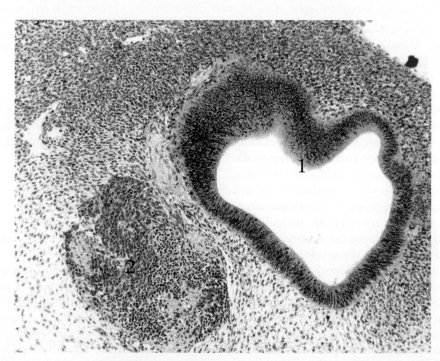

Fig. 11-8: Section through the otic vesicle (1) and statoacoustic ganglion (2) of a 16 mm bovine embryo. Courtesy Sinowatz and Rüsse (2007).

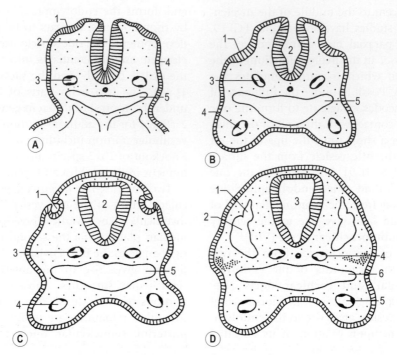

Fig. 11-9: Transverse section through the region of the rhombencephalon showing formation of the otic vesicles. A: 1: otic placode; 2; Neural groove; 3: Dorsal aorta; 4: Surface ectoderm; 5: Pharynx. B: 1: Otic pit; 2: Neural groove; 3: Dorsal aorta; 4: Ventral aorta; 5: Pharynx; C: 1: Otic vesicle; 2: Rhombencephalon; 3: Dorsal aorta; 4: Ventral aorta; 5: Pharynx; D: 1: Recessus labyrinthi; 2: Anlage of the ductus cochlearis; 3: Rhombencephalon; 4: Dorsal aorta; 5: Ventral aorta; 6: Pharynx with tubotympanic recess. Courtesy Sinowatz and Rüsse (2007).

orientated at 90° to each other. Similarly, the central area of the horizontal diverticulum undergoes apoptosis, leaving residual tissues to form the **lateral semicircular duct**. One end of each semicircular duct enlarges at its junction with the utriculus, forming an **ampulla**. In the ampullae, specialized clusters of receptor cells develop – the **cristae ampullares**. Together with the **macula utriculi** and **macula sacculi**, they represent the sensory organs of balance. Several genes guide the development of the semicircular ducts; in the absence of *Otx-1* the lateral semicircular duct fails to develop, and the homeobox transcription factor Dlx is necessary for the development of the anterior and posterior semicircular ducts.

The **cochlear diverticulum** evaginates from the ventral part of the saccule. The **cochlear duct** curls as it elongates and forms the membranous cochlea.

The epithelial cells on one surface of the duct form specialized hair cells and supporting cells of the organ of Corti, or **spiral organ**. The connection between the saccule and the cochlea becomes constricted and forms the narrow **ductus reuniens**.

The embryonic vestibular and cochlear ducts are surrounded by mesenchyme, which later forms a cartilaginous matrix. The inner lining of the cartilaginous capsule undergoes apoptosis, leaving a **perilymphatic space** between the membranous labyrinth and the cartilage. This becomes filled with fluid, **the perilymph**. Differential reshaping of the cochlea results in the establishment of two spaces beside the cochlear duct, the **scala tympani** and the **scala vestibuli**, which are separated from one another, except at the apical tip, by the cochlear duct (Fig. 11-11). The **spiral ligament** mediates the attachment of the lateral wall of the cochlear duct

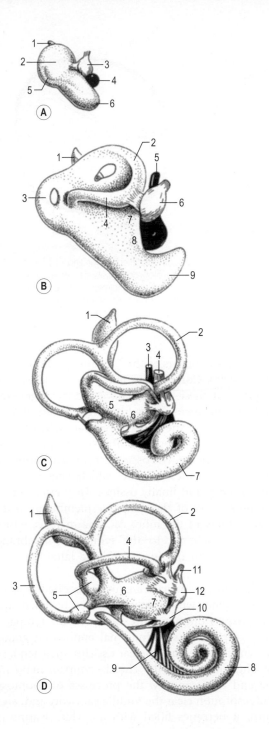

Fig. 11-10: Development of the right membranous labyrinth. A: 1: Saccus endolymphaticus 2: Utricular part of the otocyst; 3: Ganglion vestibulare; 4: Ganglion spirale (cochleare); 5: Anlage of the anterior semicircular duct; 6: Sacculus of the otocyst. B: 1: Saccus endolymphaticus; 2: Anlage of the anterior semicircular duct; 3: Anlage of the posterior semicircular duct; 4: Anlage of the lateral semicircular duct; 5: N. cochlearis; 6: Ganglion vestibulare; 7: Utriculus; 8: Sacculus; 9: Anlage of the cochlea. C: 1: Saccus and ductus endolymphaticus; 2: Ductus semicirculares; 3: Pars cochlearis of N. vestibulo-cochlearis; 4: Pars vestibularis of N. vestibulo-cochlearis; 5: Utriculus; 6: Sacculus; 7: Cochlea. D: 1: Saccus and ductus endolymphaticus; 2: Anterior semicircular duct; 3: Posterior semicircular duct; 4: Lateral semicircular duct; 5: Ampullae membranaceae; 6: Utriculus; 7: Sacculus; 8: Cochlea; 9: Pars cochlearis of N. vestibulo-cochlearis; 10: Ganglion spirale; 11: Pars vestibularis of N. vestibulo-cochlearis; 12: Ganglion vestibulare. Courtesy Sinowatz and Rüsse (2007).

to the cartilaginous capsule which serves as a template for the later formation of the osseous labyrinth.

The sensory neurons of the **vestibulocochlear nerve** (VIII), in particular the **vestibular** and **spiral ganglia**, originate from cells that migrate out from the medial wall of the otic vesicle. The cochlear part (the spiral ganglion) is formed in close association with the sensory cells of the organ of Corti which develops in the cochlea. Neural crest cells invade the developing vestibular and spiral ganglia and differentiate into satellite and supporting cells. The sensory cells of the organ of Corti also originate from the epithelium of the otic vesicle and undergo a complicated pattern of differentiation. Recent studies, based mostly on loss-of-function experiments, have indicated that Notch signalling and basic helix-loop-helix genes are involved in the regulation of hair-cell fate during cochlear development.

Development of the middle ear

Tympanic cavity and auditory tube

Development of the middle ear occurs in intimate association with the developmental changes of the first and second pharyngeal arches (Fig. 11-12). The

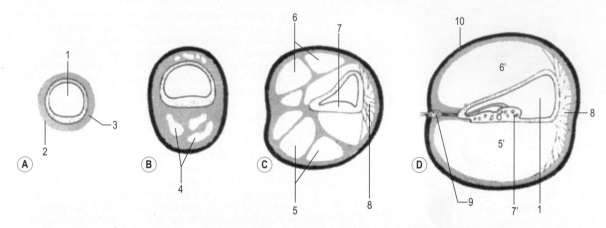

Fig. 11-11: Stages of the development of the membranous and bony labyrinth of humans (modified according to Moore, 1980). Transverse sections through the ductus cochlearis at different times of prenatal development (between week 8 and week 20, A-D) showing the differentiation of the Corti-organ. 1: Cochlear duct; 2: Wall of the otic vesicle; 3: Mesenchyme; 4: Vacuoles, forming later the perilymphatic space; 5: Anlage of the scala tympani; 5′: Scala tympani; 6: Anlage of the scala vestibuli; 6′: Scala vestibuli; 7: Anlage of the Corti-organ; 7′: Corti-organ; 8: Spiral ligament; 9: Spiral ganglion; 10: Bony labyrinth. Courtesy Sinowatz and Rüsse (2007).

tympanic cavity and the **auditory tube** (Eustachian tube) arise from an expansion of the first pharyngeal pouch, an endodermal outpocket of the foregut between the first and second pharyngeal arches (see Chapter 14). Therefore, the entire middle ear cavity and auditory tube, through which the tympanic cavity communicates with the nasopharynx, are lined with an endoderm-derived epithelium. In the Equidae, a ventral diverticulum develops from each auditory tube and gives rise to a large mucus-secreting sac, the **guttural pouch**. The blind end of the first pharyngeal pouch approaches the innermost portion of the first pharyngeal cleft, but the inner endodermal epithelium of the wall and the ectodermal lining of the pharyngeal cleft remain separated by a layer of mesenchyme. Later, the thickness of this mesenchymal layer decreases significantly and the whole complex, consisting of tissue from all three-germ layers, establishes the **tympanic membrane** (eardrum).

Middle ear ossicles (auditory ossicles) and middle ear muscles

Just dorsal to the first pharyngeal pouch, a conspicuous condensation of mesenchyme, derived from the neural crest, appears as the first anlage of the auditory ossicles. Comparative anatomical studies have shown that these ossicles have a dual origin: the **malleus** and **incus** arises from neural-crest-derived mesenchyme of the first pharyngeal arch, whereas the **stapes** originates from the second pharyngeal arch mesenchyme. The ossicles are at first composed of condensed mesenchyme, which later becomes cartilaginous and finally ossifies. They extend from the inner layer of the tympanic membrane to the oval window of the inner ear. The malleus, which becomes anchored to the tympanic membrane, articulates with the incus, and the latter with the stapes.

The auditory ossicles are first embedded in loose mesenchyme, which later becomes resorbed and gives rise to the **tympanic cavity**. As the tympanic cavity expands, its endodermal epithelium gradually envelops the middle ear ossicles, their tendons and ligaments, and the chorda tympani nerve. At the end of pregnancy, the processes of apoptosis and resorption clear the middle ear cavity and, after birth, it becomes filled with air. This clearing of the cavity leaves the auditory ossicles suspended within it covered by a thin epithelium. However, even at birth, some remaining mesenchyme

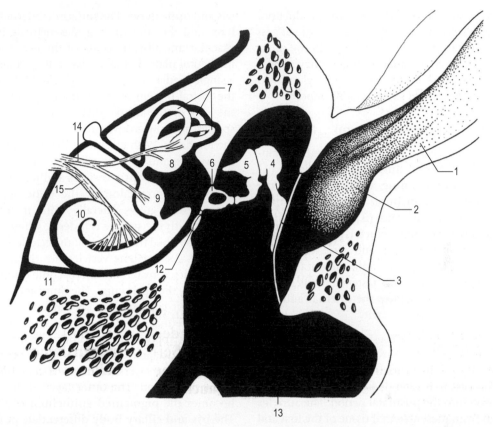

Fig. 11-12: Section through the canine ear, showing the anatomical relationships of the structures that constitute the inner, middle and external ear. 1: Auricle; 2: External ear canal; 3: tympanic membrane; 4: Malleus; 5: Incus; 6: Stapes; 7: Membranous semicircular ducts; 8: Utriculus; 9: Sacculus; 10: Cochlea; 11: Os temporale; 12: cochlear window; 13: Tympanic cavity; 14: Pars cochlearis of the N. vestibulocochlearis; 15: Pars cochlearis of the N. vestibulocochlearis. Courtesy Sinowatz and Rüsse (2007).

dampens the free movement of the auditory ossicles.

Two middle ear muscles are involved in the modulation of the transmission of auditory stimuli through the middle ear. The **tensor tympani muscle**, which is attached to the malleus, develops from first arch mesenchyme and is innervated by a branch of the nerve of this arch, the trigeminal nerve (V; see Chapter 10). The **stapedius muscle** is of second pharyngeal arch origin, is associated with the stapes, and is innervated by the facial nerve (VII, the nerve of the second pharyngeal arch).

Development of the external ear

External auditory meatus

The external auditory meatus arises from an inward expansion of the first pharyngeal cleft. Epithelial cells at the blind end of the meatus proliferate and form a solid epithelial mass, the **meatal plug**. However, late in the fetal period, a channel develops in the meatal plug, extending from the future opening of the external auditory meatus to the level of the tympanic membrane to form the **external auditory meatus**. **Sebaceous** and **modified sweat glands**, which are responsible for cerumen production, begin their development at about the middle of gestation in association with hair follicles in the outer portion of the external canal. Although they appear anatomically mature before birth, these glands do not reach full functional capacity until puberty.

Tympanic membrane (eardrum)

As has been already described, the tympanic membrane contains tissue of three different origins: (1) an **outer ectodermal lining** at the bottom of the auditory meatus, (2) an **inner endodermal lining** of the tympanic cavity, and (3) an **intermediate layer of ectomesenchyme**, which is reduced significantly during development and later forms the fibrous stratum of the tympanic membrane. The tympanic membrane is firmly fastened to the handle of the malleus and separates the external auditory meatus from the tympanic cavity.

Auricles (pinnae)

Development of the auricles is a lengthy and complex process that extends from early embryonic life until well into the postnatal period. The **auricles** are formed from mesenchymal tissue of the first and second pharyngeal arches that surround the first pharyngeal cleft. Nodular masses of mesenchyme (**auricular hillocks**) take shape along each side of the first pharyngeal cleft early in development, enlarge asymmetrically in a species-specific manner, and ultimately fuse to form the auricle which shifts from the base of the neck to its definitive location as gestation advances.

SUMMARY

Development of the eye

The eyes develop from three sources: (1) the **neuroectoderm** of the forebrain, (2) **surface ectoderm** of the head, and (3) head **mesenchyme** of **neural crest origin** between these layers. The ectodermal outgrowth from the brain gives rise to the **retina**, **iris** and **optic nerve**. The surface ectoderm forms the **lens**, and the surrounding mesenchyme forms the **vascular** and **fibrous coats** of the eye. The area of the neural plate that gives rise to the eyes is initially a single median region, the **optic field**, located near the rostral margin of the future prosencephalon. At the end of the third week of pregnancy in most species, shallow grooves are formed on the sides of the forebrain. With closure of the neural tube, these grooves expand as outpocketings of the forebrain. These are called **optic vesicles** and remain attached to the prosencephalon by the **optic stalks**. Each optic vesicle grows laterally until it comes into contact with the surface ectoderm, where it induces a circumscribed thickening of the ectoderm, the **lens placode**. As the lens vesicles are developing, the optic vesicles invaginate and become double-walled structures, the **optic cups**. The inner and outer layers of the optic cups are initially separated by a lumen, the intraretinal space. It soon disappears, and the two layers appose to each other. The **inner layer** of the optic cup later develops into the **neural retina** with its three layers of neurons that function in visual perception. The **outer layer** of the optic cup becomes the **pigmented epithelium** of the retina. The **iris** and **ciliary body** differentiate at the lip of the optic cup, where the neural and pigment layers of the retina meet. The iris develops by the peripheral extensions of both layers of the optic cup so that they cover the edges of the lens vesicle. The stroma of the iris is of neural crest origin.

The muscles of the iris, the **sphincter pupillae** and **dilator pupillae** are of neuroectodermal origin. The **ciliary muscle** develops between the iris and the neural retina. The ciliary body is connected to the lens by a set of radial elastic **zonular fibres** that constitute the suspensory ligament of the lens. The **vitreous body** arises from a loose mesenchyme that invades the cavity of the optic cup by way of the choroid fissure and forms a fibrillar mesh within the cup. The **cornea** is formed by (a) an epithelial layer derived from the surface ectoderm, (b) the primary stroma, originating from mesenchyme surrounding the optic cup, and (c) an epithelial layer (corneal endothelium) that borders the anterior chamber.

The **anterior chamber** of the eye develops from a cleft-like space within the mesenchyme located between the developing cornea and lens. The **posterior chamber** of the eye arises from a space that forms in the mesenchyme posterior to the developing iris and anterior to the developing lens. Each **eyelid** is formed from a fold of ectoderm with a mesenchymal core. Once their formation has commenced, the eyelids grow rapidly towards each other over the developing cornea until they meet and fuse with one another. The temporary fusion involves only the epithelial layer of the eyelid, resulting in a persisting epithelial lamina between them. Separation of the eyelids occurs before birth in humans (around the seventh month of gestation), horses and ruminants and at about the eight and tenth days (pups and kittens, respectively) after birth in carnivores. Around the time when the eyelids fuse, the **lacrimal glands** develop from a number of solid buds from the surface ectoderm at the dorsolateral angles of the orbits. These buds branch and become canalized to form the ducts and alveoli of the lacrimal glands.

Development of the ear

The ear is a complex organ consisting of three compartments, the **external**, **middle-** and **inner ear**, each of which has a different embryonic origin. The structures of the outer and external ear are derived from the **first** and **second pharyngeal arches** and the **intervening first pharyngeal cleft** (externally) and **pharyngeal pouch** (internally). The primordia of the inner ear are bilateral thickenings (**otic placodes**) of the surface ectoderm, located immediately adjacent of the middle of the myelencephalon. The otic placodes invaginate to form the **otic pits**, which contact the wall of the myelencephalon. After a short time, the lips of the pit close, separating the **otic vesicle** from the surface ectoderm, and a series of outpocketings from the otic vesicle establish the primordia of the **endolymphatic**, **semicircular** and **cochlear ducts**.

The **cochlear diverticulum** evaginates from the ventral part of the **saccule**. The cochlear duct curls as it elongates and forms the **membranous cochlea**. The epithelial cells on one surface of the duct form specialized hair cells and supporting cells of the organ of Corti (**spiral organ**). The embryonic vestibular and cochlear ducts are surrounded by mesenchyme, which later forms a cartilaginous matrix. The inner lining of the cartilaginous capsule undergoes apoptosis resulting in the **perilymphatic space** between the membranous labyrinth and the cartilage. This space becomes filled with **perilymph**. Differential reshaping of the cochlea results in the establishment of two spaces beside the cochlear duct, the **scala tympani** and the **scala vestibuli**.

The **tympanic cavity** and the **auditory tube** (Eustachian tube) arise from an expansion of the **first pharyngeal pouch**, an endodermal outpocketing of the foregut between the first and second pharyngeal arches. **Malleus** and **incus** ossicles arise from neural-crest-derived mesenchyme of the **first pharyngeal arch**, whereas the **stapes** originates from the second pharyngeal arch mesenchyme. The **tensor tympani muscle**, which is attached to the malleus, develops from first-arch mesenchyme and is innervated by a branch of the first pharyngeal nerve, the trigeminus (V). The **stapedius muscle** is of second-arch origin. It is associated with the stapes and is innervated by the facial nerve (VII, the nerve of the second pharyngeal arch). The **external auditory meatus** arises from an inward expansion of the first pharyngeal cleft. The **tympanic membrane** contains tissue from all three germ layers: (a) an outer ectodermal lining at the bottom of the auditory meatus, (b) an inner endodermal lining of the tympanic cavity, and (c) an intermediate layer of mesenchyme, which is reduced significantly during development and later forms the fibrous stratum of the tympanic membrane. The **auricles** are formed from mesenchymal tissue of the first and second pharyngeal arch that surrounds the first pharyngeal cleft. Early in development, nodular masses of mesenchyme (auricular hillocks) take shape along each side of the first pharyngeal cleft, enlarge asymmetrically in a species-specific manner, and ultimately fuse to form the auricle.

Box 11-1 Molecular regulation of the eye and ear

The transcription factor **Pax6** plays an leading role in the development of the **eye** and has sometimes been called the 'master gene' for eye development. Mutations in *Pax6* cause no-eye or small-eye phenotypes in mammals. *Pax6* appears to be involved in a feedback loop with another homeobox-containing gene, *Six3*, in this control. Besides being a master gene for eye development, *Pax6* plays significant roles during the induction of differentiation of the lens and retina.

Some of the molecular mechanisms of retinal patterning have been established in several species, especially the mouse. Dorsoventral patterning is initiated by the expression of Bone Morphogenetic Protein 4 (**BMP4**) dorsally and Sonic hedgehog (**Shh**) ventrally. The presence of Shh induces the production of **Otx2** in the outer layer of the optic vesicle and leads to its differentiation into the pigmented layer of the retina. In the inner, neural layer of the optic cup, Shh and the protein **ventroptin** stimulate the expression of the transcription factors **Vax2** and **Pax2** in the ventral retina. Also in this area, Shh inhibits the expression of *BMP4*. In the dorsal part of the developing retina, BMP4 stimulates the expression of *Tbx5*.

Of the many molecules that are unequally distributed within the three dimensions of the retina, opposing gradients of **ephrins** and their receptors may have the most pronounced influence on retinal patterning. As the number of cells in the inner layer of the early retina increases, the differentiation of the different neurons begins. There are two major gradients of differentiation: the first more or less vertically from the inner to the outer layers of the retina; the second more horizontally from the centre to the periphery. Differentiation in the horizontal gradient starts with the appearance of ganglion cells. As the ganglion cell layer is established, neighbouring neural precursor cells of the ganglion cells are prevented from premature differentiation by the expression of the *Notch* gene. The protein coded by *Notch* keeps these cells in an undifferentiated state that will be overcome later by differentiation signals from the neighbourhood of the neuroblasts. Differentiation of amacrine and horizontal cells establishes the inner and outer

nuclear layers of the retina. These neurons send out processes which contribute to the definition of the inner and outer plexiform layers. The bipolar neurons and receptor cells of the retina, the rod and cone cells, differentiate last. It has been shown recently in the mouse that *Otx2* is a key regulatory gene for cell fate determination amongst retinal photoreceptor cells

Recent molecular studies have revealed that numerous guidance molecules control the **development of the visual neural pathway**. Axonal projections from the ganglion cells to the optic disc are thought to depend on **adhesion molecules** and **inhibitory extracellular matrices** such as chondroitin sulphate. The formation of the optic nerve and the optic chiasma require ligand-receptor interactions between **netrin-1** and **DDC (deleted in colorectal cancer) receptor**, and **Slit** proteins and **Robo** receptors, respectively. Netrin-1 serves as a growth cone attractor and Shh plays a role as a signal counteracting axonal outgrowth. The gradient distributions of **ephrin** ligands and receptors are essential for correct ipsilateral projections at the optic chiasma and the topographic mapping of axons in the rostral colliculi. Moreover, the axon guidance activities of **Slit** and **semaphorin 5A** require the existence of heparin sulphate, which binds to numerous guidance molecules.

Mutational analyses in the mouse and studies of the expression of diffusible growth factors have greatly assisted the identification of many of the genes involved in **ear** development. Recent evidence suggests that key genes involved in the development of the inner ear have been conserved among mammals and even among vertebrates. Three categories of genes expressed during development of the inner ear have been established. In the first group are genes that are expressed in the ear and exert a general function on the overall capacity of the ear to develop (candidate genes for this group are *Eya1*, *Six1*, *Sox2*, *Gata3*, *Fgfr2b*, and *Fgf3/10* or *Fgf3/8*). The second group comprises genes that exert their effects either by affecting gene upregulation in the ear or by coding for diffusible substances secreted within or outside the ear. Diffusible factor genes or modifiers of their expression are **Wnt1/3a**, **Shh** and **Gli3**. **Kreisler**, **Gbx2**, **Hoxa**, and **Hoxb** cluster genes have been shown to regulate the production of similar diffusible factors in the brain. Genes of the third group fine tune morphogenetic effects in the inner ear by regulating fusion plate formation of the circular canals and regulating the size of the canal diameter. Examples of these genes are **BMPs**, **EphB2**, **Nor1**, and **Netrin**.

Recent evidence suggests that **Fgf19** produced in the paraxial mesoderm induces the expression of **Wnt 8c** in the rhombencephalic neuroepithelium, which in turn stimulates the secretion of **Fgf3**. Later, under the influence of Fgf3, the otic placode invaginates and separates from the surface ectoderm to form the otic vesicle (otocyst). The otic vesicle elongates and forms a dorsal vestibular and a ventral cochlear region. In the absence of **Pax2**, neither the cochlea nor the spinal ganglion develops. The formation of the semicircular canals involves the expression of the homeobox transcription factor gene **Nkx5-1**, which is important for the development of the dorsal portion of the inner ear. **Otx1** is necessary for the development of the lateral semicircular canal, and in the absence of the homeobox transcription factor **Dex5**, the anterior and posterior semicircular canals fail to develop.

FURTHER READING

Aguirre, G.D., Rubin, L.F. and Bistner, S.I. (1972): Development of the canine eye. Am. J. Vet. Res. 33:2399–2414.

Baker, C.V.H. and Bronner-Fraser, M. (2001): Vertebrate cranial placodes. I. Embryonic induction. Dev. Biol. 232:1–61.

Barishka, R.Y. and Ofri, R. (2007): Embryogenetics: gene control of the embryogenesis of the eye. Vet. Ophtalmol. 10:133–136.

Bistner, S.I., Rubin, L.F. and Aguirre, G.D. (1973): Development of the bovine eye. Am. J. Vet. Res. 34:7–12.p 3–31.

Chow, R.L. and Lang, R.A. (2001): Early eye development in vertebrates. Ann. Rev. Cell Dev. Biol. 17:255–296.

Cvekl, A. and Piatigorsky, J. (1996): Lens development and crystalline gene expression. many roles for Pax-6. Bioessays 18:621–630.

De Schaepdrijver, L., Lauwers, H., Simoens, P. and Geest, J.P. (1990): Development of the retina in the porcine fetus: a light microscopic study. Anat. Histol. Embryol. 19:222–235.

Donovan, A. (1966): The postnatal development of the cat retina. Exp. Eye Res. 5:249–254.

Fritzsch, B., Pauley, S., and Beisel KW. (2006): Cells, molecules and morphogenesis: the making of the vertebrate ear. Brain Res. 1091:151–171.

Greiner, J.V. and Weidman, T.A. (1980): Histogenesis of the cat retina. Exp. Eye Res. 30:439–453.

Lupo G., Andreazzoli M., Gestri G., Liu Y., He R.Q. and Barsacchi G. (2000): Homeobox genes in the genetic control of eye development. Int. J. Dev. Biol. 44:627–636.

Mallo, M. (1998): Embryological and genetic aspects of middle ear development. Int. J. Dev. Biol. 42:11–22.

Noden, D.M., and van de Water, T.R. (1992): Genetic analysis of mammalian ear development. Trends Neurosi. 15:235–237.

Riley, B.B. and Phillips, B.T. (2003): Ringing in the new ear: resolution of cell interactions in otic development. Develop. Biol. 261:289–312.

Rüsse, I. and Sinowatz, F. (1998): Lehrbuch der Embryologie der Haustiere, 2nd edn. Parey Buchverlag, Berlin.

Shively, J.N., Epling, G.P. and Jensen, R. (1971): Fine structure of the postnatal development of the canine retina. Am. J. Vet. Res. 32:383–392.

Zaghloul, N.A., Yan, B. and Moody, S. (2005): Stepwise specification of retinal stem cells during normal embryogenesis. Biol. Cell 97:321–337.

CHAPTER 12

Poul Hyttel

Development of the blood cells, heart and vascular system

During the early phases of development, the embryo is nourished through diffusion from the fluid secreted by the uterine glands into the uterine cavity. However, as the size and complexity of the embryo increases, it soon needs a **circulatory system** to distribute nutrients and oxygen and to remove carbon dioxide and metabolites. The circulatory system, including the **heart, arteries, veins** and **blood**, begins to develop as early as the third week of gestation to meet this need; it is the first functional organ system.

The formation of blood and blood-vessels is initiated from **haemangioblasts** in the visceral mesoderm of the yolk-sac wall. An area of blood-forming cavities is established in the visceral mesoderm in the anterior part of the embryo where it forms a horseshoe-shaped structure around the anterior and lateral portions of the neural plate (Fig. 12-1). This structure is referred to as the **cardiogenic field**, and the intra-embryonic coelom overlying it develops into the **pericardial cavity**. Gradually, the blood-forming cavities coalesce to form a horseshoe-shaped tube, the **endocardial tube**, lined by endothelial cells. This tube becomes surrounded by myoblasts (which develop from the mesenchyme) to form the **myocardium**. On the surface of the myocardium the visceral mesoderm of the pericardial cavity forms the **epicardium**, thereby completing the formation of the **cardiac tube**.

Outside the cardiogenic field, clusters of angioblasts also assemble on each side of the midline of the embryo. These bilateral assemblies develop into tubes lined by endothelial cells – the **two dorsal aortae**. Antero-posterior folding of the embryo by about 180 degrees at the front end of the embryonic

disc translocates the horseshoe-shaped cardiac tube, enclosed in its pericardial cavity, from an anterior to a ventral position (Fig. 12-2). In the process, the posterior extensions of the horseshoe-shaped cardiac tube are transformed into anterior extensions that develop into the **two ventral aortae** defining the future outlet of the heart (Fig. 12-3). Another result of the antero-posterior folding is that the cardiac tube, with the two ventral aortae extending in an anterior direction, becomes located ventral to the anterior portions of the dorsal aortae. This spatial relationship allows for the dorsal and ventral aortae on each side to become connected by **aortic arches** that correspond to the pharyngeal or branchial arches (see 'The aortic arches', this chapter). The dorsal and ventral aortae, together with the aortic arches, form the backbone of the **arterial system** whereas the initially curved portion of the cardiogenic field develops into the **heart** (Fig. 12-4). Along with these processes, bilateral collecting systems, returning blood from the arterial system to the heart, form the basis of the **venous system** which become connected to the posterior crescent of the horseshoe-shaped cardiac tube defining the future inlet to the heart (Fig. 12-3). In the following, the development of the heart, the arterial and the venous systems will be described in more detail. The lymphatic system is described in Chapter 13.

FORMATION OF BLOOD CELLS

The formation of blood cells, **haematopoiesis**, occurs in three overlapping periods. The first, or **mesoblastic period** of blood-formation, occurs in

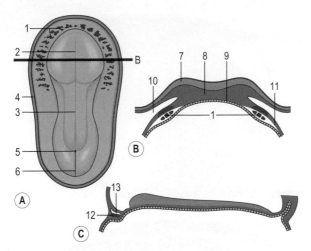

Fig. 12-1: A: Dorsal view of an embryo after removal of the amniotic folds. The cardiogenic field (1) is seen as a horseshoe-shaped structure anteriorly. 2: Neural plate; 3: Neural groove; 4: Cut edge of chorioamniotic fold; 5: Primitive node; 6: Primitive streak. **B:** Transverse section of embryo at the line 'B'. 7: Neural ectoderm; 8: Mesoderm; 9: Endoderm; 10: Intra-embryonic coelom; 11: Visceral mesoderm; **C:** Median section through the embryo. 12: Cardiogenic field; 13: Pericardial cavity.

the yolk sac. During the second, or **hepato-lienal period**, the liver and the spleen become the major blood-forming organs. This period is, in turn, overtaken by a third, or **medullary period**, in which the bone marrow takes over as the major blood-forming organ.

The mesoblastic period

The first blood cells appear in the visceral mesoderm of the yolk-sac wall very early in development (Fig. 12-5); in cattle, they can be seen in embryos at a crown-rump length of 4 mm. At first, **blood islands** are formed where larger spaces in the mesoderm become occupied with clusters of **haemangioblasts**, in which the outer cells differentiate into **angioblasts**, forming **endothelial cells**, and the inner cells into **primitive blood cells**. These blood islands coalesce into larger units and the endothelial cells form tubes establishing the first vessels. This process of spontaneous blood-vessel formation is referred to as **vasculogenesis**. Subsequently, the first generation of vessels forms new vessels by sprouting – a process

referred to as **angiogenesis**. The first blood cells to be formed are primitive nucleated erythrocytes. This primitive **erythropoiesis** depends on the formation of erythropoietic stem cells that need to be in contact with the hypoblast covering the yolk sac in order to maintain stem cell function. Primitive erythropoiesis evolves within a few days into mature erythropoiesis resulting in erythrocytes without nuclei. In cattle, primitive nucleated erythrocytes constitute 90 to 100% of the erythrocyte population at a crown-rump length of 10 to 16 mm; however, at a length of 23 to 30 mm, their contribution has decreased to 25 to 50%. More recent studies, however, have shown the yolk sac to have only limited haematopoietic potential compared with that appearing shortly after in the intra-embryonic **aorta-gonad-mesonephros (AGM) region**. It is apparently stem cells from this region that contribute to haematopoiesis in the following two periods.

Hepato-lienal period

The hepato-lienal period of haematopoiesis starts at a crown-rump length of 8 mm in cattle. By 10 mm, numerous erythropoietic stem cells as well as megakaryocytes can be recognized, and by 12 to 13 mm neutrophil granulocytes can be seen in the liver. The haematopoietic activity is based upon stem cells derived from the septum transversum and takes place at an extravascular location; the newly formed blood cells enter the vessels through diapedesis. The liver becomes the most prominent haematopoietic organ in cattle embryos from a crown-rump length of about 18 mm, and its activity persists up to a length of about 35 cm, i.e. up to the fifth month of pregnancy. During the sixth month, however, the liver's blood-forming activity declines and at birth it has ceased. The spleen is active in haematopoiesis from the third to the seventh month of pregnancy in cattle.

Medullary period

The bone marrow begins its haematopoietic activity at a crown-rump length of about 18 cm during the fourth month of pregnancy in cattle. Its haematopoietic stem cells are probably derived from the liver.

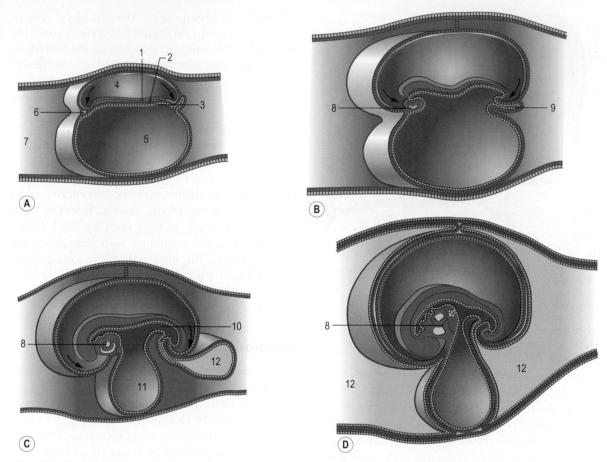

Fig. 12-2: Positioning of the developing heart. **A:** The trilaminar embryonic disc, composed of ectoderm (1), mesoderm (2), and endoderm (3), bulges into the amniotic cavity (4) and delineates the primitive yolk sac (5) ventrally. The arrows indicate the cranio-caudal folding of the embryonic disc. The cardiogenic field is seen anteriorly (6). 7: Extra-embryonic coelom. **B:** The developing heart (8) is brought ventro-caudally. 9: Allantoic bud. **C:** The primitive gut (10) has been formed through the cranio-caudal and lateral foldings of the embryonic disc and the developing heart (8) has been brought to a more ventral position. 11: Yolk sac; 12: Allantois. **D:** The developing heart (8) has achieved its more or less final position and the allantois has enlarged. Modified from Sadler (2004).

THE HEART

The heart develops from the horseshoe-shaped cardiac tube after embryonic folding has repositioned it within the pericardial cavity ventral to the embryonic disc (Fig. 12-3). The anterior extensions of the horseshoe develop into the two ventral aortae whereas the posterior crescent makes contact with the developing venous system. In parallel with the antero-posterior folding, a lateral folding moves the lateral aspects of the embryonic disc ventrally and towards each other in the midline of the embryo. This folding brings the posterior portions of the two ventral aortae gradually closer to each other ventral to the foregut; eventually portions of the two aortae fuse form to a single tube which extends the cardiac tube anteriorly (Fig. 12-3). At its anterior

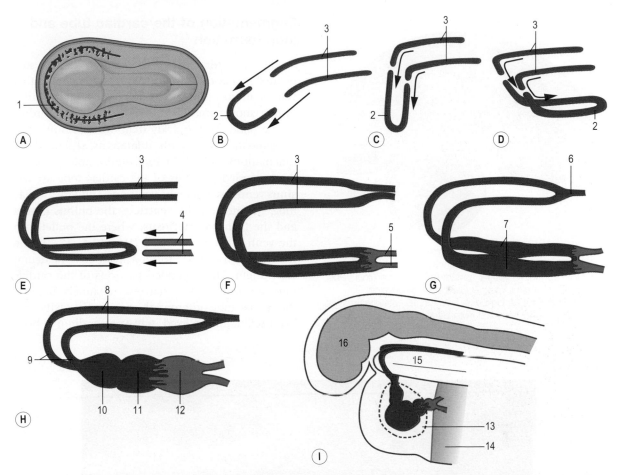

Fig. 12-3: Positioning of the heart and development of the dorsal and ventral aortae. **A:** Dorsal view of embryo with the cardiogenic field (1) anteriorly. **B:** With the cranio-caudal folding of the embryo, the cardiac tube (2) is brought caudo-ventrally. The developing dorsal aortae (3) approach the cardiogenic tube. **C–E:** The cardiogenic tube (2) is brought to a position ventral to the dorsal aortae (3) and the vitelline veins (4) approach the cardiogenic tube. **F:** The caudal portion of the cardiogenic tube fuses (5) with the cranial portion of the vitelline veins. **G:** The caudal portions of the dorsal aortae fuse (6) and the two sides of the cardiac tube fuse as well (7). **H:** The dorsal (8) and ventral (9) aortae have formed, and the developing heart has formed the bulbus cordis (10), ventricle (11) and atrium (12). **I:** Overview of the position of the developing heart and the dorsal and ventral aortae. 13: Pericardial cavity; 14: Septum transversum; 15: Primitive gut; 16: Brain vesicles. Modified from McGaedy et al. (2006).

end, the cardiac tube will be continuous with the two ventral aortae, defining the outlet of the heart; at its posterior end, the tube will be joined by the venous system, defining the inlet of the heart. The tube expands in diameter and begins to pump blood out into the ventral aortae, the aortic arch system and thence the dorsal aortae. In return it receives the venous drainage at its posterior pole. Coordinated embryonic heart beats begin at around Day 22 of pregnancy in the pig, Day 23 in the dog and cattle, and Day 24 in the horse.

At this stage of development, the heart consists of a single tube. To develop into the four-chambered mammalian heart that circulates blood to the body and the lungs separately, the cardiac tube undergoes first a **loop formation** and then an **internal division**.

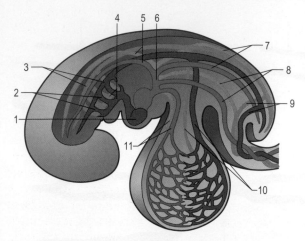

Fig. 12-4: Overview of the developing vascular system.
1: Developing heart; 2: Aortic arches on the left side;
3: Dorsal aortae; 4: Ventral aortae; 5: Cranial cardinal veins;
6: Common cardinal vein; 7: Caudal cardinal veins;
8: Umbilical veins; 9: Umbilical arteries; 10: Vitelline arteries;
11: Vitelline veins. Modified from Sadler (2004).

Segmentation of the cardiac tube and loop formation

In the pericardial cavity the cardiac tube is suspended in a dorsal mesocardium and anchored to a ventral mesocardium (the latter deteriorates after only a short time). Some portions of the cardiac tube expand more quickly than others, resulting in a segmented tube with dilatations separated by indentations (Fig. 12-3). In posterior-anterior order, the expanded portions of the cardiac tube are the **sinus venosus**, where the veins open into the cardiac tube, the **atrium**, the **ventricle**, the **bulbus cordis** and the **truncus arteriosus**, where the outlet into the ventral aortae is found (Figs 12-6, 12-7). The **truncus arteriosus** is formed from cells of neural crest origin. The expanded portions of the cardiac tube are connected by narrower channels. Because the cardiac tube outgrows the pericardial cavity, and because the tube is fixed in the pericardium at both

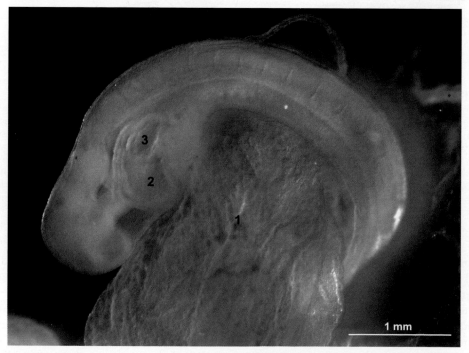

Fig. 12-5: Pig embryo at Day 16 of development showing blood vessels developing in the wall of the yolk sac (1). The developing heart, with its ventricle (2) and atrium (3), has folded to its ventral position.

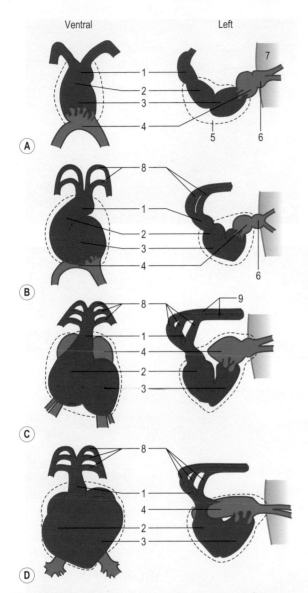

Ventral   Left

Fig. 12-6: Ventral and left aspects of the segmentation and loop formation of the heart at progressive stages of development (A-D). 1: Truncus arteriosus; 2: Bulbus cordis; 3: Ventricle; 4: Atrium; 5: Pericardial cavity; 6: Sinus venosus; 7: Septum transversus; 8: Aortic arches; 9: Dorsal aortae. Modified from McGaedy et al. (2006).

this stage of development. At least in cattle, the loop formation occurs around the 10–12 somite stage, around Day 22 of gestation. Throughout this process, the developing heart is beating at a rhythm set by pacemakers in the sinus venosus. At first, the **sinus venosus** and the **atrium** are not enclosed within the pericardial cavity, but they gradually become enveloped by the pericardium. During this enclosure, the atrium becomes positioned dorsal to the ventricle, and the **loop takes on the shape of an S** instead of a U. Again in cattle, this process occurs around the 20 somite stage, i.e. around Day 23 of gestation. The tube is smooth-walled as it begins its loop formation, but then regions on either side of the primary interventricular foramen (between the ventricle and the bulbus cordis) develop trabeculae. The trabeculated portion of the **ventricle** develops into the future **left ventricle** whereas the trabeculated portion of the **bulbus cordis** develops into the future **right ventricle**.

Formation of the four heart chambers

The developing heart becomes divided by complex septa. Although this is a continuous process in which the different septa develop in parallel, the following description follows the individual septa separately for the sake of simplicity. First though, the expansion of the atrium by its incorporation of the sinus venosus and portions of the venous system must be considered.

Incorporation of the sinus venosus into the atrium

The first veins to open into the sinus venosus are the **ompholomesenteric** or **vitelline veins** (see 'Development of the venous system', later in this chapter), followed shortly by the **umbilical** and the **cardinal veins**. The three pairs of veins are connected with the sinus venosus in such a manner that the sinus forms **right** and **left sinus horns** (Fig. 12-8). Gradually, the **right side of the venous inlet is favoured** and the opening from the sinus venosus into the atrium shifts to the right and becomes narrower. During this process, a portion of the right part of

ends, the tube becomes **U-shaped** with the loop of the U (the junction between the ventricle and the bulbus cordis) pointing ventrally. The loop is prominent and forms the heart bulge that is clearly seen on the outside of the embryo and is characteristic of

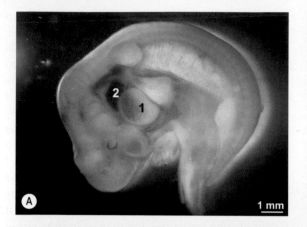

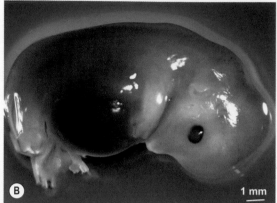

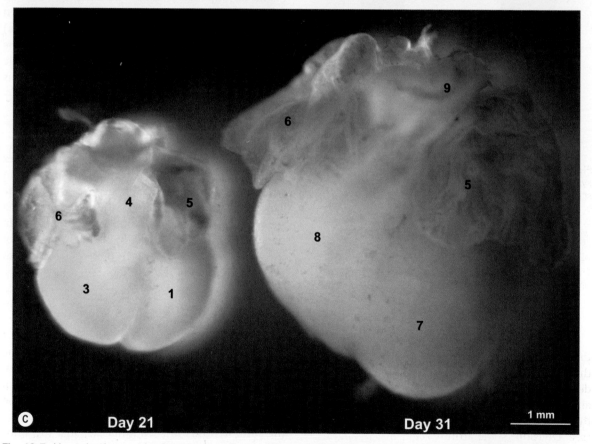

Fig. 12-7: Heart development in pig embryos at Day 21 (A) and 31 (B) of development. **A:** 1: Ventricle; 2: Atrium. **C:** Left aspect of hearts from Day 21 and 31 pig embryos. 1: Ventricle; 3: Bulbus cordis; 4: Truncus arteriosus; 5: Left auricle; 6: Right auricle; 7: Left ventricle; 8: Right ventricle; 9: Conus arteriosus.

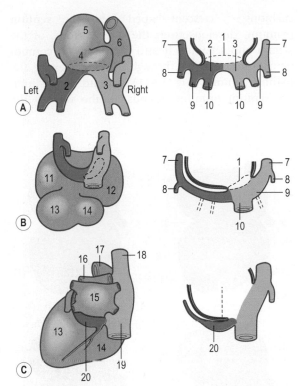

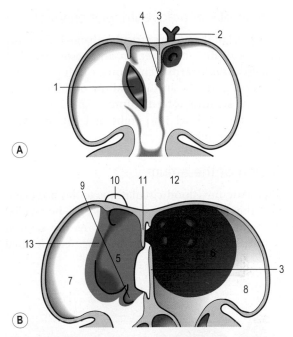

Fig. 12-8: Dorsal aspect of the development of the venous system in the heart region. 1: Sinoatrial opening; 2: Left sinus horn; 3: Right sinus horn; 4: Atrium; 5: Ventricle; 6: Bulbus cordis; 7: Left and right anterior cardinal veins; 8: Left and right posterior cardinal veins; 9: Left and right umbilical veins; 10: Left and right vitelline veins; 11: Left atrium; 12: Right atrium; 13: Left ventricle; 14: Right ventricle; 15: Left atrium; 16: Pulmonary arteries; 17: Aorta; 18: Cranial vena cava; 19: Caudal vena cava; 20: Coronary sinus. Modified from Sadler (2004).

Fig. 12-9: Incorporation of the right sinus horn and the pulmonary veins into the atrium at two stages of development (A, B). 1: Opening of right sinus horn into the atrium; 2: Opening of the pulmonary veins into the atrium; 3: Septum primum; 4: Ostium primum; 5: Incorporated portion of right sinus horn; 6: Incorporated portion of pulmonary veins; 7: Right auricle; 8: Left auricle; 9: Opening to caudal vena cava; 10: Opening to cranial vena cava; 11: Septum secundum; 12: Foramen ovale; 13: Crista terminalis. Modified from Sadler (2004).

the sinus venosus (the right sinus horn) merges into the atrium (Fig. 12-9). The lateral crest-shaped borderline between the incorporated sinus and the atrium develops into the **crista terminalis** whereas the medial one develops into the **septum secundum** (see 'Division of the atrium', later in this chapter). The anterior portion of the right sinus horn develops into the part of the **cranial vena cava** that opens into the right atrium whereas the posterior portion develops into the corresponding portion of the **caudal vena cava**. The left sinus horn eventually develops into the **coronary sinus**. The original right atrium remains as the **right auricle** whereas the smooth-walled portion of the atrium develops from the incorporated sinus venosus.

While the sinus venosus is being incorporated into the right side of the atrium, the **pulmonary veins** start to open into the left side of the atrium. At first, they do so through a single opening from the common cavity into which four pulmonary veins drain. Later, however, the common cavity is incorporated into the atrium resulting in four individual openings for the pulmonary veins (Fig. 12-9). The original left atrium remains as the **left auricle** whereas the smooth-walled portions of the atrium are formed by the incorporated parts of the pulmonary veins.

Division of the atrioventricular channel

At the level of the atrioventricular channel, the inner cardiac wall develops anterior and posterior thickenings, the **endocardial cushions**, which grow until they meet and fuse in the midline of the canal to form the **septum intermedium** (Fig. 12-10). This divides the channel into **right** and **left atrioventricular channels**.

Division of the atrium

To separate the blood circulations to the body and lungs, the cardiac tube derivatives need to be divided into right and left compartments. As the septum intermedium develops from the endocardial

cushions, a crescent-shaped fold, the **septum primum**, develops from the dorsal aspect of the atrium and separates it into right and left components connected only through a minor opening, the **ostium primum** (Fig. 12-11). Around this ostium, the septum primum extends all the way to the

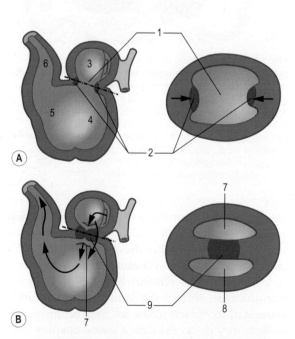

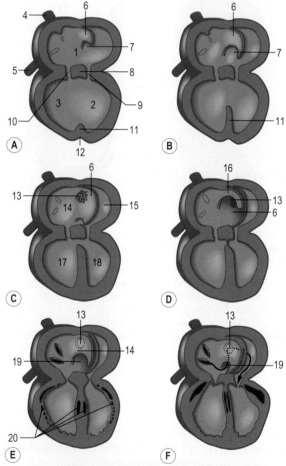

Fig. 12-10: Division of the common atrioventricular canal into left and right canals at different stages of development (A-B). Diagrams to the right are dorsal views of areas indicated by broken lines. 1: Common atrioventricular canal; 2: Endocardial cushions; 3: Atrium; 4: Ventricle; 5: Bulbus cordis; 6: Truncus arteriosus; 7: Right atrioventricular canal; 8: Left atrioventricular canal; 9: Septum intermedium. In 'A' the arrows indicate growth of the cushions, and in 'B' the arrows indicate the direction of blood flow. Modified from McGaedy et al. (2006).

Fig. 12-11: Partitioning of the heart into four chambers. 1: Atrium; 2: Ventricle; 3: Bulbus cordis; 4: Cranial vena cava; 5: Caudal vena cava; 6: Septum primum; 7: Ostium primum; 8: Septum intermedium; 9: Left atrioventricular canal; 10: Right atrioventricular canal; 11: Interventricular septum; 12: Interventricular sulcus; 13: Foramen secundum; 14: Right atrium; 15: Left atrium; 16: Septum secundum; 17: Right ventricle; 18: Left ventricle; 19: Foramen ovale; 20: Cavitations in myocardium. Modified from McGaedy et al. (2006).

endocardial cushions, thus contributing to the development of the septum intermedium. As the endocardial cushions grow towards the midline, the septum primum also grows, and when the cushions fuse, the septum also fuses ventrally, thus gradually closing the ostium primum. Before this closure, however, programmed cell death in the dorsal region of septum primum results in formation of the **ostium secundum** which allows continued blood flow from the developing right atrium to the left (Fig. 12-11). In the horse, this event occurs at a crown-rump length of 11.5–12 mm, i.e. around Day 30-32 of gestation. Shortly thereafter, a second crescent-shaped fold, the **septum secundum**, develops to the left of the septum primum. The septum secundum grows until it has completely covered the ostium secundum, but retains an oval opening, the **foramen ovale**. The dorsal portion of the septum secundum fuses with the septum primum whereas the ventral portion establishes a valve regulating the blood flow from the primitive right atrium to the left atrium.

Division of the ventricle and the bulbus cordis

When the U-shaped cardiac tube is formed, the junction between the ventricle and the bulbus cordis points ventrally. The bulbus cordis consists of a dilated portion adjacent to the ventricle and a narrower portion, the **conus cordis**, joining the truncus arteriosus. The transition between the ventricle and the bulbus cordis is marked externally by a groove and internally by a muscular fold that develops into the **muscular part** of the **interventricular septum**, which grows dorsally towards the septum intermedium (Figs 12-11, 12-12). An **interventricular foramen** persists for some time, but this opening is gradually closed by the **membranous part** of the **interventricular septum** which develops from the posterior endocardial cushion. In the horse at least, the closure of the interventricular septum occurs at a crown-rump length of 14 to 16 mm, i.e. around Day 35–36 of gestation. It is important to understand that the membranous part of the interventricular septum develops in such a way that **both the ventricle (the future left ventricle) and the dilated portion of the bulbus cordis (the future right ventricle) maintain openings into the conus cordis**. In parallel with the septum formation, the walls of the ventricle and the bulbus cordis thicken and develop a trabeculated pattern on the inside. Trabeculation results to some degree from the formation of cavitations in the wall which later open into the lumen. The expansion of the ventricle and the bulbus cordis brings their walls into apposition ventrally. There, the walls gradually fuse and add to the interventricular septum (Fig. 12-6).

Division of the conus cordis and truncus arteriosus

With the development of the septa primum and secundum, the atrium is, except for the regulated blood flow through the foramen ovale, divided into a primitive right and left atrium. In parallel, the development of the interventricular septum results in the formation of the primitive right and left ventricles. Formation of right and left atrioventricular channels results in the primitive right atrium draining into the corresponding right ventricle (except for the blood that flows through the foramen ovale to the primitive left atrium) while the primitive left atrium drains into the corresponding left ventricle. Each of the primitive ventricles expels its blood into the conus cordis which forwards it to the ventral aortae through the truncus arteriosus. To complete the division of the cardiac tube into right and left halves, the **bulbus cordis and the truncus arteriosus also need to be divided** into two channels. This is accomplished by the formation of two opposing cushions in the walls of these compartments. The cushions in the conus cordis fuse with those of the truncus arteriosus to form conu-truncal cushions. These develop spirally to direct the blood flow into the ventral aortae (Fig. 12-13). As they grow, the cushions fuse in the midline to form the **aorticopulmonary septum** dividing the blood flow into two separate channels. Hence, these developments result in separate outlets from the primitive right and left ventricles into the ventral aortae.

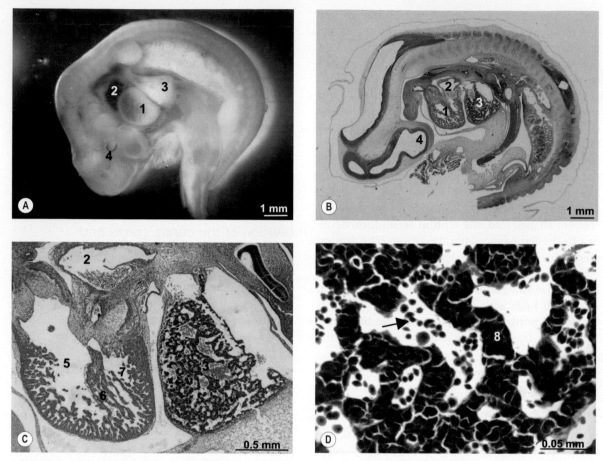

Fig. 12-12: Porcine embryo at Day 21 of development presenting heart development and a haematopoietic liver. **A, B:** Whole embryo (A) and sagittal section (B) presenting the developing heart ventricle (1) and atrium (2). 3: Liver; 4: Brain vesicles. **C:** The developing heart presenting right (5) and left (7) ventricles separated by the interventricular septum (6). 2: Atrium; 3: Liver embedded in septum transversum. **D:** Developing liver cell cords (8) with numerous nucleated erythrocytes (arrow) between them.

Development of valves

Blood in the developing heart needs to be directed from the venous inlet towards the arterial outlet. Two systems of valves, the **atrioventricular valves** and the **semilunar valves**, develop to ensure this directional flow.

The **atrioventricular valves** develop from the edges of the right and left atrioventricular channels. An important mechanism in their development is a cavitation of the myocardium of the primitive right and left ventricle beneath the septum intermedium

(Fig. 12-14). This restructuring of the ventricular wall results in the formation of valves suspended in muscular cords. On the left side, two valves form – the **bicuspid** or **mitral valves**; on the right, three valves –the **tricuspid valves**. The parts of the muscular cords that attach to the valves are replaced by connective tissue, the **chordae tendineae**; the rest of the muscular cords become the **papillary muscles**.

The **semilunar valves** develop as swellings at the outlet of the truncus arteriosus into the ventral aortae during the division of the truncus by the

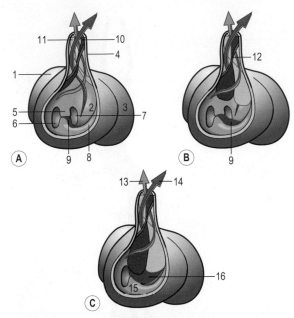

Fig. 12-13: Partitioning of the conus cordis and truncus arteriosus at successive stages of development (A-C). 1: Right atrium; 2: Bulbus cordis; 3: Ventricle; 4: Conus cordis continuing into truncus arteriosus; 5: Septum intermedium; 6: Right atrioventricular canal; 7: Left atrioventricular canal; 8: Muscular part of interventricular septum; 9: Membranous part of interventricular septum: 10: Left conu-truncal cushion; 11: Right conu-truncal cushion; 12: Aorticopulmonary septum; 13: Pulmonary channel; 14: Aortic channel; 15: Right ventricle; 16: Left ventricle. Modified from Sadler (2004).

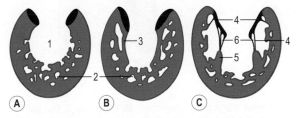

Fig. 12-14: Ventral aspect of the development of the atrioventricular valves at successive stages of development (A-C). 1: Lumen of the ventricle; 2: Cavities in the myocardium; 3: Muscular cord; 4: Atrioventricular valves; 5: Papillary muscle; 6: Chordae tendineae. Modified from Sadler (2004).

growing cushions. Upon completion of the aorticopulmonary septum, the swellings give rise to three primitive valves in each of the aortic and pulmonary outlets. The valves attain their final shape by hollowing out on the upper surface.

Development of the conducting system

Propagation of myocardial contractions becomes possible once the myocardial cells become connected through gap junctions. Specialized myocardial cells develop into a well-defined conducting system that regulates the rate and propagation of contraction. The first group of such specialized cells forms the **atrioventricular node** which, in the sheep, becomes recognizable as a medial subendocardial thickening in the primitive right atrium at a crown-rump-length of 11 to 12 mm. In cattle, the node is visible at a length of 9 mm, has grown into the septum intermedium at 13 mm, and at 23 mm has developed the **atrioventricular fasciculus** that distributes the impulses in the ventricular walls through the **Purkinje fibres**. A second node, the **sinoatrial node**, develops subepicardially at the future opening of the vena cava caudalis. In the sheep, this structure becomes recognizable at a crown-rump-length of 10 to 11 mm.

THE ARTERIAL SYSTEM

The cranial portions of the arterial system originate mainly from the **aortic arches** and the cranial parts of the **dorsal** and **ventral aortae**. Caudal elements of the system develop from **segmental arteries** arising from the more caudal regions of the dorsal aortae. At first, the latter extend caudally as a pair and then, over a certain distance, they fuse to form a single, 'unpaired', aorta (Fig. 12-3). The unpaired segment of the dorsal aorta develops into the **thoracic** and **abdominal aorta** whereas the most caudal portion, which remains paired, develops into the **internal** and **external iliac** arteries and their extensions. An unpaired **median sacral artery** continues the unpaired aorta caudally.

The aortic arches

When the pharyngeal or branchial arches form, each arch receives its own cranial nerve and its own artery. This results in the formation of, in principle, six arterial arches (aortic arches) between the dorsal and ventral aortae on each side. The ventral aortae

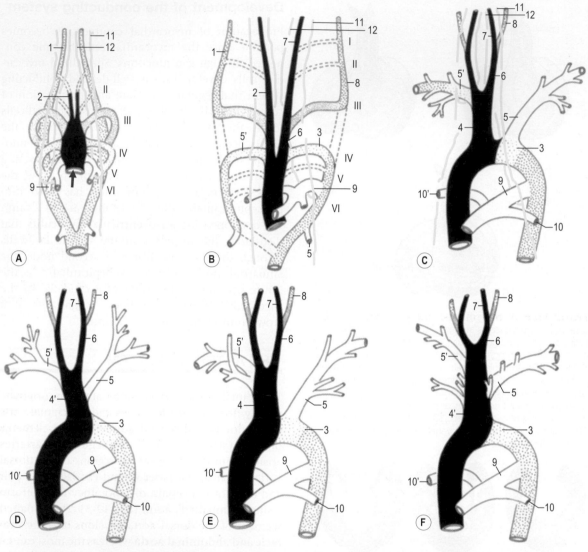

Fig. 12-15: Ventral aspect of the development of the aortic arches. **A:** Initial stage of development. **B:** Progressed, but still species-indifferent stage of development. **C:** Dog. **D:** Cattle. **E:** Pig. **F:** Horse. The red arrows indicate where the truncus arteriosus of the developing heart is attached to the ventral aortae. I-VI: Aortic arches 1-6; 1: Right dorsal aorta; 2: Right ventral aorta; 3: Aorta; 4: Truncus brachiocephalicus; 5: Left subclavian artery; 5′: Right subclavian artery; 6: Common carotid artery; 7: External carotid artery; 8: Internal carotid artery; 9: Ductus arteriosus; 10: Left pulmonary artery; 10′: Right pulmonary artery; 11: N. Vagus; 12: N. laryngeus recurrens. Courtesy Sinowatz and Rüsse (2007).

are continuous with the arterial outlet from the primitive heart, the truncus arteriosus. The ventral aortae extend cranially from the truncus arteriosus which is also where the aortic arches, extending to the dorsal aortae, originate after fusion of the heart tube in the midline (Fig. 12-15). The aortic arches develop in parallel with the gradual increase in the number of somites. Whereas all six aortic arches remain functional in fishes, the **first** and **second arches** are largely rudimentary in mammals and the

fifth arch either remains rudimentary (as in the horse and pig) or never develops at all (as in cattle). Hence, only the **third, fourth and sixth aortic arches** form components of the developing circulatory system. The aortic arches appear in a cranial to caudal sequence and they are not all present at any one time.

The **ventral aortae**, extending cranially from the truncus arteriosus, develop into the **common carotid arteries** and, in the cranial region, into the **external carotid arteries** (Fig. 12-15). The cranial portions of the dorsal aortae develop into the **internal carotid arteries**.

The **first aortic arch** largely degenerates, but a small portion remains and forms **the maxillary artery** as an extension from the external carotid artery. Likewise, despite overall degeneration of the **second aortic arch**, small portions of it do develop into the **hyoid** and **stapedial arteries**. The **third aortic arch** is prominent, but gradually becomes smaller and displaced cranially to form the connection from the common carotid artery to the internal carotid artery.

The parts of the dorsal aortae between the third and fourth aortic arches regress. The **fourth aortic arch** is retained as the **aortic arch** on the **left**, while the **right** arch forms the **right subclavian artery**.

The fate of the **sixth aortic arch** is much different. As explained above, two different flow channels evolve in the truncus arteriosus: one for the lung circulation and one for the body. The channel giving rise to the body circulation, arising from the primitive left ventricle of the heart, supplies blood to the derivatives of the third and fourth aortic arches and the ventral and dorsal aortae; the channel for the lung circulation, arising from the primitive right ventricle, supplies the sixth aortic arches. The sixth aortic arch regresses on the right but, on the left, develops into the **pulmonary trunk**. During embryonic and fetal development, the pulmonary trunk remains connected to the aortic arch through a part of the left sixth aortic arch, the **ductus arteriosus**. At birth, the lumen of the ductus arteriosus is obliterated, but the non-patent structure persists as the **ligamentum arteriosum**. This unilateral persistence of the sixth aortic arch may have a significance for

the function of the intrinsic muscles of the larynx, most of which are innervated by the recurrent laryngeal nerve from the vagus nerve (see Chapter 14). The recurrent laryngeal nerve hooks around the sixth aortic arch, but regression of the arch on the right side releases the nerve to be hooked around the right subclavian artery, under much less tension than its counterpart on the left (Fig. 12-15).

Growth of the embryo and fetus modifies the structure of the arterial system that develops from the aortic arches, the ventral aortae and the cranial portions of the dorsal aortae. Major changes result from the cephalic folding and elongation of the neck that displaces the heart caudally into the thoracic cavity. This causes a pronounced elongation of the common carotid arteries. Moreover, other vessels develop from the aortic arch complex. These include the **subclavian arteries** and their extensions such as the **axillary artery,** important for the front limb. Several species-specific alterations also occur (Fig. 12-15).

The segmental arteries

The dorsal aortae that extend caudally (initially paired, later fused into a single vessel) give rise to **dorsal**, **lateral** and **ventral segmental arteries** (Fig. 12-16).

The **dorsal segmental arteries** are paired and found in each segment along the major portion of the embryo from the most cranial somites back to the sacral region. They run dorsally and give rise to two rami; a dorsal branch that supplies the dorsal body region and the neural tube and its derivatives, and a ventral branch to the ventral body wall. The right and left ventral rami anastomose at the ventral midline and develop into the intercostal arteries in the thoracic region and into lumbar arteries in the abdominal region.

In the cervical region, seven dorsal pairs of segmental arteries are formed. The six most cranial lose their connection to the aorta but the seventh pair remains connected (Fig. 12-17). The six disconnected arteries unite with the seventh on each side to form the paired **vertebral arteries**. These extend cranially where they fuse to form the single **basilary**

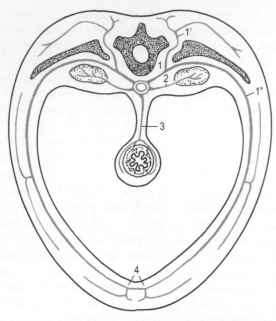

Fig. 12-16: General organization of the segmental arteries. 1: Dorsal segmental artery; 1′: Dorsal portion of dorsal segmental artery; 1″: Ventral portion of dorsal segmental artery; 2: Lateral segmental artery; 3: Ventral segmental artery. Courtesy Sinowatz and Rüsse (2007).

artery which, at the level of the developing mesencephalon, anastomoses with the internal carotid arteries (see Chapter 10).

The **lateral segmental arteries** arise from the unpaired portion of the aorta and supply organs developed from the intermediate mesoderm (Fig. 12-18). During the embryonic phase of development, the **mesonephric, adrenal,** and **genital ridge arteries** are the most prominent lateral segmental arteries (see Chapter 15). With the further development of the urogenital system, these arteries develop into the **ovarian, testicular** and **adrenal arteries,** while the **renal arteries** develop subsequently in conjunction with the formation of the metanephros.

The **ventral segmental arteries** are associated with the yolk sac and the allantois. The most cranial pair, the **omphalomesenteric** or **vitelline arteries,** arises from the unpaired portion of aorta and supply the yolk sac (Fig. 12-4). As the relative size of the

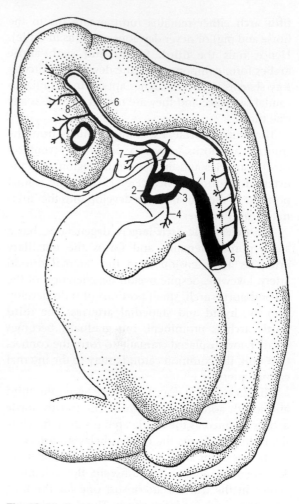

Fig. 12-17: Development of the segmental arteries in the neck region. 1: Dorsal aorta; 2: Ventral aorta; 3: Ductus arteriosus; 4: Pulmonary artery; 5: Vertebral artery; 6: Basilary artery; 7: External carotid artery; 8: Internal carotid artery. Courtesy Sinowatz and Rüsse (2007).

yolk sac diminishes and the final gut takes shape, the **left vitelline artery involutes** and disappears while the **right one develops into the coeliac artery** and the **cranial mesenteric artery** (Fig. 12-18). The coeliac artery supplies the caudal portion of the foregut including the stomach, the cranial portion of the duodenum, the liver, pancreas and spleen; the cranial mesenteric artery, through its localization in the mesentery, supplies the midgut from the

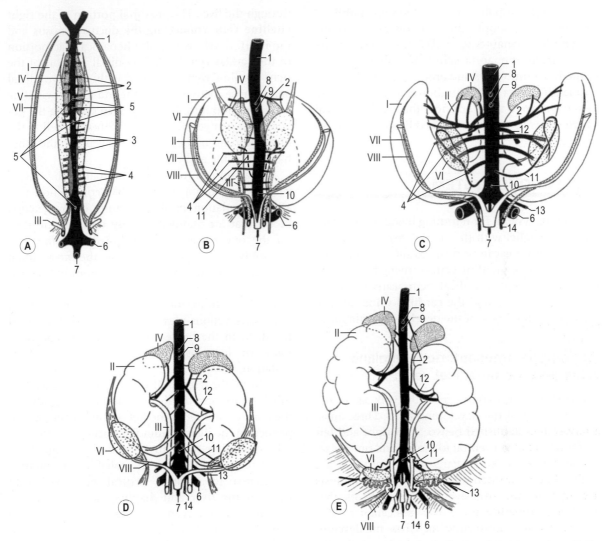

Fig. 12-18: Ventral aspect of the development of the lateral and ventral segmental arteries in the female bovine embryo (A-E). Note that the number of segmental arteries is reduced with development. I: Mesonephros; II: Metanephros; III: Ureter; IV: Adrenal gland; V: Gonadal ridge; VI: Ovary; VII: Wolffian or mesonephric duct; VIII: Müllerian or paramesonephric duct developing into the uterus; 1: Aorta; 2: Adrenal arteries; 3: Gonadal ridge arteries; 4: Mesonephric arteries; 5: Ventral segmental arteries; 6: Umbilical artery; 7: Median sacral artery; 8: Coeliac artery; 9: Cranial mesenteric artery; 10: Caudal mesenteric artery; 11: Ovarian artery; 12: Renal artery to metanephros; 13: External iliac artery; 14: Internal iliac artery. Courtesy Sinowatz and Rüsse (2007).

duodenum to the transverse colon (see Chapter 14). Rotation of the gut takes place around the cranial mesenteric artery which consequently becomes located in the root of the mesentery. Caudal to the cranial mesenteric artery, another, smaller pair of ventral segmental arteries gives rise to the **caudal mesenteric artery** supplying the hindgut from the transverse colon on. With the development of the allantois, the most caudal pair of ventral segmental arteries develops dramatically from the caudal portion of the unpaired aorta to form the **umbilical arteries** which supply the allantois and thus the **placenta** (see Chapter 9; Fig. 12-18). These arteries course from the aorta along the allantoic duct through the umbilicus and arborize in the placenta. Postnatally, parts of the umbilical arteries give rise to the **internal iliac arteries**, the **cranial vesical arteries** as well as the obliterated **ligamentum teres vesicae**.

THE VENOUS SYSTEM

The venous system, for returning blood to the heart, forms in parallel with the arterial system. Basically, three major veins can be distinguished: the **omphalomesenteric** or **vitelline veins** carrying blood from the yolk sac, the **umbilical veins** carrying blood from the placenta, and the **cardinal veins** carrying blood from the body of the developing embryo.

The omphalomesenteric or vitelline veins and the umbilical vein

The vitelline veins course from the yolk sac to the sinus venosus of the developing heart. Three anastomoses are established between the **right** and **left vitelline veins**: two ventral to the gut and one dorsal to the gut (Fig. 12-19). Parts of the right and left vitelline veins and the most cranial anastomosis develop into an extensive capillary network that forms the **sinusoids** of the liver (see Chapter 14).

Initially, the **umbilical veins** bypass the developing liver on their way to the heart. Gradually, however, the proximal portion of the right umbilical vein forms anastomoses with the developing liver sinusoid network. Subsequently this vein involutes and disappears between the umbilicus and the developing liver. Thus, only the **left umbilical vein** is left for transporting oxygenated blood from the placenta to the embryo. This vein establishes an anastomosis with the most proximal portion of the right vitelline vein, and this anastomosis persists more or less throughout embryonic and fetal development as the **ductus venosus** which functions as a shunt for oxygenated blood from the placenta

through the liver. The proximal portion of the **right vitelline vein**, connecting the ductus venosus and the heart, develops into the hepatocardiac portion of the **caudal vena cava**. The distal portion of the right vitelline vein, together with the two distal anastomoses between the right and the left vitelline veins, develop into the **portal vein** draining the gut and its derivatives. The most proximal as well as the distal portions of the left vitelline vein, on the other hand, involute and disappear.

At least in carnivores and ruminants, the ductus venosus includes a sphincter-like constriction that allows regulation of the amounts of oxygenated blood that are shunted directly through the duct on the one hand, and distributed into the liver sinusoids on the other. In the pig, the most caudal portion of the ductus venosus becomes obliterated at an early stage of development and so oxygenated blood from the placenta runs through an alternative venous plexus to the cranial portion of the duct. In the horse, too, the ductus venosus is more or less lost during the second half of gestation.

At birth, the **left umbilical vein** is obliterated and involutes to form the **ligamentum teres hepatis**. In the embryo and fetus, the left umbilical vein is suspended in the **ligamentum falciforme**, a peritoneal fold extending from the umbilicus to the liver. When the vein involutes, this falciform ligament is withdrawn to a small vertical peritoneal fold between the liver and diaphragm ventral to the caudal vena cava. A more or less pronounced fatty deposit is seen along its former line of attachment extending from the umbilicus to the sternum.

The cardinal veins

The development of the body's venous system parallels that of the arterial system and, to begin with, is associated with the prominent mesonephros. Bilaterally symmetrical **cardinal veins**, divided into caudal and cranial portions, are formed soon after the development of the dorsal aortae (Figs. 12-4, 12-20). The right and left **caudal cardinal veins** are found dorsolateral to the mesonephros and carry blood from the caudal portion of the body and the

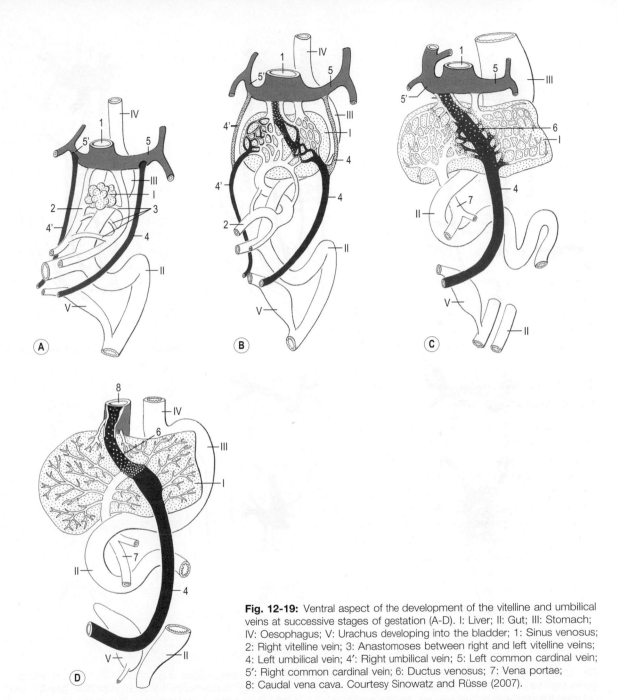

Fig. 12-19: Ventral aspect of the development of the vitelline and umbilical veins at successive stages of gestation (A-D). I: Liver; II: Gut; III: Stomach; IV: Oesophagus; V: Urachus developing into the bladder; 1: Sinus venosus; 2: Right vitelline vein; 3: Anastomoses between right and left vitelline veins; 4: Left umbilical vein; 4': Right umbilical vein; 5: Left common cardinal vein; 5': Right common cardinal vein; 6: Ductus venosus; 7: Vena portae; 8: Caudal vena cava. Courtesy Sinowatz and Rüsse (2007).

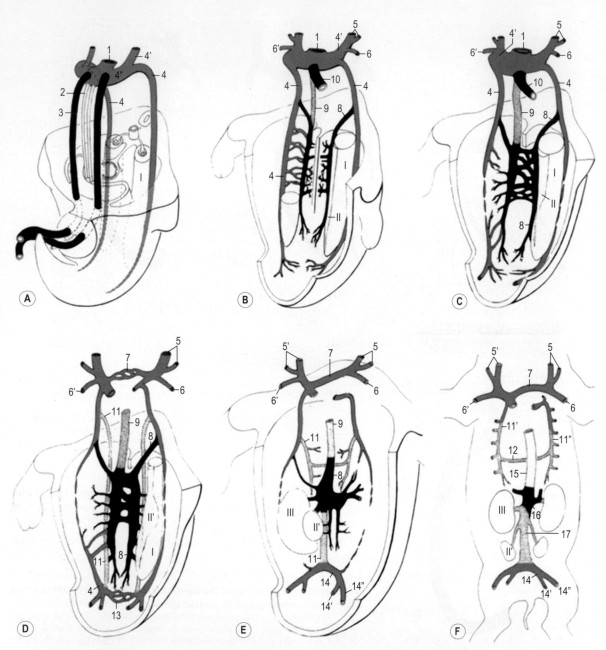

Fig. 12-20: Ventral aspect of the development of the cardinal veins at successive stages of gestation (A-F). Black: Umbilical veins; Light blue: Cardinal veins; Dark blue: Subcardinal veins; Stippled black: Supracardinal veins; Stippled blue: Anastomosis between the right subcardinal vein and hepato-cardiac portion of right vitelline vein; I: Mesonephros; II: Gonadal ridge; II': Gonad; III: Metanephros; 1: Sinus venosus; 2: Vitelline vein; 3: Umbilical vein; 4: Caudal cardinal vein; 4': Cranial cardinal vein; 4": Common cardinal vein; 5: Left internal and external jugular veins; 5': Right internal and external jugular veins; 6: Left subclavian vein; 6': Right subclavian vein; 7: Anastomosis between the cardinal veins; 8: Subcardinal vein; 9: Anastomosis between the right subcardinal vein and hepatocardiac portion of right vitelline vein; 10: Hepatocardiac portion of right vitelline vein; 11: Supracardinal veins; 12: Anastomosis between supracardinal veins; 13: Caudal anastomosis between cardinal veins; 14: Common iliac vein; 14': Internal iliac vein; 14": External iliac vein; 15: Abdominal portion of caudal vena cava; 16: Lumbar portion of caudal vena cava; 17: Pelvic portion of caudal vena cava. Courtesy Sinowatz and Rüsse (2007).

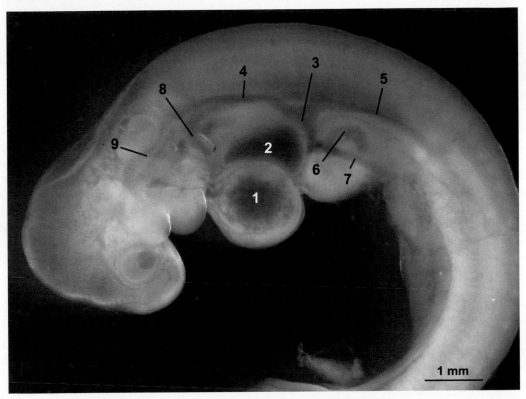

Fig. 12-21: Pig embryo at Day 18 of development displaying blood filled portions of the venous system. The yolk sac has been removed. 1: Heart ventricle; 2: Atrium; 3: Common cardinal vein; 4: Cranial cardinal vein; 5: Caudal cardinal vein; 6: Vitelline vein; 7: Umbilical vein; 8: Vein of third pharyngeal arch; 9: Jugular vein.

mesonephros to the heart. The right and left **cranial cardinal veins** carry blood from the cranial portions of the body, including the head, to the heart. At the level of the heart, the cranial and caudal cardinal veins on each side fuse to form the **common cardinal veins**. These initially open into the sinus venosus (together with the vitelline and umbilical veins) through the right and left sinus horns (Fig. 12-21).

A second venous system arises in the form of the bilateral **subcardinal veins** that run medial to the mesonephros in parallel with the caudal cardinal veins (Fig. 12-20). Cranially, the subcardinal veins drain into the caudal cardinal veins. During the second month of gestation, when the mesonephros is at its developmental peak (at least in ruminants and pigs), the cardinal and subcardinal veins become

connected through numerous anastomoses in this region of the embryo. Moreover, near the adrenal glands, the right and left subcardinal veins form an extensive network of anastomoses. Another prominent anastomosis between the cranial portion of the right subcardinal vein and the hepatocardiac portion of the right vitelline vein later develops into a portion of the **caudal vena cava**.

About two weeks after the formation of the subcardinal veins, a third venous system – the bilateral **supra-cardinal veins** – arises (Fig. 12-20). These veins run along the truncus sympathicus and open cranially into the caudal cardinal veins. The midportions of the right and left caudal cardinal veins are obliterated and the remaining caudal portions make contact with first the subcardinal veins and later the supracardinal veins.

In the final venous system, the **internal** and **external iliac veins,** as well as the **common iliac vein,** arise from the caudal portions of the caudal cardinal veins. The pelvic part of the **caudal vena cava** develops from the right supracardinal vein, the lumbar portion from the anastomoses between the right and left subcardinal vein and from the cardinal veins, the abdominal portion from the anastomosis between the right subcardinal vein and the hepatocardiac portion of the right vitelline vein. The **azygos** and **hemiazygos veins** develop from the cranial portions of the right and left cardinal and supracardinal veins. An anastomosis between the right and left supracardinal veins allows for the formation of the hemiazygos vein (the vein from one side draining into the equivalent vein on the other side). In the horse and carnivores, it is the right vena azygos and the left vena hemiazygos that persist; the opposite is true for the ruminants and pigs, the left vena azygos and the right vena hemiazygos persisting.

Cranial to the heart, the right and left cardinal veins become connected by an anastomosis that provides the functional drainage of the left head and neck region because the proximal portion of the left cranial cardinal vein disappears (Fig. 12-20). The right and left cranial cardinal veins develop into the **right** and **left internal jugular veins**; the **external jugular veins** develop as secondary structures in relation to the formation of the face. The **right** and **left subclavian veins** initially drain into the ipsilateral cranial cardinal veins but, with caudal displacement of the heart, their drainage gradually shifts to the right cranial cardinal vein. In the final venous system, the right and the left cardinal veins both drain into the right common cardinal vein, the left through the anastomosis. In the pig and carnivores, this anastomosis develops to the **left brachiocephalic** vein, with the left internal and external jugular veins and the axillary vein draining into it. The **right brachiocephalic vein** arises from the proximal portion of the right cranial cardinal vein. The right and left brachiocephalic veins unite to form the **cranial vena cava** which opens into the right atrium. In horses and ruminants, the jugular and subclavian veins open directly into the cranial vena cava.

CIRCULATION BEFORE AND AFTER BIRTH

The fetal circulation

During fetal development, the **placenta** is where oxygen and nutrients are taken in and carbon dioxide and metabolites are excreted. The oxygen-rich blood reaches the embryo and fetus through the **umbilical veins**. These veins are paired in the funiculus umbilicalis but only the left one enters the fetus (Fig. 12-22), the right one involuting between the umbilicus and the liver as explained above. The left umbilical vein runs towards the liver where most of the blood flows through the **ductus venosus** directly into the **caudal vena cava**. Only a small fraction enters the sinusoids of the liver; a fraction that can be regulated by the above-mentioned sphincter mechanism in the ductus venosus. On the other hand, the oxygenated blood in the ductus venosus receives deoxygenated blood from the liver and from the inactive digestive tract and its associated organs through the **portal vein**.

In the caudal vena cava, the relatively oxygenated blood mixes with the deoxygenated blood from the caudal portion of the body before it enters the **right atrium** (Fig. 12-23). Here, it is guided towards the foramen ovale by a valve in the caudal vena cava. The pressure in the right atrium is much greater than in the left causing most of the relatively oxygenated blood to pass through the foramen ovale to the **left atrium**. Only a small fraction of the relatively oxygenated blood remains in the **right atrium** and is mixed with the deoxygenated blood, entering from the head and front portion of the body by way of the cranial vena cava, to continue into the **right ventricle** and to be pumped into the **pulmonary trunk**.

In the left atrium, the relatively oxygenated blood mixes with the minimal amount of deoxygenated blood that arrives from the inactive lungs by way of the pulmonary veins. Subsequently, this mixture enters the **left ventricle** and thence the **aorta**. Since the coronary and brachiocephalic arteries are the first branches of the aorta, the blood received by the

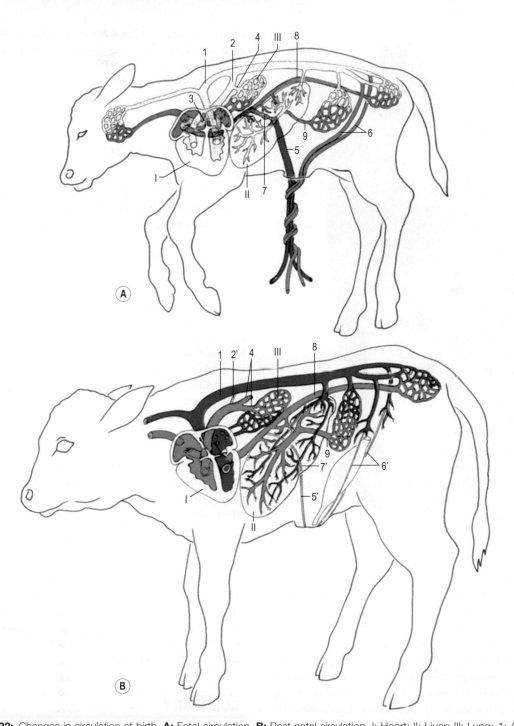

Fig. 12-22: Changes in circulation at birth. **A:** Fetal circulation. **B:** Post natal circulation. I: Heart; II: Liver; III: Lung; 1: Aorta; 2: Ductus arteriosus; 2′: Ligamentum arteriosum; 3: Foramen ovale; 4: Pulmonary arteries; 5: Left umbilical vein; 5′: Ligamentum teres hepatis; 6: Umbilical arteries; 6′: Ligamentum teres vesicae; 7: Ductus venosus; 8: Caudal vena cava; 9: Vena portae. Courtesy Sinowatz and Rüsse (2007).

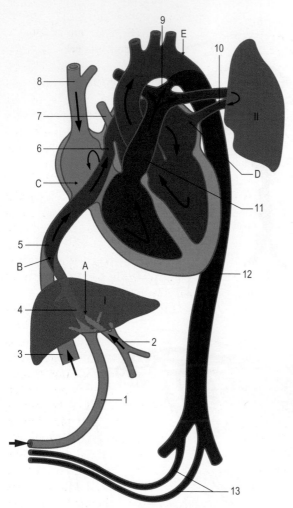

Fig. 12-23: Mixture of oxygenated and deoxygenated blood in the fetal circulation. I: Liver; II: Lung; 1: Left umbilical vein; 2: Vena portae; 3: Caudal vena cava; 4: Ductus venosus; 5: Hepato-cardial portion of caudal vena cava; 6: Foramen ovale; 7: Right pulmonary vein; 8: Cranial vena cava; 9: Ductus arteriosus; 10: Left pulmonary vein; 11: Pulmonary trunk; 12: Aorta; 13: Umbilical arteries. Note that the oxygenated blood is mixed with relatively deoxygenated blood at five locations (A–E). Modified from Sadler (2004).

heart musculature and brain comes from this relatively oxygenated source. The mixed blood in the **truncus pulmonalis** is, due to the high pressure in the fetal lung circulation, to a high degree shunted through the **ductus arteriosus** into the aorta where it mixes with the relatively oxygenated blood from

the left ventricle. This mixture results in blood of medium oxygen tension; it is this that supplies the caudal portion of the fetus. This blood mixture is also, by way of the **umbilical arteries**, returned through the umbilical cord to the placenta for oxygenation.

The changes in circulation at birth

Birth terminates the fetal-maternal association through the placenta. As a result, carbon dioxide tension in the newborn is increased. This stimulates receptors in the respiratory centre in the medulla oblongata and, thus, respiration.

The first **inspiration** expands the lung volume considerably and thus **stimulates pulmonary blood circulation** (Fig. 12-22). The resulting increased blood flow through the pulmonary veins increases the pressure in the left atrium and thereby affects the septum between the right and left atria: higher pressure in the left atrium compresses the thin septum primum against the more substantial septum secundum and **closes the foramen ovale**. Thus, the blood that has been oxygenated in the lungs as a result of the first inspiration flows into the left ventricle (instead of continuing its former diversion to the right side of the heart) and is expelled into the aorta. The **ductus arteriosus closes reflexly**, preventing deoxygenated blood from the pulmonary trunk from entering the aorta. The blood flow from the placenta to the fetus is stopped by the **contraction of the ductus venosus and left umbilical vein**. The blood flow to the placenta is stopped by **contraction of the umbilical arteries**.

The obliterated ductus arteriosus persists as the **ligamentum arteriosum**, the obliterated left umbilical artery as the **ligamentum teres hepatis**, the obliterated umbilical arteries as the **ligamentum teres vesicae**, and the closed foramen ovale remains visible as the **fossa ovalis**.

SUMMARY

The **circulatory system** is the first functional organ system to be formed and includes the **heart**, arteries, veins, and blood. Initially, mesodermal haemangioblasts in the wall of the yolk sac differentiate into angioblasts that form endothelial cells, and inner cells that form blood cells. This occurs in the anterior end of the embryonic disc in the horseshoe-shaped cardiogenic field that develops into the cardiac tube. The intra-embryonic coelom overlying this structure forms the pericardial cavity. Other angioblasts form the paired dorsal aortae, one on each side of the midline. With the antero-posterior 180° folding of the embryo, the cardiac tube is brought to a ventral position with the extensions of the horseshoe that now point anteriorly forming the paired ventral aortae. The ventral and dorsal aortae become connected by the aortic arches. The more posterior regions of the ventral aortae fuse and extend the cardiac tube anteriorly. At its anterior end, the cardiac tube is continuous with the ventral aortae; its posterior end makes contact with the developing venous system. The cardiac tube later develops into a U-shaped structure, divided into the sinus venosus, where the veins open into the cardiac tube, the atrium, the ventricle, the bulbus cordis and the truncus arteriosus, where the outlet into the ventral aortae is found. The sinus venosus becomes incorporated into the right side of the atrium, and the pulmonary veins become partially incorporated into the left side of the atrium. The atrium is divided from the ventricle by the endocardial cushions resulting in separate left and right atrioventricular channels. Subsequently, the cardiac tube is divided into two parallel channels by dividing septae. The atrium is divided by the septum primum and septum secundum leaving the foramen ovale between the two halves. The ventricle and wide posterior portion of the bulbus cordis are divided by the interventricular septum and form the left and the right ventricles, respectively. Finally, the anterior narrow portion of the bulbus cordis and the truncus arteriosus are divided into two channels by the aorticopulmonary septum. Hence, a four-chambered heart with two parallel channels has been formed. Later, the valves as well as the conducting system develop.

The third, fourth, and sixth aortic arches develop into different portions of the final vascular system, whereas the first, second and fifth arches fail to develop or are obliterated. The ventral aortae develop into the common carotid arteries and the internal carotid artery. The third aortic arch forms the connection between the common and internal carotid artery. The fourth aortic arch forms the aortic arch on the left side and the right subclavian artery on the right. The sixth aortic arch forms the pulmonary trunk and, on the left side, the ductus arteriosus connecting the pulmonary trunk and the aortic arch.

The dorsal aortae gradually fuse, and segmental arteries arise from them. Dorsal segmental arteries supply the neural tube and axial body components, lateral segmental arteries supply the urogenital system, and ventral segmental arteries supply the gastrointestinal system and form the coeliac, cranial mesenteric, and caudal mesenteric arteries.

The body's venous system develops from three major components: the vitelline veins, the umbilical veins, and the cardinal veins. The vitelline veins form the hepatocardiac portion of the caudal vena cava, the sinusoids of the liver, and the portal vein. The right umbilical vein is obliterated, but the left umbilical vein has an important function during pregnancy in transporting oxygenated blood from the placenta to the embryo. The cardinal veins and their two generations of successors, the subcardinal and the supracardinal veins, form the rest of the caudal vena cava, the internal and external iliac veins as well as the azygos and hemiazygos veins. In the anterior region of the embryo, the cardinal veins form the right and left internal jugular veins as well as the brachiocephalic veins.

The formation of blood cells, haematopoiesis, is initiated in the yolk sac during the so-called mesoblastic period, is taken over by the liver and spleen during the hepato-lienal period, and, finally, happens primarily in the bone marrow during the medullary period.

During fetal life, oxygenated blood from the left umbilical vein enters the right atrium where most of it passes through the foramen ovale to the left atrium. From there, it enters the left ventricle and the aorta. Blood passing from the right atrium into the right ventricle and into the pulmonary trunk can be shunted into the aorta through the **ductus arteriosus**. The umbilical arteries, in turn, transport the deoxygenated blood to the placenta. At birth, dramatic changes of the circulation occur: the left umbilical vein is obliterated and is retained as the **ligamentum teres hepatis**, the foramen ovale is closed, the ductus arteriosus is obliterated and retained as **ligamentum arteriosum**, and the umbilical arteries are obliterated and retained as the **ligamentum teres vesicae**.

Box 12-1 Molecular regulation of the development of the vascular system

During the process of gastrulation, lateral plate mesoderm is split into somatic (parietal) and visceral (splanchnic) portions. Visceral mesoderm, together with the underlying endoderm, forms the splanchnopleura. The first haemangiogenic mesoderm is formed in the wall of the yolk sac giving rise to both blood and blood vessels. The definitive haematopoietic stem cells in fish, amphibians, birds and mammals are, however, thought to be formed intra-embryonically, in the visceral lateral plate mesoderm closer to the aorta. This region has been called **aorta-gonad-mesonephric (AGM) region**. Haematopoietic stem cells within the AGM region express genes encoding critical regulators of their formation, like **SCL**, **Runx-1**, **c-Myb** and **LMO-2** in addition to genes encoding cell surface markers like **CD34** and the receptor molecule **c-Kit**. The proto-oncogene *c-Myb* specifically affects haematopoiesis in the para-aortic AMG region. The haematopoietic stem cells from the AGM-region later colonize the fetal liver and probably also the bone marrow, the major site of blood formation throughout adult life. A puzzling paradox, however, is that the number of pluripotent haematopoietic stem cells in the AGM region is very small. Recent data have shown that the placenta is an additional early source of blood stem cells in mammals. The murine placenta contains haematopoietic stem cells within the vascular labyrinth region. Pluripotent haematopoietic stem cells appear to be generated along with the endothelium of the placental blood vessels. This suggests that haemangioblasts are formed in the placenta as well as in the yolk sac. The numbers of these cells appear large enough to account for the population of stem cells later found in the liver. The liver may therefore receive stem cells from both the AGM region and the placenta, with a potential third contribution from yolk sac haemangioblasts.

The haemangiogenic cells become specified through **BMP** and **FGF** signalling originating from the underlying hypoblast and endoderm. Inhibitory signals from the neural tube (**Wnt proteins**) and the notochord (**Noggin** and **Chordin**) prevent the formation of cardiogenic fields in the posterior parts of the embryo. In the anterior portion of the embryo, on the contrary, hypoblast and endodermal cells within the developing foregut produce signalling molecules, including **Cerberus**, **Dickkopf** and **Crescent,** antagonizing the neural tube Wnt signalling. Cardiogenic mesoderm therefore becomes specified through BMP (and FGF) signalling in the absence of Wnt signalling. This leads to expression of *Nkx2.5*, a master gene for cardiac development.

In the chick and the mouse, it has been shown that posterior cardiac domains (the sinus venosus and atrium) become established through exposure to high concentrations of **retinoic acid**, the local accumulation of which is ultimately controlled by Hox genes. Anterior cardiac domains are specified through the action of, for example, the transcription factor **Tbx5** that later also plays an important role in cardiac septation. Heart looping and formation of heart chambers is dependent on the left-right patterning proteins (**Nodal**, **Lefty-2**; see Chapter 7). Ultimately, **Hand1** proteins become restricted to the left ventricle (overlapping with *Tbx5* expression) and **Hand2** proteins to the right. The truncus arteriosus is derived primarily from *Pax3*-expressing neural crest cells.

Blood vessels form independently from the heart, eventually linking up to it. In the first phase of vasculogenesis, mesodermal cells in the splanchnopleura form haemangioblasts under the inhibitory control of **Wnt** signalling originating from the neural tube. During the second phase of vasculogenesis, the haemangioblasts condense, giving rise to blood islands in which blood progenitor cells and endothelial cells eventually form. Vascular endothelial growth factors (**VEGF**s), a group of currently seven members (of which five are known in mammals), are involved in the formation of endothelial cells, their resultant formation of primary capillary plexuses, and the subsequent phases of angiogenesis. Three tyrosine kinase receptors for VEGF have been identified: VEGFR-1 (Flt1), VEGFR-2 (Flk1), and VEGFR-3. **VEFG-A**, also known as vascular permeability factor (VPF), bind to both VEGF-R1 and VEGF-R2. **VEGF-R2** is involved in formation, proliferation and migration of endothelial cells, while **VEGF-R1** is involved in capillary tube formation. **VEGF-B** and

Placental Growth Factor (**PIGF**) only bind to VEGF-R1. **VEGF-C** and **VEGF-D** are, in particular, known to act as lymphangiogenic growth factors acting through **VEGF-R3**.

Primary capillary plexuses contain two types of endothelial cells: arterial **ephrin-B2**-expressing endothelial cells and venous **EphB4**-expressing endothelial cells. EphB4 is a receptor for ephrin-B2, and during angiogenesis, ligand–receptor interactions ensure fusion of the venous capillaries with arterial capillaries. Maturation of newly formed vessels involves recruitment of pericytes that form the smooth muscle cells covering arteries. **Angiopoietins** and **platelet-derived growth factor** (**PDGF**) are known to be involved in this process.

FURTHER READING

Broccoli, F. and Carinci, P. (1973): Histological and histochemical analysis of the obliteration processes of ductus arteriosus Botalli. Acta Anat. 85:69–83.

Canfield, P.J. and Johnson, R.S. (1984): Morphological aspects of prenatal haematopoietic development in the cat. Zbl. Vet. Med. C. 13:197–221.

Coulter, C.B. (1909): The early development of the aortic arches of the cat, with especial reference to the presence of a fifth arch. Anat. Rec. 3:578–592.

Dickson, A.D. (1956): The ductus venosus of the pig. J. Anat. 90:143–152.

Field, E.J. (1946): The early development of the sheep heart. J. Anat. 80:75–85.

Field, E.J. (1951): The development of the conducting system in the heart of the sheep. Br. Heart J. 13:129–147.

Forsgren. S., Strehler, E. and Thornell, L.E. (1982): Differentiation of Purkinje fibres and ordinary ventricular and atrial myocytes in the bovine heart: an immuno- and enzyme histochemical study. Histochem. J. 14:929–942.

Grimes, M., Greenstein, J.S. and Foley, R.C. (1958): Observations on the early embryology of the bovine heart in embryos with six to twenty paired somites. Am. J. Vet. Res. 19:591–599.

Hammond, W.S. (1937): The developmental transformations of the aortic arches in the calf (Bos taurus), with especial reference to the formation of the arch of the aorta. Am. J. Anat. 62:149–177.

Lewis, F.T. (1906): Fifth and sixth aortic arches and related pharyngeal pouches in pig and rabbit. Anat. Anz. 28:506–513.

Los, I.A. and van Eijndthoven, E. (1973): The fusion of the endocardial cushions in the heart of the chick embryo. Z. Anat. Entwicklungsgesch. 141:55–75.

Martin, E.W. (1960): The development of the vascular system in 5–21 somite dog embryos. Anat. Rec. 137:378.

McGaedy, T.A., Quinn, P.J., FitzPatrick, E.S. and Ryan, T. (2006): Veterinary Embryology. Blackwell Publishing Ltd., Oxford, UK.

Muir, A.R. (1951): The development of the sinu-atrial node in the heart of the sheep. J. Anat. 85:430.

Muir, A.R. (1954): The development of the ventricular part of the conducting tissue in the heart of the sheep. J. Anat. 88:381–391.

Noden, D.M. and de Lahunta, A. (1985): The embryology of domestic animals. Williams & Wilkens, Baltimore, London.

Rüsse, I. and Sinowatz, F. (1998): Lehrbuch der Embryologie der Haustiere, 2nd edn, Parey Buchverlag, Berlin.

Sadler, T.W. (2006): Langman's Medical Embryology. 10th edition, Lippincott Williams and Wilkins, Baltimore, Maryland, USA.

Scavelli, C., Weber, E., Aglianò, M., Cirulli, T., Nico, B., Vacca, A. and Ribatti, D. (2004): Lymphatics at the crossroads of angiogenesis and lymphangiogenesis. J. Anat. 204:433–449.

Shaner, R. (1929): The development of the atrioventricular node, bundle of His, and sinu-atrial node in the calf, with a description of a third embryonic node-like structure. Anat. Rec. 44:85–99.

Srivastava, D. (2006): Making or breaking the heart: from lineage determination to morphogenesis. Cell 126:1037–1048.

Vitums, A. (1969): Development and transformation of the aortic arches in the equine embryos with special attention to the formation of the definitive arch of the aorta and the common brachiocephalic trunk. Z. Anat. Entwicklungsgesch. 128:243–270.

Vitums, A. (1981): The embryonic development of the equine heart. Zbl. Vet. Med. C. 10:193–211.

CHAPTER 13

Morten Vejlsted

Development of the immune system

The adult body employs multiple layers of defence against foreign materials. These defences are derived from all three embryonic germ layers. **Physical barriers,** comprising intact epithelia on external and internal body surfaces (i.e. the skin and gastrointestinal tract) serve as a first layer of defence and are derived from the ectoderm and endoderm, respectively. In contrast, cells central to the second and third layers of defence, the **innate (pre-existing) immunity** and **specific (induced/acquired) immunity** systems, are derived from the mesoderm. The **innate immunity system** can act very rapidly but **lacks any form of memory**; important components of this system are the **granulocytes** of the myeloid cell lineage that develop from haematopoietic stem cells. The **acquired or adaptive immunity system,** of the lymphoid cell lineage, on the other hand has **memory**; cells of the **lymphocyte** lineage form descendants with effector as well as memory competence. Acquired immunity is dependent on microbial colonization of the gut and is therefore a postnatal phenomenon. Potential pathogen microbes in the gut and on the external body surfaces exhibit high mutation rates. In essence, acquired immunity is all about evolution of the lymphocyte cell lineage having the ability to somatically mutate surface receptors to keep up with this continual exposure to new challenges.

During intra-uterine life, the **placenta** largely protects the embryo and fetus from exposure to foreign pathogens (see Chapter 9). This results in newborn animals being more or less immunologically naïve – equipped with the fundamentals of the acquired immune system, but still awaiting antigen stimulation for its final development. To compensate for

this, intake of antibody-laden **colostrum** from the mother protects the newborn passively during the first few weeks post partum,. Then, however, the newborn's own immune system has to mature for the animal to survive. Since this is a textbook on embryology, the focus will be on intra-uterine formation of the cells and organs of the immune system. For descriptions of the post-natal maturation of the immune system and the immune response, as well as immunological specificity and memory, textbooks such as 'Veterinary Immunology: An Introduction' by Tizard (2008) should be consulted.

THE LYMPHOCYTES

It has been customary to begin any description of the cells of the developing immune system with a discussion of haematopoietic stem cell formation in the yolk sac. Recently, however, it has been shown that the haematopoietic potential of this yolk-sac stem cell population is limited compared to that of stem cells appearing in the intra-embryonic **aorta-gonad-mesonephros (AGM) region** shortly afterwards (see Chapter 12). Thus, it is now generally accepted that first the fetal **liver,** then the **thymus and** the **spleen** (during the hepato-lienal period), and finally the **bone marrow** (during the medullary period) are seeded by haematopoietic stem cells from the AGM region, eventually giving rise to the full complement of the lymphoid, erythroid and myeloid cell lineages. It is the **lymphoid cell lineage** that gives rise to the **Natural Killer (NK) cells** and **B and T lymphocytes** whereas the **myeloid cell** lineage gives rise to neutrophil, eosinophil and the basophil **granulocytes.**

Differentiation of lymphocytes begins in the **thymus** as early as during the hepato-lienal period. Later, **gut-associated lymphoid tissue** develops, followed by the appearance of **lymph nodes**, **tonsils**, and the **spleen**. With the onset of the medullary period, the **bone marrow** becomes a site of both haematopoiesis, including lymphopoiesis, and lymphocyte differentiation. The bone marrow, the thymus, and also the gut-associated lymphoid tissue comprise the **primary lymphoid tissues**, in which cells of the lymphoid cell lineage differentiate and mature. From the primary lymphoid tissues, immune-competent lymphocytes eventually reach **secondary lymphoid tissues** where immune responses to antigens occur in the newborn animal. Secondary lymphoid tissues include the **lymph nodes**, **spleen**, **mucosa-associated lymphoid tissues (MALT)** and **skin associated lymphoid tissues (SALT)**.

Differentiation of the lymphoid cell lineages

Based on function and specific cell-surface molecules, the **lymphoid cell lineage** may be divided into large lymphocytes with a granular cytoplasm and small lymphocytes with almost no cytoplasm. The **large granular lymphocytes** are, together with the granulocytes, effector cells in the innate immune system, and are also known as **Natural Killer** or **NK cells**. The **small lymphocytes** comprise several sublineages, the two major ones being the **T** and **B lymphocytes.** T and B lymphocytes differ in function, depending on their various cell-surface receptors (see below). Functionally, **T lymphocytes** are said to mediate a **cellular immune response** to foreign macromolecules either directly (by killing virus-infected cells, for example) or indirectly, through activation of specialized phagocytes, including tissue macrophages. **B lymphocytes**, in contrast, are said to mediate a **humoral immune response** through their differentiation into antibody-producing **plasma cells**. The antibodies bind to set areas on foreign macromolecules (**antigens**) known as **epitopes**, which may be parts of cell-surface proteins, polysaccharides, or glycosaminoglycans on invading bacteria or viruses. The binding mediates phagocytosis of the intruders and this mechanism is known as **opsonization**. Antibodies may also activate certain serum proteins (collectively known as the complement system) thereby mediating cell lysis, or may bind to and neutralize bacterial toxins or viruses.

The T lymphocyte

As outlined above, T lymphocytes differentiate from common haematopoietic stem cells initially formed in the AGM region. From there, a small population seeds the **Thymus** (hence the name) early in fetal development. In the thymus, progenitor T lymphocytes proliferate, mature and form cells each of which is committed to recognizing a single epitope on either self- or non-self antigens. The basis of this specificity lies in the **T cell receptor (TCR)**. Each mature T lymphocyte carries only one type of TCR on its cell surface (around 10^5 of that particular type per cell). The thymus harbours a huge number of **clones**, i.e. individual T lymphocyte populations, and all T lymphocytes within a clone share the same TCR characteristics.

In contrast to antibodies, the TCR only recognizes epitopes associated with **major histocompatibility complex (MHC)** molecules. These are special types of cell-surface molecules and are sites for presentation of an animal's own or foreign epitopes. There are two classes of MHC molecules: **MHC class I** molecules, expressed by all nucleated cells except nerve cells; and **MHC class II** molecules, expressed on special antigen-presenting cells and on B lymphocytes. **CD4** and **CD8** are other types of cell-surface molecules, defined and grouped through the use of specific antibodies (CD is an acronym for 'Cluster Defined'). During maturation in the thymus, clones of T lymphocytes differentiate into either CD4-expressing T helper lymphocytes (Th cells) or CD8-expressing cytotoxic lymphocytes (Tc cells). **CD4-expressing Th cells** only recognize epitopes presented by **MHC class II** molecules. Such epitopes are presented by antigen-presenting cells or B lymphocytes, which characteristically present epitopes that are parts of **exogenous** peptides from foreign particles or from pathogens that have invaded the organism and been subjected to endocytosis. **CD8-expressing Tc cells**, on the other hand, only recognize epitopes presented by **MHC class I** molecules; these are characteristically **endogenous**, reflecting peptides synthesized within the cell. Virus-infected cells or tumour cells for example, in which protein synthesis is altered, may be recognized in this way by Tc cells through presentation of these epitopes of 'non-self' proteins by MHC class I molecules.

During the **maturation of the T lymphocytes** in the thymus, about 98% of the cells are eliminated through the process of apoptosis. This elimination includes **two selection rounds**, the first ensuring that only those T lymphocytes that recognize MHC molecules survive, and the second making sure that all T lymphocytes recognizing 'self' epitopes are eliminated. Before their maturation, the T lymphocytes express neither CD4 nor CD8. These immature T lymphocytes are mainly located in the subcapsular thymic areas where the surrounding reticular cells are rich in both MHC class I and MHC class II molecules. During maturation, T lymphocytes move into deeper parts of the cortex, where expression of both CD4 and CD8 is initiated. The consequent 'double positive' T lymphocytes, i.e. those expressing both CD4 and CD8, then undergo an initial, or **positive selection** in which their TCRs are tested against the MHC molecules on surrounding reticular cells. Only T lymphocytes recognizing 'self' MHC molecules will survive this process. The positive selection forms the basis of the **MHC restriction** that results in T lymphocyte acceptance of 'self' MHC molecules only. The selected T lymphocytes then move deeper into the thymus where, upon reaching the cortico-medullary junction, the selected 'double positive' T lymphocytes undergo the second, or **negative selection** for 'self' reactivity. This results in the elimination of T lymphocytes carrying TCRs recognizing epitopes of 'self' antigens. In this way, 'self' is accepted, forming the basis of **immunological tolerance**.

One problem inherent to these selections is that during the positive selection, T lymphocytes recognizing 'self' MHC molecules are selected *for*, whereas during the negative selection, T lymphocytes recognizing 'self' MHC, and other, molecules are selected *against*. The reason for this paradoxical process, which would ultimately leave no surviving T lymphocytes, is still an enigma. One favoured hypothesis to explain the contradiction is that the positive selection results in populations of T lymphocytes with receptors having a range of affinities, from low to high, for 'self' MHC molecules. Through the negative selection, T-lymphocytes with high affinity receptors are weeded out while those with low affinity survive. Thus, instead of using an 'either/or' criterion, the second, negative selection occurs according to 'more or less' guidelines.

Only T lymphocytes that have survived both positive and negative selection move into the medulla, and then as either CD4-positive, MHC class II-restricted T helper (Th) lymphocytes or CD8-positive, MHC class I-restricted cytotoxic (Tc) lymphocytes. The end result is a selection for TCRs (on either Th or Tc cells) specifically recognizing a combination of 'self' MHC molecules and foreign or altered epitopes. The T lymphocytes, however, are functionally naïve when they leave the thymus. Subsequently, they circulate in the blood, lymphatic tissues, and lymph to perform what may be termed 'immunological surveillance'. Only upon TCR recognition of foreign or altered epitopes presented by the MHC class I or II molecules will the T lymphocytes undergo final differentiation, perform their role in the cellular immune response, and establish memory.

The B-lymphocyte

As is true of T lymphocytes, it is generally accepted that B lymphocytes differentiate from a common haematopoietic stem cell. In many species, B lymphocyte development and maturation takes place in the **Bone marrow**. However, at least in the sheep, the major site for these processes appears to be in an ileal **Peyer's patch.** This intestinal primary lymphoid organ appears to be a mammalian equivalent of the avian bursa of Fabricius. Like the thymus (see later), it involutes around puberty and B lymphocytes take up residence in the bone marrow and secondary lymphoid tissues and organs, including other Peyer's patches found in the intestines of the adult animal.

Progenitor B lymphocytes, like T lymphocytes, initially proliferate and mature to form clones of cells individually committed to recognize only one epitope on either 'self' or 'non-self' antigens through their **B cell receptors (BCRs)**. The BCRs are immunoglobulins of the IgM type representing membrane-bound antibodies. In contrast to the TCR, the BCR is able to recognize epitopes without involving MHC molecules. B lymphocytes express both MHC class I and II molecules, the latter being characteristic of antigen-presenting cells. B lymphocytes are selected, like T lymphocytes, through positive and negative selection eliminating B lymphocytes recognizing 'self' epitopes. Eventually, mature, naïve B lymphocytes, like the T lymphocytes, leave their primary lymphatic organ (either the ovine ileal Peyer's patch or the bone marrow), circulate in the blood and lymph, and colonize secondary lymphatic tissues.

The circulation and final differentiation of lymphocytes

The T and B lymphocytes circulate throughout the organism once or twice a day, spending most time in special areas of the **secondary lymphoid tissues** known as the **T and B dependent zones**. In the adult, these zones are where **immune reactions** to foreign macromolecules most commonly take place because the zones contain special antigen-presenting cells, expressing MHC class II molecules. In utero, however, such an immune reaction cannot occur because it requires both cellular T lymphocyte-mediated and humoral B lymphocyte-mediated elements, a combination that does not materialize until after birth. Put simply, an immune reaction depends on activation of CD4-positive Th cells, which depends on the epitopes being 'properly' presented by the MHC class II antigen-presenting cells. In the specialized microenvironment of the second-

ary lymphatic tissues, naïve lymphocytes become activated as a result so that they can form lymphoblasts.

The T lymphoblasts eventually differentiate into **memory T lymphocytes** and **effector cells**, whereas B lymphoblasts differentiate into **memory B lymphocytes** and **plasmablasts**. As their names imply, these lymphocytes carry immunological memory. In contrast to the naïve B lymphocytes, memory B lymphocytes express, in addition to IgM, BCRs of the IgG, IgA and IgE type directed towards the specific epitope selected for. Plasmablasts eventually differentiate into **plasma cells**. In contrast to the membrane-bound BCRs on their progenitor plasmablasts, plasma cells will produce a specific BCR molecule, an **antibody**, for secretion. Initially, only antibodies of the IgM type will be secreted. Later, other types of antibodies will also be produced.

LYMPHOID ORGANS AND TISSUES

Lymphoid organs and tissues may be classified according to their roles in the generation of lymphocytes, regulation of lymphocyte production, and provision of environments for trapping foreign antigens. Organs that regulate the initial development and maturation of lymphocytes, including the positive and negative selections, are called **primary lymphoid organs**. T lymphocytes develop and mature in the <u>thymus</u>. B lymphocytes may mature in a variety of organs, depending on the species: in birds, in the <u>bursa of Fabricius</u> associated with the cloaca; in most mammals in the **bone marrow**; in the sheep at least, in the intestinal lymphoid tissues known as the ileal **Peyer's patch**. It is important to stress again that there is no presentation of foreign antigens in primary lymphoid organs and, therefore, no immune responses related to acquired immunity.

Thymus

The thymus is a primary lymphoid organ where T lymphocytes mature. In ruminants, the thymus forms around Day 40 of gestation, in carnivores around Day 30, and in the horse around Day 60. It is located in the neck and thoracic inlet regions, depending on the species. As a proportion of body mass, its size is greatest in the newborn animal in which the full complement of (naïve) T lymphocytes has already been produced. Around puberty, the thymus involutes and the parenchyma is gradually replaced by adipose tissue although it appears to remain functional even in the adult animal.

When fully formed the thymus is a paired organ composed of lobules of loosely packed epithelial cells covered by a connective tissue capsule. An abnormally thick basement membrane underlying a continuous layer of epithelial cells surrounding the blood vessels in the thymus forms the **blood-thymus barrier**, protecting the maturing T lymphocytes from exposure to foreign antigens. No lymphatic vessels leave the thymus.

The **thymic reticulum** develops from the ventral **endodermal** part of the **third pharyngeal pouches**, closely linked to the development of the parathyroid glands from the dorsal parts of these pouches (Fig. 14-11). In contrast, the **thymic capsule** and connective tissue septae originate from the neural-crest-derived **mesenchyme** of the third branchial arch surrounding the thymic primordium (see Chapter 14). The fact that an epithelium forms the reticulum of a lymphoid organ is unique for the thymus and palatine tonsil; in other lymphoid organs, primary and secondary, the whole framework is thought to be of pure mesenchymal origin, derived from the neural crest or the mesoderm.

The ventral portion of the third pharyngeal pouches is hollow at first, but continued development separates the pouch from its attachment to the pharyngeal cavity, and a solid body of endodermal cells is formed that expands as it migrates ventrally and caudally (Fig. 14-11). As the heart migrates into the thoracic cavity (see Chapter 12), parts of the thymus are drawn caudally into the cranial mediastinum. Thus, the thymus as a whole forms a Y-shaped structure, fused at its caudal end and with its bilateral cranial end still attached to the developing pharynx. In the newborn, this overall structure is best conserved in ruminants where an unpaired thoracic part and left and right cervical parts can be recognized. Both cervical and thoracic parts also form in pigs, but to a lesser degree, and in the horse and dog only the thoracic parts develop.

Eventually, the endoderm-derived reticulated stroma of the thymus is **infiltrated by parenchyma consisting of T lymphocyte precursors** of haematopoietic stem cell origin (see above) and other cells of mesodermal origin. T lymphocyte progenitors, initially negative for both CD4 and CD8 molecules, seed the cortex, especially the subcapsular areas where epithelial reticular cells are rich in molecules, both MHC class-I and class-II molecules. These epithelial cells are also known as 'nurse cells' because they regulate initial T-lymphocyte proliferation and maturation. They do so by secreting signalling molecules together known as 'thymic hormones', some of which depend on zinc for their function. Thus, zinc-deficient animals may bear progeny deficient in T lymphocytes. The further maturation of the T lymphocytes and their migration into the deeper portions of the thymus and into the blood stream and the secondary lymphatic organs has been described above.

Bone marrow/ileal Peyer's patch

In newborn ruminants and pigs, lymphoid tissue is present in the aboral portion of the small intestine. Pre-natally, however, at least in the sheep, an ileal **Peyer's patch** exists and is regarded as a **primary lymphoid organ** for B lymphocyte maturation – functionally equivalent to the bursa of Fabricius in birds. Whether this is true of other ruminants and the pig is unclear. In the sheep, the size of the ileal Peyer's patch as a proportion of body mass is greatest around birth. The lymphoid structures seen postnatally in the small intestine of ruminants and pigs are *secondary* lymphoid organs (part of GALT, see below) that contain both B and T lymphocytes and persist throughout life.

For now, in domestic species other than the sheep, the **bone marrow** is to be regarded as the primary lymphoid tissue where positive and negative selection among B lymphocytes is thought to occur in the outer region. In all domestic animal species, the bone marrow later functions as a **secondary lymphoid tissue.**

Lymphatic vasculature, lymph nodes and other secondary lymphoid tissues

Blood vessels originate from mesoderm-derived endothelial cell precursors (**angioblasts**) that proliferate and organize into primitive vascular channels (vasculogenesis; see Chapter 12). Channels grow, remodel and form primitive networks by endothelial sprouting and splitting (angiogenesis). The lymphatic vasculature develops in parallel with the blood vasculature but more slowly.

Whereas the blood vasculature forms a continuous loop, with arteries and veins connected through capillaries, the lymphatic system is an **open-ended, one-way transit system,** consisting of tissue capillaries, collecting vessels and ducts, that finally drains into the venous circulation through the jugular vein or the cranial vena cava. The embryonic lymphatic endothelial cells are generally considered to arise from veins, bud off and form **primary lymphatic sacs.** From primary lymphatic sacs, additional budding of cells gradually extends capillary networks surrounding tissues and organs. The lymphatic system first appears as **six primary lymph sacs** forming in an anterior-posterior sequence (Fig. 13-1): the **paired jugular lymph sacs** in the cervical region; a **retroperitoneal lymph sac** on the dorsal

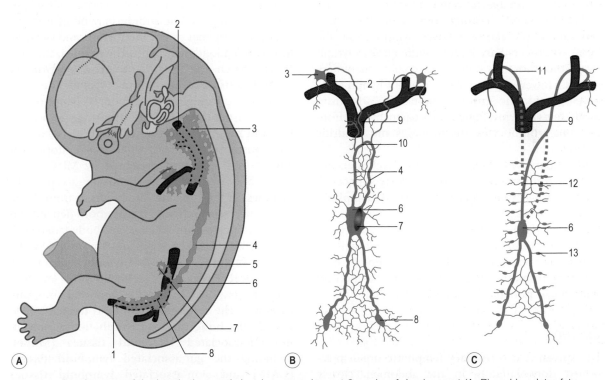

Fig. 13-1: Development of the lymphatic vessels in a human embryo at 9 weeks of development (A, B) and in a later fetus (C). 1: Femoral vein; 2: Internal jugular vein; 3: Jugular lymph sac; 4: Thoracic duct; 5: Caudal vena cava; 6: Cisterna chyli; 7: Retroperitoneal lymph sac; 8: Posterior lymph sac; 9: Cranial vena cava; 10: Anastomosis; 11: Right lymphatic duct; 12: Final thoracic duct; 13: Lymph node. Dotted lines in "D" indicate involuted structures. Modified from Carlson (2004).

body wall at the root of the mesentery in the abdominal cavity; the **cisterna chyli** in the same region, but later and more dorsally at the level of the dorsal aortae; and the paired **posterior lymph sacs** at about the same time as the cysterna chyli. Lymphatic vessels connect these lymph sacs. Two major lymphatic vessels connect the cisterna chyli with the jugular lymph sacs, and an anastomosis forms between these two vessels. The **thoracic duct** develops from these structures with the right-hand vessel forming the caudal portion and the left-hand vessel forming its cranial portion.

The **lymph nodes** are **secondary lymphoid organs**, inserted into the course of the collecting lymph vessels, and serving as local filters in the lymph stream as it makes its way towards the blood circulation. The nodes tend to arise in groups, **lymph centres**, at strategically important sites. For example, the medial retropharyngeal lymph centre receives all lymph draining from the head, the deep cervical lymph centre receives lymph from the neck, and the axillary lymph centre receives lymph from the thoracic limb and cranial mammary glands. However, little is known about lymph node development. The stroma is thought to arise from local mesenchyme, and the parenchyma from invading lymphocytes, macrophages and dendritic cells.

Secondary lymphatic organs also develop in conjunction with internal or external body surfaces in the form of the **mucosa-associated lymphoid tissues** (MALT), comprising the **gut-associated lymphoid tissue (GALT)**, and the **skin-associated lymphoid tissues (SALT)**. One component of MALT is the **palatine tonsil**, the reticulum of which develops from the endoderm within the **second pharyngeal pouch** (see Chapter 14).

Spleen

The **spleen** is a **secondary lymphatic organ** positioned dorso-laterally in the abdomen, closely attached to the ventricle by the gastrolienal ligament, a part of the dorsal mesogastrium (see Chapter 14). Like the lymph nodes, the spleen functions as a filter with specialized antigen-presenting cells catching inflowing antigens. However, in contrast to the lymph nodes, the spleen is **inserted into the blood stream** and so filters blood-borne antigens. The primordium of the spleen, like that of the lymph nodes, arises from local mesenchyme derived from mesoderm. In the second trimester, the complex vascular structure of the **red pulp** has formed. As described in Chapter 12, the spleen overlaps with, and succeeds, the fetal liver as a principal organ of haematopoiesis. The **white pulp** forms following infiltration of the organ by lymphocytes, macrophages and dendritic cells.

SUMMARY

The parenchyma of the immune system is of mesodermal origin, tracing back to the **haematopoietic stem cells** appearing in the aorta-gonad-mesonephros (AGM) region. The stroma may be of ectodermal, mesenchymal or (in the thymus and palatine tonsil) of endodermal origin. The **thymus**, the ileal **Peyer's patch** and the **bone marrow** are **primary lymphoid tissues** where lymphocytes mature independently of antigen stimulation. **T lymphocytes** mature in the thymus where they undergo a **positive** and **negative selection** to make them competent, postnatally, to react to foreign epitopes (or altered 'self' epitopes) presented by MHC molecules, but, on the other hand, to accept 'self' epitopes. In the fetus they are hindered from doing so by the placenta. Hence, the newborn depends on a supply of **colostrum**, the first antibody-laden milk that it drinks. T lymphocytes are responsible for the **cellular immune response**. **B lymphocytes** mature in the ileal Peyer's patch or in the bone marrow, and are responsible for the **humoral immune response**. The **secondary lymphoid tissues**, which include the **bone marrow**, **lymph nodes**, **spleen**, **mucosa-associated lymphoid tissues** (MALT), including **the gut-associated lymphoid tissues (GALT)** and **skin-associated lymphoid tissues (SALT)**, are sites where antigens are presented and where immune responses are elicited in the animal after birth. In the fetus, an immune reaction is not elicited.

FURTHER READING

Blackburn, C.C. and Manley, N.R. (2004): Developing a new paradigm for thymus organogenesis. Nature Rev. Immunology 4:278–289.

Carlson, B.M. (2004): Human embryology and developmental biology. Mosby, Philadelphia, PA USA.

Felsburg, P.J. (2002): Overview of immune system development in the dog: comparison with humans. Human Exp. Toxicology 21:487–492.

Kindt, T.J., Goldsby, R.A. and Osborne, B.A. (2007): Kuby Immunology. W.H. Freeman and Co., New York, USA.

Ling, K.-W. and Dzierzak, E. (2002): Ontogeny and genetics of the hemato/lymphopoiteic system. Current Opinion in Immunology 14:186–191.

Mebius, R.E. (2003): Organogenesis of lymphoid tissues. Nature Rev. Immunology 3:292–303.

Oliver, G. (2004): Lymphatic vascululature development. Nature Rev. Immunology 4:35–45.

Oliver, G. and Harvey, H. (2002): A stepwise model of the development of lymphatic vasculature. Ann. N.Y. Acad. Sci. 979:159–165.

Sinkora, J., Rehakova, Z., Sinkora, M., Cukrowska, B. and Tlaskalova-Hogenova, H. (2002): Early development of immune system in pigs. Vet. Immunol. Immunopath. 87:301–306.

Tizard, I.R (2008): Veterinary Immunology – an Introduction. 8th edn, W B Saunders Co., Philadelphia, Pennsylvania, USA.

Yasuda, M., Jenne C.N., Kennedy, L.J. and Reynolds J.D. (2006): The sheep and cattle Peyer's patch as a site of B-cell development. Vet. Res. 37:401–415.

CHAPTER 14

Development of the gastro-pulmonary system

Poul Hyttel

With the cranio-caudal and lateral foldings of the trilaminar embryonic disc, the primitive yolk sac, lined by the endoderm dorsally and by the hypoblast laterally and ventrally, is divided into an **intra-embryonic tube lined by endoderm** and an **extra-embryonic yolk sac lined by hypoblast** (Fig. 14-1). These two compartments initially communicate through a wide opening at the developing umbilicus; later, this communication becomes narrowed to a thin vitelline duct that persists for as long as the yolk sac is present (see Chapter 9). The intra-embryonic tube, lined by endoderm and covered by splanchnic mesoderm, is referred to as the **primitive gut**.

The primitive gut is divided into three parts. The cranial portion, the **foregut**, is blind, closed cranially by the oro-pharyngeal membrane which is lined by endoderm on the inside and covered by ectoderm on the outside (see Chapter 7). The caudal portion, the **hindgut**, is also blind, being closed by the cloacal membrane, similarly lined by endoderm and covered by ectoderm. A connecting portion, the **midgut**, opens into the yolk sac. An ectodermal depression at the location of the oro-pharyngeal membrane, the **stomodeum**, later develops into the oral cavity, while a similar depression at the site of the cloacal membrane, the **proctodeum**, develops into the anus and the opening of the uro-genital system.

The primitive gut is suspended from the dorsal and ventral body walls by mesenteries consisting of double layers of peritoneum developed from the mesoderm. The **dorsal mesentery** extends from the caudal end of the developing oesophagus to the cloacal region of the hindgut and gives rise to the greater omentum and the mesentery of the gut. The **ventral mesentery** develops from the septum transversum, and becomes restricted to the caudal portion of the foregut, i.e. the caudal oesophagus, the stomach and the initial portion of the duodenum. The developing liver grows into the ventral mesenterium and the septum transversum, and the former develops into the lesser omentum. One part of the ventral mesenterium, the falciform ligament, carries the left umbilical vein from the umbilicus to the liver (see Chapter 12).

The primitive gut gives rise to a number of endodermal derivatives (Fig. 14-2). From the foregut come **derivatives of the pharyngeal arches, pouches and clefts**, the **respiratory system**, the **oesophagus**, the **stomach** as well as the **liver** and **pancreas**. The midgut forms most of the **intestine**, and the hindgut gives rise to caudal parts of the intestine and also the **allantois** (see Chapter 9).

Finally, it should be mentioned that the gastrointestinal system develops an extensive nerve supply referred to as the **enteric nervous system**; numerous neural crest cells invade the investments of the gastrointestinal system and form ganglia in the **submucosal** and **myenteric plexuses** (see Chapter 10).

THE ORAL AND NASAL CAVITY AND PALATE

The primary oral cavity develops from the **stomodeum** as the oro-pharyngeal membrane regresses to connect the endodermally-lined primitive gut to the ectodermally-lined stomodeum (Fig. 14-2). The demarcation between the ectoderm- and

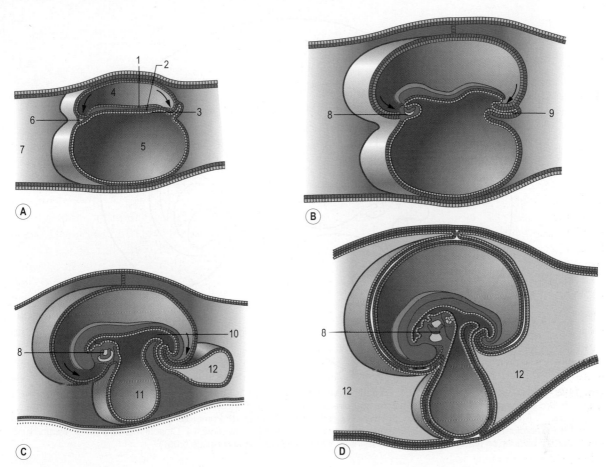

Fig. 14-1: Development of the primitive gut with advancing stages of gestation (A-D). **A:** The trilaminar embryonic disc composed of ectoderm (1), mesoderm (2), and endoderm (3) protrudes into the amniotic cavity (4). The arrows indicate the cranio-caudal folding of the embryonic disc. The primitive yolk sac (5) is lined dorsally by the endoderm and elsewhere by the hypoblast (6). 7: Trophectoderm; 8: Extra-embryonic coelom; 9: Allantoic bud. **B:** The allantoic bud hindgut develops further (9). **C:** The primitive gut is formed through the cranio-caudal and lateral foldings of the embryonic disc and a foregut (10), midgut (11), and hindgut (12) can be defined. The midgut communicates with the yolk sac (13), the hindgut with the allantois (14). The foregut is closed by the oro-pharyngeal membrane (15) and the hindgut by the cloacal membrane (16). **D:** The liver bud (17) is visible and the allantois (14) has occupied most of the extra-embryonic coelom. Modified from Sadler (2004).

endoderm-derived portions of the definitive oral and nasal cavities cannot be distinguished.

The primary nasal and oral cavities

The first recognizable facial structures are the **fronto-nasal prominence** and the paired **maxillary** and **mandibular prominences**. These develop dorsally, laterally and ventrally, respectively, to the entrance to the stomodeum (Fig. 14-3). The maxillary and mandibular prominences are derived from the first pharyngeal arch (see later). The ectoderm of the fronto-nasal prominence differentiates into the paired **nasal (olfactory)** and **lens placodes**. The latter develop into the lenses of the eyes (Chapter 11). **Medial** and **lateral nasal prominences** subsequently develop at each side of the nasal placodes. Gradually, the nasal placode invaginates to form the **nasal pit** which develops into the **primary nasal cavity**, which is separated from the **primary oral**

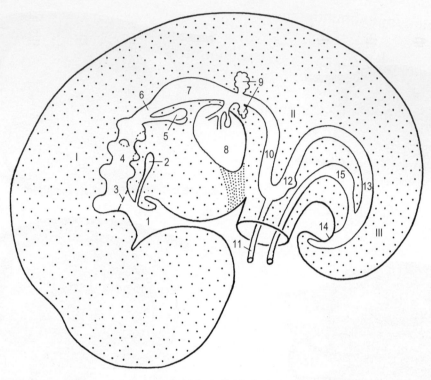

Fig. 14-2: Derivatives of the primitive gut. I: Foregut; II: Midgut; III: Hindgut; 1: Stomodeum; 2: Primordium of the thyroid gland; 3: Oro-pharyngeal membrane; 4: Pharynx and pharyngeal pouches; 5: Respiratory diverticulum. 6: Primordium of the esophagus; 7: Primordium of the stomach; 8: Liver bud; 9: Pancreatic buds; 10: Primordium of the small intestine; 11: Vitelline duct; 12: Primordium of the caecum; 13: Primordium of the rest of the large intestine; 14: Cloacal membrane; 15: Primordium of the urinary bladder on urachus connecting to allantois. Courtesy Sinowatz and Rüsse (2007).

cavity, developed from the stomodeum, by the **oronasal membrane** (Fig. 14-4). With the regression of the caudal aspects of this membrane, the **primary choanae** connecting the developing nasal and oral cavities are formed, and the oronasal membrane itself forms the **primary palate**.

Construction of the facial structures around the entrance to the developing nasal and oral cavities starts from the prominences described above (Fig. 14-5). The maxillary prominence increases in size, extends further medially, and fuses with the medial nasal prominence. This lays the foundation for formation of the bones of the upper jaw (the maxilla and incisive bones) and the upper lip. The final shape of the upper lip depends upon the degree of midline fusion between the medial nasal prominences: in **carnivores and small ruminants**, incom-

plete fusion leaves a medial groove, the **philtrum**; in **horses, cattle, and pigs,** the fusion is complete and results in a **continuous upper lip**.

The maxillary and medial nasal prominences are separated by the **nasolacrimal groove** extending dorso-laterally towards the optic placode. With development, the ectoderm at the bottom of this groove forms a solid cord that sinks into the underlying mesenchyme. Later, the cord develops a lumen and forms the **nasolacrimal duct** connecting the conjunctiva of the developing eye with the nasal cavity.

The shaping of the face varies from species to species, and even within a species, as is especially obvious in the dog (see Chapter 16). Horses, cattle, and pigs have relatively long skulls due to the growth of the bones defining the oral and nasal cavities; they are described as being **dolichocephalic**. Pri-

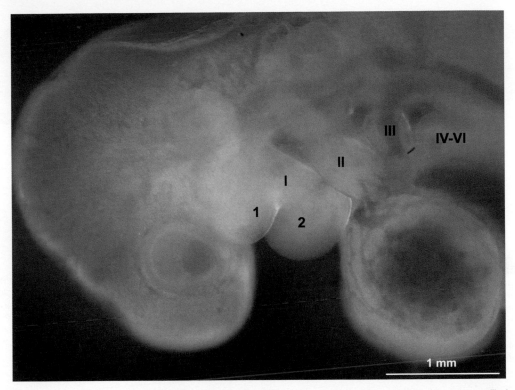

Fig. 14-3: Pig embryo at Day 18 of development. The first pharyngeal arch is divided into maxillary (1) and mandibular (2) processes. I–VI: Pharyngeal arches.

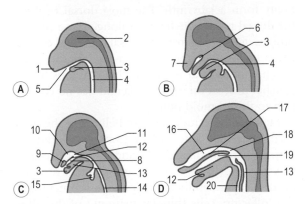

Fig. 14-4: Development of the oral and nasal cavities presented as median sections at successive stages (A-D). 1: Nasal placode; 2: Brain vesicle; 3: Mandibular prominence; 4: Foregut; 5: Stomodeum; 6: Nasal pit; 7: Frontonasal prominence; 8: Primary oral cavity; 9: Maxillary process; 10: Primary nasal cavity; 11: Primary choana; 12: Oronasal membrane; 13: Tongue; 14: Oesophagus; 15: Lung bud; 16: Secondary nasal cavity; 17: Secondary palate; 18: Choana; 19: Secondary oral cavity; 20: Trachea. Modified from McGaedy et al. (2006).

mates and humans, on the other hand, have short skulls and are **brachycephalic**. In the dog, some breeds are dolichocephalic, others brachycephalic, and yet others, between these extremes, are referred to as being **mesocephalic**.

The nasal cavity

The oronasal membrane (or primary palate) becomes replaced by the secondary palate which develops from primordia in the **palate processes** extending from the maxillary bones (Fig. 14-6). In parallel, the **nasal septum** develops from the dorsal aspect of the nasal cavity and grows ventrally. Eventually, the developing nasal septum fuses with the palate processes, partially separating the developing nasal and oral cavities (Fig. 14-7). The palate processes are membranous at first, but later intramembranous ossification in their rostral two-thirds forms the bones of the **hard palate** (see

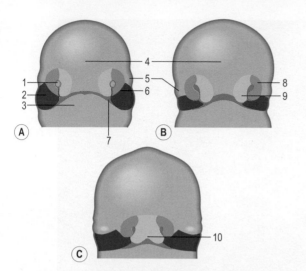

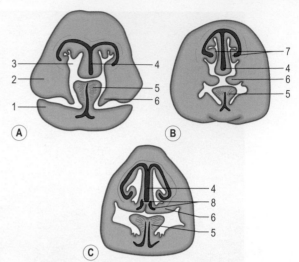

Fig. 14-5: Development of the facial structures related to the oral and nasal cavities (A-C). 1: Nasal placode; 2: Maxillary prominence; 3: Mandibular prominence; 4: Frontonasal prominence; 5: Lens placode; 6: Nasolacrimal groove; 7: Stomodeum; 8: Lateral nasal prominence; 9: Medial nasal prominence; 10: Site of species-dependent fusion between the bilateral medial nasal prominences. Modified from McGaedy et al. (2006).

Fig. 14-6: Development of the secondary oral and nasal cavities presented as cross sections (A-C). 1: Mandibular prominence; 2: Maxillary prominence; 3: Primary nasal cavity; 4: Developing nasal septum; 5: Tongue; 6: Palate process; 7: Developing conchae; 8: Developing vomeronasal organ. Modified from McGaedy et al. (2006).

Chapter 16). The secondary palate closes around Day 32 of development in the cat, around Day 33 in dog and pig, between Days 49 and 56 in horse, and between Days 56 and 63 in cattle. Caudally, mesenchyme covered by the ectoderm develops into the **soft palate** (which is particularly long in the horse) and, in the process, the **secondary choanae** and the **arcus palatopharyngeus** are formed. Rostrally, the secondary palate fuses with the remnants of the primary palate except for the paired **incisive ducts**. These ducts maintain the communication between the oral and nasal cavities, except in the horse where the oral opening of the duct is obliterated by the mucosa.

Conchae

The **conchae** are formed from processes extending from the lateral aspect of the developing nasal cavity (see Chapter 16). They first consist of a mesenchymal core covered with ectodermal epithelium; later, endochondral ossification transforms the conchae

into scroll-like structures. Conchae developed from the ethmoid bone in the caudal region of the nasal cavity form a labyrinth. The most dorsal of these, the **dorsal nasal concha**, is prolonged by a conchal process developing from the nasal bone and extends rostrally through the nasal cavity. Another large concha, the **ventral nasal concha**, develops from a conchal process on the maxilla and has no connection to the ethmoid bone.

Most of the ectodermal epithelium of the nasal cavity develops into pseudostratified epithelium with goblet and ciliated cells and forms the **respiratory region**. However, in the most caudal region, a portion of the epithelium develops the neurosensory olfactory cells (bipolar neurons) of the **olfactory region**. In both regions, the ectodermal epithelium also gives rise to **nasal glands**.

Vomeronasal organ

As mentioned, the fusion of the secondary palate is incomplete and leaves the incisive duct as an opening between the oral and nasal cavity. A sec-

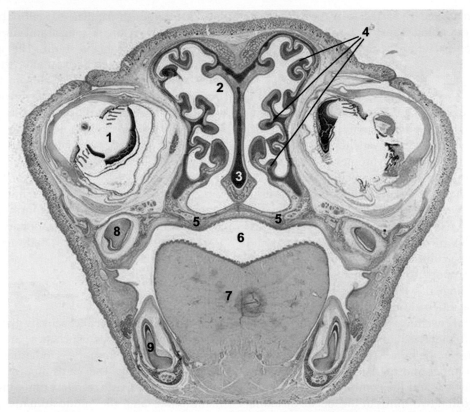

Fig. 14-7: Cross section of fetal cat head. 1: Eye; 2: Secondary nasal cavity; 3: Developing nasal septum; 4: Developing conchae; 5: Palatine processes; 6: Secondary oral cavity; 7: Tongue; 8: Dental primordium in the maxilla; 9: Dental primordium in the mandible.

ondary duct develops in the ventral mucosa of the nasal cavity and forms the paired **vomeronasal organ** (Fig. 14-6). The duct is lined by ectodermal epithelium differentiating into respiratory as well as olfactory regions.

Paranasal sinuses

The ectodermal epithelium lining the nasal cavity forms solid outgrowths that penetrate the bones of the skull. The outgrowths subsequently develop a lumen and gradually form the **paranasal sinuses** which remain connected to the nasal cavity (see Chapter 16). The paranasal sinuses are so poorly developed at birth that they are scarcely recognizable. The final anatomy of the sinuses is species-specific and of clinical significance. For example, in

the horse, the maxillary sinus is closely associated with the roots of the premolars and molars; in cattle, the frontal sinus extends into the horn processes.

The oral cavity

With the formation of the secondary palate and choanae, the nasal and oral cavities as well as the pharynx are established. Ectodermal thickenings on the developing jaws form upper and lower **labio-gingival laminae**. Subsequently, a loss of cells and tissues in the intermediate portions of these laminae results in the formation of **lips** and **gums** as well as the **vestibulum oris** between them. Lateral fusion between the upper and lower labio-gingival laminae results in development of the **cheeks**, thereby defining the aperture of the mouth. Caudally, the oral cavity is demarcated on each side by the **palatoglossal arches** extending from the border between the hard and soft palate to the root of the tongue.

Tongue

The tongue develops at the bottom of the oral cavity from a portion of the first pharyngeal arch (see later) and from myoblasts that invade the tongue primordium from the occipital myotomes. The first sign of tongue development is a medial prominence, referred to as the **tuberculum impar**, derived from the first pharyngeal arch (Fig. 14-8). The ingrowth that will give rise to the thyroid gland is found just caudal to this prominence (see later). Rostral and lateral to tuberculum impar, paired **lateral lingual swellings** develop from the first pharyngeal arch. The lateral lingual swellings fuse with each other and with the tuberculum impar. The midline fusion of the lateral swellings gives rise to the **lingual septum** and the **lyssa** in carnivores or **cartilago dorsi linguae** in the horse. The borders between the tuberculum impar and the lateral lingual swellings are gradually lost and the combined structures give rise to the rostral two-thirds of the tongue including its apex and body. The radix (root) of the tongue is developed from a median prominence, the **copula**, arising from the second pharyngeal arch and from the **eminentia hypobranchialis** from the third and fourth pharyngeal arch. The cupola atrophies and is overgrown by material from the rostral portion of the eminentia hypobranchialis that forms most of the root of the tongue. The muscle of the tongue is derived from **occipital myotomes** and is innervated by the **hypoglossal nerve** (XII).

Most of the stratified squamous epithelium of the tongue is of endodermal origin; only the apex is covered by ectoderm-derived epithelium. Axons from visceral afferent neurons induce the development of the gustatory papillae. The first to form are the **fungiform papillae,** induced by axons from the chorda tympani of the **facial nerve (VII)**. Later, axons from the **glossopharyngeal nerve (IX)** induce the development of the **vallate papillae** and **foliate papillae**. Serous gustatory glands develop from the endodermal epithelium in connection with the latter two types of papillae. Gustatory papillae are formed elsewhere on the tongue and gums, but their primordia atrophy before birth. The **mechanical papillae** of the tongue develop after the gustatory ones have formed. The general somatic afferent innervation of the tongue is derived from the contributions it receives from the various pharyngeal arches. Thus, the rostral two-thirds (developed from the tuberculum impar and lateral lingual swellings of the first pharyngeal arch) are innervated by the trigeminal nerve (V; the nerve of this arch) while the caudal third (developed from the eminentia hypobranchialis of the third and fourth pharyngeal arches) is innervated by the glossopharyngeal nerve (IX; the nerve of the third arch) and vagus nerve (X; from the fourth arch).

Salivary glands

Both the greater and smaller salivary glands develop as solid epithelial cords, which grow into the underlying mesenchyme from the ectodermal epithelium of the oral cavity. The cords branch, develop a lumen, and give rise to secretory units, the **acini**. The **mandibular** and the **monostomatic sublingual salivary glands** are the first to develop, at around a crown-rump length of 21 mm in cattle and pigs. These two glands retain long excretory ducts which open on the paired sublingual carunculae. The **parotid** and the **polystomatic sublingual salivary glands** develop shortly thereafter.

Teeth

The teeth develop from ectodermal and mesenchymal components (in the head region, the mesenchyme, being of neural crest origin, is also derived from the ectoderm). The basic components of the tooth are **enamel**, **dentin** and **cementum**. The enamel is produced by cells originating in the ectodermal gingival epithelium whereas the rest of the tooth is produced from cells coming from the underlying mesenchyme. There are two main types of teeth in domestic animals, **brachydont** and **hypsodont**, but despite their different morphology and histology, their embryology is not very different.

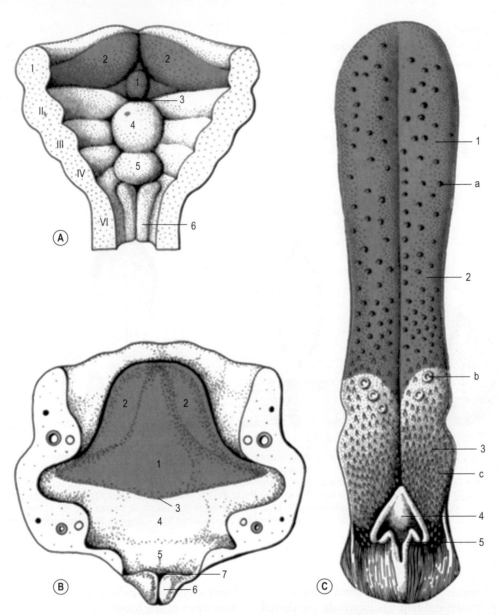

Fig. 14-8: Development of the tongue and the larynx. Red: Components developed from the first pharyngeal arch. **A:** I–VI: Pharyngeal arches I–VI, 1: Tuberculum impar; 2: lateral lingual swellings; 3: Primordium of the thyroid gland; 4: Copula; 5: Eminentia hypobranchialis; 6: Arytenoid swelling. **B:** Later developmental stages of the structures defined in A. 7: Laryngeal orifice. **C:** Tongue of the dog. 1: Apex linguae; 2: Corpus linguae; 3: Radix linguae; 4: Epiglottis; 5: Arytenoid; a: Papillae fungiformes; b: Papillae valatae; c: Papillae filiformes. Courtesy Sinowatz and Rüsse (2007).

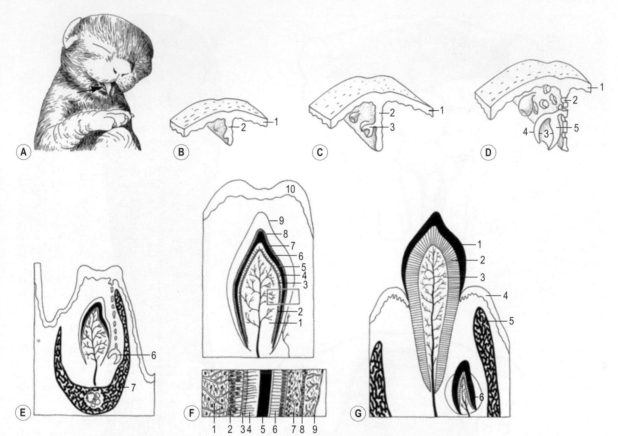

Fig. 14-9: Development of the brachydont tooth. **A:** Location of the gingiva (arrow) with tooth development in cat fetus.
B: 1: Ectodermal epithelium of the gingiva; 2: Dental lamina. **C:** 1: Epithelium; 2: Dental lamina; 3: Cap-shaped dental bud.
D: 1: Epithelium; 2: Remnant of dental lamina; 3: Inner enamel epithelium; 4: Outer enamel epithelium; 5: Stellate reticulum;
E: 6: Primordium of the permanent tooth; 7: Developing mandibula. **F:** 1: Dental pulp: 2: Ondontoblasts; 3: Predentin;
4: Dentin; 5: Enamel; 6: Ameloblasts; 7: Stellate reticulum; 8: Outer enamel epithelium; 9: Dental sac. **G:** 1: Enamel; 2: Dentin;
3: Pulp; 4: Gingival epithelium; 5: Mandibula; 6: Primordium of the permanent tooth. Courtesy Sinowatz and Rüsse (2007).

The first step in tooth development is the formation of an ectodermal laminar ingrowth, the **dental lamina**, from the gingival epithelium (Fig. 14-9). Small **cap-shaped dental buds** develop on the side of this lamina and, with development, enclose a core of mesenchyme known as the **dental papilla**. Each cap-shaped dental bud has an **outer** and **inner enamel epithelium** and forms a structure known as the **enamel organ** (Fig. 14-10). The mesenchyme between the outer and inner enamel epithelium is known as the **stellate reticulum**. The shaping of the inner enamel epithelium determines the shape of the crown of the tooth.

Although formation of the enamel organ is the first step in tooth development, the first dental component to be produced is **dentin**. The mesenchyme adjacent to the inner enamel epithelium organizes into a columnar epithelium made up of **odontoblasts**. These cells produce **predentin**, which is deposited between the odontoblasts and the inner enamel epithelium. The predentin is subsequently mineralized and turned into bone-like **dentin**.

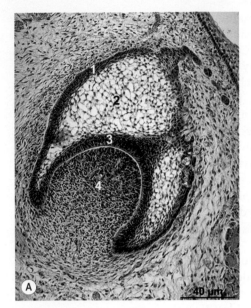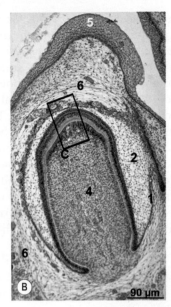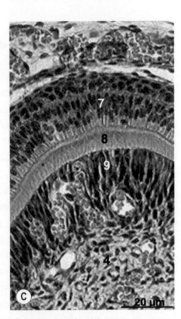

Fig. 14-10: Tooth development in a cat fetus at an early (A) and later (B) stage of gestation. The box 'C' is enlarged in C.
1: Outer enamel epithelium; 2: Stellate reticulum; 3: Inner enamel epithelium; 4: Dental papilla; 5: Gingival surface epithelium;
6: Dental sac; 7: Ameloblasts; 8: Predentin; 9: Odontoblasts.

However, whereas in the formation of bone osteocytes become encapsulated by the extracellular bone matrix, in tooth formation the odontoblasts withdraw from the inner enamel epithelium as increasing amounts of predentin and dentin are deposited; only long slender cytoplasmic projections from the odontoblasts remain in contact with the inner enamel epithelium and become embedded in the dentin, which is laid down concentrically around the cytoplasmic projections. Dentin production starts at the tip of the dental pulp. Odontoblasts remain active throughout life and their continuous production of predentin and dentin reduces the size of the dental pulp, which carries blood vessels and nerves.

Shortly after dentin production has begun, the production of **enamel** is also initiated. Stimulated by the dentin, the inner enamel epithelium differentiates into a columnar epithelium composed of **ameloblasts**. These cells produce the enamel (again starting at the tip of the developing tooth) which is deposited outside the dentin. As the enamel is laid down the ameloblasts are displaced peripherally,

thereby reducing the thickness of the stellate reticulum.

At the base of the cap-shaped enamel organ, the inner and outer enamel epithelia meet. From their junction, the epithelium proliferates and extends deeper into the mesenchyme as the **root sheath** which is responsible for the architecture of the **root** (the number and shape of root projections). The root sheath induces the adjacent mesenchyme to differentiate into the odontoblasts that produce the dentin of the root of the tooth. There is no stellate reticulum at this location and so the inner enamel epithelium never differentiates into ameloblasts. Consequently, the **root of the brachydont tooth** is **not covered with enamel**. With increasing dentin production in the root, the pulp is gradually reduced in size and the narrow **root channel** is formed. In anelodont teeth (i.e. those in which growth stops) the root sheath atrophies; in the elodont tooth (which continues its growth – the tusks in boars, for example) there is no atrophy and the tooth is rootless.

The mesenchyme around the cap-shaped enamel organ condenses to form the **dental sac**. Around the root of the tooth, the mesenchyme of the dental sac differentiates into **cementoblasts** producing cementum, another bone-like substance similar to dentin. The cementoblasts, unlike odontoblasts, become embedded in the intercellular substance, as in bone. The more peripheral portions of the dental sac around the developing root form the tough collagen-rich fibres which become organized into the **periodontal ligament** that fixes the tooth in the bone of the jaw.

Formation of the **hypsodont tooth** follows basically the same pattern. However, the shaping of the crown is more complex and, because the enamel organ is not restricted to the crown of the tooth, more of the tooth becomes covered by enamel. Furthermore, because the dental sac differentiates into cementoblasts around the complete tooth (rather than just the root), the enamel is covered with a layer of cementum. Consequently, as the erupted hypsodont tooth wears away, it is replaced by more tooth pushed out of the gingiva. Hence, instead of having a fixed crown, the hypsodont tooth is said to have a **clinical crown** – that portion of the tooth that is exposed at any particular time.

A first set of enamel organs is responsible for the formation of the **deciduous teeth** while a secondary set forms the **permanent teeth** (Fig. 14-9).

THE FOREGUT

The most cranial portion of the foregut gives rise to the **pharynx** including the **pharyngeal arches** and **pouches** and their derivatives. Caudal to the pharynx, the foregut develops into the **larynx**, **trachea**, **bronchi**, **lungs**, **oesophagus**, **stomach** and the oral portion of the **intestine**, up to where the **liver** and **pancreas** (also foregut-derivatives) bud off.

The pharynx

In the pharyngeal region, the foregut becomes involved in the formation of **pharyngeal arches** also referred to as the **branchial arches** from the Greek term 'branchia' meaning gill. In principal, six pharyngeal arches are prepared for. However, the fifth

arch is rudimentary and never develops and the sixth remains part of the neck and does not become distinct. Consequently, only four pharyngeal arches are clearly visible. Just caudal to each arch, an **internal pouch** develops (Figs. 14-11, 14-12) and an **external pharyngeal cleft** corresponds to each pouch. Due to the loss of the fifth arch, the fifth pouch becomes incorporated into the fourth. Thus, often only four clefts and pouches are referred to. The pharyngeal arches and clefts/pouches are lined by ectodermal epithelium on the outside and endodermal epithelium on the inside. The mesenchyme, which is derived from neural crest cells, is thick in the arches and thin where the clefts/pouches form. However, the clefts and pouches of mammals, unlike those of fish, do not fuse to form gill slits, at least under normal conditions. The pharyngeal arches and clefts/pouches give rise to a number of organs (Table 14-1).

The pharyngeal clefts

The first pharyngeal cleft develops into the **external auditory meatus** (Fig. 14-11). The second, third and fourth clefts are overgrown by a caudal extension from the second pharyngeal arch. The **cervical sinus** is formed as a result of the initial overgrowth but closes later.

The pharyngeal arches

The pharyngeal arches consist of mesenchyme originating from the neural crest. In each arch, the mesenchyme gives rise to particular cartilage or bone derivatives, muscles, and an aortic arch (artery), and becomes associated with a particular nerve (Fig. 14-11). The arteries are described in Chapter 12.

The first pharyngeal (mandibular) arch. This arch consists of a dorsal portion, the **maxillary process**, and a ventral portion known as the **mandibular process** (Fig. 14-3). From the maxillary process come the **maxilla**, the **zygomatic bone**, and a portion of the **temporal bone** as well as the **secondary palate** by intramembranous ossification. The mandibular process contains a plate of cartilage referred to as **Meckel's cartilage**. Most of this structure disappears, but its most dorsal portions give rise

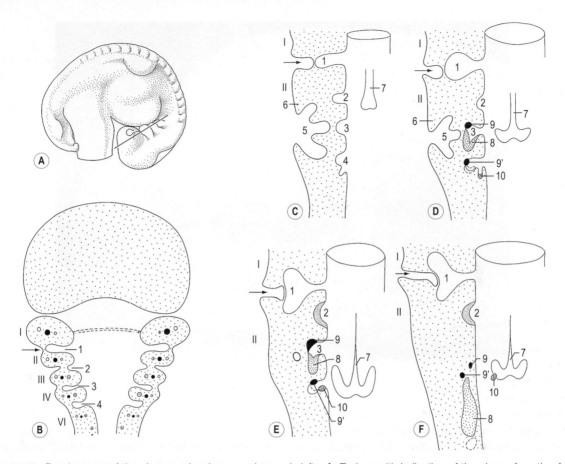

Fig. 14-11: Development of the pharyngeal arches, pouches and clefts. **A:** Embryo with indication of the plane of section for 'B'. **B:** I–VI: Pharyngeal arches, each with its cartilage, artery and nerve components. 1–4: Pharyngeal pouches. The first pharyngeal cleft, which will form the external auditory meatus (arrow) associates with the first pouch. **C:** The cervical sinus (5) is defined by a caudal extension (6) from the second pharyngeal arch. 7: Primordium of thyroid gland. **D–F:** The pharyngeal pouches differentiate. 2: Palatine tonsil. 8: Primordium of thymus; 9: Primordium of external parathyroid gland; 9': Primordium of internal parathyroid gland; 10: Ultimobranchial body. Courtesy Sinowatz and Rüsse (2007).

to the **incus** and **malleus** of the middle ear. The mandibular process also gives rise to the **mandible** through intramembranous ossification. The muscular derivatives of the first pharyngeal arch include the **muscles of mastication** (temporalis, masseter and pterygoids) as well as the **mylohyoid, rostral belly of digastricus, tensor tympani**, and **tensor veli palatini**. The first pharyngeal arch and its derivatives are supplied by the **trigeminal nerve (V)**.

The second pharyngeal (hyoid) arch. This arch is smaller than the first and contains **Reichert's cartilage**, remnants of which give rise to the **stapes** of

the middle ear. The mesenchyme from the second arch also differentiates into the **lesser horn** and the **upper portion of the body of the hyoid bone**, and the **styloid process of the temporal bone**. The muscles developing from the second pharyngeal arch include the **muscles of facial expression** as well as the **stapedius, stylohyoid, caudal belly of digastricus**, and **auricular** muscles. The second pharyngeal arch and its derivatives are supplied by the **facial nerve (VII)**.

The third pharyngeal arch. The cartilage of this arch gives rise to the **greater horn** and **lower part of the**

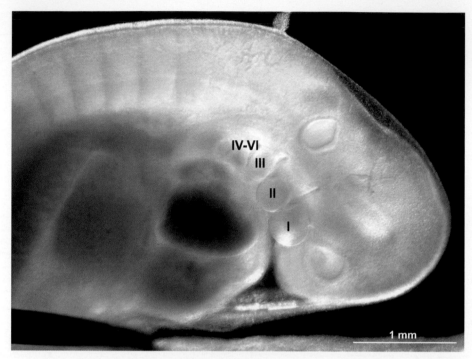

Fig. 14-12: Sheep embryo at Day 19 of development. I–VI: Pharyngeal arches.

body of the hyoid bone; muscular derivatives include the **stylopharyngeus**; the arch and its derivatives are supplied by the **glossopharyngeal nerve (IX)**.

The fourth and sixth pharyngeal arches. Major portions of the larynx including the **epiglottic, thyroid, cricoid,** and **arytenoid cartilages** (the latter including the corniculate and cuneiform processes) are formed from the cartilage of these arches. Derived muscles include the **cricothyroid, levator palatini, constrictors of pharynx,** and the remaining **intrinsic muscles of larynx.** The arches are supplied by the **vagus nerve (X)** from which the **recurrent laryngeal nerve** supplies all the intrinsic muscles of larynx except for the cricothyroid muscle which is supplied by the **cranial laryngeal nerve.** The cranial laryngeal nerve takes a direct course to the larynx at the site where the vagus nerve passes this structure. The recurrent laryngeal nerve, on the other hand, splits off from the vagus nerve much later and hooks around the sixth aortic arch on each side before making its way back cranially to the larynx (see

Chapter 12, Fig. 12-15). On the right side the sixth aortic arch is obliterated, and so the recurrent nerve is released and hooks around the fourth aortic arch instead (the fifth is rudimentary). On the left, however, the sixth aortic arch is retained as the ductus arteriosus (developing postnatally into the ligamentum arteriosum) and the recurrent laryngeal nerve remains hooked around the sixth aortic arch. In the horse, this long course of the nerve on the left side may result in hemiplegia of the intrinsic laryngeal muscles in this side causing a condition referred to as 'roaring' where the left vocal fold is left paralyzed in the respiratory tract. The left recurrent laryngeal nerve of the giraffe is said to be the longest cell in any (land) mammal!

The pharyngeal pouches

The organs developing from the pouches are collectively referred to as the **branchiogenic organs** (Fig. 14-11).

Table 14-1: Derivatives of the pharyngeal arches, pouches and clefts and their associated nerves.

	ARCH DERIVATIVES						
Pharyngeal arch	**Cartilage**	**Bone**	**Connective tissue**	**Muscles**	**Pouch derivatives**	**Cleft derivatives**	**Nerve**
First (mandibular)	Meckel's	Maxilla Mandible Zygomatic bone Temporal bone Malleus Incus	Ligament of malleus Spheno-mandibular ligament	Muscles of mastication Mylohyoid Rostral belly of digastricus Tensor tympani Tensor veli palatini	Auditory tube Guttural pouches	External auditory meatus	Trigeminal (V)
Second (hyoid)	Reichert's	Stapes Lesser horn and upper part of body of hyoid bone Styloid process of temporal bone	Stylohyoid ligament	Muscles of facial expression Stapedius Stylohyoid Caudal belly of digastricus Auricular	Palatine tonsil	None	Facial (VII)
Third	None	Greater horn and lower part of body of hyoid bone Styloid process of temporal bone	None	Stylopharyngeus	External parathyroid gland Thymus	None	Glosso-pharyngeal (IX)
Fourth and sixth	Epiglottic Arytenoid Thyroid Cricoid		None	Intrinsic muscles of larynx Levator palatini Constrictors of pharynx	Internal parathyroid gland Ultimo-branchial body	None	Vagus (X)

The first pharyngeal pouch. This pouch initially forms a diverticulum referred to as the **tubotympanic recess** which extends to become closely opposite the first pharyngeal cleft. This cleft, as already mentioned, forms the external auditory meatus and, correspondingly, the tubotympanic recess gives rise to both the dilated **middle ear cavity** and the **auditory (Eustachian) tube**. In the horse, the auditory tubes form voluminous dilations, the **guttural pouches**. The wall between the cleft and the pouch develops into the **tympanic membrane** covered by ectodermal epithelium on the outside and endodermal epithelium on the inside.

The second pharyngeal pouch. This pouch persists only in carnivores and cattle where it forms the **tonsilar fossa** and **sinus**, respectively. The endodermal epithelium of the pouch forms the reticulated stroma of the **palatine tonsil**. These structures are later invaded by immune competent cells.

The third pharyngeal pouch. Dorsal and ventral primordia develop from this pouch. The dorsal primordium gives rise to the **external parathyroid gland** while the ventral one forms a reticulated stroma, the structural basis of the **thymus**, invaded later by cells of the lymphocyte lineage destined to become **T lymphocytes** (see Chapter 13). The external parathyroid gland maintains its relationship to the thymus and, with it, migrates caudally to become located lateral to the thyroid cartilage (in the horse and carnivores) or at the division of the common carotid artery (in ruminants and pigs). During the caudal growth and migration of the thymus, a slim **cervical portion** and a more rounded **thoracic portion** are formed. In the horse and carnivores, the initial connection to the pharyngeal region is rapidly lost. In ruminants and pigs, however, the cervical portion of the thymus persists. The direct open connection of the thymus to the pharyngeal pouch is lost in all species. In the caudal part of the cervical portion and in the thoracic portion, the two parts of the initially bilateral organ fuse into a single structure. In the thoracic portion, this becomes located in the cranial mediastinum. The final location of the thymus in the newborn varies with species: in ruminants and pigs distinct cervical and thoracic portions are seen; in the horses the cervical portion is reduced in size; and in carnivores the cervical portion is completely lost. The thymus becomes populated by lymphocytes derived from the bone marrow. Upon arrival through the vascular system, the lymphocytes proliferate vigorously in the network formed by the reticular cells developed from the original endodermal primordium and establish the T-lymphocyte population of the body. The T-lymphocytes later spread to other locations, notably the lymph nodes, to establish T-dependent zones. At birth, the thymus is fully developed but it starts to involute soon afterwards and involution becomes especially marked during puberty.

The fourth pharyngeal pouch. Like the third, this pouch develops dorsal and ventral primordia. The dorsal primordium develops into the **internal parathyroid gland** which, like its external counterpart, also migrates caudally with the thymus and becomes located lateral to the thyroid cartilage, embedded in the thyroid gland. The ventral primordium may, depending on the species, be involved in formation of the **thymus**, but is generally considered to be of minor importance.

The fifth pharyngeal pouch. This pouch, often considered as being incorporated into the fourth, gives rise to the **ultimobranchial body** that is later incorporated into the thyroid gland where it forms the parafollicular cells, i.e. the C-cells.

The thyroid gland. The **thyroid gland** develops from a ventral epithelial thickening in the pharyngeal portion of the foregut. For this reason it makes sense to describe it in relation to the branchiogenic organs (Fig. 14-11). The thickening grows into the underlying mesenchyme where it forms the long slender **thyroglossal duct** which, at its distal end, forms a horseshoe-shaped bilobed structure. The slender portion of the duct is lost and the bilobed part moves further caudally to the cranial end of the trachea where the two lobes of the thyroid gland develop from the lobes of the primordium. In the pig, the **two lobes** maintain a physical connection through a well-developed **isthmus** but this is either less developed or absent in other species. Initially, the thymus consists of solid epithelial strands, but these later develop into the **thyroid follicles**.

The larynx

In the cranial portion of the foregut just caudal to the developing pharynx, an internal **laryngo-tracheal groove** forms and deepens while, externally, the developing oesophagus becomes separated from the larynx and trachea by the **tracheo-oesophageal groove** (Fig. 14-13). Internally, further development of the external groove results in the formation of the **tracheo-oesophageal septum** defining the **respiratory diverticulum**.

At first, the laryngeal opening into the pharynx is in the form of a slit, but the slit later develops into at T-shaped opening that becomes surrounded by three swellings (Fig. 14-8). Cranially to the opening, the **epiglottal swelling** develops from the eminentia hypobranchialis, mainly originating from the third and fourth pharyngeal arches, and caudo-laterally, the paired **arytenoid swellings** form from the sixth arch (the fifth arch is rudimentary). The mesenchyme in these swellings, which is of neural crest origin, forms the **epiglottic** and **arytenoid cartilages** (Table 14-1). The mesenchyme of the fourth and sixth pharyngeal arch caudo-lateral to the ary-

tenoid cartilages consolidates to form the **thyroid cartilage**; even further caudally, the mesenchyme of the sixth arch forms the **cricoid** cartilage.

The **intrinsic laryngeal muscles** are also developed from the mesenchyme of the pharyngeal arches: the **crico-thyroid muscles** from the fourth arch, innervated by the **cranial laryngeal nerve** from the vagus; the **remaining intrinsic muscles** from the sixth pharyngeal arch, innervated by the **caudal laryngeal nerve** from the recurrent laryngeal nerve, a ramification of the vagus nerve.

As the laryngeal cartilages and muscles develop, the **vocal folds** are formed. In the horse and dog, and to a minor degree in pigs, the endodermal epithelium forms a lateral outpocketing resulting in the **laryngeal ventricles**. In the process, the well-defined **vestibular folds** are formed rostral to the vocal folds in the horse and the dog.

The trachea

Caudally, the developing larynx opens into the primitive trachea which quickly grows in a caudal direction. The mesenchyme around its endodermal lining is of neural crest origin, at least in the cervical region, and gives rise to the cartilaginous **tracheal rings** progressing cranio-caudally. It is the mesenchyme that also forms the smooth **tracheal muscle** while endodermal epithelium specializes into a ciliated, pseudostratified, **respiratory epithelium,** rich in goblet cells. Tracheal glands are associated with the epithelium.

The bronchi and lungs

The development of the bronchi and lungs can be divided into sequential periods: the **embryonic period**, when the primordium of the bronchi and lungs is formed; the **fetal period**, when the ramified bronchi are formed and the preliminary structures for gas exchange are established; and the **postnatal period**, when the definitive structures for gas exchange, the alveoli, are developed and the lungs assume their adult form. The fetal period can be subdivided into overlapping **pseudo-glandular, canalicular, saccular** and **alveolar** periods.

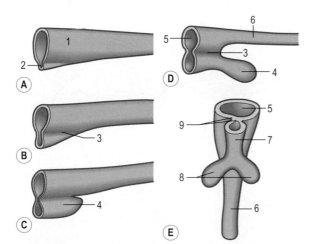

Fig. 14-13: Development of the respiratory diverticulum. 1: Foregut; 2: Laryngo-tracheal groove; 3: Tracheo-oesophageal groove; 4: Respiratory diverticulum; 5: Pharynx; 6: Primordium of oesophagus; 7: Primordium of trachea; 8: Primordia of principal bronchi; 9: Tracheo-oesophageal septum. Modified from McGaedy et al. (2006).

The embryonic period

After its initial caudal growth, the primitive trachea forms the lung buds that fork caudo-laterally as the **principal bronchi** (Fig. 14-14). The smaller left bud grows in a more lateral direction than does the larger right one. The principal bronchi, in turn, bud into the **lobar bronchi** defining how the lungs will divide into lobes – species-specific patterns that become discernable at the end of the embryonic period. The lobes protrude into the developing pleural cavity and become surrounded externally by mesenchyme that forms the **pleura**. In cattle and pigs, a particular **tracheal bronchus** develops directly from the trachea and supplies the right cranial lobe. As the lobar bronchi are formed, the first subsequent budding into the **segmental bronchi** begins. The pulmonary arteries (developing from the sixth aortic arches; see Chapter 12) and veins develop in parallel with the ramification of the bronchial tree.

The pseudo-glandular period

This period of lung development takes its name from the gland-like ramification that is seen in the

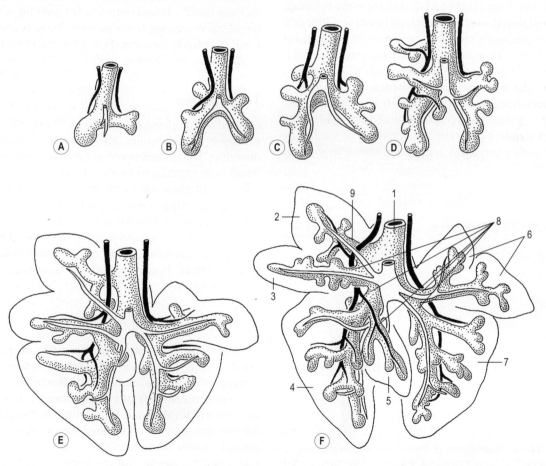

Fig. 14-14: Ventral aspect of development of the bronchial tree in the pig at a crown-rump length of the embryo of 7.5 mm (A), 10 mm (B), 12 mm (C), 13.5 mm (D), 15 mm (E), and 18.5 mm (F). Black: arteries; White: veins; 1: Trachea; 2: Right cranial lobe; 3: Middle lobe; 4: Right caudal lobe; 5: Accessory lobe; 6: Left cranial lobe; 7: Left caudal lobe; 8: Lobar bronchi; 9: Bronchus trachealis. Courtesy Sinowatz and Rüsse (2007).

bronchial tree. The lobar bronchi give rise to the **segmental bronchi** that undergo up to 20 bifurcations depending on the species. At this stage, the bronchi present themselves as tubules lined by a columnar endodermal epithelium. The bronchi ramify in the surrounding mesenchyme and eventually give rise to the **terminal bronchioles**.

The canalicular period

This period is characterized by the formation of the primordia of those portions of the lungs that will later be engaged in gas exchange. The terminal bronchioles, formed during the pseudo-glandular period, ramify further by bifurcation and each terminal bronchiole gives rise to a tubule system included in a **pulmonary lobule**. Hence, by two to three bifurcations, the terminal bronchioles give rise to **respiratory bronchioles**, each of which undergoes three to four more bifurcations in forming secondary tubules, the **canalicules**, for which this period is named. The ends of the canalicules form sets of short **terminal saccules,** also referred to as the primitive alveoli. The canalicules are lined by a columnar epithelium surrounded by a developing network of capillaries. The epithelial height is reduced where capillaries make close contact with the epithelium.

The saccular period

During this period the terminal branching of the air conducting system results from three to four further bifurcations of the terminal saccules. With the last bifurcation, **blind saccules** are formed.

The alveolar period

This is the period when the final compartments for gas exchange, the **alveoli**, are formed. The formation of alveoli occurs in a centripetal direction, the most distal ones first. In cattle, this process starts at about 240 days of gestation. The endodermal epithelium in the developing alveoli differentiates into squamous **type I alveolar cells**, which cover most of the alveolar surface, and the more cuboidal **type II alveolar cells**, which specialize in the production of surfactant, a phospholipid that reduces surface

tension in the alveoli. The first phospholipid-producing cells are established earlier, during the canalicular period. Type II alveolar cells also serve as stem cells for regenerating alveolar cells of type I. During the fetal period, the lumen of the complete respiratory system is filled with fluid secreted from the developing glands of the system, supplemented by additional amniotic fluid aspirated as a result of prenatal respiratory movements.

The postnatal period

Although the alveolar period provides primitive alveoli that allow the neonate to breath, **mature alveoli** are not formed until the lungs become functional after birth. In the early postnatal period, there is a marked longitudinal growth of the respiratory bronchioles and the alveolar saccule, as well as additional alveolar development from the walls of these structures. At birth, most of the fluid in the respiratory system is expelled through the mouth and nose. The first inspiration fills the system with air; remaining fluid is removed by absorption by the epithelial cells and transported into the blood and lymph systems.

The oesophagus

The oesophagus extends from the developing pharynx, where it opens dorsal to the larynx, to the spindle-shaped primordium of the stomach. The oesophagus is wide and short at first but, with the growth of the thorax and the development of the heart and lungs, it becomes more extended and narrow and embedded in the mediastinum. The endodermal epithelium of the oesophagus develops into a **stratified squamous epithelium** with glands extending into the submucosa. The distribution of the **oesophageal glands** is species-specific. The mesoderm surrounding the endodermal epithelium gives rise to the investments of the esophagus: the **lamina propria**, **lamina muscularis mucosae**, **tela submucosa**, **tunica muscularis**, and **tunica adventitia** or **serosa**. The structure of the tunica muscularis also displays important species-specific differences: in the ruminants and dogs, it is composed of striated muscle; in the pig, the most caudal portions carry smooth muscle; and in the horse and cat, the muscle of the caudal one-third is smooth. While the smooth muscle cells develop from the mesenchyme surrounding the endoderm, the striated muscle cells apparently migrate from the pharyngeal arches.

The stomach

The stomach develops as a spindle-shaped dilation of the more caudal portion of the foregut, becoming evident during the third week of gestation in the pig. The development of the stomach differs between species; in the following, the **simple stomach**

and the **ruminant stomach** will be described separately.

The simple stomach

The dorsal portion of the spindle-shaped stomach primordium grows more rapidly than the ventral part with the result that a dorsal convex and a ventral concave curvature are formed. The dorsal curvature will later develop into the **greater curvature** and the ventral to the **lesser curvature** of the stomach.

In order to assume its final transverse position in the abdominal cavity, the stomach completes **two rotations**: one around a cranio-caudal axis and the other on a dorso-ventral axis (Fig. 14-15). The **first**

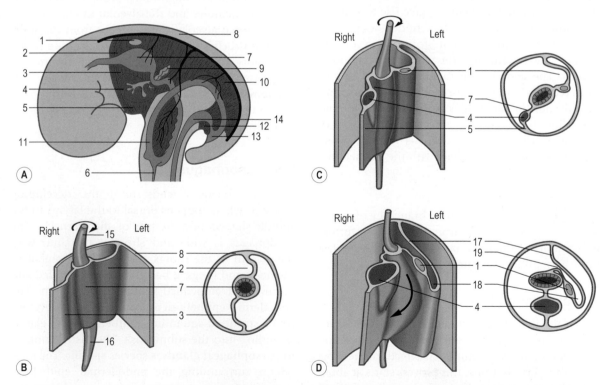

Fig. 14-15: Rotation of the primordium of the stomach and formation of the lesser and greater omentum. The first rotation is 90° clockwise around a cranio-caudal axis (B–C). The second rotation is 45° counter-clockwise around a dorso-ventral axis (D). 1: Primordium of the spleen; 2: Dorsal mesogastrium; 3: Ventral mesogastrium; 4: Primordium of the liver; 5: Falciform ligament; 6: Vitelline duct; 7: Primordium of the stomach; 8: Dorsal body wall; 9: Dorsal pancreatic bud; 10: Dorsal mesentery; 11: Midgut loop; 12: Primordium of the median ligament of the bladder; 13: Cloaca; 14: Urachus; 15: Primordium of the oesophagus; 16: Primordium of the duodenum; 17: Greater omentum; 18: Omental bursa; 19: Foramen omentale. Modified from McGaedy et al. (2006).

rotation (90° clockwise around a cranio-caudal axis) brings the dorsal portions of the developing stomach to the left, and the ventral portions to the right. As a result, the left vagus nerve assumes a ventral position and the right vagus a dorsal position. At the **second rotation**, the stomach turns about 45° clockwise around a dorso-ventral axis, positioning it largely transversely in the abdominal cavity with the caudal portions to the right and the cranial parts to the left (Fig. 14-16). With the further growth, the left-hand (cranial) portions develop into the **cardia** and the **fundus**, the middle part into the **corpus**, and the right-hand (caudal) portion into the **pylorus**. The cardia and fundus become voluminous, particularly in the horse, forming the **saccus caecus ventriculi**.

Those parts of the dorsal and ventral mesentery that are attached to the stomach are referred to as the **dorsal** and **ventral mesogastrium** (Fig. 14-15). The dorsal mesogastrium is initially wide, and cavities develop in its mesenchyme. Later, these cavities coalesce to a single space, referred to as the pneumo-enteric recess, which later becomes connected to the peritoneal cavity. With the development of the septum transversum into the centrum tendineum of the diaphragm, a portion of this cavity becomes trapped in the thoracic cavity adjacent to the oesophagus where it forms the bursa infracardiaca.

The portion of the pneumo-enteric recess that remains in the abdominal cavity participates in the formation of the **bursa omentalis**. With the first

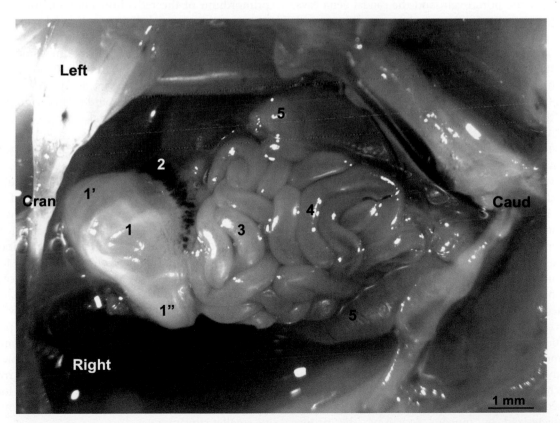

Fig. 14-16: Ventral aspect of the abdominal cavity of a pig fetus at Day 44 of development. The large primordium of the liver has been removed. The stomach (1) has assumed its more or less transverse location. Cran: Cranial; Caud: Caudal; 1': Fundus; 1": Pylorus; 2: Spleen; 3: Jejunum; 4: Colon ascendens forming the spiral loop; 5: Mesonephros.

rotation of the stomach, the insertion of the dorsal mesogastrium moves from a dorsal to a left position and a sac, including the abdominal portions of the pneumo-enteric recess, is gradually formed. This sac later develops into the **bursa omentalis**. The spleen develops in the dorsal mesogastrium which also accommodates the left lobe of the pancreas. With the second rotation, the insertion of the dorsal mesogastrium on the stomach assumes a more or less caudal position and further development of the mesogastrium itself results in the formation of the final **greater omentum**, comprising a superficial and a deep layer with the bursa omentalis in between. The access to the bursa from the peritoneal cavity persists on the right side as the **foramen omentale**. This opening is found at the free margin of the ventral mesogastrium (i.e. the lesser omentum) bordered by the portal vein and the caudal vena cava. Further growth of the greater omentum varies with species: in the carnivores it extends a long way caudally, covering all the intestines; it is smaller in the pig and horse.

The first rotation of the stomach takes the insertion of the ventral mesogastrium to the right, joining the developing stomach to the ventral body wall and the septum transversum. The liver bud grows into the ventral mesogastrium and the septum transversum. With the second rotation of the stomach, the ventral mesogastrium becomes more cranially directed, towards the septum transversum. Later, the liver is released from the septum transversum again, as the ventral mesogastrium develops into the **lesser omentum** while the **coronary, triangular and falciform ligaments** of the liver are formed from the septum.

The differentiation of the **mucosa** of the stomach varies with species. In the carnivores, the entire mucosa develops **glands,** whereas in the pig and, in particular, the horse, a non-glandular region is formed, characterized by multilayered squamous epithelium. The glandular mucosa develops into specialized regions each with its characteristic type of secretion: the **cardiac** and the **pyloric glands** are characterized by mucous secretions; the **proper gastric glands** by secretion of substances for digestion, including HCl and pepsinogen. In the pig, the

proper gastric glands are recognizable at around 2 months of gestation, when their mucus-secreting cells develop. Soon after, the parietal cells start to appear followed, at around 3 months of gestation, by the chief cells.

The ruminant stomach

As in the development of the simple stomach, the faster growth of the dorsal portion of the ruminant stomach primordium results in the formation of a convex dorsal curvature and a less convex ventral curvature, evident in the bovine embryo at around 30 days of gestation (Figs 14-17, 14-18). In the cranial part of the dorsal curvature, **a greater right and a smaller left ruminal bud** develop. At the same time, just caudal to these ruminal buds, the primordium of the **reticulum** buds off the dorsal curvature in a cranial direction. Caudal and more ventral to the primordium of the reticulum, the primordia of the **omasum** and **abomasum** soon become established and, by around 40 days of gestation, all four compartments are visible in the bovine embryo. The grooves and pilae dividing the rumen into its dorsal and ventral sacs also appear at this stage.

With the **first rotation** of the stomach system (90° clockwise around a cranio-caudal axis), the ruminal buds and the primordium of the reticulum are taken to the left, and the primordia of the omasum and the abomasum to the right. As an additional component of the first rotation, the ruminal buds rotate about 150°, changing their orientation from pointing cranio-dorsally to the final location with the dorsal and ventral saccus cecus pointing caudally. Along with this rotation, the reticulum is brought to a cranial location towards the developing diaphragm, the omasum to a position on the right, and the abomasum to a ventral position on the right side of the abdominal cavity. Only the abomasum participates in the **second rotation** of the stomach which results in a ventral location of its greater curvature and a dorsal location of its smaller curvature.

During the third month of gestation, the relative sizes of the four compartments of the bovine

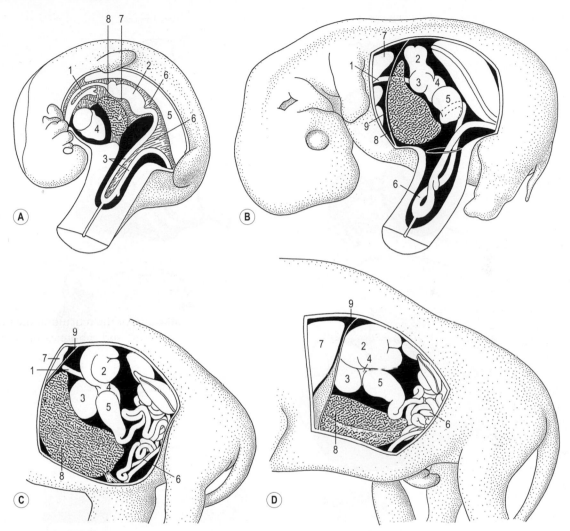

Fig. 14-17: Development of the stomach in cattle embryos/fetuses at a crown rump length of 10 mm (A), 22 mm (B), 80 mm (C), and 110 mm (D). **A**: 1: Primordium of the oesophagus; 2: Primordium of the stomach; 3: Primordium of the intestine; 4: Primordium of the heart; 5: Mesonephros; 6: Dorsal mesogastrium; 7: Ventral mesogastrium; 8: Primordium of the liver. **B–C:** 1: Oesophagus; 2: Rumen; 3: Reticulum; 4: Omasum; 5: Abomasum; 6: Intestine; 7: Lung; 8: Liver; 9: Diaphragm. Courtesy Sinowatz and Rüsse (2007).

stomach system in the fetus are comparable with those seen in the adult. Subsequently though, the abomasum develops at a higher rate and at birth accounts for about half of the total volume of the stomach system. This is because the abomasum is needed to make use of the liquid diet during the first weeks after birth; liquids more or less bypass the rumen, reticulum and omasum by means of the **sulcus reticuli** and **sulcus omasi** to gain direct

access to the abomasum. With the dietary change from liquids to solids, the rumen, reticulum and omasum become functional and increase in size.

The attachment of the **dorsal** and **ventral meso-gastrium** to the stomach system becomes reorganized in a complicated manner with the development of the ruminant stomach. In short, because the ruminal buds develop from the dorsal portion of the spindle-shaped stomach primordium, the dorsal

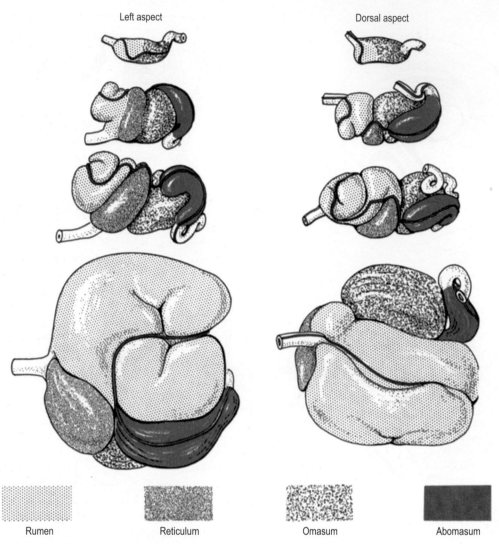

Left aspect

Dorsal aspect

Rumen

Reticulum

Omasum

Abomasum

Fig. 14-18: Development of the ruminant stomach. The red line indicates the insertion of the greater omentum. Courtesy Sinowatz and Rüsse (2007).

mesogastrium, which forms the **greater omentum**, inserts on the rumen. The line of insertion stretches from the oesophagus along the right longitudinal groove, around the caudal groove and further along the left longitudinal groove onto the greater curvature of the abomasum (Fig. 14-18). On the other hand, the ventral mesogastrium, forming the **lesser omentum**, has an insertion line from the oesophagus, over the omasum and along the minor curvature of the abomasum.

Initially, all four compartments of the ruminant stomach system are lined by a columnar endodermal epithelium. However, the **linings of the rumen, reticulum and omasum** are gradually changed into a **multilayered squamous epithelium**, whereas the **abomasum retains its columnar epithelium**. Midway through the second month of gestation, the plicae of the omasum are formed; towards the end of the second month the spiral mucosal folds of the abomasum develop; early during the third month the cristae reticuli form; towards the end of the third month, the ruminal papillae develop; and subsequently the differentiation of the typical regions of the glandular mucosa is seen.

The liver

The liver and the pancreas both develop from **dorsal** and a **ventral endodermal buds** that originate from the most caudal region of the foregut, which ends up forming the most oral portion of the duodenum. The liver and a minor portion of the pancreas develop from the ventral bud, the major portion of the pancreas from the dorsal bud (Fig. 14-19).

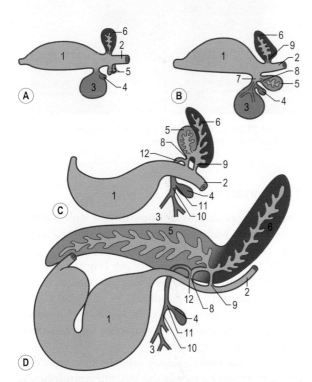

Fig. 14-19: Development of the liver and pancreas in the dog. 1: Primordium of the stomach; 2: Primordium of the duodenum; 3: Primordium of the liver; 4: Primordium of the gall bladder; 5: Ventral pancreatic primordium; 6: Dorsal pancreatic primordium; 7: Hepatopancreatic duct; 8: Pancreatic duct; 9: Accessory pancreatic duct; 10: Hepatic ducts; 11: Cystic duct; 12: Common bile duct. Courtesy Sinowatz and Rüsse (2007).

The hepatogenic part of the ventral endodermal bud develops into a larger cranial and a smaller caudal portion. The caudal or **cystic portion** develops into the **gall bladder** and **cystic duct**. The cystic portion fails to develop in certain species such as the horse, rat and whale, all of which lack a gall bladder. The cranial or **hepatic portion** develops into the **liver tissue** and the remaining **bile ducts**. The endodermal cells of the hepatic bud portion grow through the ventral mesogastrium into the septum transversum where they interact with the surrounding mesenchyme to form other cellular components of the liver including connective tissue, endothelial cells, Kupffer cells, and the blood-forming cells characteristic of the embryonic and fetal liver.

The relatively large endodermal cells differentiate into **hepatocytes** and become arranged in rods or plates with intervening **sinusoids**. The sinusoids develop from parts of the right and left vitelline veins and the most cranial anastomosis between them (see Chapter 12). Later, the hepatocyte plates become oriented in a radial fashion around the **central vein**. Even later, the connective tissue becomes organized around the **lobules**. In the pig, this is a rather late phenomenon, not being completed until early postnatally.

The liver grows quickly and expands to occupy most of the abdominal cavity, creating the so-called liver prominence on the outside of the embryo (Fig. 14-20). Mesenchyme from the septum transversum gives rise to the **liver capsule** and the **liver ligaments**. Hence, with the caudal growth of the liver, the organ gradually becomes almost detached from the septum transversum, but remains attached to the developing diaphragm by the **coronary**, **triangular**, and **falciform ligaments**. Initially, the liver develops a **left** and a **right lobe**, but subsequent outgrowths from the right lobe form the **quadrate** and **caudate lobes**. This, in turn, is followed by species-specific division of the lobes. The final position and orientation of the liver in the abdominal cavity is influenced by the species-specific situation of other organs: in carnivores and the pig, the liver remains more or less horizontally attached to the diaphragm in the midline; in the horse the intestinal system displaces the liver by 45°

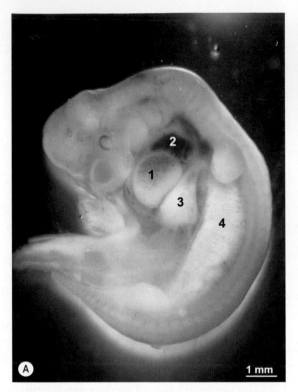
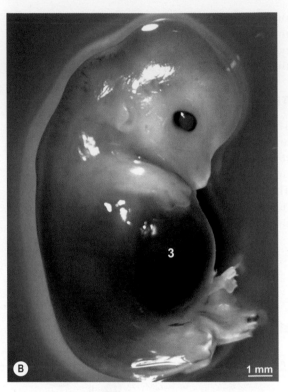

Fig. 14-20: Development of the liver in the pig embryo at Days 21 (A) and 31 (B) of development. Note the marked enlargement of the organ. 1: Heart ventricle; 2: Atrium; 3: Primordium of the liver; 4: Mesonephros.

to the right; and in ruminants the stomach system pushes the liver 90° to the right.

During its growth, the liver is of great significance as a blood-forming structure; haematopoietic stem cells, derived from the mesenchyme of the septum transversum, establish **haematopoietic islands** in the liver. With the development of these islands, the first period of blood-formation (in the yolk sac, the mesoblastic period) comes to an end and the second period, the hepato-lienal period begins. This period is, in turn, overtaken by a third period, the medullary period, in which the bone marrow develops as the major blood-forming organ.

The smaller caudal portion of the liver bud, the cystic portion, develops into the **gall bladder** and the **cystic duct** (Fig. 14-19). The remaining portion of the gall duct system develops from the hepatic duct. Each duct system appears as a solid strand of cells that later develops a lumen.

The pancreas

The pancreas develops from **dorsal** and **ventral endodermal buds** off the caudal end of the foregut (Fig. 14-19). The two buds are clearly recognizable by 19 days of gestation in the pig (Fig. 14-21) and by Day 26 in cattle. With the first rotation of the stomach around a longitudinal axis, the ventral pancreatic bud is moved dorsally, close to the dorsal bud, and with further development the two buds fuse to form a single organ.

The **dorsal bud** develops into the major portion of the pancreas including the **left** and **right lobes** as well as a portion of the **body**; the **ventral bud** develops into a **portion of the body** of the pancreas and also the liver (as described above). The dorsal bud gradually grows into the mesoduodenum in an arboreal fashion as endodermal cell cords that later develop a lumen. The main duct of the dorsal bud

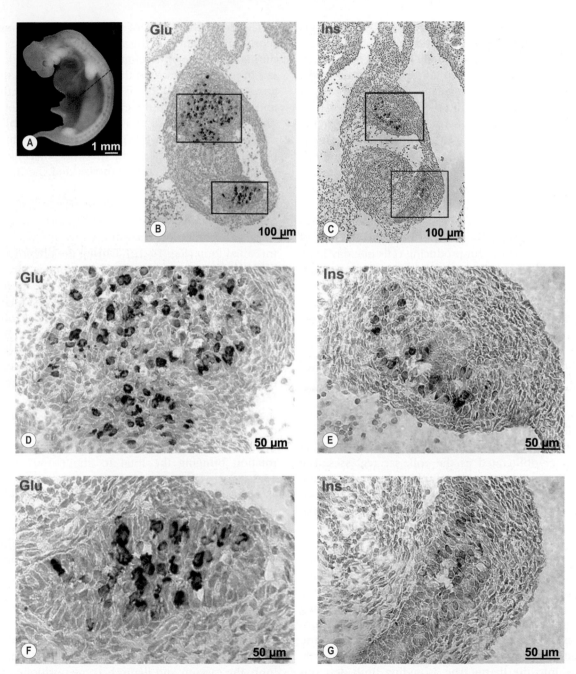

Fig. 14-21: Immunohistochemical stainings for glucagon (Glu) and insulin (Ins) in a pig embryo at Day 19 of development (**A**). Broken line represents the position of the transverse sections shown in 'B' and 'C'. (**B**) Dorsal and ventral pancreatic primordia (boxed) with glucagon-stained cells. (**C**) Dorsal and ventral pancreatic primordia (boxed) with insulin-stained cells. (**D**) Upper boxed area from 'B', showing the scattered glucagon-stained cells of the dorsal pancreatic primordium. (**E**) Upper boxed area from 'C', showing insulin-stained cells of the dorsal pancreatic primordium. (**F**) Lower boxed area from 'B', showing ventral pancreatic primordium with glucagon-stained cells. (**G**) Lower boxed area from 'C', showing ventral pancreatic primordium with insulin-stained cells. Courtesy Sinowatz and Rüsse (2007).

develops into the accessory pancreatic duct which is later obliterated in the cat and small ruminants.

The main duct of the smaller **ventral bud**, which develops into a portion of the pancreatic body, develops into the pancreatic duct which is later obliterated in the ox and pig.

The budding endoderm gives rise to both the **exocrine acini** and the **endocrine islets of Langerhans**. The latter are formed from endodermal cell clusters that gradually lose their connection to the exocrine system. In the pig, scattered glucagon- and insulin-producing cells can be found as early as at 19 days of gestation (Fig. 14-21); in cattle, glucagon-producing cells may be found at 26 days of gestation and insulin-producing cells one day later. Initially, some cells may produce both hormones, but this capability is lost later in pregnancy. Somatostatin-producing cells appear slightly later, at 31 and 45 days of gestation in pigs and cattle, respectively.

THE MIDGUT

The midgut is initially in open connection with the yolk sac. However, body foldings gradually narrow this connection down to the **vitelline duct**, and that is later obliterated as the yolk sac regresses. The midgut grows more rapidly than the body overall, and soon it forms a **loop** suspended in a **dorsal mesentery** (Fig. 14-22) consisting of a cranial descending and a caudal ascending limb.

The caudal part of the foregut, which, as already mentioned, develops into the oral portion of the duodenum, is positioned more or less horizontally and is connected to the descending limb of the intestinal loop. The first portion of the descending loop develops into the aboral portion of the **duodenum**, the subsequent portion into the **jejunum**, and the tip of the loop, where it connects to the yolk sac, into the **ileum**. The ascending limb develops into the **caecum** as well as part of the **transverse colon**. The more horizontal hindgut develops into the remaining portion of the transverse colon, **descending colon**, and **rectum** as well as the **allantois** and its derivatives.

The descending limb of the midgut loop grows more rapidly than does the ascending limb. Because, during this phase of development, the haematopoietic liver occupies most of the abdominal cavity, the growing intestinal loop is displaced out of the abdominal cavity into the extra-embryonic coelom. This process is referred to as **physiological umbilical herniation** (Fig. 14-23). Later, when the third period of haematopoiesis in the bone marrow is initiated, the liver decreases in size and the intestines return into the abdominal cavity.

The right vitelline artery gives rise to, among others, the cranial mesenteric artery (see Chapter 12) that becomes localized in the mesentery of the intestinal loop (Fig. 14-22). During the physiological umbilical herniation, this loop **rotates clockwise around a dorso-ventral axis** with the cranial mesenteric artery located in the axis. The first phase of rotation, which occurs when the intestinal loop forms the hernia, accounts for 180°. Hence, the formerly caudal descending limb is brought to a location cranial to the descending limb. Later, during the reduction of the hernia, an additional rotation augments the rotation to about 270°. At the return of the intestinal loop to the abdominal cavity the final species-specific positioning of the intestines occurs; a process that includes yet more rotation bringing the total to about 360° (Fig. 14-22).

Perhaps due to the additional mass imposed by the caecum, the ascending limb is the last to re-enter the abdominal cavity. Hence, the caudally located descending loop enters first, and the ascending portion of the duodenum and the jejunum become positioned to the left of the median plane and the cranial mesenteric artery where they push the descending colon (from the hindgut) even further to the left. The long coils of the jejunum occupy a major portion of the ventral abdominal cavity. With the return to the abdominal cavity of the ascending limb, the caecum and ileum become positioned to the right of the median plane. The ileum opens into the junction between the caecum and the ascending colon. This feature is modified in the carnivores (where the ileum finally opens into the ascending colon) and in the horse (where the ileum opens into

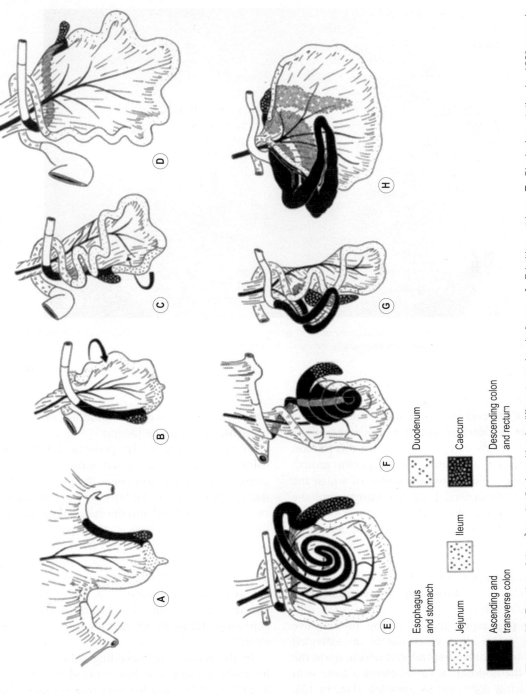

Fig. 14-22: Rotation of the gut to its final position in different species. Left view. **A:** Primitive gut loop. **B:** Clockwise rotation by 180° around a dorso-ventral axis. **C:** Clockwise rotation by 270°. **D:** Final location of the gut in the dog after clockwise rotation by 360°. **E:** Final location of the gut in ruminants. **F:** Final location of the gut in the pig. **G:** Location of the gut after clockwise rotation by 270° in the horse. **H:** Final location of the gut in horse after clockwise rotation by 360°. Courtesy Sinowatz and Rüsse (2007).

Esophagus and stomach

Jejunum

Ascending and transverse colon

Duodenum

Ileum

Caecum

Descending colon and rectum

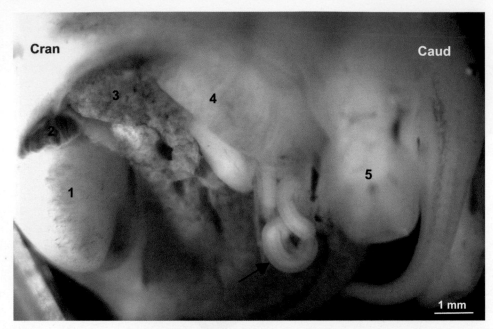

Fig. 14-23: Oblique aspect of the abdominal cavity of a pig embryo at Day 31 of development showing the physiological umbilical herniation (arrow). The liver has been partly removed. 1: Ventricle of the heart; 2: Atrium; 3: Liver; 4: Mesonephros; 5. Limb bud.

the base of the caecum; see below). The ascending colon also becomes localized to the right of the median plane but, except in carnivores, this portion of the intestine undergoes species-specific growth and relocation. The transverse colon, of which the oral portion is derived from the midgut and the aboral from the hindgut, always becomes localized in a right to left orientation just cranial to the cranial mesenteric artery. It continues into the descending colon, extending caudally to the left.

In the **horse, pig and ruminants** a growth and repositioning of the **ascending colon** and **caecum** occurs.

In the **pig**, rapid growth of the presumptive ascending colon soon gives rise to an extended portion that becomes a **spiral coil** which, upon the return to the abdominal cavity, forms a cone with its base facing right and its apex left (Fig. 14-16). These rearrangements occur during the second month of gestation, leaving the caecum positioned to the left with the apex pointing caudally into the

pelvic cavity. The outer longitudinal muscle layer condenses to form the taeniae.

In the **ruminants**, the presumptive ascending colon also has an increased growth rate and is arranged in a **spiral coil**. As in the pig, the coil initially forms a cone, but it later develops into a more two-dimensional coil and the mesocolon fuses with the mesojejunum. Hence, the ascending colon becomes localized centrally in the same mesentery that carries the jejunum in its periphery. Finally, **proximal** and **distal loops** are formed oral and aboral to the spiral loop, respectively. Due to the growth of the rumen, the intestines localize to the **supraomental recess** to the right in the abdominal cavity.

In the **horse**, the ascending colon exhibits an increased growth rate but, instead of forming a spiral coil, it builds a **long narrow U-shaped loop** in which the two limbs are kept tightly apposed by a narrow mesocolon. The loop grows cranially in the right side of the abdominal cavity, turns at the developing diaphragm and continues caudally on the left side to the pelvic inlet. Hence, right and left dorsal and ventral portions are formed. The final equine caecum is formed by contribution from the ascending colon. As a result, **an oral portion of the ascending colon forms the base of the caecum**, and the ileum, which according to its embryonic origin should have opened into the junction between the caecum and the ascending colon, opens into the base of the caecum instead. The caecum exhibits continued growth, and due to a higher growth rate caudo-ventrally, a cranio-dorsal lesser curvature and a caudo-ventral greater curvature with the apex pointing cranio-ventrally are formed. Consequently, the body and apex of the caecum become positioned between the right and left segments of the ascending colon. The descending colon elongates as well and, with the extension of its mesentery, it assumes a very mobile location allowing for extensive rectal palpation. As in the pig, the outer longitudinal muscle layer condenses to form the taeniae.

HINDGUT

As already described, the oral portion of the hindgut gives rise to the aboral portion of the **transverse colon** and the **descending colon**. The more aboral portion of the hindgut gives rise to the **rectum**, and to the **allantois** and its derivatives. By the third week of gestation, the allantois is visible as an extensive bud from the hindgut extending into the extra-embryonic coelom. It is first seen as an anchor-shaped extension just caudal to the embryo proper (Fig. 14-24). The allantoic duct enlarges as the primitive urogenital sinus which forms the primordium of the urinary bladder. These derivatives of the allantois will be described in conjunction with the urogenital system (see Chapter 15).

The hindgut terminates in the **cloaca**, a caudal cavity lined by endoderm and sealed from the amniotic cavity by the cloacal membrane which is lined by endoderm and covered by ectoderm on the

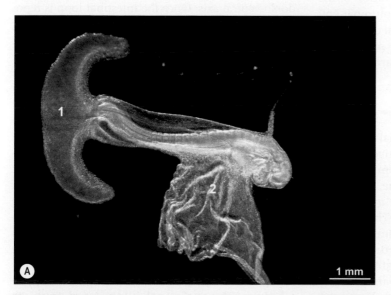
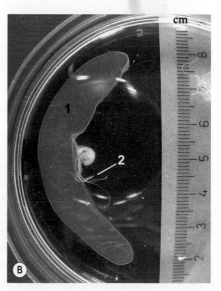

Fig. 14-24: Development of the allantois (1) from the hindgut in the sheep embryo by Day 17 (A) and 19 (B) of development. Note that the yolk sac (2) is rudimentary at Day 19.

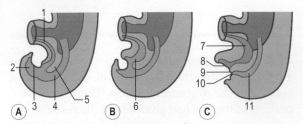

Fig. 14-25: Development of the hindgut. 1: Allantoic duct opening into the allantois; 2: Cloaca; 3: Cloacal membrane; 4: Hindgut; 5: Urorectal septum; 6: Primitive urogenital sinus; 7: Primordium of urinary bladder; 8: Urogenital membrane; 9: Perineal body; 10: Anal membrane; 11: Rectum. Modified from Sadler (2004).

outside (Fig. 14-25). The allantoic duct and the hindgut are separated by a layer of mesoderm referred to as the **urorectal septum**. With the cranio-caudal folding of the embryo, this septum approaches the **cloacal membrane**. Eventually, this membrane is divided into an **anal membrane** and a **urogenital membrane**. Both membranes rupture, connecting the hindgut to the amniotic cavity via the future anus, and opening a hole from the urogenital sinus to the amniotic cavity. The urorectal septum develops into the **perineal body**.

The **anal canal** is formed by proliferation of the ectoderm. The endoderm, forming a columnar epithelial lining of the rectum, and the anal canal, lined by a stratified squamous epithelium, meet at the **anorectal line** where the anal canal starts.

SUMMARY

The **epithelium** of the gastrointestinal system as well as the **parenchyma** of its derivatives, such as the liver and pancreas, are derived from the **endoderm** whereas the **connective tissue**, **muscular components**, **serosal coverings** and **mesenteries** are all derived from the **mesoderm**. The **nervous components** are derived from the **neural crest**.

The primitive mouth, the **stomodeum**, and the primitive **nasal cavity** are lined by epithelium of ectodermal origin and become separated by a **primary** and later a **secondary palate**. They communicate through first **primary** and later **secondary**

choanae. From the primitive nasal cavity, the conchae, **vomeronasal organ** and **paranasal sinuses** develop. In relation to the oral cavity, the **salivary glands** develop from ectodermal epithelial cords, the **tongue** develops from swellings of the pharyngeal arches covered by endodermal epithelium, and the **teeth** develop from the enamel organs, derived from the oral cavity ectodermal epithelium, and the ameloblasts and odontoblasts that originate in the mesenchyme from the neural crest.

The gastrointestinal tract extends from the **oro-pharyngeal membrane** to the **cloacal membrane** and comprises the **foregut**, **midgut** and **hindgut**. The **foregut** gives rise to the **pharynx** and its derivatives, the **respiratory system**, **oesophagus**, **stomach**, and the **oral portion of the duodenum**, as well as the derivatives of the duodenal endoderm, the **liver** and **pancreas**. The latter two organs develop from a dorsal bud that forms most of the pancreas and a ventral bud that gives rise to a smaller portion of the pancreas as well as the liver and bile duct system.

The **midgut** forms an **intestinal loop** which, over a certain period of development, extends out of the umbilicus of the embryo into the extra-embryonic coelom as a physiological umbilical herniation. The intestinal loop turns 360° clockwise around a dorso-ventral axis. Once the intestinal loop is repositioned in the abdominal cavity, the **descending loop** forms the **aboral portion of the duodenum**, **jejunum** and the **oral portion of the ileum**, while the **ascending loop** gives rise to the **aboral portion of the ileum**, **caecum**, **ascending colon** and portion of the **transverse colon**. The ascending colon and the caecum in particular become positioned in a species-specific orientation.

The **hindgut** gives rise to a portion of the **transverse colon**, the **descending colon**, and **rectum**. The hindgut initially opens into the endodermal **cloaca** from which the allantoic duct extends to the allantois. The cloaca is closed by the **cloacal membrane**. A **urorectal septum** later separates the rectum from the allantoic duct and, with the rupture of the cloacal membrane, openings are created from the hindgut, developing into the **anus**, and the **urogenital sinus**. The **anal canal** is developed from the ectoderm.

Box 14-1 Molecular regulation of the development of the primitive gut and its derivatives

The **endoderm** forms the epithelial lining of the respiratory and digestive tracts and is a major component of many glands, including the thyroid, thymus, pancreas and liver. Development encompasses stages of **tube formation**, **bud formation** and **organ-specific cytodifferentiation**. Muscular and connective tissues associated with the endoderm are formed from the visceral mesoderm surrounding it, except for the pharyngeal region in which these components are derived from the neural crest.

The molecular regulation of endoderm differentiation is to a high degree determined by overlapping patterns of gene expression; the **Hox genes** (see Chapter 2) and related genes are of particular importance (Fig. 14-26). The *Hox* genes, including the **Nkx** and **Pax** genes, are expressed in a well organized pattern along the developing gut and, at certain overlapping regions, sphincters are formed in the associated mesoderm. The *Hox* genes are considered master genes within certain regions of the developing gut, regulating a cascade of downstream genes that instruct further differentiation of its various components. The **Cdx2** and **Pdx1** genes are close relatives to the *Hox* genes, belonging to the so-called Parahox gene cluster. *Cdx2* is involved in formation of posterior structures. *Pdx1* is initially expressed in posterior foregut, but later it becomes important for the development of the pancreas (see below). In the following, the developmental regulation will be exemplified by the development of the foregut in the mouse into the pharyngeal region, the region around the respiratory diverticulum, and the caudal region forming the stomach and the liver and pancreatic primordia.

The pharyngeal region

The pharyngeal region extends from the buccopharyngeal membrane to the respiratory diverticulum. In the developing pharynx, muscular and connective tissues are formed primarily by neural crest cells. These cells migrate into the pharyngeal arches from hindbrain rhombomeres, carrying a **Hox code** with them. As an example, the genes *Hox-a2/Hox-b2*, *Hox-a3/Hox-b3*, and *Hox-a4/Hoxb-4* are expressed in neural-crest-derived mesenchyme of the second, third and fourth pharyngeal arch, respectively. Acting upon this code, pharyngeal pouch endoderm controls further differentiation of the various components of each pharyngeal arch through expression of **BMP7** caudally, **FGF8** cranially, and **Pax1** dorsally in each pouch. In addition, **Sonic hegdehog** (**Shh**) is expressed caudally in the endoderm of pharyngeal pouches 2 and 3.

The region around the respiratory diverticulum

Among many others, the transcription factors **Foxa1** and **Foxa2**, **Gata4** and **Gata6** have been shown to be crucial for the early development of the foregut. Expression of **HNF3α** and **β** is also found in the foregut endoderm and is maintained in the lung epithelium throughout embryonic, fetal and adult life. Several studies have demonstrated HNF3β to be of significance in lung differentiation and regulation of surfactant protein gene expression. Interestingly, once the lungs have formed, *Gata6*, but not *Gata4*, continues to be expressed in the lung epithelium. In particular, *Gata6* appears to be an important transcription factor for lung development and may be required for activation of the lung developmental programme in the foregut endoderm.

The genetic programs that determine axis and branching patterns of bronchi are defined at an early developmental stage. For example, the **left-right axis** of the lung appears to be specified well before there is any sign of the organ as such. Left-right differences in patterning are first seen when secondary buds form. These differences continue to develop as airways undergo branching and are assembled into lobes by the visceral pleura (lobation), which result in more lobes in the right lung. The basis for left-right asymmetry in the lungs and other viscera lies in genes such as **Lefty-1** and **-2**, **nodal**, and **Pitx-2**.

Although only few aspects of the molecular regulation of early development of the mammalian lung are clear, specification of lung tissue probably depends on FGF signalling from cardiac mesoderm as also described for the development of the liver (see below). Collectively, the data are compatible with the idea that **FGF-10** locally induces and

Continued

guides the outgrowth of lung buds to proper positions during lung branching morphogenesis. There is also genetic evidence that the chemotactic response and lung bud induction, elicited in the epithelium by FGF-10, result from local activation of FGFR-2. The process by which saccules transform into alveolar units involves formation of secondary septae from the pre-existing walls and represents the final major morphogenic event of the developing lung. Recent data suggest that **retinoic acid** signalling is involved in alveolization of the lung.

The caudal foregut region

Special for the foregut endoderm is the inherent ability to differentiate into liver tissue unless inhibited from doing so. Inhibiting molecules (including the TGF-β member **activin**) are secreted by neighbouring mesoderm, ectoderm and the notochord outside the hepatic field. Cranial to the hepatic field, Sry-like HMG box transcription factor **Sox2** is expressed in endoderm forming the oesophagus and the ventricle. Around the hepatic field, liver development is stimulated by **FGF2** and bone morphogenetic proteins (**BMPs**) from the cardiac mesoderm and septum transversum, respectively (Fig. 14-27). For further development of the hepatocyte and biliary cell lineages, expression of hepatocyte nuclear transcription factors (**HNF3** and **4**) is necessary. The expression of liver-specific genes, such as the genes for albumin or alpha-fetoprotein, can in principle occur in any region of the gut tube that is exposed to the inductive influence of the cardiogenic mesoderm secreting FGFs. Developing heart cells are not the only mesodermal derivative needed to form the liver; endothelial cells from blood vessels secreting FGFs are also involved. If endothelial cells are not present around the hepatic field of the gut tube, the liver bud fails to form. In order to respond to the FGF signals, the gut epithelium has to become competent. This competence is achieved by the expression of forkhead transcription factors in the endoderm. Mouse embryos lacking **Foxa1** and **Foxa2** expression in the endoderm fail to develop a liver bud. Later in liver development, other forkhead transcription factors, such as HNFs, become important.

Both pancreatic and duodenal development depend on expression of the pancreatic and **duodenal homeobox 1 (Pdx1)** in the endoderm (Fig. 14-27). Differentiation of endocrine, as opposed to exocrine, progenitor cells depends on expression of **Ngn3**. Differential expression of **Arx** and **Pax4** leads to formation of either the α- or the β-/δ cell lineages. Formation of α-cells later depends on expression of **Pax6** whereas formation of β-cells depends on expression of **Nkx6.1** in addition to **Pax4**. The differential events leading to the formation of PP, δ and ε-cells are less clear.

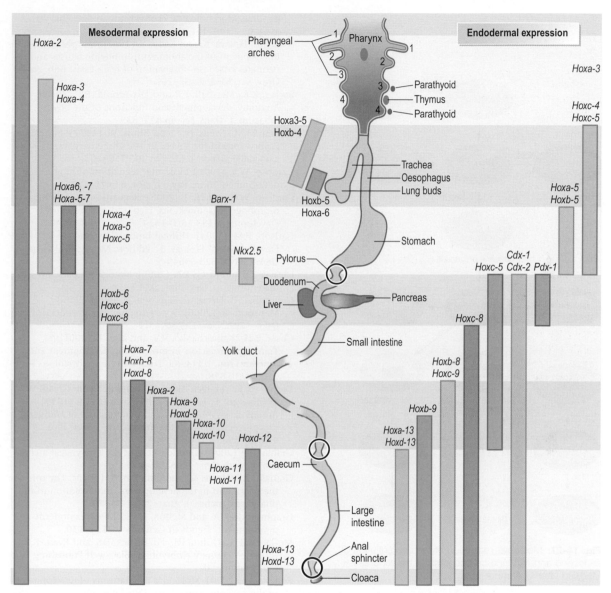

Fig. 14-26: The expression of *Hox* genes along endoderm (right panel) and associated mesoderm (left panel) of the developing gastro-pulmonary tract in the mouse. The circles indicate where sphincters develop. Modified after Carlson (2004).

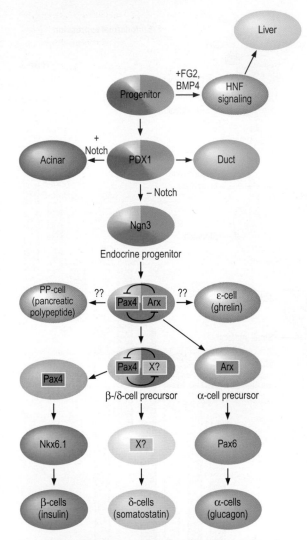

Fig. 14-27: Molecular regulation of the differentiation of endocrine and exocrine components of the pancreas. Modified after Collombat et al. (2006).

FURTHER READING

Alumets, J., Hakanson, H. and Sundler, F. (1983): Ontogeny of endocrine cells in porcine gut and pancreas. Gastroenterology 85:1359–1372.

Arias, J.L., Cabrera, R. and Valencia, A. (1978): Observations on the histological development of the bovine rumen papillae. Morphological changes due to age. Zbl. Vet. Med. C. 7:140–151.

Asari, M., Fukaya, K. and Kano, Y. (1981): Morphological development of the abomasum in bovine fetuses and neonates based on observation of resin casts. Bull. Azabu Univ. Vet. Med. 2:257–261.

Becker, R.B., Marshall, S.P. and Dix Arnold, P.T. (1963): Anatomy, development and functions of the bovine omasum. J. Dairy Sci. 46:835–839.

Bryden, M.M., Evans, H.E. and Binns, W. (1972): Embryology of the sheep. II. The alimentary tract associated glands. J. Morph. 138:187–205.

Cardoso, W.V. (2001): Molecular regulation of lung development. Ann. Rev. Physiol. 63:471–494.

Cardoso, W.V. and Lü, J. (2006): Regulation of early lung morphogenesis: questions, facts and controversies. Development 133:1611–1624.

Carlson, B.M. (2004): Human Embryology and Developmental Biology. 3rd edition. Mosby, Philadelphia, USA. ISBN 0-323-03649-X.

Cleaver, O. and Krieg, P.A. (2001): Notochord patterning of the endoderm. Dev. Biol., 234:1–12.

Collombat, P., Hecksher-Sørensen, J., Serup, P. and Mansouri, A. (2006): Specifying pancreatic endocrine cell fates. Mech. Dev. 123:501–512.

Costa, R.H., Kalinichenko, V.V. and Lim, L. (2001): Transcription factors in mouse lung development and function. Am. J. Physiol. Lung Cell Mol. Physiol. 280:L823-L838.

Dechamp, J., Van Den Akker, E., Forlani, S., De Graaff, W., Oosterveen, T., Roelen, B. and Roelfsema, J. (1999): Initiation, establishment and maintenance of Hox gene expression patterns in the mouse. Int. J. Dev. Biol. 43:635–650.

Graham, A. (2003): Development of the pharyngeal arches. Am. J. Med. Gen., 119A:251–256.

Graham, A., Okabe, M. and Quinlan, R. (2005): The role of the endoderm in the development and evolution of the pharyngeal arches. J. Anat. 207:479–487.

Grapin-Botton, A. and Melton, D.A. (2000): Endoderm development. Trends in Genetics 16:124–130.

McGaedy, T.A., Quinn, P.J., FitzPatrick, E.S. and Ryan, T. (2006): Veterinary embryology. Blackwell Publishing Ltd., Oxford, UK.

Roberts, D. (2000): Molecular mechanisms of development of the gastrointestinal tract. Dev. Dynamics 219:109–120.

Rüsse, I. and Sinowatz, F. (1998): Lehrbuch der Embryologie der Haustiere, 2nd edn, Parey Buchverlag, Berlin.

Sack, W.O. (1964): The early development of the embryonic pharynx of the dog. Anat. Anz. 115:59–70.

Sadler, T.W. (2006): Langman's Medical Embryology. 10th edition, Lippincott Williams and Wilkins, Baltimore, Maryland, USA.

Trahair, J. and Robinson, P. (1986): The development of the ovine small intestine. Anat. Rec. 214:294–303.

Warburton, D., Schwarz, M., Tefft, D., Flores-Delgado, G., Anderson, K.D. and Cardoso W.V. (2000): The molecular basis of lung morphogenesis. Mech. Dev. 92:55–81.

Warner, E.D. (1958): The organogenesis and early histogenesis of the bovine stomach. Am. J. Anat. 102:33–63.

Wells, J.M. and Melton, D.A. (1999): Vertebrate endoderm development. Annu. Rev. Cell Dev. Biol. 15:393–410.

Williams, R.C. and Evans, H.E. (1978): Prenatal dental development in the dog, *Canis familiaris*. Chronology of tooth germ formation and calcification of decidous teeth. Zbl. Vet. Med. C. 7:152–163.

CHAPTER 15

Fred Sinowatz

Development of the urogenital system

The **urogenital system** can be functionally divided into two entirely different components, the **urinary system** and the **genital system**, but the embryonic developments of the two are intimately interwoven. Both are derived from the nonsegmented **intermediate mesoderm**, which is also referred to as the nephrogenic plate, and the neighbouring mesodermal coelomic epithelium. Early proliferation of this portion of the mesoderm causes a longitudinal swelling – termed the **urogenital plate** – along the dorsolateral aspect of the abdomen.

DEVELOPMENT OF THE URINARY SYSTEM

Mammalian kidney formation, **nephrogenesis**, commences with the successive appearances of three generations of kidney primordia: the **pronephros**, **mesonephros**, and **metanephros** (Fig. 15-1). These primordia arise in an anterior-posterior wave of cellular differentiation in the so-called **nephrogenic cord** which is part of the urogenital plate. As these primordia develop, their excretory ducts become localized parallel to the nephrogenic cord. The duct associated with the second kidney primordium, the mesonephros, becomes particularly well-developed and is referred to as the the **mesonephric** or **Wolffian duct**.

Pronephros

Significant function of the **pronephros** is limited to the **lower vertebrates**, fish for example. In most **mammals the pronephros is rudimentary** and consists of seven or eight pairs of pronephric tubules that appear briefly at the level of somites seven to 14. In the intermediate mesoderm of this region, a duct, the **pronephric duct**, develops and grows caudally to the cloaca. In the sheep, pronephric tubules become quite well developed and connect to the pronephric duct.

Mesonephros

The **mesonephros** is fully operational in lower vertebrates like amphibians. In **mammals**, the mesonephros is a vestige of the nephrogenic cord, and its appearance is **transitory**. The mesonephros and its mesonephric duct are derived from intermediate mesoderm that extends from upper thoracic to upper lumbar segments. In domestic animals, 70–80 pairs of **mesonephric tubules** appear approximately between the levels of somites nine through 26. Each tubule is apposed to a blood vessel on one end, and connects into the posterior end of the pronephric duct on the other. The duct grows towards the cloaca and forms the **mesonephric** or **Wolffian duct**. The mesonephric tubules lengthen rapidly, form an S-shaped loop, and acquire a tuft of capillaries that later form the **glomerulus** at their medial extremity. The glomeruli are supplied by a rich vascular plexus, composed of numerous lateral branches of the dorsal aorta, within the mesonephros. Around each glomerulus, the tubulus forms a **Bowman's capsule**. Together these structures constitute a **renal corpuscle**. Laterally, the tubules join the longitudinal collecting duct, the mesonephric duct.

The fully developed mesonephros is of considerable size in domestic animals, forming an ovoid

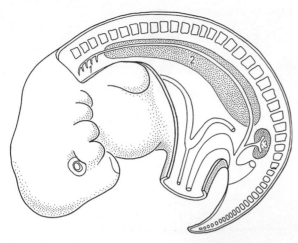

Fig. 15-1: Subdivision of the intermediate mesoderm into areas that will form the pronephros (1), mesonephros (2), and metanephros (3). Courtesy Sinowatz and Rüsse (2007).

organ on each side of the midline (Figs 15-2, 15-3). Due to its size, it is partly responsible for the physiological herniation of the growing intestinal loop (see Chapter 14). The size of the mesonephros correlates to some extent with the type of placenta and

how well the placenta cleans the blood. Thus, it is largest in species with a six-layered placental barrier (epitheliochorial placenta; see Chapter 9) such as the pig and sheep, and smallest in carnivores with a four-layered barrier (endotheliochorial placenta). Soon after their formation, most of the **mesonephric tubules start to degenerate**. Degeneration of the cranial portion of the mesonephros occurs around the eighth and ninth week of gestation in the horse, and tenth week in cattle.

Metanephros

It is the third generation of urinary organs, the **metanephros**, that matures to form the **permanent kidney** (Figs 15-4, 15-5). In cattle, its development begins at the level of somites 26 through 28, when the embryo is about 6–7 mm in length. The metanephros is derived from two primordial structures: the **ureteric bud**, an outgrowth of the mesonephric duct, and the **metanephric blastema**, which is located in the sacral region and originates from the posterior end of the nephrogenic cord. In forming

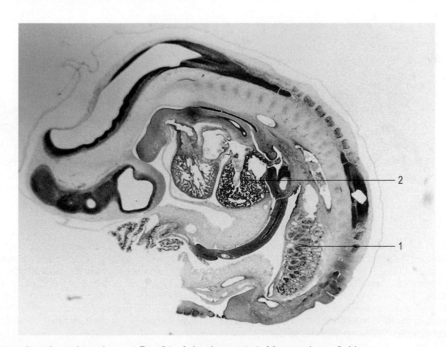

Fig. 15-2: Mesonephros in a pig embryo at Day 21 of development. 1: Mesonephros; 2: Liver.

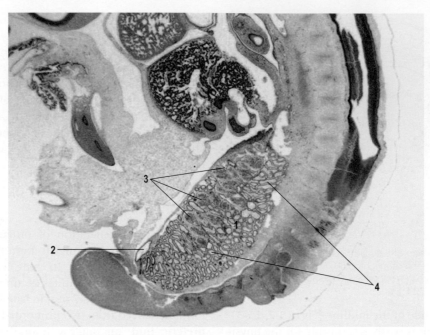

Fig. 15-3: Higher magnification of the mesonephros in a pig embryo at Day 21 of development. 1: Mesonephros; 2: Mesonephric (Wolffian) duct; 3: Glomeruli of the mesonephros; 4: Mesonephric tubuli.

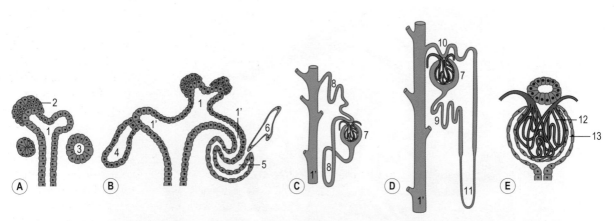

Fig. 15-4: Stages in the development of a metanephric tubule. A: As the terminal bud of the metanephric duct branches, the surrounding mesenchyme cells split into parts. A single condensation of mesenchymal cells goes through a defined series of stages to form a renal tubule.1: Ureteric bud with two ampullae; 2: cap of metanephric tissue; 3: Renal vesicle. B: The renal vesicle gives rise to small S-shaped tubules. Capillaries (6) grow into the pocket (5) at one end of the S and differentiate into glomeruli. 1: Ampulla; 1′: Collecting tubule; 4: Renal tubule. C: At the points where the collecting tubule (1′) splits, numerous nephrons consisting of corpuscula renales (7) and renal tubules (8) develop. D: The nephron forms proximal (9) and distal (10) convoluted tubules, which are connected by the Henle's loop (11). E: Differentiated corpusculum renis. 12: Glomerulus; 13: Bowmans capsule. Courtesy Sinowatz and Rüsse (2007).

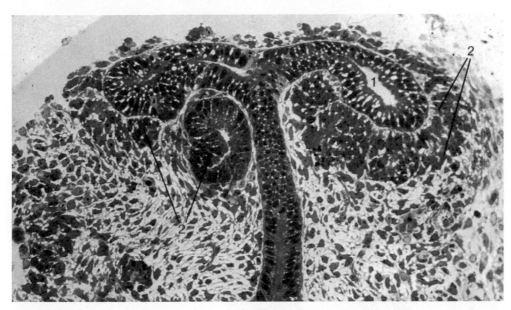

Fig. 15-5: Development of a metanephrogenic excretory unit in a bovine embryo of 17 mm CRL. 1: Ureteric bud; 2: Caps of metanephric tissue.

the metanephros, the ureteric bud grows anteriodorsally into the overlying posterior intermediate mesoderm where it interacts with this loosely organized mesenchyme, the metanephric blastema, located on the lateral aspect of the aorta. This epithelial-mesenchymal interaction leads to a dramatic **transformation of the mesenchyme into an epithelial phenotype**, which reciprocates by inducing the ureteric bud to undergo arborization and generation of **nascent nephrons**.

Collecting system

The combination of **elongation** and **branching** (up to 14 or 15 dichotomous branching divisions) of the ureteric bud plays a central role in the development of the metanephros (Fig. 15-6). Outgrowth of the ureteric bud from the mesonephric duct is induced by the secretion of alial-derived neurotrophic factor (GDNF) by glial cells derived from the undifferentiated mesenchyme of the metanephrogenic blastema. GDNF secretion is controlled by WT-1, a transcription factor that makes the mesenchyme competent to respond to induction by the

ureteric bud. The inductive signal GDNF is bound by c-Ret, a member of the tyrosine kinase receptor superfamily, which is located in the plasma membrane of the epithelial cells of the ureteric bud. In response to GDNF, the epithelial cells of the ureteric bud produce fibroblast growth factor 2 (FGF2), BMP1/BMP2, and leukaemia inhibitory factor (LIF), which stimulate the surrounding metanephric mesenchyme to form precursors of renal tubules.

The formation of functional nephrons in the developing metanephros involves **three cell lineages**, all derived from the mesoderm: **epithelial cells** from the ureteric bud, **mesenchymal cells** of the metanephric blastema, and ingrowing **endothelial cells**. The first step of nephron formation is the condensation of mesenchymal blastema cells around terminal buds of the branching ureteric bud. As the mesenchymal cells condense, the expression of several proteins typically found in mesenchymal cells (like collagen I, collagen III, and fibronectin) is lost and replaced by epithelial-type proteins like collagen IV, syndecan-1, and laminin, which ultimately contribute to the basal membrane around the tubular cells.

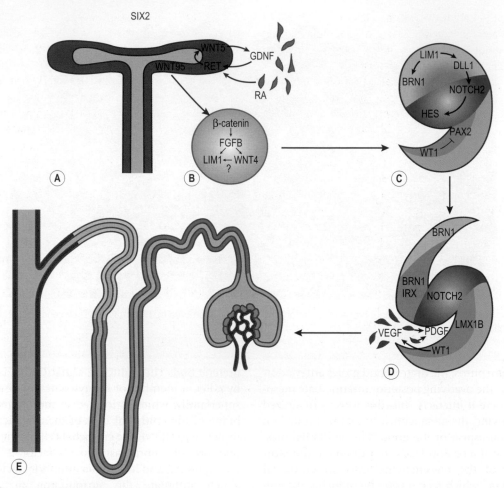

Fig. 15-6: Nephron induction and patterning.

A: Glial-derived neurotrophic factor (GDNF) released from mesenchymal cells (blue) surrounding the ureter binds to the RET receptor at the tip of the ureter (red) and induces growth and branching. RET signalling activates WNT11, which is required in a positive-feedback loop to maintain expression of *GDNF* in the metanephric mesenchyme. Retinoic acid signalling (RA) from stromal cells (pink) is required to maintain *RET* expression in the ureteric bud. Sine oculis homeobox homologue 2 (SIX2) suppresses tubulogenesis in renal precursor cells (purple), which reside at the outer cortex of the developing kidney.

B: WNT9B released from stalk regions of the ureter induces canonical β-catenin signalling in the metanephric mesenchyme, which activates a molecular cascade involving fibroblast growth factor 8 (FGF8), the LIM homeobox protein LIM1 (also known as LHX1) and WNT4. WNT4 induces the mesenchyme-to-epithelial transition and the formation of the renal vesicle (brown).

C: LIM1 is required to induce the initial stages of patterning in the renal vesicle, by controlling the expression of the POU-domain transcription factor BRN1 and Delta-like protein 1 (DLL1) at the pole of the vesicle that lies in close proximity to the ureter. Expression of the Wilms tumour transcription factor (WT1) becomes restricted to the presumptive podocyte layer of the comma-shaped body, where it suppresses paired-box protein 2 (PAX2).

D: The comma-shaped body extends to form an S-shaped structure. Under the control of transcription factors, distal segments further extend and differentiate towards distal tubule segments (with a high concentration of BRN1) and intermediate tubule segments. NOTCH2 controls proximal tubule fate. Podocyte cells mature under the control of transcription factors such as WT1 and LIM homeobox transcription factor 1B (LMX1B), and release signals (vascular endothelial growth factor (VEGF)) that attract endothelial cells (red), which in turn produce factors (for example, platelet-derived growth factor (PDGF) that support the differentiation of mesangial cells.

E: A patterned nephron showing the vascular loop (red), podocytes (dark green), Bowman's capsule (light green), proximal convoluted tubule (blue), intermediate segments with Henle's loop (orange), distal convoluted tubule (yellow) and collecting duct (dark red). Modified from Schedl (2007).

The mesenchymal condensations of the metanephric blastema around the terminal buds of the branches develop into a renal tubule in stages. The aggregates of metanephric blastema cells organize into an **epithelial cord** that canalizes to form a **tubule** (Fig. 15-4). The primordium of the tubule first assumes a **comma shape**, with a central lumen at its distal end and a basal lamina assembled on its outer surface. These events mark the transformation of mesenchymal cells into an epithelium. Subsequently, a slit-like space develops outside the transforming **podocyte** precursors in the tubular primordium, and precursors of vascular endothelial cells migrate into this space. These vascular endothelial cells ultimately form the capillaries of the **glomerulus**, which are connected with branches of the lateral segmental arteries arising from the aorta. Between the cells of the glomerular endothelium and the neighbouring podocytes, a thick basal lamina is formed that later serves as an important component of the **renal filtration barrier**.

As the glomerular component of the nephron takes shape, the comma-shaped tubular primordium is transformed into an **S-shaped structure**. During this process the rest of the tubule primordium acquires the characteristics of epithelial cells. The cells now express E-cadherin, which seals the lateral border of the cells, and laminin is deposited at their basal surfaces. A characteristic pattern of gene expression can be observed along the length of the S-shaped tubules: near what will later be the glomerular end of the tubule, *WT-1* becomes strongly expressed, whereas *Pax2* expression declines. At the other end (the future distal convoluted tubule) expression of both *Wnt-4* and *E-Cadherin* remain prominent. In the middle part of the S-shaped tubule (the future proximal convoluted tubule) *K-cadherin* expression remains high. Later, differentiation of the renal tubule progresses from the proximal to the distal convoluted tubule. The middle part of each tubule develops into an elongated, thin, hairpin-like loop that extends into the medulla of the kidney and is referred to as the tubulus attenuatus or the **loop of Henle**. During the differentiation, the tubular epithelial cells also acquire molecular features characteristic of mature kidney cells, including expression of brush border antigens or the Tamm-Horsfall protein. The mature nephrons each consist of a renal corpuscle located in the outer cortical portion of the kidney, and an elongated tubular loop that extends centrally and contributes to the medulla of the kidney.

Development of the kidney involves the formation of approximately **15 successive generations of nephrons** in the peripheral cortical zone (Figs 15-7, 15-8, 15-9). The first renal corpuscles to form are located at the corticomedullary junction. Many of the early nephrons become apoptotic during later fetal stages. Collecting tubules elongate and new generations of nephrons are induced and form at progressively more superficial levels. Thus, the outermost nephrons are less mature than are those located deeper in the cortex. Depending on the species, nephrogenesis ceases at or shortly after birth; nephrogenesis continues during the first weeks post partum in the dog, and for the first three weeks in the pig. The number of nephrons formed differs between the species: about 200 000 nephrons form in the feline kidney, 300 000–500 000 in the dog, and 1.5–4 million in ruminants and pigs.

The variations in macroscopic appearance of the mature kidney result from differences in the branching of the ureteric bud and the arrangement of nephrons associated with these branches (Fig. 15-9). In **cattle**, the ureteric bud, from which the ureter is derived, forms two major branches (primary branches) that subdivide into 12 to 25 minor (secondary) branches. Consequently, the bovine kidney develops 12–25 separate **lobes,** each retaining its distinct pyramid-forming papillae. The bovine kidney is therefore often referred to as a **multipyramidal kidney**. The papillary ducts within each lobe drain into a **calyx**. The bovine kidney differs from that of the other domestic animals in having **no renal pelvis**.

In the **pig**, although the **cortex is not lobated**, the **medulla is subdivided into renal pyramids forming papillae** and so the porcine kidney is also **multipyramidal**. Each papilla consists of nephric loops and the collecting tubules and ducts that empty into terminal branches of a **minor calyx**. The dilated end of the porcine ureteric bud forms the **renal pelvis**. From the two major divisions of

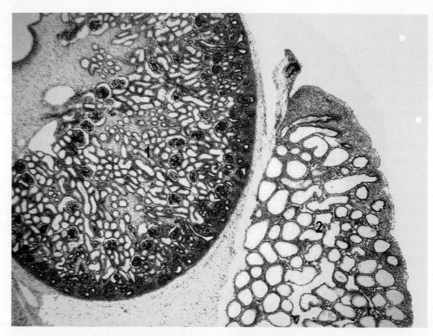

Fig: 15-7: Metanephros and regressing mesonephros of a bovine fetus with a CRL of 30 cm. 1: Metanephros; 2: Mesonephros.

the renal pelvis (**major calyces**) up to ten funnel-shaped minor calyces originate. Despite it superficially smooth appearance, the multilobular structure of the porcine kidney reveals itself in both its multipyramidal appearance and the separate drainage of each lobe through minor calyces.

In the **horse**, **small ruminants**, and **carnivores** no calyces are formed and the papillary duct drains directly into a **common pelvis**. In the horse, the renal pelvis possesses two long, thin-walled processes (**terminal recesses**) in which the urine is collected. The terminal recesses are lined by the same epithelium as the collecting ducts and may be regarded as fusions of collecting ducts originating from the nephrons located near the poles of the kidney. The **cortex** undergoes a complete fusion resulting in a **non-lobated**, smooth surface of the kidney. Moreover, fusion of the apical regions of the medullary pyramids results in the formation of a ridge-like common papilla, the **renal crest**. All collecting ducts open into the pelvis on this ridge which runs on the roof of the pelvis. The deep lateral recesses of the canine pelvis do not collect urine, but

segregate the medullary regions into wedge-shaped structures called renal pyramids

The metanephric kidney develops first in the pelvic region of the embryo. However, due to the extensive growth and elongation of the posterior portion of the fetus, in a relative sense the kidney ascends a short distance into the abdomen and in most species becomes situated ventral to the cranial lumbar vertebrae. The ureter elongates accordingly, commensurate with fetal growth.

Bladder and urethra

During development of the hindgut, the cloaca is subdivided by the urorectal septum into the **rectum** (dorsally) and the **urogenital sinus** (ventrally). The latter comprises an anterior pelvic region and a posterior phallic region (Fig. 15-10). Cranially, the urogenital sinus is connected to the allantoic cavity through the **urachus** which is continued in the allantoic stalk. After degeneration of the cloacal membrane the allantoic stalk opens caudally into the amniotic cavity through the **urogenital orifice**.

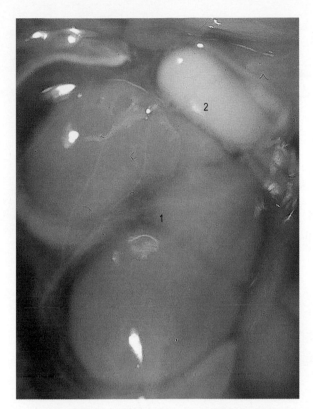

Fig. 15-8: Metanephros (1) and adrenal gland (2) of a bovine fetus with a CRL of 12.7 cm.

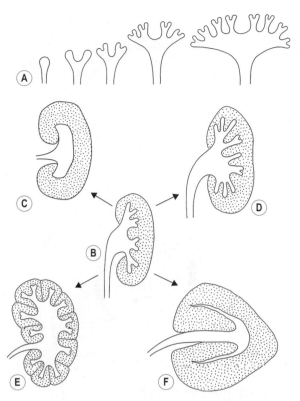

Fig. 15-9: Development of the renal pelvis, calyces and collecting tubules of the metanephros. A: Splitting of the ureteric bud in the metanephrogenic blastema. B: Indifferent stage of the metanephros: C–F: Differentiation of the metanephros in carnivores (C), pig (D), bovine (E), and horse (F). Courtesy Sinowatz and Rüsse (2007).

The **bladder** forms from the **proximal portion of the urachus and the pelvic region of the urogenital sinus** (Figs. 15-10, 15-11). The attenuated distal end of the urachus solidifies into a cord-like structure, which is suspended in a peritoneal fold that ultimately forms the **median umbilical ligament**, leading from the bladder to the umbilical region. As the bladder grows, its expanding wall incorporates the terminal portions of mesonephric ducts and the ureteric buds, and each duct system develops its own separate openings into the developing bladder. Initially, the mesonephric ducts open anterior to the ureteric buds, but gradually the positions of these orifices shift, so that the ends of the ureteric buds finally open into the bladder laterally and anterior to the mesonephric ducts. A triangular area in the dorsal wall of the neck of the bladder and the cranial urethra represents the region of mesonephric duct and ureteric bud incorporation. The base of this trigone is delineated anteriorly by the entrance of the forming ureters. The apex is located where the mesonephric ducts each enter to form the ductus deferens on either side of a small swelling referred to as the urethral crest. **The trigone in the dorsal wall of the bladder is lined by epithelium of mesodermal origin whereas the rest of the bladder epithelium is derived from the endoderm**. The non-epithelial components of the bladder wall (connective tissue and smooth muscle) are derived from the visceral mesoderm.

In the female, the **urethra** develops from the anterior portion of the pelvic urogenital sinus and the remainder of the sinus forms the **vestibule**. In the male, the caudal urogenital sinus gives rise to the **penile urethra**.

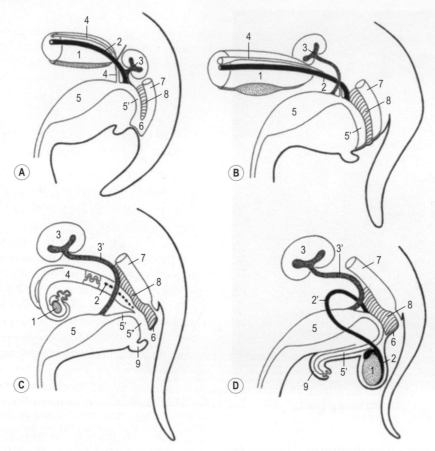

Fig. 15-10: Differentiation of the Wolffian and Müllerian ducts and dislocation of the urethra during the development of male and female genital organs.
A and B: Indifferent stage: 1: Mesonephros and genital ridge (stippled); 2: Wolffian duct; 3: Ureteric bud; 4: Müllerian duct; 5: Sinus urogenitalis (later urinary bladder) with primary urethra (5'). 6: Cloaca; 7: Rectum; 8: Septum urorectale.
C: Female genital organs: 1: Ovary; 2: Gardner's duct (remainings of the mesonephric duct); 3: Metanephros with ureter (3'); 4: Uterus; 5: Urinary bladder with urethra (5') and vestibulum (5''); 6: Perineum; 7: Rectum; 8: Septum urorectale; 9: Clitoris.
D: Male genital organs: 1: Testis; 2: Epididymis; 2': Ductus deferens; 3: Metanephros with ureter (3'); 5: Urinary bladder with urethra (5'); 6: Perineum; 7: Rectum; 8: Septum urorectale; 9: Penis. Courtesy Sinowatz and Rüsse (2007).

DEVELOPMENT OF THE MALE AND FEMALE GENITAL ORGANS

Sex determination

Chromosomal sex is established at fertilization, when a **Y-** or an **X-chromosome-bearing sperma-tozoon** fuses with the oocyte to determine the **genetic sex** of the zygote. The *sex determining region*

of the *Y gene (Sry)*, a member of the Sox family of transcription factors, is the testis-determining gene. It is located within a 35-kilodalton region on the short arm of the Y-chromosome. In the mouse, *Sry* encodes a 223 amino acid DNA-binding protein of the high mobility group (HMG) box class. It presumably regulates the expression of other genes, which then confer the cellular phenotype. Additional evidence that *Sry* is the Y-encoded

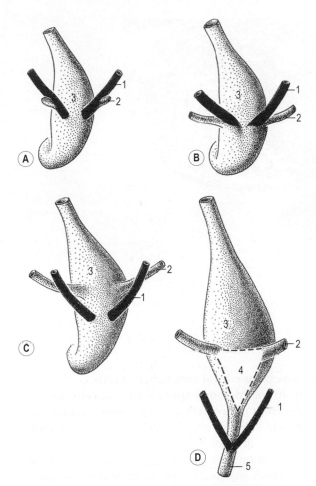

Fig. 15-11: Dorsal view of the bladder showing the relation of the ureters and the mesonephric ducts during development. A: Initially the ureters are formed by an outgrowth of the mesonephric duct, but with time they assume a separate entrance into the urinary bladder (B-D). 1: Mesonephric duct; 2: Ureteric bud; 3: Urinary bladder; 4: Trigone of the bladder (trigonum vesicae); 5: Urethra. Courtesy Sinowatz and Rüsse (2007).

sex-specific phenotype is not apparent until after 4 to 7 weeks of development, depending on the species. Subtle differences, however, are expressed much earlier as it has been demonstrated that the rate of development up to the blastocyst stage is faster in males than in females.

Primordial germ cells and indifferent stage of gonadal development

During the **indifferent stage of gonadal development, primordial germ cells (PGCs) migrate from the yolk sac into the gonadal primordium** (see Chapter 4). The PGCs are the source of germ cells in the adult gonad. PGCs can first be identified in the epiblast, where their formation, at least in mice, is dependent upon the expression of BMP4 by the extraembryonal ectoderm (see Chapter 20). The extraembryonic ectoderm is formed during development of the amnion in mice, and, because amniogenesis is basically different in the domestic animals and the mouse, it is uncertain whether a similar mechanism operates in the domestic species. PGCs can be identified histochemically by their high alkaline phosphatase activity and by their expression of pluripotency transcription factors such as Oct4. These cells pass through the early primitive streak and become located as a small cluster of cells in the extraembryonic mesoderm, near the base of the allantois. They then become incorporated into the endoderm of the posterior wall of the yolk sac, where they are apparently further dislocated from the embryonic disc. Subsequently, the PGCs shift to a site in the mesoderm along the yolk sac and allantois stalks. From there they apparently migrate in the wall of the hindgut and through the dorsal mesentery until they reach the newly formed genital ridge (Fig. 15-12).

Studies in mutant mice have demonstrated that the **passage of PGCs to the dorsal mesentery and into the genital ridges probably requires active locomotion.** This, especially the initial stages of migration, is accomplished by active amoeboid movement of the cells in response to molecular clues form the extracellular matrix. In avian species, PGCs reach the genital ridge via the blood stream.

testis-determining gene has come from experiments with transgenic mice: sex reversal from female to male was found after a small genomic fragment carrying the mouse *Sry* gene was introduced as a transgene into XX embryos. These results demonstrate not only that Sry is involved in testis determination, but that it is the *only* gene of the Y chromosome that is required for this process. Although the genetic sex of the embryo is fixed at fertilization, the gross

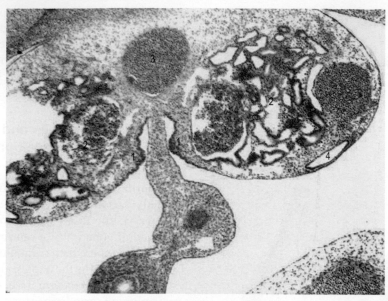

Fig. 15-12: Cross section through a sheep embryo of 17 mm CRL. 1: Genital ridge; 2: Mesonephros; 3: Aorta; 4: Wolffian duct.

PGCs divide during migration to the gonadal primordia in response to mitogenic factors such as LIF and Steel factor and many remain linked to one another through long cytoplasmic processes. They also express the transcription factor Oct4, which is involved in the maintenance of their pluripotent state (see Chapter 4) and is the same gene that maintains the undifferentiated state of blastomeres and the ICM in developing embryos (see Chapter 6). PGCs can be found in the genital ridge by Day 16 in the pig, Day 21 in dogs, Day 22 in sheep, Day 25 in cattle, and Day 28 in humans. Approximately 1000 to 2000 PGCs enter the genital ridge. A few days after colonizing the genital ridges, PGCs undergo mitotic arrest. **In the testis primordium the PGCs do not enter meiosis until puberty whereas meiosis is initiated during fetal development in the ovary primordium.**

The gonads develop from an elongated region of steroidogenic mesoderm along the ventromedial border of the mesonephros. As already described, the mesonephros is a primitive kidney developing from unsegmented, intermediate mesoderm. The early genital ridge consists of three major cell populations: **local mesenchymal cells, cells derived from the coelomic epithelium**, and **cells originating from the regressing mesonephric tubules** that invade the presumptive gonadal tissue. Recently, some of the molecular mechanisms of gonadal differentiation have been established. One of the earliest genes required for the formation of the gonads is *WT-1* which is expressed throughout the intermediate mesoderm and also plays an important role in the development of kidneys. *Lim-1* is another major gene involved in the early phase of gonadal development: in its absence no gonads form. Another gene, *steroid factor 1*, is expressed in the early indifferent gonad as well as in the developing adrenal medulla, which forms from cells in the cranial part of the steroidogenic mesoderm.

Although the sex of a mammalian embryo is determined genetically at the time of fertilization, the genital ridges remain morphological indifferent during the first weeks of gestation. When the PGCs arrive in the **gonadal ridge**, the resident mesenchymal cells and the coelomic epithelium proliferate and, consequently, the developing gonadal ridges project into the coelomic cavity (Figs. 15-12, 15-13).

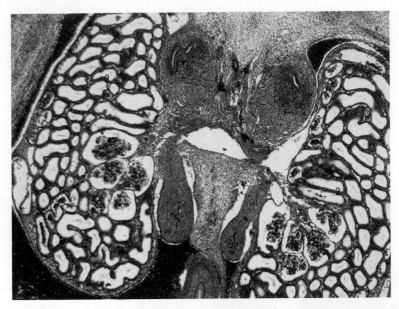

Fig. 15-13: Cross section through a bovine fetus of 11.3 cm CRL. 1: Gonad; 2: Mesonephros.

This ridge forms in embryos of approximately 9–10 mm CRL and grows quickly when the PGCs arrive. Cords of epithelial cells from the mesonephric tubules and regressing glomerular capsules penetrate the mesenchyme of the genital ridge and form a number of irregularly shaped cords – the **primitive sex cords** or gonadal cords – that incorporate PGCs. In both sexes these cords are temporarily connected to the surface epithelium. At this time it is still **impossible to differentiate the male and female gonad morphologically** and they are therefore referred to as **indifferent gonads**.

Differentiation of the testis

Differentiation of the testis (Figs 15-14, 15-15) occurs under the influence of the *Sry* gene (testis-determining factor) on the Y-chromosome. Without the expression of products of this gene, the indifferent gonad develops somewhat later into an ovary. In male embryos, transcripts of the *Sry* gene only become detectable in the genital ridge just at the

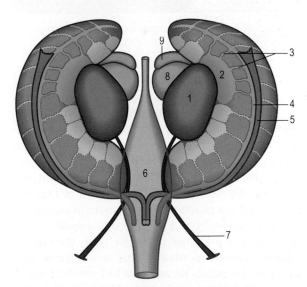

Fig. 15-14: Schematic drawing showing the topography of the urogenital system after the differentiation of the gonads. 1: Gonad; 2: Giant glomerulus; 3: Tubules of the mesonephros; 4: Mesonephric (Wolffian duct); 5: Paramesonephric (Müllerian) duct; 6: Sinus urogenitalis; 7: Gubernaculum testis; 8: Metanephros; 9: Adrenal gland. Courtesy Sinowatz and Rüsse (2007).

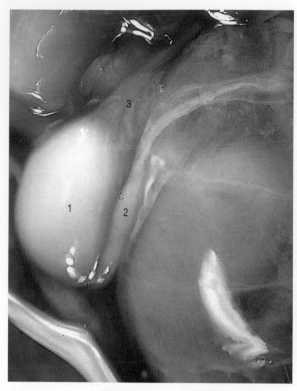

Fig. 15-15: Testis (1) and epididymis (2) of a bovine fetus with a CRL of 12 cm. 3: Plexus pampiniformis.

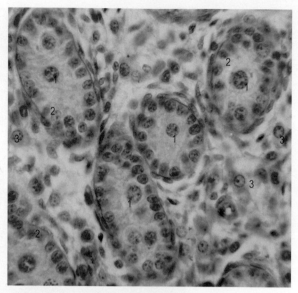

Fig. 15-16: Testis of a bovine embryo of 10 weeks gestation. The testicular cords consist of primordial germ cells (1) and presumptive Sertoli cells (2). Between the cords mesenchymal cells form the first generation of androgen-secreting Leydig cells (3).

onset of testis differentiation. Neither the expression of the *Sry* gene in the testis primordium, nor subsequent testicular development, is dependent on the presence of germ cells. *Sry* triggers testis formation by inhibiting *Dax-1*, a member of the nuclear receptor family, which is also expressed in the indifferent gonad at the same time. The inhibition of *Dax-1* is necessary for a genetically male gonad to express its sex phenotypically and develop into a testis.

Under the influence of the *Sry* gene, the cells of the primitive sex cords continue to proliferate and penetrate deep into the medulla to form the **testicular** or **medullary cords** (Figs 15-16, 15-17). The subsequent development of the indifferent gonad into a testis is initiated in the medullary region of the gonadal ridge. The testicular cords transform into solid **tubules** composed of **primitive germ cells** centrally and presumptive sustentacular cells or **Sertoli cells** peripherally. These tubules are arranged in **horseshoe-like loops** connected at both ends to a network of tiny cells strands, the later **rete testis**. The testicular tubules develop a lumen at the time of puberty and become the **seminiferous tubules**. The rete testis eventually joins the **efferent ductules**, which are derived from remaining mesonephric tubules. They link the rete testis to the mesonephric or Wolffian duct, which becomes the **ductus epididymidis** and the **ductus deferens**.

The developing male gonad also produces a chemoattractive substance that stimulates the migration of mesonephric cells to the gonad, where they surround the testicular cords and differentiate into the contractile **myoid cells**. As the testicular cords differentiate, a dense layer of fibrous connective tissue, the **tunica albuginea**, forms as a capsule surrounding the testicular cords beneath the surface epithelium of the gonad. A tunica albuginea is first seen in cattle at Day 41 (CRL 20 mm), sheep at Day 31 (17 mm CRL), the horse at Day 30 (16 to 17 mm CRL), and the dog at Day 29 (19 to 20 mm CRL).

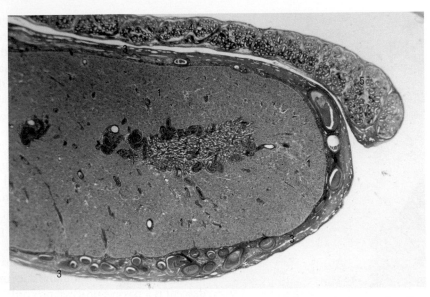

Fig. 15-17: Testis and epididymis of a newborn calf. 1: Testicular parenchyma; 2: Mediastinum testis with rete testis; 3: Tunica albuginea; 4: Corpus epidiymidis; 5: Cauda epididymidis.

In the mesenchyme between the testicular cords, the first generation of androgen-producing **Leydig cells** develop in cattle at a CRL of 30 mm (Day 42) and in pigs at 33 mm. During the next two days, these cells initiate an **increasing production of testosterone and androstendione**. This endocrine activity is important for the differentiation of the male sexual duct system, the development of the external male genitalia, and differentiation of the sexual centres in the brain, which are important for the development of male behaviour. After several weeks to months (7 months of gestation in cattle), the **first (fetal) generation of Leydig cells gradually involutes**, to be replaced later by a **second generation of Leydig cells** before puberty. The second generation cells differentiate from connective tissue cells and are responsible for initiation and further stimulation of spermatogenesis.

Descent of the testes

This refers to the migration of the testes from their intra-abdominal site of development into the scrotum, usually located in the inguinal region (Fig. 15-18). In mammals, this process is subject to species variation. For instance, in aquatic mammals, elephants, and armadillos, the testes remain within the abdominal cavity and descent does not occur. In most mammals, however, including all our domestic species, the testes migrate to an extra-abdominal location. In these species, a temperature of 2–4°C below the core body temperature is required for normal spermatogenesis.

Like the kidney, the testes develop in a retroperitoneal position. Before their descent, the testes are anchored cranially by a **suspensory ligament**, derived from the diaphragmatic ligament of the mesonephros, and caudally to the inguinal ligament of the mesonephros, which later becomes the **gubernaculum testis**. As the mesonephros degenerates, the ligaments supporting the gonads and ducts remain attached to the wall of the peritoneal cavity. The site of attachment of these folds shifts from dorsolateral to ventrolateral as the ducts pass caudally.

Testicular descent occurs in three phases. The first is associated with the **enlargement of the testes** and the concomitant regression of the mesonephros. Under the influence of androgens, the anterior **suspensory ligament regresses** and the testis is released

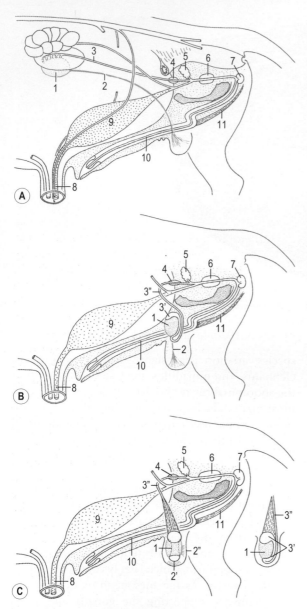

Fig. 15-18: Descent of the testis in cattle. A: The testis is located in the abdominal cavity. B: Testis passing the inguinal canal. C: Testis within the scrotum. 1: Testis; 2: Gubernaculum testis; 2': Lig. testis proprium and Lig. caudae epididymidis; 2": Lig. inguinale testis; 3: Wolffian duct; 3': Epididymis; 3": Ductus deferens: 4: Ampulla ductus deferentis; 5: Vesicular gland; 6: Prostate; 7: Bulbourethral gland; 8: Urachus; 9: Urinary bladder; 10: Urethra; 11: M. retractor penis. Courtesy Sinowatz and Rüsse (2007).

from its location near the diaphragm. During the second phase, usually called **transabdominal descent**, the **testes move down to the level of the inner opening of the inguinal canal**, mainly as a result of growth and elongation of the body while the testis remains at an approximately constant distance from the urogenital sinus. Recent data show that, at least in mice, this phase of testicular descent depends on the expression of *Insl-3* in the testis. Without Insl-3 the testes remain in their cranial location. The third phase is termed **transinguinal descent** which moves the testes into the scrotum. This phase is androgen dependent and involves the guidance of the gubernaculum testis. Whether the gubernaculum actively pulls the testis into the scrotum, or just acts as a guiding structure, has not been finally resolved but many data indicate that the descent is a passive process; no contractile tissue can be demonstrated in the gubernaculum.

Although the mechanisms of testicular migration into the scrotum are not clear, the time frame of the event is well established. The testes are located at the internal opening of the inguinal canal in dogs at Day 50, in cattle at Day 90, in pigs at Day 70, and in horses at Day 240. As the testis approaches the inguinal opening, the tail of the epididymis enters the inguinal canal. Once the testis is positioned adjacent to the inguinal canal, changes occur that reduce the size disparity between the canal and the gonad; an increase in intercellular fluid causes **the gubernaculum to swell** at the level of the canal, thereby facilitating the entry of the testis into the canal. **Once the testis has entered the inguinal canal, contraction of the internal opening together with contractions of the abdominal muscles force the testis along the canal and through the external inguinal opening**. The time of passage through the inguinal canal is species-dependent – rapid in cattle and pigs, but slow in horses. As the testis leaves the inguinal canal, the gubernaculum testis regresses, facilitating the final descent of the testis into the scrotum. The transinguinal descent is androgen-dependent. The approximate times of testicular descent are shown in Table 15-1.

Failure of normal testicular descent is termed **cryptorchidism**. It is seen most frequently in horses

Table 15-1: Descent of the testis

Species	Beginning of testicular descent	Testis within the inguinal canal	Testis within the scrotum
Cattle	15.8 cm CRL	22 cm CRL	40 cm CRL
Sheep	15 cm CRL	17.5 cm CRL	25 cm CRL
Pig	Day 65 p.c.	Day 85–90 p.c.	At birth
Horse	Day 45 p.c.	Before birth	At birth
Dog	–	Day 3–4 p.p.	Day 35–40 p.p.

CRL = crown-rump length; p.c. = post coitum; p.p = post partum

and pigs, and also in miniature dogs. Several pathological conditions, like abnormal testicular development, abnormal development of the vaginal process, abnormal development of the gubernaculum testis, or endocrine disorders have been associated with cryptorchidism, but its aetiology is still not clear. There are many indications that cryptorchidism is an inherited condition. Bilateral cryptorchidism causes infertility, but as the Leydig cells are unaffected by the higher core body temperature, the animals usually have the phenotype and behavioural characteristics of a typical male. In dogs there is also an increased frequency of neoplastic changes of abdominal testes compared to scrotal testes.

Postnatal differentiation of Sertoli cells and formation of the blood-testis barrier

During postnatal differentiation primitive Sertoli cells undergo extensive morphological and biochemical differentiation to give rise to mature **Sertoli cells**. These developmental changes appear to be mediated to a large extent by FSH and are accompanied by a marked stimulation of protein synthesis in the Sertoli cells. Experimental transplantation of testicular tissue to normal and hypophysectomized mice has demonstrated that the pituitary gland strongly influences the postnatal maturation of Sertoli cells with specific effects on nucleolar differentiation and formation of intercellular tight junctions.

Among the morphological changes that occur during the postnatal differentiation of Sertoli cells, the formation of occlusive **tight junctions** between them is of great functional importance. Studies on the adult testes of numerous species have shown that Sertoli cell junctions are the main component of the **blood-testis barrier** – the barrier that divides the seminiferous epithelium into a basal compartment containing spermatogonia and preleptotene spermatocytes and an adluminal compartment accommodating the more advanced stages of spermatogenic cells (see Chapter 4). In the domestic animals, formation of occlusive tight junctions between neighbouring Sertoli cells and the establishment of the blood-testis barrier occur around puberty. The blood-testis barrier has several important effects on spermatogenesis. There are immunological differences between the spermatogonia and preleptotene spermatocytes (found beneath the blood- barrier) and the more advanced spermatocytes and spermatids of the adluminal compartment. These differences are established during the initial spermatogenic cycle. It is only after the passage of spermatocytes into the adluminal compartment that autoantigenic molecules are synthesized and/or inserted into the plasma membrane of the spermatocytes.

Main features of the adult testis

The **testis** is covered by a fibrous capsule, the **tunica albuginea**, from which small trabeculae of connective tissue extend inwards. The two major compartments of the testis are the interstitial or intertubular compartment and the seminiferous

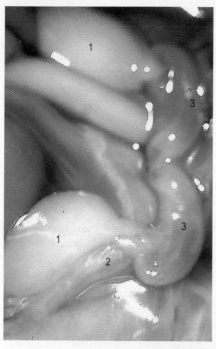

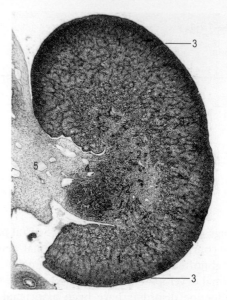

Fig. 15-20: Longitudinal section through the ovary of a sheep fetus with a CRL of 30 cm. In the cortex numerous cortical cords penetrating the underlying mesenchyme can be seen. 1: Cortex of the ovary; 2: Medulla of the ovary. 3: Superficial epithelium of the ovary. 4: Hilus of the ovary; 5: Mesovarium.

Fig. 15-19: Ovary (1), oviduct (2) and uterus (3) of a bovine fetus with a CRL of 18.6 cm. Left is cranial.

tubule compartment. The **interstitial compartment** contains the androgen-producing **Leydig cells**, blood vessels, lymphatic vessels, nerve fibres, and macrophages. The endothelium of the testicular capillaries is continuous and no fenestrations can be seen. The lymphatic vessels are irregular and only incompletely lined by endothelium. The Leydig cells possess a roundish nucleus and, in their cytoplasm, abundant smooth endoplasmic reticulum and long mitochondria with tubular cristae where the enzymes associated with steroid synthesis are located. The seminiferous epithelium of the convoluted **tubuli seminiferi contorti** contains the somatic **Sertoli cells** and the different generations of **germ cells**. Sertoli cells are tall columnar cells, which extend from the basal lamina to the tubular lumen and form the structural framework of the seminiferous epithelium. They have numerous and important interrelationships with the germinal cells (see Chapter 4). The seminiferous tubule compartment is bounded by 'boundary tissue' made up of a

basement membrane, the **contractile myoid cells**, and the lymphatic endothelium. Contractions of the myoid cells provide the propulsive forces that transport spermatozoa and tubular fluid towards the excurrent duct system.

Differentiation of the ovaries

In female animals, the expression of *Dax-1*, in the absence of *Sry*, suppresses the formation of a testis and allows the indifferent gonads to develop into ovaries (Fig. 15-19). Contrary to testicular development, the presence of viable germs cells is necessary for ovarian differentiation; if PGCs fail to reach the genital ridges, the gonadal anlagen regress and streak ovaries result.

After the PGCs have reached the genital ridge, they remain concentrated in the outer (cortical) region of the future ovary (Figs 15-19, 15-20, 15-21). The medullary region also contains some PGCs that become enclosed in primitive sex cords, but in a far

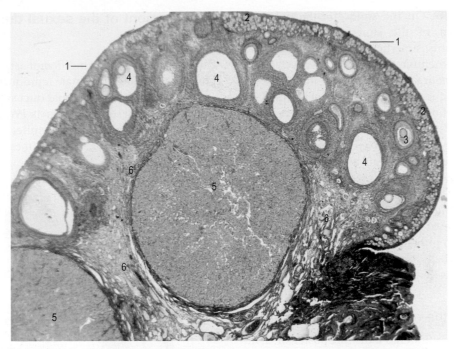

Fig. 15-21: Ovary of an adult cat showing the different generations of follicles and corpora lutea. 1: Superficial epithelium; 2: Primordial follicles; 3: Secondary follicle; 4: Antral (tertiary) follicle; 5: Corpus luteum; 6: Ovarian stroma.

less well developed state than in the testis. The more abundant PGCs in the cortex also become associated with somatic cells, but the origin of these so-called **follicle cells** is still disputed. Three sites of origin of follicle cells have been proposed: (1) cells of the **coelomic epithelium**, (2) **primitive sex cords of mesonephric origin**, and (3) a **combination** of both.

The primary germ cells that are surrounded by presumptive follicle cells are called **oogonia**. They proliferate by **mitoses** for some time and later enter the **prophase of meiosis**, possibly under the influence of meiosis-stimulating factor from the mesonephros. With the **beginning of the prophase of the first meiotic division**, the germ cells are called **primary oocytes** and, together with the follicle cells, they form **primordial follicles**. Oogonia and oocytes are connected by intercellular cytoplasmic bridges that play a role in the synchronization of their development. The primary oocytes continue the first

meiotic division until they reach the **diplotene stage, when division is arrested**. The primary oocytes remain at this stage until the block is removed as a result of the follicle being selected for ovulation during postnatal folliculogenesis (see Chapter 4). Therefore, many months to years may elapse between imposition of the prenatal meiotic block during embryonic life and its lifting near the time of ovulation.

At the medullary-cortical junction of the fetal ovary, an inconspicuous tunica albuginea is formed, separating the cortex and medulla. The cortex contains the majority of the oocytes. In the central part of the ovary, the germ cells disappear, replaced by a vascular stroma that forms the ovarian medulla. The connective tissue and the blood vessels of the medulla are derived from the mesonephros. The developing ovary does not maintain a relationship with the mesonephros and, other than a few remnants, **all mesonephric tubules degenerate in the** female embryo. On the surface of the ovary the cuboidal form of the superficial epithelium is retained. As this superficial epithelium does not revert to mesothelium, the ovary is not covered with typical peritoneum in the adult. In the ovaries of bitches and queens, narrow channels lined by surface epithelium protrude into the cortex of the ovary.

In the ovary of the **horse, the development of the follicles is confined to a small central area**, which corresponds to the **medulla ovarii** of other species. The non-follicular area is peripherally located. During prenatal development, the unattached surface of the ovary becomes concave and the coelomic epithelium is retained in this point. Therefore, in the horse, ovulation occurs only in this site, which is called the **ovulation fossa**.

Descent of the ovaries

The ovaries also undergo a distinct **posterior dislocation**, varying with species. As they grow and cross over the Müllerian ducts, the ovaries move posteriorly and laterally. In dogs and cats, the migration is not very pronounced and the ovaries occupy a position in the sublumbar region caudal to the kidney. In the mare, the ovaries become positioned midway between the kidneys and the pelvic inlet. In pigs and cattle, the descent is more pronounced and the ovaries finally occupy a position much nearer the pelvic inlet. The final position of the ovaries is stabilized by ligaments, which are remnants of structures associated with the mesonephros. Cranially, the diaphragmatic ligament of the mesonephros becomes the **suspensory ligament of the ovary**. As already described, the inguinal ligament of the mesonephros is later called the **gubernaculum**. Its cranial portion, located between the ovary and the Müllerian duct, forms the **proper ligament of the ovary** between the ovary and the tip of the uterine horn. The remainder of the gubernaculum gives rise to the **round ligament of the uterus**. In the bitch, the most caudal ends of the round ligaments continue through the inguinal canal and can be identified outside the canal. This may predispose bitches to inguinal herniation.

Development of the sexual duct system

Indifferent stage

During the sexually indifferent stage, embryos posses both male and female reproductive tract primordia. The **indifferent sexual duct system** consists of the **paired mesonephric ducts (Wolffian ducts)** and **paramesonephric ducts (Müllerian ducts;** Fig. 15-22). The development of the mesonephric duct

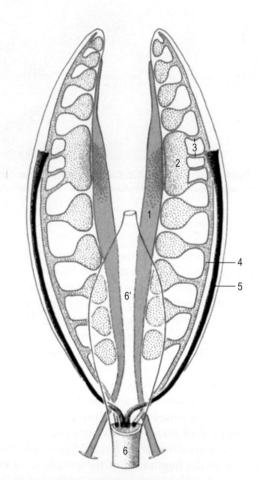

Fig. 15-22: Schematic drawing showing the relative positions of the Wolffian and Müllerian ducts during the indifferent stage of genital development. 1: Genital ridge (red); 2: Giant glomerus (seen in cattle); 3: Mesonephric tubules; 4: Wolffian (mesonephric) duct; 6: Müllerian (paramesonephric) duct; 6: Sinus urogenitalis; 6': Urinary bladder. Courtesy Sinowatz and Rüsse (2007).

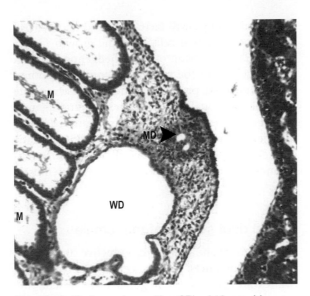

Fig. 15-23: Bovine embryo with a CRL of 18 mm. M: Mesonephros; MD: Müllerian duct; WD: Wolffian duct.

has been described in the previous paragraphs on the formation of the mesonephros. The **paramesonephric ducts** form bilaterally in both male and female embryos on the lateral side of the mesonephros, close to the mesonephric duct (Fig. 15-23). Initially, a longitudinal paramesonephric invagination develops in the coelomic mesothelium. This deepens and, finally, separates from the peritoneal lining to form a solid cord of cells that grows caudally along the lateral and then ventral wall of the mesonephros. Subsequently, a lumen is formed in the cord. **Anteriorly, the paramesonephric duct opens into the abdominal cavity with a funnel-like structure.** Posteriorly, it first runs laterally to the mesonephric duct, then crosses it ventrally to grow posteriomedially and meet the paramesonephric duct from the opposite side. The two tubes fuse and extend further posteriorly. **The posterior tip of the combined ducts projects into the posterior wall of the urogenital sinus**, where it causes a small swelling, the paramesonephric or Müllerian swelling. The mesonephric duct opens into the urogenital sinus on either side of the paramesonephric tubercle. The fate of the indifferent genital ducts depends on the sex of the gonad.

Sexual duct system of the male

As mentioned previously, development of the genital duct system in the male depends on hormones from the testis. **Müllerian inhibiting substance (MIS)**, produced by the embryonic Sertoli cells, suppresses the development of the Müllerian ducts (paramesonephric ducts), leaving only remnants at their anterior and posterior ends (appendix testis and part of the utriculus prostaticus). MIS is a glycoprotein of the Transforming Growth Factor-β (TGF-β) family. It primarily affects the mesenchymal cells surrounding the paramesonephric duct; these cells express a gene encoding a serine/threonine kinase membrane-bound receptor, which binds MIS. Under its influence the surrounding mesenchymal cells cause the epithelial cells of the paramesonephric duct to regress.

As the mesonephros regresses, a few excretory tubules (epigenital tubules) make contact with the cords of the rete testis and are eventually transformed into the **efferent ductules**. Excretory tubules along the posterior pole of the testis (paragenital tubules) do not join the rete testis. Their vestiges are collectively called the paradidymis.

Under the influence of testosterone from the embryonic Leydig cells, the **mesonephric duct** continues to develop and becomes the main drainage system for the testis. Testosterone enters cells of target tissues where it may be converted by a 5α-reductase to dihydrotestosterone. Testosterone and dihydrotestosterone bind to a specific intracellular androgen receptor and the hormone-receptor complex is translocated to the nucleus where it binds to DNA to regulate transcription of tissue-specific genes. Testosterone and its main metabolite, 5α-dihydrotestosterone, mediate the differentiation of the mesonephric duct to form the **epididymis, the ductus deferens, the ejaculatory ducts, and the seminal vesicles**. Immediately below the entrance of the efferent ductules, the mesonephric duct becomes highly convoluted, forming the **ductus epididymidis**. From the epididymis to the outbudding of the seminal vesicle, the mesonephric duct is invested by a thick layer of smooth muscle cells and forms the **ductus deferens**. The regions of the mesonephric ducts posterior to the primordium of the seminal vesicles become the **ejaculatory ducts**. The blind anterior end of the mesonephric duct persists as the appendix testis.

The regional development of the male genital ducts is influenced by *Hox* genes. *Hoxa-10*, for example, is expressed along the mesonephric duct from the cauda epididymis to the point where the ductus deferens joins the urethra. Mice with mutants of both the *Hoxa-10* and *Hoxa-11* genes exhibit a homeotic transformation, resulting in the partial transformation of the ductus deferens to epididymis.

Male accessory sex glands

Closely associated with the development of the male genital duct systems is the formation of the **male accessory sex glands (seminal vesicles, ampulla ductus deferentis, prostate, and bulbourethral glands)**. The bull, ram, boar, stallion, and most small laboratory animals have prostate, bulbourethral, and seminal vesicle glands as well as ampullae ductus deferentis. The cat lacks seminal vesicles, and in the dog only a prostate gland is found. The male accessory glands develop as **epithelial evaginations** from the epithelium of the **mesonephric duct** (seminal vesicles, ampulla ductus deferentis) and the **sinus urogenitalis** (prostate, bulbourethral glands). Their formation requires androgen stimulation and epithelio-mesenchymal interactions. The androgens stimulate the mesenchymal cells to cause the associated epithelium to develop the gland-specific characteristics.

The development of the prostate is controlled by androgens, growth factors, and epithelio-mesenchymal interactions. Underlying all these molecular actions is the expression of the transcription factors Hoxa-13 and Hoxd-13. They determine, at least in the mouse, at which site of the urogenital sinus a prostate will form. The parenchyma of the prostatic complex is derived from prostatic buds. These are solid epithelial outgrowths which emerge from the endodermal urogenital sinus immediately below the developing bladder and grow into the surrounding mesenchyme. Dihydrotestosterone, acting through receptors in the mesenchymal cells, induces the secretion of growth factors (FGF10 and TGFβ1) by the mesenchymal cells, and the growth factors regulate the expression of sonic hedgehog (Shh) in the epithelium of the urogenital sinus. In response to Shh signalling, prostatic epithelial buds evaginate from the urogenital sinus into the surrounding mesenchyme. The extent of budding is controlled by the inhibitory action of BMP4. The developing prostatic epithelium also induces some cells of the surrounding mesenchyme to differentiate into smooth muscle cells.

Sexual duct system of the female

The mammalian female reproductive tract comprises the **oviducts, uterus, cervix and vagina**. If ovaries are present, or if gonads are absent, the sexual duct system differentiates into a female phenotype. The absence of Müllerian inhibiting substance (MIS) allows the Müllerian duct to develop into the major structures of the female reproductive tract. Initially, three parts can be recognized in each duct: (a) an anterior portion that opens into the abdominal cavity, (b) a transverse part that crosses the mesonephric duct, and (c) a posterior portion that fuses with the corresponding part of the paramesonephric duct of the opposite side. With the descent of the ovary, the first two portions develop into the oviduct and the third forms the uterus and the cranial portion of the vagina. The mesonephric ducts regress, leaving only rudimentary structures.

A number of genes that appear to be essential for the development of the female reproductive tract have been identified recently. Among them, *Lim 1*, *Pax2*, *EMx2*, *Wnt-4*, and *Wnt-7* are indispensable for the development of the paramesonephric duct. In particular, *Lim1*, which codes for a LIM-domain-containing transcription factor, has been shown to be crucial for the initial formation of the duct.

Pax2, a member of the Pax gene family, possesses a highly conserved paired box which encodes a 128 amino acid DNA-binding domain – the Paired domain – at the N-terminus. Knockout of the *Pax2* gene in the mouse resulted in defects in the formation of the kidney, ureters and genital tract in addition to defects in ear and brain development. In contrast to what occurs in *Lim1* null embryos, both the mesonephric and paramesonephric ducts form initially in *Pax-2* null mutants, but both soon degenerate.

Emx2 is expressed in the intermediate mesoderm. In the mouse, *Emx2* null mutants completely lack the urogenital system; the paramesonephric ducts never form. *Emx2* expression is only seen during the very early stages of paramesonephric and mesonephric duct formation. These results suggest that this gene is only required in a specific window of time during development of the intermediate mesoderm, possibly providing a survival signal.

The mammalian *Wnt* genes encode secreted signalling glycoproteins that influence multiple processes during development. *Wnt4* null females exhibit a complete loss of the female reproductive tract, whereas male mutants appear normal. This phenomenon is due to the failure of paramesonephric duct formation in both sexes; in the absence of Wnt-4, the paramesonephric duct simply fails to form. *Wnt-7*, which plays an important role in the setting up of the dorsoventral axis of the developing limb, is expressed in the epithelium of the paramesonephric ducts and is required for their normal development. Wnt-7 appears to be involved in maintaining the expression of certain Hox-genes (*Hoxd 10* through *Hoxd 13*) as well as the Hoxa paralogues that are spread along the female reproductive tract. It has been shown in mice that *Hoxa-9* is expressed in the oviduct, and *Hoxa-10* in the uterus and cervix as well as the upper vagina. Mutations of the *Hox* genes cause a homeotic transformation.

As already mentioned, in the female, the mesonephric duct regresses due to the absence of male hormones. The cells of the **paramesonephric duct** proliferate and differentiate rostro-caudally, forming the **oviduct**, **uterus**, **cervix**, and the **cranial portion of the vagina**. Concomitantly, the single layered Müllerian duct epithelium differentiates and gives rise to the distinct morphologies that characterize the different regions of the female reproductive tract. Classical tissue recombination experiments have demonstrated that the differential fate along the anteroposterior axis requires reciprocal inter-

actions between the epithelium of the paramesonephric duct and the underlying mesenchyme.

The anterior portions of the Müllerian ducts become the **oviducts** (Figs 15-24, 15-25). The anterior end of each paramesonephric duct is referred to as the funnel field and develops into the **infundibulum** of the oviduct, which forms fimbriae and opens into the coelomic cavity. Towards their posterior ends, the paramesonephric ducts approach the midline and cross the mesonephric ducts ventrally. This crossing and ultimate fusion of the posterior portions of the paramesonephric ducts is caused by the entire urogenital ridges of both sides moving medially and gradually coming to lie in a transverse plane. After fusion of the paramesonephric ducts in the midline, a broad transverse pelvic fold is established. This fold, which extends from the lateral sides of the fused ducts toward the wall of the pelvis, is the **broad ligament of the uterus**.

The morphology of the uterus varies considerably among mammals and reflects the extent of fusion between the two paramesonephric ducts (Fig. 15-26). Most rodents and lagomorphs (for example the rabbit) have a **uterus duplex**, which means that both cervices of the uterus open separately into a common vagina. Primates, including the human, by contrast, display extensive fusion of the paramesonephric ducts resulting in a **uterus simplex** with the oviducts opening into a common uterine cavity. In domestic species, the posterior ends of the paramesonephric ducts fuse to varying extents. All domestic animals have a **bicornuate uterus** in which the uterine horns join to form a uterine body that opens into the vagina by a single cervix (Fig. 15-27). The openings of the two horns into the body may be largely (as in the cow) or partially separated internally by an intercornual septum. The portions cranial to the region of fusion remain distinct and are the primordia of uterine horns and oviducts.

Unlike the oviducts, the uterus in all mammals possesses glands. In most mammals studied so far, **uterine gland** development occurs postnatally. The timing of uterine gland formation is highly species-specific. In rodents, epithelial invagination is seen on Day 5 after birth, and mature glands can be detected at Day 15. In ungulates, development of

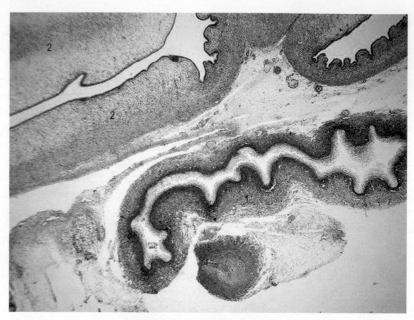

Fig. 15-24: Oviduct (1) and uterus (2) of a sheep fetus at 30 weeks of gestation. No glands are found in the uterus at this stage of development and no distinct folds are found in the oviduct.

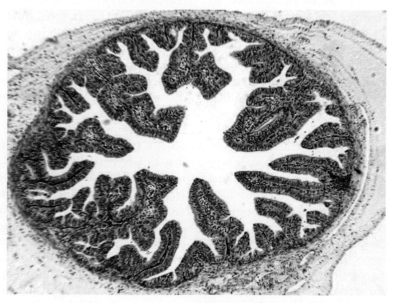

Fig. 15-25: Cross section through the oviduct of a bovine fetus with a CRL of 74 cm. Note that primary and secondary mucosal folds are well developed.

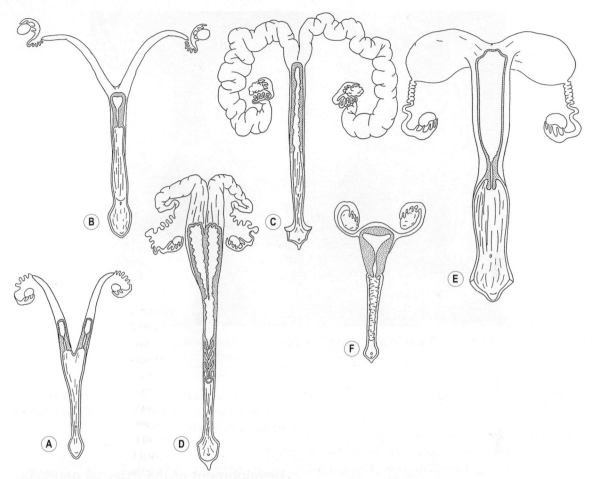

Fig. 15-26: Different shapes of the uterus in several species resulting from differences in the fusion of the Müllerian ducts. A: rabbit (uterus duplex, vagina simplex); B: Carnivores; C: Pig; D: Bovine; sheep; E: horse (uterus bicornis); F: Human (uterus simplex). Courtesy Sinowatz and Rüsse (2007).

glands begins right after birth and is completed by Days 12 and 56 in pigs and sheep, respectively. In primates, including humans, formation of uterine glands begins in utero, continues after birth and reaches histological maturity at puberty.

Uterine gland formation includes epithelial invagination, bud formation, branching, and coiling. The cellular and molecular mechanisms controlling uterine gland formation are not fully understood but new data indicate that epithelial-mesenchymal interactions, tissue remodelling factors, steroid hormones and their receptors, and prolactin are all involved in the process. For example,

it has been shown that Wnt-signalling is important in uterine gland formation. *Wnt7a* is exclusively expressed in the uterine luminal epithelium and not in glandular epithelium. In contrast, *Wnt5a* is mainly expressed in the uterine stroma during postnatal development. Both *Wnt7a* and *Wnt5a* mutant uteri fail to form uterine glands, indicating that Wnt signalling is essential for uterine gland formation. Uterine gland development also involves endometrial gland remodelling. Matrix metalloproteinases (MMPs) and their inhibitors (TIMPS) have been shown to be key regulators of branching of glands, including those of the uterus.

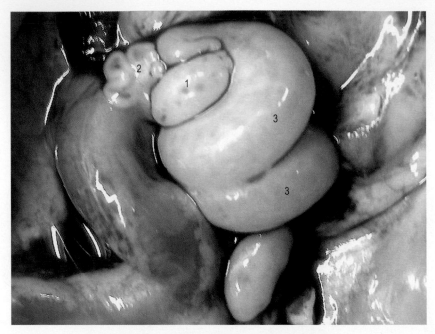

Fig. 15-27: Bovine embryo at a CRL of 58 cm. 1: Ovary; 2: Oviduct; 3: Uterus bicornis.

Development of the vagina

It is generally agreed that at least the anterior portion of the vagina arises from the posterior portions of the fused paramesonephric ducts but to what extent the urogenital sinus contributes to the rest of the vagina is still disputed. At the point where the paramesonephric ducts join the urogenital sinus, the blind ends of the paramesonephric ducts fuse with the epithelial lining of the urogenital sinus to form the epithelial **vaginal plate**. Proliferation continues at the anterior end of the plate, increasing the distance between the uterus and the urogenital sinus. Subsequently, **cannulation** of these solid structures forms the lumen of the vagina. Thus, **the vagina has a dual origin: its anterior portion derived from the paramesonephric ducts, and the posterior portion from the urogenital sinus**. The caudal portions of the urogenital sinus also form the **vestibule**. The lumen of the vagina is separated from the urogenital sinus by a thin membrane, the **hymen**, which consists of the epithelial lining of the sinus and a thin layer of vaginal cells.

In domestic animals, the hymen breaks down during subsequent development and remnants of it persist only rarely.

Development of the external genitalia

The external genitalia are derived from three complexes of mesodermal tissue located around the cloaca (Figs 15-28, 15-29). At the anteroventral end of the cloacal membrane, the **genital tubercle** is formed. Lateral to the cloacal membrane, extending most of its length, are the **cloacal (urogenital) folds**. These are soon subdivided into **urethral folds** anteriorly and **anal folds** posteriorly. Distances between the anus and the base of the genital tubercle are commonly used to differentiate male from female fetuses; a disparity is first detected at Day 30 in canine and Day 42 in bovine embryos. After that time, the anogenital distance remains constant in the female and increases in the male. Peripheral to the urogenital folds and posterolateral to the cloacal membrane, are the **genital and labioscrotal**

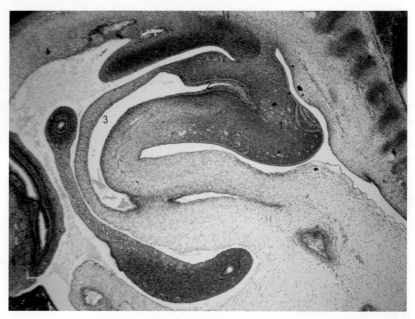

Fig. 15-28: Indifferent stage of the external genitalia of a bovine embryo with a CRL of 19 mm. 1: Phallus; 2: Urethra; 3: Urinary bladder.

swellings. These are present and similar in both sexes prior to sex differentiation.

Shortly after the appearance of the genital tubercle, and prior to the completion of the development of the urorectal septum, the epithelial lining of the floor of the urogenital sinus expands anteroventrally along the ventral margin of the elongating genital tubercle. These endodermal cells form the **urethral plate**, a solid cord of cells extending inward from the ventral surface of the tubercle. Later, the urethral plate hollows to form a canal: the urogenital folds enlarge by proliferation of mesenchymal cells on both sides of the urethral plate and a median urethral groove becomes established on the ventral surface of the genital tubercle.

External genital organs of the female

In the female, the **urogenital folds** that border the urogenital orifice fuse only at their dorsal and ventral ends and form the **labia (minora) of the vulva**. They overgrow the genital tubercle, which becomes internalized in the floor of the vestibule. Another consequence of the failure of the urogenital folds to fuse is that the urogenital sinus opening does not become incorporated into the phallus and the genital tubercle does not enlarge into a penile structure, as in the male. Instead, it gives rise to the **clitoris**, which appears vestigial in most domestic animal species. However, the genital tubercle does form a glans, and therefore the small clitoris has both a body and a glans. The **genital swellings** shift cranially to the genital tubercles and **disappear** during fetal development. Therefore (with few exceptions) no labia majora are formed in domestic animals as they are in humans. The urogenital sinus remains as the **vestibule**, with openings from both the vagina and **urethra**. The female urethra, which develops from the more cranial part of the urogenital sinus is homologous to the prostatic urethra of the male, which has a similar origin.

External genital organs in the male

Development of the external genitalia in the male is controlled by androgens from the fetal testis. Under the influence of dihydrotestosterone, a rapid

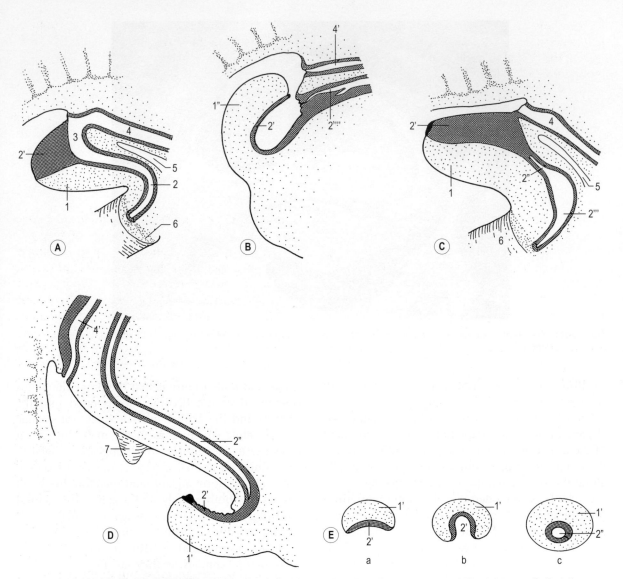

Fig. 15-29: Development of the external genitalia and the urethra (sheep). A: Female embryo, CRL of 14 mm; B: Female embryo, CRL of 36 mm; C: Male embryo, CRL of 19 mm; D: Male embryo, CRL of 39 mm; E: Cross sections of the penis demonstrating the formation of the urethra: a: urogenital plate; b: urogenital furrow; c: urethra. 1: Genital tubercle; 1′: Penis; 1″: Clitoris; 2: Sinus urogenitalis; 2′: Urethral plate; 2″: Urethra; 2‴: Urinary bladder 2⁗: Vestibulum vaginae 3: Cloaca; 4: Hindgut; 4′: Rectum; 5: Coelom; 6: Funiculus umbilicalis; 7: Scrotum. Courtesy Sinowatz and Rüsse (2007).

elongation **the genital tubercle** occurs, turning it into the **phallus**. As it grows, the **penile urethra** takes shape by ventral folding and **midline fusion of the urogenital folds**. This process proceeds in a proximo-distal direction and leads to the formation of a midline epithelial cord located in the **urethral groove** on the ventral face of the elongating phallus. The midline cord detaches from the ventral surface epithelium and becomes canalized to form the epithelium of the urethra proper. The site of fusion of the urogenital folds is indicated by the **genital raphe**.

The **glans penis** originates from the apex of the genital tubercle. From a shallow invagination at the apex of the genital tubercle, a cord of epithelial cells grows into the tubercle and then fuses with the urethral groove. Subsequently, this cord becomes canalized and forms the **distal portion of the penile urethra**.

In most domestic mammals (with exception of the cat), the body of the penis remains extensively attached to the abdominal body wall. Thus, its growth is directed anteriorly under the skin along the ventral surface of the body wall defining the position of the future penis. In ungulate fetuses a band of muscles (the umbilical sphincter) forms a sling that pulls the penis against the body wall.

Separation of the distal body of the penis from a superficial ring of skin occurs secondarily. A circular plate of ectodermal cells forms at the distal tip of the phallus and invaginates into the mesenchyme of the tubercle. This epithelial lamina later splits, giving rise to a cleft, the **preputial cavity**. The folds are transformed into flaps of skin covering the glans. This is the **prepuce**, and the opening formed by the edges of the flaps (the preputial opening) allows the glans to protrude from the skin. The bovine preputial cavity is not completed until 4–9 months after birth. The ectodermal plate does not initially form a complete ring, but leaves a ventral connection between the body of the penis and the prepuce, the **frenulum**. This is normally the last structure to degenerate to complete the preputial cavity. Loss of the major portion of the frenulum is necessary for normal protrusion of the penis. If a bull calf is castrated too soon after birth, the formation of the preputium is incomplete and the frenulum often persists.

In the **horse** and **ruminants**, proliferation of mesenchymal tissue around the orifice of the urethra extends the urethral opening beyond the glans penis. This **urethral process** is short in the stallion, but can reach a length of several centimetres in the ram. Mesenchyme in the glans and body of the penis of the **dog** ossifies and forms the **os penis**

The genital swellings form the **scrotum**. In several species (the dog, horse, and cattle) they dislocate anteriorly and remain closely apposed to the genital tubercle. In cats and pigs, however, the swellings remain beneath the anus.

SUMMARY

The urogenital system can be functionally divided into two entirely different components, the **urinary system** and the **genital system**, but their embryonic developments are intimately interwoven.

Kidney

Mammalian kidney formation, nephrogenesis, commences with the successive appearance of three generations of kidney primordia: the **pronephros**, **mesonephros**, and **metanephros**. These primordia arise as an anteroposterior wave. In most mammals the pronephros is rudimentary and consists of seven or eight pairs of pronephric tubules. The appearance of the mesonephros is also transitory. In domestic animals, 70–80 pairs of mesonephric tubules appear. These lengthen rapidly, form an S-shaped loop, and acquire a tuft of capillaries that later form the glomerulus at their medial extremity. Laterally, the tubules join the longitudinal collecting duct, the **mesonephric duct**. It is the third generation of urinary organs, the metanephros, that matures to form the permanent kidney. The **metanephros** is derived from two primordial structures, the **ureteric bud**, an outgrowth of the mesonephric duct, and the **metanephric blastema**, which is located in the sacral region and originates from the posterior end of the nephric ridge. The formation of functional **nephrons** in the developing metanephros involves three cell lineages, all derived from the mesoderm: epithelial cells from the ureteric bud, mesenchymal cells of the metanephric blastema, and in-growing endothelial cells. The mesenchymal condensations of the metanephric blastema located around the terminal buds of the branches undergo a series of developmental changes to form a **renal tubule** that develops into a nephron. The variations in macroscopic appearance of the mature kidney result from differences in the branching of the ureteric bud and the arrangement of nephrons associated with these branches.

Bladder and urethra

During development of the hindgut, the cloaca is subdivided by the **urorectal septum** into the rectum (dorsally) and the **urogenital sinus** (ventrally). The latter includes an anterior pelvic region and a posterior phallic region. The urogenital sinus is connected cranially to the allantoic cavity through the **urachus**, which is continued into the allantoic stalk. The **bladder** develops from the proximal portion of the urachus and the pelvic region of the urogenital sinus. As the bladder grows, its expanding wall incorporates the terminal portions of mesonephric ducts and the ureteric buds, with each duct system developing its own separate openings into the bladder.

Development of the male genital organs

Chromosomal sex is established at fertilization, when a Y- or X-chromosome-bearing spermatozoon fuses with the oocyte. There is now substantial evidence that the so-called *sex determining region of the Y gene (Sry)* is the testis-determining gene. The gonads develop from an elongated region of mesoderm along the ventromedial border of the mesonephros – the **genital ridge**. During the indifferent stage of gonad development, **primordial germ cells (PGCs)** migrate from the yolk sac into the ridge. During their migration, many PGCs are linked to one another through long cytoplasmic processes. When the PGCs arrive in the gonadal ridges, the resident mesenchymal cells and the coelomic epithelium proliferate, making the ridges project into the coelomic cavity. Cords of epithelial cells from the mesonephric tubules and regressing glomerular capsules penetrate the mesenchyme of the genital ridge and form a number of irregularly shaped cords, the **primitive sex cords,** that incorporate PGCs. Differentiation of the **testis** occurs under the influence of the *Sry* gene (testis-determining factor) on the Y-chromosome. The cells of the primitive sex cords continue to proliferate and penetrate deep into the medulla to form the testicular or medullary cords. The testicular cords transform to solid tubules composed of **primitive germ cells** located centrally and presumptive sustentacular cells or **Sertoli cells** located peripherally. These tubules are arranged in horseshoe-like loops that are connected on both ends to a network of tiny cellular strands, the later **rete testis**. At puberty the testicular tubules develop a lumen and develop into the **seminiferous tubules**. The rete testis eventually joins the **efferent ductules**, which are derived from remaining mesonephric tubules. They link the rete testis and the mesonephric duct, which becomes the **ductus epididymidis** and the **ductus deferens**. Mesonephric cells migrate into the gonad, where they surround the testicular cords and differentiate into the contractile myoid cells. In the mesenchyme between the testicular cords, the androgen-producing **Leydig cells** develop. The fetal Leydig cells are later replaced by a second generation of Leydig cells before puberty. Androgens produced by the Leydig cells are important for the differentiation of the male sexual duct system and the development of the external male genitalia.

Development of the female genital organs

In females, the expression of *Dax-1*, in the absence of *Sry*, suppresses the formation of a testis and allows the indifferent gonads to develop into ovaries. After the **PGCs** have reached the genital ridge, they remain concentrated in the outer (cortical) region of the future ovary. The PGCs become associated with somatic cells, but the origin of these so-called follicle cells is still disputed. Three sites of origin have been proposed for the **follicle cells**: (1) the coelomic epithelium, (2) primitive sex cords of mesonephric origin, and (3) a combination of both. The primary germ cells that are surrounded by presumptive follicle cells are called **oogonia**. They proliferate by mitoses for some time and later enter the prophase of meiosis. With the beginning of the prophase of the first meiotic division, the germ cells are called **primary oocytes** and, together with the follicle cells, they form **primordial follicles**.

In the female, the mesonephric duct regresses due to the absence of male hormones. The cells of a parallel **paramesonephric duct** proliferate and differentiate rostro-caudally, forming the **oviduct**, **uterus**, **cervix**, and the **cranial portion** of the **vagina**. During this time, the single layered Müllerian duct epithelium differentiates and gives rise to morphologically distinct regions of the female reproductive tract. The anterior portions of the two Müllerian ducts become the **oviducts**. In domestic species, the posterior ends of the paramesonephric ducts fuse to a varying extent resulting in a **bicornuate uterus**, in which the **uterine horns** join to form a **uterine body** that opens into the vagina by a single **cervix**. The **vagina** has a dual origin: its anterior portion is derived from the paramesonephric ducts, whereas the posterior portion originates from the urogenital sinus. The caudal portions of the urogenital sinus also form the vestibule

Development of the external genitalia

The external genitalia are derived from three complexes of mesodermal tissue located around the cloaca. At the anteroventral end of the cloacal membrane, the **genital tubercle** is formed. Lateral to the cloacal membrane, extending over most of its length, are the **cloacal** (urogenital) **folds**. They are soon subdivided into **urethral folds** anteriorly and **anal folds** posteriorly. Peripheral to the urogenital folds and posterolateral to the cloacal membrane, are the **genital** and **labioscrotal swellings**. Prior to sex differentiation these are present and similar in both sexes. In the **female**, the urogenital folds that border the urogenital orifice fuse only at their dorsal and ventral ends and form the **labia (minora) of the vulva**. The genital swellings shift cranial to the genital tubercles and disappear during fetal development. Therefore (with few exceptions) no labia majora are formed in domestic animals. Development of the external genitalia in the **male** is controlled by androgens from the fetal testis. A rapid elongation the genital tubercle occurs, transforming it into the **phallus**. As its growth continues, the penile urethra takes shape by ventral folding and midline fusion of the urogenital folds. The **glans penis** originates from the apex of the genital tubercle. The genital swellings form the **scrotum**.

Box 15-1 Molecular regulation of urogenital development

Molecular regulation of kidney development

Induction of the kidney occurs through reciprocal interactions between an epithelial component (the mesonephric or Wolffian duct) and the metanephric mesenchyme (or blastema). The kidney anlagen (or metanephrogenic mesenchyme) are specified at the caudal end of the nephrogenic cord in a process that involves gene activation by the transcription factors ***odd skipped-related (ODD1)***, ***Eyes absent homologue 1 (EYA1)*** and members of the ***paired-box (Pax)*** gene family.

One of the most crucial events in kidney formation is the first signalling process that induces the outgrowth of the ureter from the mesonephric bud. ***WT1***, expressed by mesenchymal cells of the metanephros, makes the metanephrogenic blastema responsive to induction by the ureteric bud. Central to the induction process is the expression of the signalling molecule **glial-derived neurotrophic factor (GDNF),** which is released from the mesenchyme and binds to its receptors RET and GDNF-family receptor a1 (GFRA1) in the mesonephric duct. The activation of GDNF in the metanephric blastema is controlled by a complex molecular network that includes regulation by **EYA1** and **PAX2**. In addition, members of the *HOX11* paralogous genes and the signalling molecule **growth and differentiation factor 11 (GDF11)** are required for *GDNF11* expression in the metanephric mesenchyme. Recent studies have shown that the extracellular matrix protein **nephronectin** is also of importance for renal development. It is expressed in epithelial cells and interacts directly with the α8β1 integrin on the surface of mesenchymal cells. Mice lacking nephronectin or integrin α8β1 fail to express *GDNF* and do not develop kidneys.

Continued

Interactions between the branching uteretic bud and the mesenchyme are mediated by the production of **GDNF** and **HGF** by the mesenchymal cells and the expression of the tyrosine kinase receptors RET and MET by the ureteric epithelium. **PAX2** and **WNT4** produced by the ureteric bud cause the epithelial-mesenchyme transition, which is necessary for excretory tubule differentiation.

Although interactions between the mesenchyme and the ureter are crucial, stromal cells represent a third cellular component with an equally important contribution to ureter branching. In this context, stromal cells are defined as mesenchymal cells that do not undergo a mesenchyme-to-epithelium transition. They can be found scattered between forming nephrons. The earliest known marker for stromal cells is the **winged-helix transcription factor FOXD1**.

The nephron is organized along the proximal-distal axis into distinct regions: the glomerulus, the proximal tubule, Henle's loop, and the distal tubule. Nephron segments fulfil particular physiological functions such as blood filtration, pH regulation and reabsorption of solutes. These functions are reflected in segment-specific gene expression patterns. A recently defined set of *solute carrier (SLC)* **genes** can serve as markers for the various segments of the nephron.

Probably the most complex segment in the nephron is the glomerulus. It is composed of an intricate arrangement of endothelial, mesangial and podocyte cells. A key role for glomerular assembly falls to the developing podocyte precursors. These cells begin to express high levels of *vascular endothelial growth factor (VEGF)* which attracts endothelial cells. The endothelial cells in turn express *platelet derived growth factor (PDGF)* and specific extracellular matrix proteins such as laminin α3 that are necessary for the formation of mesangial cells. Differentiation into podocytes requires several transcription factors, including **WT1** and **LIM homeobox transcription factor 1b (LMX1B)**.

For the formation and specification of the proximal tubules the **Notch** signalling pathway occupies a central role. Besides its role in distal tubule development, **BRN1** is required for the formation of the Henle's loop. In the mouse, a subset of *Irx*

genes marks the future intermediate tubule compartment in the S-shaped bodies of the developing metanephros. One of the first genes to be induced by WNT-β-catenin signalling in the renal vesicle is *FGF8*. It is required for the activation of a genetic cascade involving **LIM1** and the POU-domain transcription factor **BRN1** specifying the distal tubules. *BRN1* knockout mice show disrupted development of Henle's loop and the distal convoluted tubules

Molecular regulation of gonadal development

In recent years, some of the molecular mechanisms of gonadal differentiation have been established. One of the earliest genes required for the formation of the gonadal primordia is *WT-1*. This gene is expressed throughout the intermediate mesoderm and also plays an important role in the development of the kidneys. The other major gene involved in the early phase of gonadal development is *LIM1*; in the absence of LIM1 no gonads form. Another gene, *steroid factor 1,* is expressed in the early indifferent gonad as well as in the developing adrenal medulla, which forms from cells in the cranial part of the steroidogenic mesoderm.

There is now substantial evidence that the so-called *sex-determining region of the Y gene (Sry)* is the testis-determining gene. *Sry* is a member of the Sox family of transcription factors and is located within a 35-kilodalton region on the short arm of the Y-chromosome. Without the expression of products of this gene, the indifferent gonad develops somewhat later into an ovary. In male embryos, transcripts of the *Sry* gene can only be detected in the genital ridge just at the onset of testis differentiation. Neither the expression of the *Sry* gene in the testis primordium, nor later testicular development, is dependent on the presence of germ cells. Under the influence of the *Sry* gene, the cells of the primitive sex cords continue to proliferate and penetrate deep into the medulla to form the testicular or medullary cords. Sry triggers testis formation by inhibiting *Dax-1*, a member of the nuclear receptor family, which is also expressed in the indifferent gonad at the same time. The inhibition of *Dax-1* is necessary for a genetically male gonad to express its phenotypic sex and develop into a testis. Genes downstream from *Sry*, like **SOX9** and *steroidogenesis factor 1*

(SF1) stimulate the differentiation of Sertoli and Leydig cells. Expression of *Sry* is also important for the formation of the tunica albuginea and failure of the cortical cords in the ovary to develop.

The development of the genital duct system in the male depends on hormones from the testis. **Müllerian inhibiting substance (MIS)**, produced by the embryonic Sertoli cells, suppresses the development of the Müllerian ducts (paramesonephric ducts), leaving only remnants at their anterior and posterior ends (the appendix testis and part of the utriculus prostaticus). MIS is a glycoprotein of the Transforming Growth Factor-β (TGFβ) family. It primarily affects the mesenchymal cells surrounding the paramesonephric duct. The mesenchymal cells express a gene encoding a serine/threonine kinase membrane-bound receptor, which binds MIS. Under its influence the surrounding mesenchymal cells cause the epithelial cells of the paramesonephric duct to regress. **Testosterone** from the embryonic Leydig cells stimulates the development of the mesonephric (Wolffian) duct which becomes the main drainage system for the testis. Testosterone and its main metabolite, 5α-dihydrotestosterone, mediate the differentiation of the mesonephric duct to form the epididymis, the ductus deferens, the ejaculatory ducts, and the seminal vesicles. The regional development of the male genital ducts is also influenced by *Hox* genes. **Hoxa-10**, for example, is expressed along the mesonephric duct from the cauda epididymis to the point where the ductus deferens joins the urethra. Mice with mutants of both the *Hoxa-10* and *Hoxa-11* genes exhibit a homeotic transformation, resulting in the partial transformation of the ductus deferens to epididymis.

The development of the prostate is controlled by androgens, growth factors, and epithelio-mesenchymal interactions. Underlying all these molecular actions is the expression of the transcription factors **Hoxa-13** and **Hoxd-13**. They determine at which site in the urogenital sinus a prostate will form. The parenchyma of the prostatic complex is derived from prostatic buds. Dihydrotestosterone, acting through receptors in the mesenchymal cells, induces the secretion of growth factors (**FGF10** and **TGFb-1**) by the mesenchymal cells, which regulate the expression

of **Sonic hedgehog (Shh)** in the epithelium of the urogenital sinus. In response to Shh signalling, prostatic epithelial buds evaginate from the urogenital sinus into the surrounding mesenchyme. The extent of budding is controlled by the inhibitory action of **BMP4**. The developing prostatic epithelium also induces some cells of the surrounding mesenchyme to differentiate into smooth muscle cells.

The master gene for ovarian development is **WNT4**. It causes the upregulation of **DAX1** that inhibits the expression of **SOX9**. In contrast to testicular development, ovarian development requires the presence of viable germ cells; if primary germ cells fail to reach the genital ridges, the gonadal anlagen regress and streak ovaries result. *WNT4*, in cooperation with several other downstream located genes, is important for the formation of cortical cords in the ovary, the disappearance of medullary cords, and prevention of the development of a tunica albuginea in the periphery of the organ.

A number of genes that appear to be essential for the development of the female reproductive tract have recently been identified. Among them, **LIN1, PAX2, EMx2, Wnt-4**, and **Wnt-7** are indispensable for the development of the paramesonephric duct. In particular, *LIM1*, which codes for a LIM-domain-containing transcription factor, has been shown to be crucial for the initial formation of the duct.

PAX2, a member of the *Pax* gene family, possesses a highly conserved paired box which encodes a 128 amino acid DNA-binding domain, the Paired domain, at the N-terminus. Knockout of the *PAX2* gene in the mouse resulted in defects in the formation of the kidney, ureters and genital tracts in addition to defects in ear and brain development. In contrast to what happens in *LIM1* null embryos, in *PAX2* null mutants both the mesonephric and paramesonephric ducts form initially but both soon degenerate.

EMx2 is expressed in the intermediate mesoderm. In the mouse, *EMx2* null mutants completely lack the urogenital system; the paramesonephric ducts never form. *EMx2* expression is only seen during the very early stages of paramesonephric and mesonephric duct formation. These results suggest

Continued

that this gene is only required in a specific window of time during development of the intermediate mesoderm, possibly providing a survival signal.

The mammalian **Wnt** genes encode secreted signalling glycoproteins that influence multiple processes during development. **Wnt4** null females exhibit a complete loss of the female reproductive tract, whereas male mutants appear normal. This phenomenon is due to the failure of paramesonephric duct formation in both sexes. In the absence of Wnt-4, the paramesonephric duct simply fails to form. **Wnt-7**, which plays an important role in the setting up of the dorsoventral axis of the developing limb, is expressed in the epithelium of the paramesonephric ducts and is required for their normal development. Wnt-7 appears to be involved in maintaining the expression of certain **Hox** genes (*Hoxd 10* through *Hoxd 13*) as well as the *Hoxa* paralogues, which are spread along the female reproductive tract. It has been shown in mice that *Hoxa-9* is expressed in the oviduct, *Hoxa-10* in the uterus and cervix as well as in in the upper vagina. Mutations of the *Hox* genes cause a homeotic transformation. The absence of MIS in females allows the Müllerian duct to develop into the major structures of the female reproductive tract. Under the influence of oestrogens, cells of the paramesonephric duct proliferate and differentiate rostro-caudally, forming the oviduct, uterus, cervix, and the cranial portion of the vagina. They also stimulate the differentiation of the female external genitalia, including the labia and caudal portions of the vagina. The mesonephric duct regresses due to the absence of male hormones. It has also been shown that Wnt-signalling is important in uterine gland formation. **Wnt7a** is exclusively expressed in the uterine luminal epithelium but not in glandular epithelium. In contrast, **Wnt5a** is mainly expressed in the uterine stroma during postnatal development. Both *Wnt7a* and *Wnt5a* mutant uteri fail to form uterine glands. This indicates that Wnt signalling is essential for uterine gland formation. Uterine gland development also involves endometrial gland remodelling. **Matrix metalloproteinases (MMPs)** and their inhibitors (**TIMPS**) have been shown to be key regulators of glandular branching, including the branching of uterine glands.

FURTHER READING

Abd-Elmaksoud, A. and Sinowatz, F. (2005): Expression and localization of growth factors and their receptors in the mammalian testis. Part I: Fibroblast growth factors and insulin-like growth factors. Anat. Histol. Embryol. 34:319–334.

Abd-Elmaksoud, A., Vermehren, M., Nützel, F., Habermann, FA. and Sinowatz, F. (2005): Analysis of fibroblast growth factor 2 (FGF2) gene transcription and protein distribution in the bovine testis. Growth Factors 23:295–301.

Aitgen, R.N.C. (1959): Observations on the development of the seminal vesicles, prostate and bulbourethral glands in the ram. J. Anat. 93:43–51.

Amselgruber, W. (1983): Licht- und elektronenmikroskopische Untersuchungen zur Oogenese der Katze (Felis catus). Anat. Histol. Embryol. 12:193–229.

Amselgruber, W. and Sinowatz, F. (1992): The microvascularization of the penis of the steer (Bos taurus)]. Anat. Histol. Embryol. 21:285–305.

Berisha, B., Sinowatz, F. and Schams, D. (2004): Expression and localization of fibroblast growth factor (FGF) family members during the final growth of bovine ovarian follicles. Mol. Reprod. Dev. 67:162–171.

Baumans, V., Dijkstra, G. and Wensing, C.J.G. (1981): Testicular descent in the dog. Anat. Histol. Embryol. 10:97–110.

Bouchard, M., Souabni, A., Mandler, M., Neubuser, A. and Busslinger, M. (2002): Nephric lineage specification by PAX2 and PAX8. Genes Dev. 16:2958–2970.

Bouchard, M. (2007): PAX2 and PAX8 regulate branching morphogenesis and nephron differentiation in the developing kidney. J. Am. Soc. Nephrol. 18:1121–1129.

Bragulla, H. (2005): The development of the metanephric kidney in the pig. Anat. Histol. Embryol. 34:7.

Brophy, P.D., Ostrom, L., Lang, K.M. and Dressler, G.R. (2001): Regulation of ureteric bud outgrowth by PAX dependent activation of the glial derived neurotrophic factor gene. Development 128:4747–4756.

Canfield, P. (1980): Development of bovine metanephros. Anat. Histol. Embryol. 9:97–107.

Canfield, P.J. (1981): Electron microscopic examination of the developing bovine glomerular filtration barrier. Anat. Histol. Embryol. 10:46–51.

Costantini, F. and Shakya, R. (2006): GDNF/RET signalling and the development of the kidney. Bioessays 28:117–127.

Dudley, A.T., Godin, R.E. and Robertson, E.J. (1999): Interaction between FGF and BMP signaling pathways regulates development of metanephric mesenchyme. Genes Dev. 13:1601–1613.

Eickhoff, R., Jennemann, G., Hoffbauer, G., Schuring, M.P., Kaltner, H., Sinowatz, F., Gabius H.J., and Seitz J. (2006): Immunohistochemical detection of macrophage migration inhibitory factor in fetal and adult bovine epididymis: release by the apocrine secretion mode? Cells Tissues Organs. 182:22–31.

Esquela, A.F. and Lee, S.J. (2003):Regulation of metanephric kidney development by growth/differentiation factor. Dev. Biol. 257:356–370.

Hullinger, R.I. and Wensing, C.J.G. (1985): Descent of the testis in the fetal calf. Acta. anat. 121:63–68.

Josso, N.B., Picard, J.V., Dachieux, J.L. and Courot, M. (1985): Initiaton of production of anti-Müllerian hormone by the fetal gonad. Arch. Anat. Microscop. Morphol. Exp. 74:96–100.

Kano, Y. and Mochizucki, K. (1982): Development of the external genitalia in bovine fetuses. Jap. J. Vet Sci. 44:489–496.

Kenngott, R.A. and Sinowatz, F. (2007): Prenatal development of the bovine oviduct. Anat. Histol. Embryol. 36:272–283.

Knospe, C. (1998): Zur Entwicklung des Pferdehodens. Anat. Histol. Embryol. 27:219–222.

Knospe, C. and Budras, K.-D. (1992): Zur praenatalen Entwicklung des Pferdeovars. Anat. Histol. Embryol. 21:306–313.

Kölle, S., Dubois, C.S., Caillaud, M. Lahuec, C., Sinowatz, F. and Goudet, G. (2007): Equine zona protein synthesis and ZP structure during folliculogenesis, oocyte maturation, and embryogenesis. Mol. Reprod. Dev. 74:851–859.

Kurtz, A., Jelkmann, W., Sinowatz, F. and Bauer, C. (1983): Renal mesangial cell cultures as a model for study of erythropoietin production. Proc. Natl. Acad. Sci. U S A. 80:4008–4011.

Leimeister, C., Schumacher, N. and Gessler, M. (2003): Expression of Notch pathway genes in the embryonic mouse metanephros suggests a role in proximal tubule development. Gene Expr. Patterns 3:595–598.

McMahon, A.P. (1997): GDNF induces branching and increased cell proliferation in the ureter of the mouse. Dev. Biol. 192:193–198.

Martin, E. and Rodriguez-Martinez, H. (1993): Changes in the peritoneum during the development of the testis, epididymis and ductus deferens in the pig. Anat. Histol. Embryol. 22:201–211.

Merchant-Larios, H. (1979): Ultrastructural events in horse gonadal morphogenesis. J. Reprod. Fert. Suppl. 27:479–485.

Paula-Lopes, F.F., Boelhauve M., Habermann F.A., Sinowatz F. and Wolf E. (2007): Leptin promotes meiotic progression and developmental capacity of bovine oocytes via cumulus cell-independent and -dependent mechanisms. Biol. Reprod. 76:532–541.

Pedersen, A., Skjong, C. and Shawlot, W. (2005): Lim1 is required for nephric duct extension and ureteric bud morphogenesis. Dev. Biol. 288:571–581.

Pelliniemi, L.J. (1976): Ultrastructure of the indifferent gonad in male and female pig embryos. Tissue Cell 8:163–174.

Pelliniemi, L.J. (1985): Sexual differentiation of the pig gonad. Arch. Anat. Microsc. Morph. Exp. 74:76–80.

Reischl, J., Prelle, K., Schol, H., Neumuller, C., Einspanier, R., Sinowatz, F. and Wolf, E. (1999): Factors affecting proliferation and dedifferentiation of primary bovine oviduct epithelial cells in vitro. Cell Tissue Res. 296:371–383.

Rüsse, I. (1981): Blastemzellen zwischen Mesonephros und Ovaranlage. Verh. Anat. Ges. 75:475–477.

Rüsse, I. and Sinowatz, F. (1998): Lehrbuch der Embryologie der Haustiere, 2nd edn. Parey Buchverlag, Berlin.

Sajithlal, G., Zou, D., Silvius, D and Xu, P.X. (2005): EYA1 acts as a critical regulator for specifying the metanephric mesenchyme. Dev. Biol. 284:323–336.

Wellik, D.M., Hawkes, P.J. and Capecchi, M.R. (2002): HOX11 paralogous genes are essential for metanephric kidney induction. Genes Dev. 16:1423–1432.

Schedl, A. (2007): Renal abnormalities and their developmental origin. Nature Rev. Genetics, 8:791–802.

Schultheiss, T.M. (2006): Odd-skipped related 1 is required for development of the metanephric kidney and regulates formation and differentiation of kidney precursor cells. Development 133:2995–3004.

Sinowatz, F. and Wrobel, K.H. (1981): Development of the bovine acrosome. An ultrastructural and cytochemical study. Cell Tissue Res. 219:511–524.

Sinowatz, F. and Amselgruber, W. (1986): Postnatal development of bovine Sertoli cells. Anat. Embryol. (Berl). 174:413–423.

Sinowatz, F. and Friess, A.E. (1983): Uterine glands of the pig during pregnancy. An ultrastructural and cytochemical study. Anat. Embryol. (Berl): 166:121–134.

Stark, K., Vainio, S., Vassileva, G. and McMahon, A.P. (1994): Epithelial transformation of metanephric mesenchyme in the developing kidney regulated by WNT-4. Nature 372:679–683.

Tiedemann, K. (1976): The mesonephros of cat and sheep. Adv. Anat. Embryol. Cell Biol. 53:7–119.

Tiedemann, K. (1979): Architecture of the mesonephric nephron in pig and rabbit. Anat. Embryol. 157:105–112.

Wrobel, K.H., Sinowatz, F. and Mademann, R. (1981): Intertubular topography in the bovine testis. Cell Tissue Res. 217:289–310.

CHAPTER 16

Musculo-skeletal system

Fred Sinowatz

The musculoskeletal system consists of **bones**, **cartilage**, **muscles**, **ligaments**, and **tendons**. The main functions of the musculoskeletal system are support of the body, provision of motion, and protection of vital organs, especially the brain and thoracic and abdominal viscera. The skeletal system also serves as the main storage system for calcium and phosphorus.

THE DEVELOPMENT OF BONES (OSTEOGENESIS)

Skeletal tissue is present in almost all regions of the body. The individual skeletal elements are quite diverse in morphology and tissue structure. Three distinct lineages generate the skeleton: the somites provide the **axial (vertebral) skeleton**; the lateral plate mesoderm generates the **limb skeleton**; and the cranial neural crest gives rise to the **branchial arches** and **craniofacial bones** and **cartilage**.

Despite this diversity, there are some fundamental embryological commonalities in the development of the skeleton. Skeletal tissue arises from cells with a mesenchymal morphology, but the origins of the mesenchyme vary in different regions of the body. In the trunk the mesenchyme that gives rise to the **segmented axial skeleton** (vertebral column, ribs and sternum) is derived from the sclerotomal portion of the somites (Figs 16-1, 16-2). The **appendicular skeleton** (the bones of the limbs and their respective girdles) originates from the mesenchyme of the lateral plate mesoderm. The origins of the **head skeleton** are more complex. Some cranial bones (e.g. those making up the roof and much of

the base of the skull) are mesodermal in origin, but the facial bones and some of the bones covering the brain arise from mesenchyme derived from the ectodermal neural crest.

There are two major modes of bone formation, **intramembranous** and **endochondral ossification**. Both involve the transformation of mesenchymal tissue into bone. The direct conversion of mesenchymal cells into bone tissue is called intramembranous or desmal ossification. Endochondral ossification on the other hand involves the formations of cartilaginous models from aggregated mesenchymal cells, and the subsequent replacement of cartilage by bone tissue.

Intramembranous bone formation

Direct conversion of mesenchymal cells into bone is called intramembranous (or desmal ossification; Fig. 16-3). In the skull, neural-crest-derived mesenchymal cells proliferate and condense into compact aggregates. The condensation phase of bone formation is typically accompanied by the up-regulation of N-cadherin and N-CAM, molecules that mediate adhesion of the bone-forming cells and promote the establishment of a preskeletal condensation. Some of the mesenchymal cells change their shape to become **osteoblasts** that secrete **osteoid**, an extracellular matrix consisting of collagen and proteoglycans, which is able to bind calcium. Intramembranous bone formation involves bone morphogenetic proteins (especially BMP-2, BMP-4, and BMP-7) from the head epidermis that instruct the neural-crest-derived mesenchymal cells to become osteoblasts and to express a transcription factor CBFA1 (core

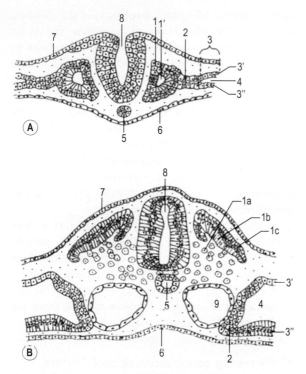

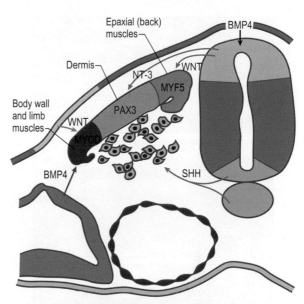

Fig. 16-1: Successive stages in the development of a somite. **A:** Mesenchymal cells are arranged into a bloc-like structure (somite) with a small cavity. 1: Somite; 1': Myocoel; 2: Intermediate mesoderm; 3: Lateral mesoderm; 3': Parietal layer of the lateral mesoderm; 3": Visceral layer of the lateral mesoderm; 4: Coelom; 5: Notochord (Chorda dorsalis); 6: Endoderm; 7: Surface ectoderm; 8: Neural groove.
B: Cells of the ventromedial wall of the somite lose their epithelial arrangement. They migrate in the direction of the notochord. These cells collectively form the sclerotome 1a. Cells at the dorsolateral portion of the somite form the myotome (1b) and the dermatome (1c). Courtesy Sinowatz and Rüsse (2007).

Fig. 16-2: Gene expression pattern during somite differentiation. Sonic hedgehog (Shh), secreted by the floor plate and notochord, causes the ventromedial part of the somite to differentiate to sclerotomal cells. They express *PAX1*, which in turn controls chondrogenesis and vertebrae formation. WNT proteins released from the dorsal part of the neural tube activate *PAX3*, which demarcates the dermomyotome from the sclerotome. WNT proteins also cause the dorsomedial portion of the somite to form epaxial muscles and to express the muscle specific gene *MYF5*. Neurotropin 3 (NT-3) secreted from the dorsal neural tube directs the middorsal portion of the somite to become the dermal layer of the skin. Hypaxial (limb and body wall) musculature originates from the dorsolateral portion of the somite under the influence of activating WNT proteins and inhibitory BMP-4 protein, which cooperate in the activation of *MYOD* expression. Modified from Sadler (2006). Reproduced with permission from Lippincott Williams & Wilkins.

binding factor 1), also called Runx2. CFBA1 activates the genes for osteocalcin, osteopontin and other bone-specific extracellular matrix proteins.

When the osteoblasts become completely surrounded by the osteoid they are called **osteocytes**. As calcification proceeds, small bony spicules radiate out from the region where ossification started and fuse with neighbouring spicules. Furthermore, several compact layers of mesenchymal cells, which form the **periosteum**, surround the entire region where intramembranous bone formation occurs. The cells of the inner layer of the periosteum are also

able to transform into osteoblasts which deposit osteoid parallel to the existing spicules.

Endochondral bone formation

In endochondral ossification the mesenchymal cells first differentiate into cartilage, which is later replaced by bone tissue (Fig. 16-4). Endochondral ossification is seen predominantly in the vertebral column, ribs, pelvis and limbs.

Endochondral ossification of a long bone consists of a characteristic sequence of events that are

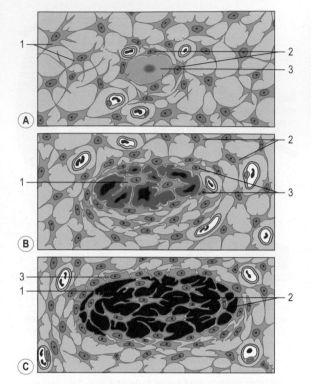

Fig. 16-3: Intramembranous ossification is the source of most flat bones. **A:** Mesenchymal cells (1) proliferate and condense into compact aggregates. Some of the mesenchymal cells change their shape. They become osteoblasts (2) and secrete osteoid (3), an extracellular matrix consisting of collagen and proteoglycans: **B:** When osteoblasts (3) are surrounded by osteoid, they become osteocytes (1); 2: Mesenchymal cell; **C:** Osteoid is able to bind calcium and becomes calcified (1). As calcification proceeds, small bony spicules radiate out from the region where ossification started and fuse with neighbouring spicules; 2: Osteocyte; 3: Osteoblast.

more fully described in histology textbooks. Here, we want to give only a short overview. Initially, a **cartilage model** of the bone is formed. Then, around its middle part, a hollow bone cylinder is formed, the **bone collar**, which is produced by intramembranous ossification within the local perichondrium. In this part of the cartilage model, the chondrocytes undergo a degenerative process with cell enlargement (hypertrophy) and matrix calcification, resulting in a 3-dimensional structure formed by the remnants of the calcified matrix. This process

starts in the middle part (**diaphysis**) of the cartilage model, where blood vessels penetrate the bone collar, bringing **osteoblasts** and **chondroclasts** to the region. The chondroclasts degrade the calcified matrix and the osteoblasts produce a continuous layer of primary bone around the cartilaginous matrix remnants. In this way, the **primary ossification centre** is established. **Second ossification centres** appear at the end of the cartilage model, the **epiphyses**. During the expansion and remodelling of the ossifying bone, the primary and secondary ossification centres produce cavities that are gradually filled with **bone marrow**.

In the two epiphyses, cartilage remains in two regions: the **articular cartilage**, which persists through adult life, and the **epiphyseal cartilage** (epiphyseal plate), which connects each epiphysis to the diaphysis. Histologically, the epiphyseal cartilage can be divided in 5 zones starting from the epiphyseal side of the cartilage:

- The **resting zone** consists of chondrocytes without signs of proliferative activity;
- The **proliferative zone** consists of chondrocytes that divide and form columns of stacked cells parallel to the long axis of the bone;
- The **hypertrophic zone** contains large chondrocytes with cytoplasm apparently filled with glycogen, and with the matrix between them reduced to thin septa;
- The **resorption zone** is characterized by death of chondrocytes and resorption and calcification of the cartilage matrix;
- The **ossification zone** consists of new bone tissue formed by osteoblasts. Blood vessels and osteoblasts derived from cells of the periosteum have invaded the cavities left by degenerated chondrocytes. The osteoblasts are distributed in a discontinuous layer over the remnants of the calcified cartilage septa. Ultimately, the osteoblasts secrete osteoid over the 3-dimensional remnants of the calcified cartilage matrix, which becomes ossified by the deposition of hydroxylapatite.

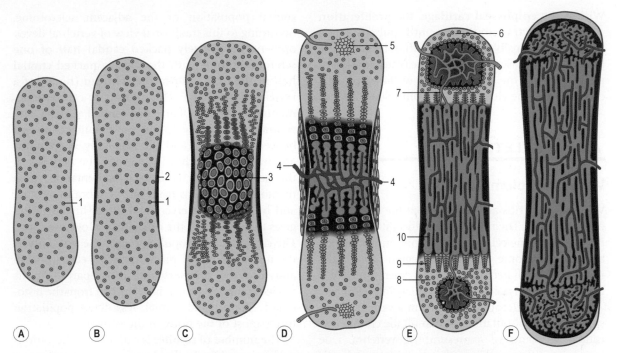

Fig. 16-4: Formation of a long bone on a model made by cartilage. **A**: Initially, a cartilage model (1) of the respective bone is formed. **B**: Around its middle part, a hollow bone cylinder is formed, the bone collar (2), which is produced by intramembranous ossification within the local perichondrium; 1: Hyaline cartilage; **C**: In the middle part of the cartilage model, the chondrocytes undergo a degenerative process with cell enlargement (hypertrophy) and matrix calcification (3), resulting in a 3-dimensional structure formed by the remnants of the calcified matrix. **D**: In the diaphysis of the cartilage model, blood vessels penetrate the bone collar (4), bringing osteoblasts and chondroclasts to this region. The chondroclasts degrade the calcified matrix and the osteoblasts produce a continuous layer of primary bone around the cartilaginous matrix remnants. In this way, the primary ossification centre is established. Secondary ossification centres (5) appear at the end of the cartilage model, the epiphyses. **E**: In the two epiphyses, cartilage remains in two regions: the articular cartilage (6), which persists through adult life, and the epiphyseal cartilage (7), which connects each epiphysis to the diaphysis. Histologically, the epiphyseal cartilage can be divided in 5 zones starting from the epiphyseal side of the cartilage:

- The resting zone consists of chondrocytes without signs of proliferative activity (8)
- In the proliferative zone (9), chondrocytes divide and form columns of stacked cells parallel to the long axis of the bone.
- The hypertrophic zone contains large chondrocytes in which the cytoplasm appears to be filled with glycogen. The matrix between the chondrocytes is reduced to thin septa.
- The resorption zone where the death of the chondrocytes occurs concomitant with that the thin septa of cartilage matrix become calcified.
- In the ossification zone (10) new bone tissue is formed by osteoblasts. Blood vessels and osteoblasts derived from cells of the periosteum have invaded the cavities left by degenerated chondrocytes. The osteoblasts are distributed in a discontinuous layer over the remnants of the calcified cartilage septa and secret osteoid over the 3-dimensional remnants of the calcified cartilage matrix, which becomes ossified by the deposition of hydroxylapatite.

F: Adult bone. Within the epiphyseal cartilage, the proliferation of chondrocytes continues until puberty. It is therefore responsible for the growth in length of the bone. The increase in sex hormone concentration causes the disappearance of the epiphyseal cartilage and the closure of the epiphyses.

Within the epiphyseal cartilage, the proliferation of chondrocytes continues until puberty. It is therefore responsible for the growth in length of the bone. The increase in sex hormone concentration at puberty causes the disappearance of the epiphyseal cartilage and the closure of the epiphyses.

AXIAL SKELETON

Vertebral column and ribs

Vertebrae and ribs are derived from the **sclerotome** of the somites. The notochord induces its surrounding mesenchyme cells to secrete epimorphin, which attracts sclerotome cells to the region around the notochord and neural tube. The sclerotome cells begin to condense and to differentiate into cartilage.

Before the sclerotome cells form a vertebra, they split into two populations which fill the cranial and caudal segments of a presumptive vertebra. Due largely to differential growth rates, the caudal cells of each sclerotome become contiguous with the cranial population of the adjacent sclerotome. According to this traditional view of vertebral development, the **densely packed caudal half of one sclerotome joins with the loosely packed cranial half of the next to form the centrum (body) of a vertebra** (Fig. 16-5). This process is called **resegmentation** and explains why spinal ganglia and ventral roots of the spinal nerves are positioned between vertebrae, and the originally intersomitic arteries subsequently run between the pedicles of the vertebral arch. Due to resegmentation, each myotome then spans from one vertebra to another and bridges the intervertebral disc. This alteration gives the myotomes the capacity to move the spine. The caudal, dense population give rise primarily to the **neural arch** and related parts of each vertebra and also the **intervertebral disc** apart from its nucleus pulposus which is a remnant from the notochord. The original cranial, less dense population forms most of the **body** of the vertebra.

The number of somites is different in the various domestic species. In the dog, for instance, there are more than 40 somites. The first four are called

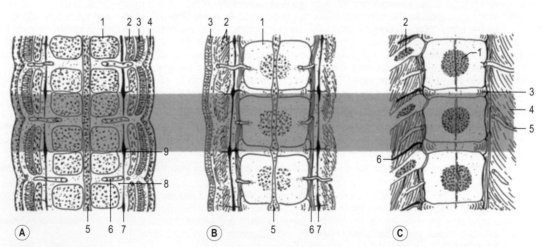

Fig. 16-5: A: The densely packed caudal half of one sclerotome joins with the loosely packed cranial half of the next to form the centrum (body) of a vertebra. This process is called resegmentation. 1: Sclerotome; 2: Myotome; 3: Dermatome; 4: Surface ectoderm; 5: Notochord; 6: Intersomitic artery; 7: Nerve; 8: Intersomitic space; 9: Intrasomitic cleft. **B and C:** Due to resegmentation, each myotome then spans from one vertebra to another and bridges the intervertebral disc. This alteration gives them the capacity to move the spine. **B:** 1: Cartilage primordium of a vertebra. 2: Segmental muscles; 3: Surface ectoderm; 5: Nucleus pulposus within a intervertebral disc; 6: Artery; 7: Nerve. **C:** Ossification centre with a vertebral body; 2: Ossification centre of a rib; 3: Intervertebral disc. 4: Segmental muscles; 5: Artery; 6: Nerve. Courtesy Sinowatz and Rüsse (2007).

occipital somites; they fuse with mesenchyme of the skull to form the occipital cartilages of the skull. The remaining somites take part in the formation of the vertebral column and the ribs. The development of sclerotomes proceeds in a craniocaudal sequence, as does chondrification of vertebrae. The pattern of ossification of vertebrae is less precise and thoracic vertebrae may begin to ossify before the cervical segments do. Vertebral ossification begins during the sixth week of gestation in the dog, and slightly later in the large domestic animals. Primary ossification centres are found in the middle of each vertebral body and laterally in the base of each neural arch. In altricial domestic animals, like the cat and dog, these ossification centres do not fuse dorsally before birth; secondary ossification centres appear during postnatal development in the periphery of

the body to form epiphyses and distal parts of the transverse processes.

The vertebral column can be divided into five areas: (1) the **cervical region**, which includes the highly specialized **atlas** and **axis** that link the vertebral column to the skull; (2) the **thoracic region**, from which the **true ribs** arise; (3) the **lumbar region**; (4) the **sacral region**, in which the vertebrae are fused into the single **os sacrum**; and (5) the **caudal region**, which represents the tail in most mammals. Patterning of the shapes of the different vertebrae is regulated by *Hox* genes.

A typical vertebra consists of a **vertebral body**, a **vertebral arch** and **foramen** (through which the spinal cord passes), **transverse processes** and usually a **spinous process**, and it arises from the fusion of several cartilaginous primordia (Fig. 16-6).

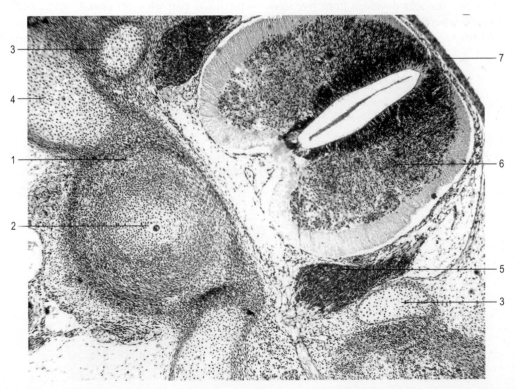

Fig.16-6: Cross section through a feline fetus of 26 mm CRL. 1: Cartilage primordium of a vertebral body; 2: Remnant of the notochord; 3: Cartilage primordium of a vertebral arch; 4: Primordium of a rib; 5: Spinal ganglion; 6; Spinal cord; 7: Epidermis.

The body, which is derived from the ventromedial sclerotomal portions of the paired somites, surrounds the notochord and serves as a bony floor for the spinal cord. The neural arches, arising from lateral sclerotomal cells, fuse on both sides with the centrum, and along with other neural arches, they form a protective roof over the spinal cord. The costal process forms the true ribs at the level of the thoracic vertebrae. At other levels along the vertebral column the costal processes become incorporated into the vertebrae proper.

The first two vertebrae of the vertebral column, the **axis** and **atlas,** have a special morphology and distinctive origin. At the cranial end of the vertebral column, a mesenchymal aggregate associated with the fifth somite, which, based on its position, should form the body of the atlas, becomes part of the surface of the axis and forms the dens of the axis. The body of the atlas is therefore deficient and is penetrated by the dens of the axis (odontoid process of the axis). Thus, the axis develops from five ossification centres, whereas the reduced body of the atlas has only one.

Formation of the intervertebral disc

Later in development the **notochord** disappears from the bodies of the vertebrae. Between the vertebrae the notochord expands into the condensed mesenchymal primordia of the intervertebral discs. In the adult animal parts of the notochord persists as the **nucleus pulposus**, which constitutes the soft core of the intervertebral disc. The bulk of the **intervertebral disc** consists of layers of fibrocartilage that differentiate from the rostral half of the sclerotome in the somite. *Pax-1* is expressed continuously during the development of intervertebral discs.

Development of ribs and sternum

The **ribs** arise from segmental **sclerotome**-derived condensation of mesenchymal cells lateral to the anlagen of the thoracic vertebrae, located between the developing myotomes (Figs 16-7, 16-8). The proximal part of a rib (head, neck, and tubercle) originates from the ventromedial sclerotome. Because of the resegmentation of the somites as they

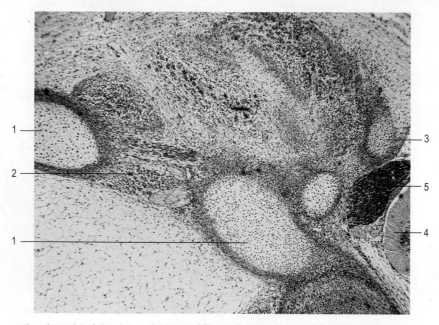

Fig. 16-7: Cross section through a feline fetus of 26 mm CRL. 1: Cartilage primordium of a rib; 2: Intercostal muscles; 3: Cartilage primordium of a vertebral arch; 4: Spinal cord; 5: Spinal ganglion.

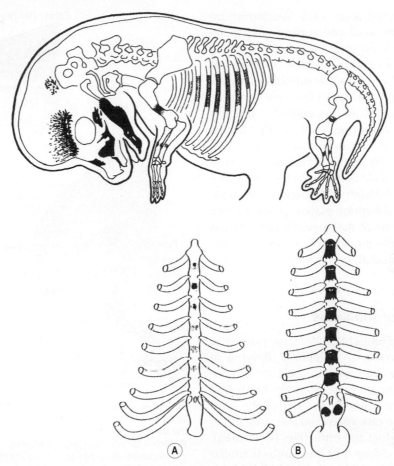

Fig. 16-8: Ossification centres of a Day 33 dog fetus. **A:** Early endochondral ossification of the sternum; **B:** Advanced endochondral ossification of the sternum. Courtesy Sinowatz and Rüsse (2007), modified after Evan and Christensen (1979).

form the vertebrae, the distal part (shaft) of the rib is derived from the ventrolateral part of the adjacent cranial somite. By the time ossification begins in the vertebrae, the ribs separate from the vertebrae. Accessory ribs, especially in the upper lumbar and lower cervical levels, are common.

The distal ends of the first nine cartilaginous ribs grow towards the midline and make contact on each side with a longitudinal aggregation of somatic mesoderm called the **sternal bar**. The sternum arises from this pair of cartilaginous bands that converge at the ventral midline as the ventral body wall consolidates. The two bars fuse in the ventral midline and undergo a secondary subdivision into a series

of **sternebrae** (Fig. 16-8). Usually a total of 8 sternebrae form, although it is not uncommon for the caudal sternebrae to remain paired. The sternebrae ultimately fuse as they ossify to form the common unpaired body of the sternum. Several common anomalies of the sternum, such as a split xiphoid process, are readily understood from its embryological development.

APPENDICULAR SKELETON

The appendicular skeleton consists of the bones of the **limbs** and **limb girdles**. There are fundamental differences in organization and developmental control between the axial and appendicular skeleton. The axial skeleton forms a protective casing around soft internal tissues like the brain, spinal cord, and pharynx, and it is these surrounded organs that induce the mesenchyme to form the bones. In contrast, the bones of the appendicular skeleton form a **central supporting core of the limbs**. Although interaction with an epithelium (the apical ectodermal ridge of the limb bud) is required for the formation of skeletal elements in the limb, morphogenetic control of the limb is inherent in the mesoderm, with the epithelium playing a stimulatory role. All components of the appendicular skeleton begin as cartilaginous models, which convert to true bone by endochondral ossification later during embryogenesis.

Development of the limbs

Forelimbs and hind limbs of the domestic mammals, as in all other terrestrial vertebrates, develop at defined positions in the cervicothoracic and lumbosacral regions of the body, respectively. **Limb bud** development begins towards the end of the third week of gestation in cats, sheep and pigs, and during the fourth week in dogs and cattle (Figs 16-9, 16-10). Development of the fore- and hind limbs is similar except that morphogenesis of the hind limbs is approximately 1 to 2 days behind that of the forelimbs.

Limb bud

Limb formation begins with the activation of a group of **mesenchymal cells** in the **somatic lateral mesoderm**. It is assumed that signals from the axial structures lead to the expression of fibroblast growth factor-10 (FGF-10) and retinoic acid in the prelimb lateral mesoderm. The prelimb mesoderm also expresses the T-Box factors *Tbx-4* and *Tbx 5*, which specify whether a forelimb or a hind limb will develop. The prelimb mesoderm also expresses *Hoxb-8*, which is necessary to establish a major signalling centre in the early limb bud – the zone of polarizing activity (ZPA, see below).

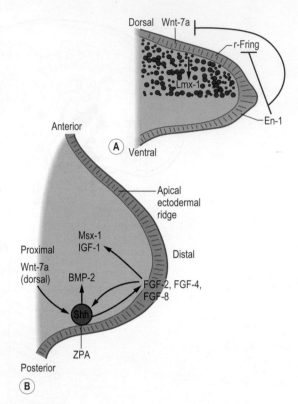

Fig. 16-9: Schematic diagram of molecular regulation of limb development (Carlson, 2004). **A:** Molecular control of the dorsoventral axis: En-1 inhibits both Wnt-7a and r-Fring. **B:** Molecular control along the anteroposterior and proximodistal axes. r-Fring: Radical fringe; ZPA: Zone of polarizing activity.

Each limb then develops from an encircled outgrowth of mesenchyme at the ventrolateral aspect of the embryo, which is covered with ectoderm. At the tip of the limb bud the ectoderm is thickened to the **apical ectodermal ridge (AER)**, which plays a pivotal role in the organization of the limb during development (Fig. 16-9). In the earliest stages of limb development, the limb mesoderm is the prime mover. It secretes Fgf-10, which stimulates the overlying ectoderm to produce Fgf-8. An AER is found in all tetrapod vertebrates and its position corresponds exactly to the border between the dorsal ectoderm that expresses the signalling molecule radical fringe, and ventral ectoderm, which expresses the transcription factor Engrailed-1 (En-1).

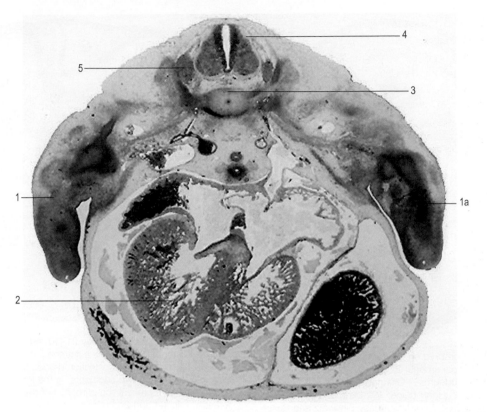

Fig. 16-10: Cross section through a bovine embryo of 16 mm CRL. 1 Left limb bud; 1a: Right limb bud; 2: Left ventricle; 3: Cartilage primordium of a vertebral body; 4: Spinal cord; 5: Spinal ganglion.

Experimental studies in mice have shown that removal of the AER results in arrest of limb development, leading to truncation of the limb.

The AER exerts an inductive influence on the neighbouring mesenchymal cells, causing them to remain as a population of rapidly proliferating, undifferentiated cells, which constitute the progress zone. Recent studies have demonstrated that the outgrowth-promoting signal produced by the AER is a fibroblast growth factor.

The mesoderm of the early limb bud consists of mesenchymal cells embedded in an intercellular matrix consisting of a loose meshwork of collagen fibres and amorphous ground substance. The limb bud contains a well-developed vascular network but is devoid of nerves. Its mesenchymal cells originate from different sources: initially they are derived exclusively from lateral plate mesoderm which later give rise to the skeletal elements, connective tissue and blood vessels of the limb; in a second phase, mesenchymal cells from the somites migrate into the limb bud and serve as precursors of striated muscle cells. Cells immigrating from the neural crest ultimately form Schwann cells of the nerves and melanocytes.

Epithelio-mesenchymal interactions during limb morphogenesis

Extensive epithelio-mesenchymal interactions occur during limb development. The **AER** stimulates the outgrowth of the limb bud by promoting mitoses in the mesenchyme and by preventing differentiation. As the limb grows, the cells further away from the

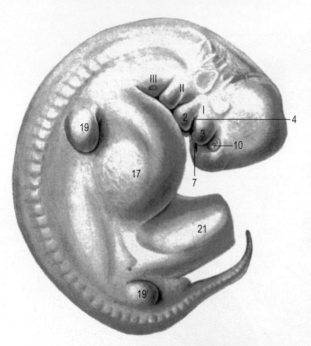

Fig. 16-11: Cat embryo on Day 20 (9 mm CRL). I, II, III: 1st, 2nd, 3rd pharyngeal arches; 2: Mandibular arch; 3: Maxillary process; 4: Stomodeum; 7: Olfactory placode; 19: limb bud of the forelimb; 17: Heart bulge; 19': Limb bud of the hindlimb; 21: Umbilical cord. Courtesy Sinowatz and Rüsse (2007).

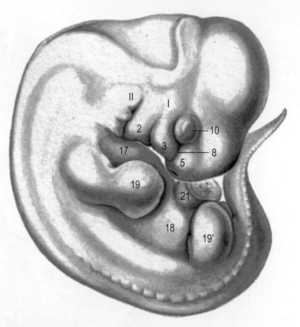

Fig. 16-12: Cat embryo on Day 21 (10 mm CRL). As the limb bud elongates, it becomes flattened in the dorsoventral plane of the embryo. A constriction divides the cylindrical proximal region into two segments. In the forelimb, these two segments represent the primordia of the arm and forearm. I, II: 1st and 2nd pharyngeal arches; 2: Mandibular arch; 3: Maxillary process; 10: Eye; 18: Liver bulge; 19: Limb bud of the forelimb; 17: Heart bulge; 19': Limb bud of the hindlimb; 21: Umbilical cord. Courtesy Sinowatz and Rüsse (2007).

AER escape from its inductive influence, start to differentiate into cartilage and striated muscle, and limb development proceeds proximodistally. The existence of the AER is reciprocally controlled by signals from the mesenchyme of the limb bud.

Establishing of the limb axes

Limb buds display three obvious axes of asymmetry: **proximodistal**, **craniocaudal**, and **dorsoventral** (Figs 16-11, 16-12). At a molecular level, it is now possible to define the signals that control patterning of each of these axes, signals that must be integrated so that formation of the various limb elements, relative to the three axes, is coordinated.

Three key organizing centres produce primary signals to regulate patterning along the three axes of the embryonic limb. **Proximodistal** growth is regulated by the apical ectodermal ridge (AER), which produces proteins of the Fibroblast Growth Factor (FGF) family that act on the underlying limb mesenchyme. **Craniocaudal** patterning is controlled by a population of cells that secrete the Sonic hedgehog (Shh) protein in the posterior aspect of the limb mesenchyme (Fig. 16-9). **Dorsoventral** patterning requires localization of the WNT7a signalling protein to the dorsal limb ectoderm via repression by the Engrailed-1 (En1) transcription factor, localized in the ventral ectoderm.

Integration of three-dimensional patterning occurs as a result of complex interplay amongst these three signalling centres as they communicate with one another to position and refine the expression domains of their key signals.

Zone of polarizing activity (ZPA)

Patterning of the craniocaudal axis of the limb is regulated by the **zone of polarizing activity (ZPA)**, a cluster of cells at the caudal border of the limb near the flank. The ZPA is already established by the time the limb buds begin to grow out from the body wall. The cells of the ZPA secrete retinoic acid, which stimulates the expression of Sonic hedgehog (Shh), a protein that controls the establishment of the craniocaudal axis of the limb and maintains the structure and function of the AER. In the absence of the ZPA or Shh, the apical ridge regresses. Besides Shh, members of the Gli family of zinc-finger transcription factors have recently been shown to play an important role in controlling the morphogenesis of the limb bud along its craniocaudal axis. *Gli-1* is expressed adjacent to the ZPA and is a mediator of the Shh signal. *Gli-3*, on the other hand, is expressed at the cranial aspect of the limb bud and represses Shh signalling.

Progress zone

The progress zone is a mesenchymal area just beneath the AER, several hundred micrometres thick, where the cells divide intensely but are not morphogenetically determined. As the limb bud grows, these cells escape the influence of the AER, differentiate, and express the *Msx-1* gene. Cells leaving the progress zone stop expressing *Msx-1* and become fixed in their ultimate morphogenetic fate; those leaving early form the proximal skeletal elements of the limb (humerus, femur), cells leaving later give rise to the more distal bones (radius, ulna, tibia, fibula, etc.).

Development of the basic limb structure

As the limb bud elongates, it becomes flattened in the dorsoventral plane of the embryo, and the **distal part becomes paddle-shaped** whereas the **proximal part appears cylindrical** (Fig. 16-13). As distal outgrowth continues, the limb bud bends ventrally and its originally ventral surface becomes the medial surface. Subsequently, the limbs **rotate approximately 90°** (clockwise in the left limb and

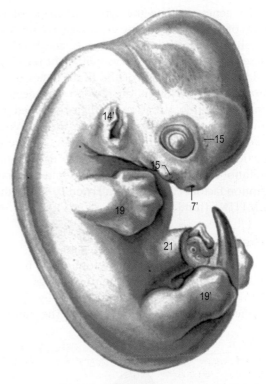

Fig. 16-13: Cat embryo on day 25 (16 mm CRL). As the limb bud elongates, the distal part becomes paddle shaped. 7': Olfactory placode; 14': Auricular hillock; 15: Developing sinus hairs; 19: Forelimb bud; 19': Hindlimb bud; 21: Umbilical cord. Courtesy Sinowatz and Rüsse (2007).

counter clockwise in the right limb) along the proximodistal axis, which moves the cranial margins of the paddle-shaped distal parts of the limbs medially.

Later, a constriction divides the cylindrical proximal region into two segments. In the forelimb, these two segments represent the primordia of the arm and forearm, and in the hind limb the thigh and leg. At defined positions between these segments, the elbow and stifle joints are formed and define the outlines of the respective limb structures. As the limb grows, mesenchymal cells condense into forms that approximate the various bones of the limbs. These mesenchymal templates are replaced by cartilaginous models which subsequently undergo endochondral ossification and form the bones of the limb.

Hox genes regulate the type and shape of the bones of the limb. *Hox* gene expression is controlled by collective expression of *Shh*, *Fgfs*, and *Wnt7a* in phase and in places that correspond to the proximal, middle and distal parts of the limb. Genes of the *Hoxa* and *Hoxd* clusters are the primary determinants in the limb. Variations in their combined patterns of expression may cause some of the differences in forelimb and hind limb structures. As already described, other important factors in determining forelimb versus hind limb structure are the transcription factors TBX5 (forelimb) and TBX4 together with PITX1 (hind limbs).

Development of digits

The basic pattern of limb development is initially the same for all domestic mammals (Figs. 16-14, 16-15, 16-16) but becomes modified by species-specific changes during development. The standard

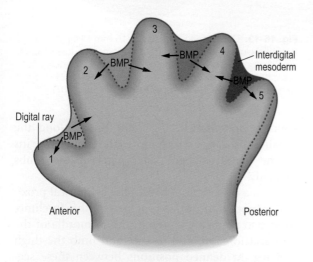

Fig. 16-14: The default construction of the distal part of forelimbs and hind limbs consisted of five radiating digits, with digit 1 in a medial and digit 5 in a lateral position. During evolution, in many mammalian species, including horse and cattle, a reduction in the number and size of digits occurred. The concentration of BMP in the interdigital mesenchyme determines the identity of the adjacent digits. In the normal limb, the highest concentration of BMP (darkest colour) specifies that the digit first will form. Modified after Carlson (2004).

pattern for the foot is the five-digit arrangement, characteristic for plantigrade animals.

As limb development progresses, the **AER** begins to break up, leaving intact segments of thickened apical ridge epithelium covering only the emerging digital ray. Between the digits, the AER regresses and as a result, the interdigital spaces are sculptured by **apoptosis**. The exact mechanisms of interdigital cell death are still not entirely clear, but bone morphogenetic proteins (BMPs) obviously play an important role. *BMP-2*, *BMP-4*, and *BMP-7* as well as the transcription factors *Msx-1* and *-2* are strongly expressed in the mesenchyme of the interdigital spaces. FGFs secreted by the AER may also play a role in interdigital cell death.

Well before the sculpting of the interdigital spaces by apoptosis becomes evident, other events in the paddle-shaped end of the developing limbs presage the formation of digits characteristic of the species. The future digits first become recognizable as longitudinal condensed aggregations of mesenchymal cells, which soon begin to secrete a precartilaginous matrix. The early digital rays then undergo species-specific segmentation to form characteristic phalangeal segments. The default construction of the distal part of forelimbs and hind limbs consisted of **five radiating digits**, with digit 1 in a medial and digit 5 in a lateral position. In many mammalian species, like horses and cattle, evolution resulted in a **reduction in the number and size of digits** as locomotion changed from plantigrade to digitigrade. This occurred in a characteristic sequence: digit 1 disappeared first, followed by digit 5 and then digits 3 and 4. Among the domestic animals, the equine foot shows the strongest reduction with only a single weight-bearing digit (digit 3) remaining. In artiodactyls (even-toed ungulates) like ruminants and the pig, digits 3 and 4 are weight-bearing, while digits 2 and 5 are small and non-weight-bearing. In carnivores, digits 2, 3, 4 and 5 are weight-bearing, while digit 1 (dew-claw) is non-weight-bearing and much reduced in size. Additional adaptations in the limbs of ungulates are partial or complete fusion of the radius and ulna, of the tibia and fibula and of metacarpal and metatarsal bones, due to the fusion

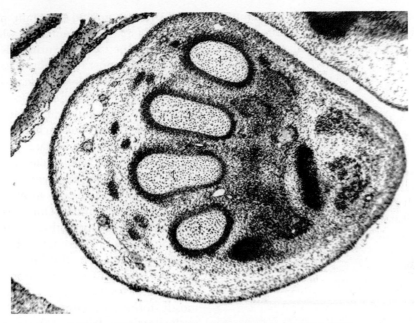

Fig. 16-15: Paw of a cat fetus of 26 mm CRL showing the cartilage primordia (1) of the digits.

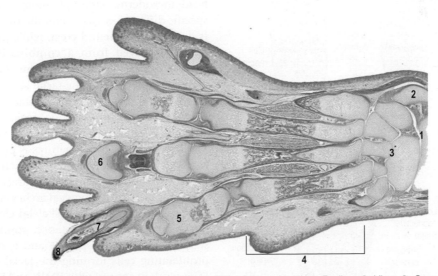

Fig. 16-16: Dorsal view of the right paw of a cat fetus with a CRL of 8 cm (d 42). 1: Radius; 2: Ulna; 3: Ossa carpi; 4: Ossa metacarpales; 5: Phalanx prima; 6: Phalanx secunda; 7: Phalanx tertia; 8: Claw.

of their respective mesenchymal primordia. In ruminants, the distal part of the cartilaginous fibular mesenchymal blastema forms a fibrous band rather than a bone.

Joints

Joints are **preformed in the cartilaginous condensations** when chondrogenesis is arrested, and a joint interzone is induced (Fig. 16-17). A **joint cavity** is then formed by **apoptotic cell death**. Surrounding mesenchymal cells differentiate into the **joint capsule**. The mechanisms determining the positions of joints are not clear, but recent studies suggest that the signalling molecule WNT 14 may play a role as inductive signal.

SKULL

The developing head skeleton can be divided into two parts: the **neurocranium**, which builds a

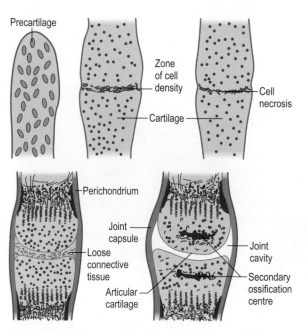

Fig. 16-17: Sequence of the formation of joints of the limbs. From Carlson (2004).

protective case around the brain, and the **viscerocranium** (splanchnocranium), which forms the skeleton of the face and surrounds the oral cavity, pharynx, and upper respiratory passages.

The bones of the skull originate from several different sources, which can be placed into three basic groups. The **first group** is derived from the **branchial arches** and the **ectomesenchymal swelling of the face area** (i.e. the frontonasal prominences) and forms most of **the facial skeleton**. The bone of the facial skeleton is therefore derived from the ectomesenchyme, which originates from neural crest cells, and is formed by **intramembranous ossification**. The **second group** comprises the **flat bones of the calvarium**. They too are formed by **intramembranous ossification**. The **third group** originates from **occipital mesenchyme**. These bones build the **floor** and **ventral walls of the cranial vault** and are mostly formed by **endochondral ossification** of cartilaginous models.

While the neural crest origin of the viscerocranium is well documented, the contribution of neural crest cells to the skull vault is more controversial. Using transgenic mice it has been recently shown that most of the skull is derived from neural crest cells but the parietal bone appears to be made from head mesoderm. Although there may be species-specific differences, in general the **front of the head is derived from neural crest**, while the **back of the head is derived from a combination of neural crest cells and head mesoderm**. Given that the neural crest cells form the facial skeleton of a vertebrate, then the rates and directions of movement of neural crest cells in the cranial region of an embryo strongly influence the shape of the facial skeleton. The regulation of facial features is probably significantly determined by paracrine growth factors. FGFs from the pharyngeal endoderm attract cranial neural crest cells into the pharyngeal arches and are responsible for the patterning of skeletal elements within the arches. FGF8, for instance, contributes to the survival of cranial crest cells and is critical for the proliferating cells forming the facial skeleton. The FGFs work in concert with BMPs and Shh, which are especially important for the neural crest derivatives of the head.

Neurocranium

Basic primordia of the cartilagenous neurocranium

The **cartilaginous neurocranium (chondrocranium)** forms the floor, the rostral wall and part of the lower walls of the cranial vault (Fig. 16-18). It consists of several pairs of cartilages and the fundamental pattern of the chondrocranium has been

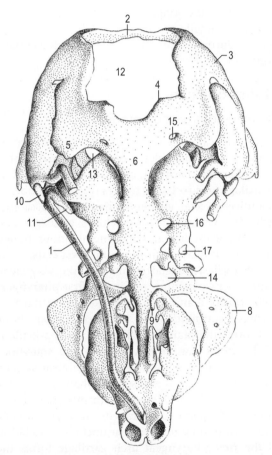

Fig. 16-18: Ventral view of the chondrocranium of a dog (from Rüsse and Sinowatz, modified after Olmstead, 1911). 1: Meckel's cartilage; 2–11: cartilage primodia of the skull: 2: Tectum posterius; 3: Os occipitale with 4: Condylus occipitalis and 5: Processus paracondylaris; 6: Basal plate; 7: Septum interorbitale; 8: Ala orbitalis; 9: Os ethmoturbinale; 10: Incus; 11: Malleus; 12: Foramen magnum; 14: Foramen opticum; 15: Canalis n. hypoglossi; 16: Canalis caroticus; 17: Canalis alaris. Courtesy Sinowatz and Rüsse (2007).

remarkably preserved in the course of phylogeny. The most caudal of these centres are the **parachordal cartilages** derived from the occipital somites and the mesenchyme on either side of the rostral part of the notochord. The parachordal cartilage and the occipital somites are collectively referred to as the basal plate cartilage.

The **prechordal cartilages** are situated just rostral to the parachordal chordal cartilages. Their caudal ends lie on either side of the hypophyseal pouch and the neurohypophyseal bud (**hypophyseal cartilage**). The rostral extensions of the prechordal cartilages fuse at an early stage of development to form the **trabecular cartilage**.

More laterally, the chondrocranium is represented by pairs of cartilages of the special sense organs (**nasal cartilaginous capsule** around the olfactory organ, **otic capsules** around the auditory organ, **optic capsules** around the eyes). The optic capsules do not form adult skeletal structures in mammals, but in birds they become incorporated into the sclera of the eyeball to form scleral cartilages.

Fates of the basic primordia

The individual primordial elements of the chondrocranium undergo several patterns of growth and fusion to form the structurally complex bones of the **basicranium** (the occipital, sphenoid, and temporal bones as well as much of the deep bony support of the nasal cavity). In addition, some of these bones (e.g. the occipital and temporal bones) incorporate membranous components during their development making them truly composite in their final form.

Endochondral ossification transforms the **basal plate cartilage** into the **basal** and **lateral parts of the occipital bone**, and the **occipital somites** to the **condyles of the os occipitale**. The **otic capsule**, which surrounds the developing inner ear, gives rise to the **petrous part of the temporal bone**. As the growing cartilages of the basal plate and the otic capsule approach each other they entrap the vagus nerve (X) and spinal accessory nerves (XI). The space around the nerves becomes the foramen lacerum.

The **hypophyseal cartilages** fuse and two pairs of ossification centres appear in the resulting cartilaginous mass. The caudal pair, surrounding the primordium of the pituitary, give rise to the **basisphenoid**. The basisphenoid contains the hypophyseal fossa, which contributes to the formation of the sella turcica. From the rostral pair the **presphenoid** takes its origin. With these processes, the trochlear (IV), abducent (VI) and ophthalmic (V) nerve become entrapped. In the adult, the space remaining around these nerves is called the orbital fissure.

The **trabecular cartilage** of the prechordal cartilage is situated close to the chondral nasal capsules and its rostral portion becomes the **osseous and cartilaginous part of the nasal septum**. The caudal part of the nasal capsule ossifies and forms spongy bone, the **ethmoid turbinates** that become remodelled by the olfactory mucosa. Also, the caudal aspect of the nasal capsule and the trabecular cartilage increase in size and finally abut. The cartilaginous connection between them is sieve-like, because the cartilage grows between the nerve fibres of the olfactory nerve (I), which extend between the developing olfactory mucosa and the olfactory bulbus of the brain. This cartilage sieve ossifies and becomes the **cribriform plate** of the **ethmoid bone**.

Membranous neurocranium (desmocranium)

The bones of the membranous neurocranium develop by means of **intramembranous ossification** centres that appear in the embryonic skin that covers the dorsal aspects of the brain and forms the roof of the cranial vault. The paired **parietal** and **frontal bones** and the **interparietal part** of the **occipital bone** arise as flat, plate-like aggregations of bony spicules (trabeculae) from mesenchyme that has been induced by specific parts of the developing brain. These spicules progressively radiate from the primary ossification centres toward the periphery. With further growth, the membranous bones enlarge by apposition of new layers of bone on the outer surface, and simultaneous osteoclastic resorption from the inner aspect. These intramembranous bones remain separate during fetal development and, even at birth, they are separated by connective tissue **sutures**, which are probably derived from two sources: neural crest cells (the **sagittal suture**) and paraxial mesoderm (the **coronal suture**).

The time of the closure of the various sutures postnatally influences the shape of the skull. Since most of the growth of the cranial vault takes places at suture lines, closure of suture stops growth at this site. In **brachycephalic** species, transverse sutures close before the longitudinal ones, thus reducing growth in length but not in width. The opposite occurs during development of **dolichocephalic** skulls.

Viscerocranium

Cartilaginous viscerocranium

Phylogenetically, the viscerocranium shows a strong relationship to the skeleton of the **branchial** or **pharyngeal arches**. Each branchial arch is supported by a **cartilaginous rod**, which gives rise to a number of definitive skeletal elements characteristics of that arch. The visceroskeleton includes cartilages and both endochondral and intramembranous bones, which are all derived from **neural crest cells**.

The earliest skeletal element of the viscerocranium is a cartilaginous rod in **the first pharyngeal arch**, called **mandibular (Meckel's) cartilage**. It becomes surrounded by intramembranous bone and forms the **mandible**. The processus articularis of the lower jaw articulates with the squamous portion of the temporal bone. The dorsal skeletal primordia of the first and second pharyngeal arches have been highly modified to transmit sound waves from the tympanic membrane to the perilymphatic fluid surrounding the cochlear duct. The caudal tip of **the first pharyngeal arch cartilage** forms the **malleus** and the **incus**; the tip of the cartilage of the **second pharyngeal arch cartilage** forms the **stapes**. Two other endochondral bones that may be derived from pharyngeal arch cartilage are the orbitosphenoid and the bulla tympanica. Neural-crest-derived cartilage from the **second pharyngeal arch (Reichert's cartilage)** gives rise to the **stapes** of the middle ear (see below). The cartilage from the second arch also differentiates into the lesser horn (**ceratohyoid**) and the upper portion of the body (**basihyoid**), of the hyoid bone. That of the **third arch** gives rise to the greater horn (**thyrohyoid**) and the lower portion of the body of the hyoid bone. Based on apparent homologies, it is assumed that **laryngeal cartilages** are derived from neural crest cells of the **fourth to sixth pharyngeal arches**.

Membranous viscerocranium

The bones of the membranous viscerocranium are derived from the neural-crest-derived mesenchyme of the **frontonasal prominences** and the **first pharyngeal arch**. They are formed by **intramembranous ossification**. As described in Chapter 14, the first pharyngeal arch forms cranially to the first pharyngeal pouch. The neural-crest-derived mesenchymal cells forming the first arch establish two processes: the **mandibular process** ventromedially and the **maxillary process** rostrally. It has been proposed that the growth of the maxillary process is the result of the establishment of a secondary signalling centre, possibly involving FGF-8, in the first pharyngeal arch. The mandibular process expands towards the ventral midline of the pharynx. Eventually the left and right mandibular processes fuse and form the lower jaw. The maxillary process grows and expands beneath the optic vesicles and contacts the lateral nasal process. The furrow between the nasal and the maxillary process is called the **nasolacrimal groove**. As the two processes merge, the ectodermal lining of the furrow becomes buried in the mesenchyme as a cord of epithelial cells that will later hollow out to form the **nasolacrimal duct** connecting the conjunctival sac with the nasal cavity.

Continuous growth causes the **maxillary processes** to expand medially and rostrally beneath the nasal elevations. Eventually they fuse near the midline with the **medial nasal process**, forming the **rostral bones of the upper jaw (maxilla, incisive)** and the **lip**. After establishing this basic relationship, all of these processes show an extensive rostral elongation, which is most prominent in horses and

least distinct in brachycephalic breeds of cats and dogs.

The **second pharyngeal arch** (hyoid arch) is also formed by neural crest cells that have emigrated from the cranial neural folds, located immediately beneath the otic placode. The second pharyngeal arch expands ventromedially and eventually fuses beneath the pharynx with the corresponding arch from the other side. The deep furrow between the first and second arch is called **first pharyngeal cleft**. The mesenchyme on both sides of this cleft forms several small swellings called **auricular hillocks**. From the hillocks on the first pharyngeal arch the **tragus** and the **rostral part of the pinna forms**. The rest of the external ear originates from mesenchyme of the second pharyngeal arch. The dorsal part of the first pharyngeal cleft becomes the **external auditory meatus**, which is filled with an epithelial plug almost until birth. It remains the only opening on the lateral aspect of the skull. The second pharyngeal arch grows caudoventrally and covers the more caudal pharyngeal groves. Active proliferation of mesenchymal cells in the second pharyngeal arch causes it to overlap the third and fourth arches. Finally, it merges with the epicardial ridge in the lower part of the neck. Thus, the second, third and fourth pharyngeal clefts lose contact with the outside. The clefts form a cavity lined with ectodermal epithelium (**cervical sinus**), which normally disappears during later development.

Establishment of facial processes

The **stomodeum** is the rostral cavity established by the formation of the cranial and lateral body foldings and the subsequent cranial flexure. It is first separated from the pharyngeal cavity by the **oropharyngeal membrane**, which breaks down when the left and right mandibular arches fuse. Due to the growth of the maxillary, mandibular and nasal processes, the oral cavity becomes greatly elongated. The epithelial lining of the mouth is largely of ectodermal origin.

On both sides of the frontonasal prominence, local thickenings (**nasal placodes**) of the surface ectoderm are established under the inductive influence of the ventral portion of the forebrain. The nasal placodes then invaginate to form nasal pits. In this manner they create a ridge of tissue that surrounds each pit and forms the nasal prominences. The prominences on the inner edge of the pits are the **medial nasal prominences**; those on the outer edge of the pits are termed **lateral nasal prominences**. These processes are continuous over the nasal pits dorsally, giving them a horseshoe-like appearance. The region between the medial nasal processes, which extends dorsally over the forebrain, is termed the **frontal prominence**.

The nasal pits deepen and subsequently contact the roof of the stomodeum. The contact zone is called **oronasal membrane**, which soon degenerates. The external nares and epithelial linings of the nasopharynx can therefore be traced back to the nasal (olfactory) placodes. Later, the ectodermal lining of the nasal pits will expand and form part of the olfactory epithelium. Most parts of the oral and nasal cavities and the palate shelves are therefore covered by ectoderm. The endoderm of the pharynx will form the caudal part of the mouth and oropharynx.

The **maxillary processes** expand medially and rostrally beneath the nasal elevations and finally fuse with the medial nasal process near the midline. Together, these components form the **maxilla** and the **incisive**. All of the processes show intense cell proliferation and undergo considerable rostral elongation.

Formation of the palate (palatogenesis)

Primary palate. Mesenchymal cells located between the nasal cavities (one cavity from each nasal pit invagination) aggregate in the rostral midline and form the medial palate process, part of which will become the **primary palate**. Later, the incisive (premaxillary) bone forms within this rostral mesenchyme. Soon after the formation of the primary palate, the floor of the midcaudal parts of the nasal sac becomes thinned and the nasal and oral cavities are separated only by a thin membrane (**oronasal membrane**) consisting of the two epithelial linings of the cavities. The oronasal membrane soon

becomes perforated and eventually ruptures. The nasal cavities then communicate with the oral cavity and also indirectly with each other. The openings at the caudal end of the primary palate are called **primary choanae**.

Secondary palate. The **secondary palate** forms later in development. Although the primary palate is derived from the incisive segment, the main part of the definitive palate originates from the **two shelf-like outgrowths of the maxillary prominence**. Formation of the secondary palate involves the following processes: growth of the palate shelves, elevation of the palate shelves (**palatine processes**), their fusion, and the removal of the epithelial seam at the site of fusion. When the palatine processes first appear, the tongue completely fills the oral cavity. As a result, the body of the tongue separates the palatine processes from each other and causes them to project ventrally. As the oral cavity enlarges, the tongue recedes along with the floor of the mouth. The palatine processes can now elevate to a horizontal position and grow towards the midline, where they eventually fuse. **Rostrally, the palatine processes not only fuse with each other but also with the nasal septum.** In this way, the fusion of the palatine processes not only separates the oral from the nasal cavity, but also partitions the nasal cavities from each other.

With the formation of the secondary palate, the position of the choanae (**secondary choanae**) moves caudally. Now the nasal cavities communicate with the pharynx. The relocated choanae become the internal nares of choanae of the adult. The more rostral parts of the palatine ossify and become the **palatine processes of the maxilla** and the **horizontal lamina of the palatine bones** in the adult. These bony structures and their associated soft tissue, and the derivatives of the primary palate, form the **hard palate**.

The lateral palatine processes are the precursors of the secondary palate. They are outgrowths of the maxillary processes, which at first grow downwards on either side of the tongue. Their formation involves ectodermal-mesenchymal interactions and specific growth factors. Studies in the mouse have shown that the expression of **Msx-1** in the palatal shelf mesenchyme stimulates a downstream cascade of BMP-4 signalling in the mesenchyme, leading to Shh signalling in the apical ectoderm.

MUSCULAR SYSTEM

Three types of musculature, **skeletal**, **cardiac**, and **smooth muscle**, are formed during embryonic development, mostly derived from the paraxial mesoderm, specifically the somites. However, the musculature of the heart (cardiac muscle) and the smooth musculature of the gut and respiratory tract arise from the splanchnic mesoderm. Other smooth muscle cells, such as those of the blood vessels and the arrector pili muscles, originate from local mesoderm.

Generation of muscle: myogenesis

The development of muscles can be studied at several different levels of organization, ranging from the determination and differentiation of individual muscle cells, to the histogenesis of muscle tissue, and finally to the formation (morphogenesis) of entire muscles. Skeletal muscle will be used as an example to illustrate how development occurs and is controlled at these different levels of organization.

There is increasing evidence that certain cells of the epiblast are already destined to become myogenic cells even before the somites are completely formed, but the conventional way to describe myogenesis is to begin with the emergence of muscle precursor cells in the **somites**. For many decades the origin of the skeletal musculature was in question, with the somites and lateral mesoderm being likely candidates. This issue was finally resolved by tracing studies using involving cellular markers, and it is now known that **virtually all of the skeletal muscle originates in somites** and somitomeres.

Proliferation and migration of myogenic cells

Myogenic cells pass through several additional mitotic divisions before becoming **post-mitotic**

myoblasts, which are committed muscle cell precursors. Proliferation of myogenic cells is caused through the action of growth factors, such as FGFs and transforming growth factor-β. As long as these growth factors are present, the myoblasts proliferate without differentiating. With the accumulation of myogenic regulatory factors during proliferation, myogenic cells upregulate the synthesis of the cell cycle protein p21, which irreversibly removes them from the cell cycle. Then, under the influence of other growth factors, such as insulin-like growth factor, the post mitotic myoblasts begin to transcribe the mRNAs for the major contractile proteins actin and myosin.

In the development of skeletal and cardiac muscle the major event in the life cycle of a post mitotic myoblast is its **fusion** with other similar cells into a multinucleated **myotube**.

Fusion of myoblasts

The **fusion** of myoblasts is a precise process involving their lining up and **adhering** (by Ca^{++}-mediated recognition mechanisms involving molecules such as M-cadherin) and the ultimate union of their plasma membranes (Figs 16-19, 16-20, 16-21). Muscle cell fusion begins when myoblasts exit the cell cycle. They secrete fibronectin onto their extracellular matrix, and bind to it through $\alpha 5\beta 1$ integrin, their major fibronectin receptor, and it appears that the signal from the integrin-fibronectin attachment is critical for instructing the myoblasts to differentiate into muscle cells.

The second step is the **alignment** of the myoblasts together into chains. This step is mediated by cell membrane glycoproteins, including several cadherins and CAMs. Recognition and alignment between cells takes place only if the two cells are myoblasts. The third step is the **cell fusion** event itself. As in most membrane fusions, calcium ions are critical. Fusion appears to be mediated by a set of metalloproteinases called meltrins. One of these meltrins (meltrin-α) is expressed in myoblasts at about the same time as fusion begins. Antisense RNA to the *meltrin-α* message inhibits fusion when added to myoblasts.

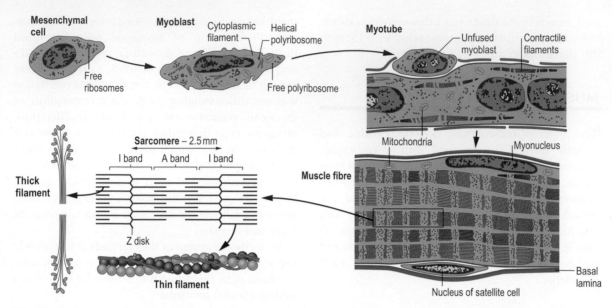

Fig. 16-19: Stages in the morphological differentiation of a skeletal muscle fibre (from Carlson, 2004). Myogenic mesenchymal cells pass through several mitotic divisions before becoming post mitotic myoblasts, which are committed muscle cell precursors. The second step is the alignment of the myoblasts together into chains. The third step is the cell fusion event itself. The fusion of myoblasts is a precise process involving their lining up and adhering by Ca++-mediated recognition mechanisms, involving molecules such as M-cadherin, and the ultimate union of their plasma membranes.

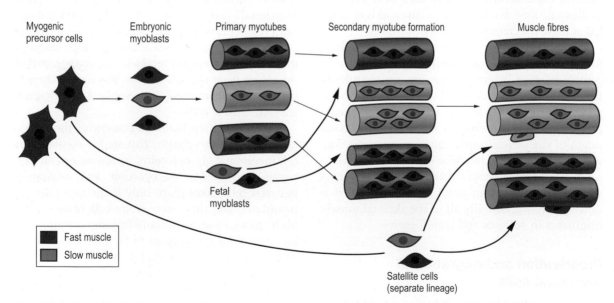

Fig. 16-20: Stages in the formation of primary and secondary muscle fibres. A family of embryonic myoblasts fuses to the primary myotubes, and fetal myoblasts contribute to secondary myotubes and satellite cells. From Carlson (2004).

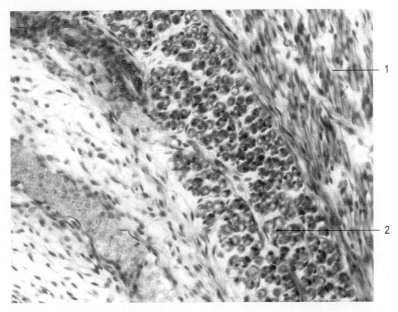

Fig. 16-21: Cat fetus with a CRL of 46 mm, Golder staining. Myoblasts fuse to primary and secondary myotubes. 1: Longitudinal sectioned myotubes; 2: Cross sectioned myotubes. Note the centrally located nuclei and the small diameter of the primary myotubes.

Synthesis of muscle proteins

Myotubes are intensively involved in mRNA and protein synthesis. In addition to forming **actin** and **myosin**, they synthesize a wide variety of other proteins, including the regulatory proteins of muscle contraction: **troponin** and **tropomyosin**. These proteins assemble into **myofibrils**, which are precisely arranged, forming contractile units, the **sarcomeres**. As the number of myofibrils increases, the nuclei of the myotubes, which had been arranged in regular central chains, migrate to the periphery of the myotube and become located directly beneath the sarcolemma. At this stage the myotube is considered to have differentiated into a **muscle fibre**, the final stage in the differentiation of the skeletal muscle cell.

Muscle fibre growth

Muscle fibre growth is accomplished by means of a population of myogenic cells, called **satellite cells**, that take up positions between the plasmalemma of the muscle fibre and the basal lamina in which each muscle fibre encases itself. Satellite cells **divide slowly** during the growth of an individual. Some of the daughter cells **fuse with the muscle fibre** so that the fibre contains an adequate number of nuclei to direct the continuing synthesis of contractile proteins required for muscle function. After muscle damage, satellite cells proliferate and fuse to regenerate fibres.

A typical muscle is not composed of a homogeneous population of muscle fibres; usually several fibre types can be distinguished according to their contractile properties, their morphology and by their possession of different isoforms of the contractile proteins. For instance, muscle fibres can exhibit either fast or slow contraction.

Histogenesis of muscle

Muscle as a tissue consists not only of muscle fibres but also of connective tissue, blood vessels, and nerves. Even the muscle fibres themselves are not homogeneous but can be separated into functionally and biochemically different types.

As muscles first form, the myoblasts are intermingled with future connective tissue mesenchyme. The arrangement of the **connective tissue** plays a decisive role in the morphogenesis of a muscle. **Capillary** sprouts grow into the developing muscle for nourishment, and **somatic efferent motor nerve fibres** enter shortly after the first myoblasts begin to form myotubes.

At one time, it was thought that all myoblasts were essentially identical and that their different characteristics (e.g. **fast** or **slow**) were imposed on them by their motor innervation. Recent research, however, has shown that distinct populations of fast and slow muscle cells are present as early as at the myoblast stage, well before nerve fibres reach the developing muscles.

Not only are there fast and slow myoblasts, but there are also early and late cellular isoforms of myoblasts, which have different requirements for serum factors and nerve interactions in their differentiation. When the earliest myoblasts fuse into myotubes, they give rise to **primary myotubes**, which form the initial basis for an embryonic muscle (Fig. 16-20). The differentiation of primary myotubes occurs before motor nerve axons have entered the newly forming muscle. Subsequently, smaller **secondary myotubes**, which arise from late myoblasts, form alongside the primary myotubes. By the time secondary myotubes form, early motor axons are present in the muscles, and it appears that the presence of nerves is required for the formation of secondary myotubes. A primary muscle tube and its associated secondary muscle tubes are initially contained within a common basal lamina and are electrically coupled. These muscle fibres actively synthesize a wide variety of contractile proteins.

Innervation of striated muscle

Embryonic muscle fibres are innervated by **general somatic efferent motor neurons** quite early in development. Although it has long been assumed that fast and slow motoneurons impose their own functional characteristics on the developing muscle

fibres, it now appears that the neurons contacted muscle fibres of a compatible type through information contained on fibre cell surfaces. Initially, a motor nerve may terminate on both fast and slow muscle fibres but, ultimately, inappropriate connections are broken, so fast nerve fibres innervate only fast muscle fibres, and slow transducing nerves innervate only slow muscle fibres.

Phenotypes of muscle fibres

The phenotypes of muscle fibres depend on the nature of the specific proteins that make up their contractile apparatus. There are qualitative differences between **fast** and **slow muscle fibres** in many of the contractile proteins. Within each type of muscle fibre, there is also a succession of isoforms of major proteins during embryonic development. The **isoform transitions of myosin** in a developing muscle fibre have been especially studied. The myosin molecule is complex, consisting of two heavy chains (HCs) and a series of four light chains (LCs). Mature fast fibres have one LC1, two LC2, and one LC3 subunits; slow muscle myosin contains two LC1 and two LC2 subunits. In addition, there are fast and slow forms (MHCf and MHCs) of the myosin heavy chain subunits. The myosin molecules possess adenosine triphosphatase activity, and differences in this activity partly account for differences in the speed of contraction between fast and slow muscle fibres.

The myosin molecule undergoes a succession of isoform transitions during development. From the fetal period to maturity a fast muscle fibre passes through a series of three developmental isoforms of the myosin heavy chain (embryonic [MHCemb], neonatal [MHCneo], and adult fast [MHCf]). Other contractile proteins of muscle fibres (e.g., actin, troponin) pass through similar isoform transitions. After injury to muscle in the adult the regenerating muscle fibres undergo sets of cellular and molecular isoform transitions that closely recapitulate those occurring in normal ontogenesis.

The phenotype of muscle fibres is not irreversibly fixed. Even postnatal muscle fibres possess a remarkable degree of plasticity. They respond to exercise by undergoing hypertrophy or becoming more resistant to fatigue. On the other hand, they adapt to inactivity or denervation by becoming atrophic. All these changes are accompanied by various changes in gene expression. Many other types of cells can also modify their phenotypes in response to changes in the environment, but the molecular changes are not always as striking as those seen in muscle fibres.

Morphogenesis of muscle

At a higher level of organization, muscle development involves the formation of **anatomically identifiable muscles**. Principally it is the **connective tissue framework,** rather than the myoblasts themselves, that determines the overall form of a muscle. Experiments have shown that myogenic cells from somites are essentially interchangeable. For example, myogenic cells from somites that would normally form muscles of the trunk can participate in the formation of normal leg muscles. In contrast, the

cells of the **connective tissue** component of the muscles appear to be imprinted with the **morphogenetic blueprint**.

Muscles of the trunk and limbs

The myogenic cells are separated into a small dorsal portion, the **epimere**, innervated by a dorsal primary ramus of a spinal nerve, and a larger ventral portion, the **hypomere**, innervated by a ventral primary ramus (Fig. 16-22). Myoblasts from the epimere fuse to form the **extensor muscles of the vertebral column**, while those of the hypomere form **limb and body wall muscles**.

Quail/chick grafting experiments have clearly shown that the major groups of skeletal muscles in the trunk and limbs arise from **myogenic precursors** located in the **somites**. In the thorax and abdomen, the intrinsic muscles of the back (the epaxial muscles) are derived from cells arising in the dorsal myotomal lip, whereas ventrolateral muscles

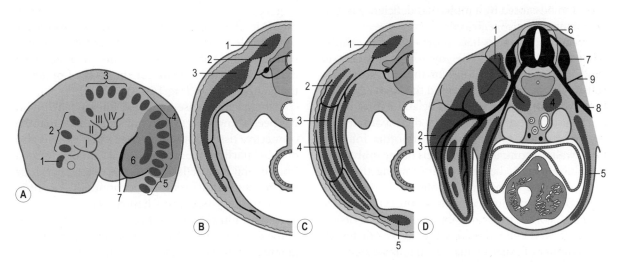

Fig. 16-22: Development of musculature in the head, limb and body wall. **A:** Myotomes in the head, neck, and thoracic region. 1: Preotic myotomes (external muscles of the eye); 2: Pharyngeal arch musculature; 3: Occipital myotomes; 4: Cervical myotomes; 5: Thoracic myotomes; 6: Limb bud; 7: Apical epithelial ridge; I-IV: Pharyngeal arches. **B:** Transverse section through the thoracic region of a 5-week embryo. 1: Epimere; 2: Intermuscular septum; 3: Hypomer. **C:** Development of skeletal muscles of the abdominal wall. 1: Extensor muscles of spine; 2: M. obliquus abdominis externus; 3: M. obliquus abdominis internus; 4: M. transversus abdomini; 5: M. rectus abdomini. **D:** Development of skeletal muscles of the thoracic wall and in the forelimb. Transverse section through the region of attachment of the limb bud. Note the extensor (dorsal) and flexor (ventral) muscular components of the limb. 1: Thoracic extensor muscles of spine; 2: Extensor muscles of the forelimb; 3: Flexor muscles of the forelimb; 4: Prevertebral muscles; 5: Intercostal muscles; 6: Medulla spinalis (spinal cord); 7: Spinal ganglion; 8: Ventral ramus of a spinal nerve; 9: Dorsal ramus of a spinal nerve. From Rüsse and Sinowatz (1998), modified after Sadler (2004).

(hypaxial muscles) arise from epithelially organized ventral buds of the somites. In the **limb regions**, myogenic cells migrate from the ventrolateral dermomyotome early during development. More cranial myogenic cells originating from similar regions of the occipital somites migrate into the developing **tongue** and **diaphragm**. At the lumbar levels, precursors of the **abdominal muscles** also move out of the epithelium of ventrolateral somitic buds. Early specification of the future hypaxial musculature within the epithelial somite is initially regulated by dorsalizing (possibly a member of the Wnt family) and lateralizing (BMP-4) signals from the ectoderm and lateral mesoderm, respectively. This leads to a more intense expression of *Pax-3* and the expression of *Lbx-1*, a homeobox gene that is exclusively expressed in the lateral dermomyotomal lips. Lbx-1 may prevent the premature differentiation of the hypaxial musculature. It is highly likely that the prune-belly syndrome, which is characterized by the absence of the abdominal musculature, will be found to be caused by a molecular deficiency in this population of myogenic cells.

Recent experiments have shown different cellular behaviour in areas of the myotomes adjacent to limb and nonlimb regions. In thoracic segments, cells of the dermatome surround the lateral edges of the myotome. This is followed by an increase in the number of myotubes formed in the myotome and the penetration of the muscle primordia into the body wall. In contrast, at the levels of the limb buds, dermatome cells die before surrounding the early myotubes that form in the myotome.

After their origin from the somites, the muscle primordia of the trunk and abdomen become organized into well-defined groups and layers. The results of a number of experiments have demonstrated fundamental differences in cellular properties between the cellular precursors of limb muscles and axial muscles.

The **skeletal muscle of the head and neck is largely of mesodermal origin**. Quail/chick grafting experiments have shown that the paraxial mesoderm, specifically the somitomeres, constitutes the main source of the cranial musculature, although some question still remains about the origin of the extraocular muscles. At least some of the cells that make up the extraocular muscles arise from the prechordal plate of the early embryo. There is increasing evidence that in some aspects, myogenesis in the head differs significantly from that in the trunk. Different controls at the level of myogenic determination between the head and the trunk have already been discussed. Also, a number of the craniofacial muscles have different phenotypic properties from trunk muscles (e.g., myosin isoforms and possibly elements of neuromuscular control of phenotype).

As with muscles in the trunk and limb, muscles in the head and neck arise by the movement of myogenic cells away from the paraxial mesoderm through mesenchyme (derived either from the neural crest or mesoderm) on their way to their final destination. Morphogenesis of muscles in the cranial region appears to be determined by information inherent in the connective tissues that ensheath the muscles. There is no early level specificity in the paraxial myogenic cells. This has been determined by grafting somites or somitomeres from one craniocaudal level to another. In these cases, the myogenic cells that leave the grafted structures form muscles normal for the region into which they migrate rather than muscles appropriate for the level of origin of the grafted somites (Fig 16-23).

Using recombinase-mediated lineage labelling it has been shown recently in transgenic mice that the connective tissue of the branchial muscles, and also of their attachment points on the skeleton, is formed from neural crest cells, irrespective of whether these attachment points ossify endochondrally or intramembranously (see also Chapter 14).

Certain muscles of the head, in particular those of the tongue, arise from the occipital somites in the manner of trunk muscles and undergo extensive migration into the enlarging head. Their more caudal level of origin is evidenced by the innervation by the hypoglossal nerve (XII), which, according to some comparative anatomists, is a series of highly modified spinal nerves. Like the myogenic cells of the limb, precursor cells of the tongue musculature express *Pax-3* while they are migrating into the head. Despite their final location in the head, these muscles are subjected to the same types of

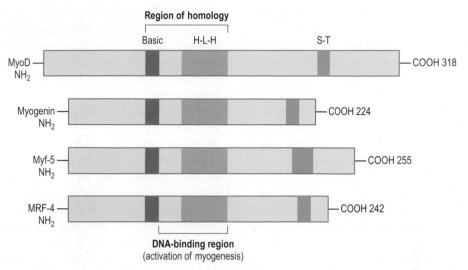

Fig. 16-23: Structural comparison of several myogenic regulatory factors. H-L-H: Homologous helix-loop-helix region; S-T: Homologous serine/threonin-rich region. From Carlson (2004).

early molecular regulation of myogenesis as trunk muscles.

Formation of tendons

In addition to the sclerotome, myotome and dermatome, two further regions of the somites have been recently postulated: the **syndetome**, from which the tendons arise, and a fifth compartment that contains **somite cells that will form the vascular walls** of the aorta and the intervertebral blood vessels. These cells can be distinguished from other cells of the somites by their possession of activated Notch proteins. The syndetome is located in the most dorsal portion of the sclerotome, an area that is adjacent to the muscle-forming myotome. The tendon-forming cells of the syndetome are characterized by the expression of the *scleraxis* gene that distinguishes them from other sclerotomal cells, which express another molecular marker, the *Pax1* gene.

The myotome's secretion of the growth factor FGF8 onto the immediately subjacent sclerotome cells induces the syndetome. Other transcription factors restrict the expression of the *scleraxis* gene to the cranial and caudal portion of the syndetome, causing two stripes of *scleraxis* gene expression.

Meanwhile, the developing cartilage cells synthesize the transcription factors Sox5 and Sox6 that inhibit the transcription of the *scleraxis* gene. In this way, the cartilage restricts the spread of the FGF8 signal. The developing tendons establish a firm association with the elements of the skeleton (including the ribs) on the one side and with skeletal muscles directly above them, thereby connecting muscles to bones.

SUMMARY

Skeletal tissue arises from cells with a mesenchymal morphology, but the origins of the mesenchyme vary in different regions of the body. In the trunk the mesenchyme that gives rise to the **segmented axial skeleton** (i.e. the vertebral column, ribs, and sternum) is derived from the **sclerotomal portion of the somites**. The **appendicular skeleton** (the bones of the limbs and their respective girdles) originates from the **mesenchyme of the lateral plate mesoderm**. The origins of the head skeleton are more complex. Some **cranial bones** (e.g. those making up the roof and much of the base of the skull) are **mesodermal in origin**, but the facial bones and some of the bones covering the brain arise from mesenchyme derived from the **ectodermal neural crest**.

There are two major modes of bone formation, **intramembranous** and **endochondral ossification**. Both involve the transformation of mesenchymal tissue into bone. The direct conversion of mesenchymal cells into bone tissue is called intramembranous or desmal ossification. Endochondral ossification on the other hand involves the formations of cartilage models from aggregated mesenchymal cells, and the subsequent replacement of cartilage by bone tissue.

Vertebrae and **ribs** are derived from the sclerotome of the somites, and the **sternum** develops from the mesoderm in the ventral body wall. The **appendicular skeleton** consists of the bones of the limbs and limb girdles. Forelimbs and hind limbs of the domestic mammals, as in all other terrestrial vertebrates, develop at defined positions in the cervicothoracic and lumbosacral regions of the body, respectively. Each limb develops then from an encircled outgrowth of mesenchyme at the ventrolateral aspect of the embryo, which is covered with ectoderm and called a **limb bud**. At the tip of the limb bud the ectoderm is thickened and forms the **apical ectodermal ridge (AER)**, which plays a pivotal role in the organization of the limb during development. Patterning of the craniocaudal axis of the limb is regulated by the **zone of polarizing activity (ZPA)**, a cluster of cells at the caudal border of the limb near the flank. **Joints** are preformed in cartilaginous condensations when chondrogenesis is arrested and a joint interzone is induced. Then a **joint cavity** is formed by apoptotic cell death. Surrounding mesenchymal cells differentiate into the **joint capsule**.

The vertebrate skull (**cranium**) is composed of the **neurocranium** (skull vault and base) and the **viscerocranium** (jaws and other pharyngeal arch derivatives). The bones of the skull originate from several different sources, which can be placed into three basic groups. One group is derived from the **branchial arches** and the **ectomesenchymal swelling of the face area** (i.e. the frontonasal prominences) and forms most of the **facial skeleton**. The bone of the facial skeleton is therefore derived from the ectomesenchyme, which originates from neural crest cells, and is formed by intramembranous ossification. The second group comprises the **flat bones of the calvarium**. They are also formed by intramembranous ossification. The third group originates from the **occipital mesenchyme**. These bones build the **floor** and **ventral walls of the cranial vault** and are mostly formed by endochondral ossification of cartilaginous models.

Three types of musculature, **skeletal**, **cardiac**, and **smooth muscle**, are formed during embryonic development, mostly derived from the paraxial mesoderm, including (a) somites, which gives rise to muscles of the axial skeleton, body wall and limbs, and (b) somitomeres, which develop into the muscles of the head. Progenitor cells for skeletal muscles originate from the ventrolateral and dorsomedial lips (edges) of the prospective **dermatomyotome**. Cells from both regions contribute to the formation of the **myotomes**. The molecular basis for this commitment is the action of members of families of **myogenic regulatory proteins (MRPs)** that, acting as master genetic regulators, turn on muscle-specific genes in the premuscle mesenchymal cells. The myogenic cells are separated into a small dorsal portion, the **epimere**, innervated by a dorsal primary ramus of a spinal nerve, and a larger ventral portion, the **hypomere**, innervated by a ventral primary ramus. Myoblasts from the epimere fuse to form the **extensor muscles of the vertebral column**, while those of the hypomere form **limb and body wall muscles**. Connective tissue derived from somites, somatic mesoderm, and neural crest cells (in the head region) provide a template for the establishment of the muscle patterns.

In addition to the sclerotome, myotome and dermatome, two further regions of the somites have been recently postulated: the **syndetome**, from which the tendons arise and a fifth compartment that contains **somite cells that will form the vascular walls** of the aorta and the intervertebral blood vessels. The syndetome is located to the most dorsal portion of the sclerotome, an area that is adjacent to the muscle-forming myotome. The tendon-forming cells of the syndetome are characterized by the expression of the scleraxis gene.

Box 16-1 Molecular regulation of musculo-skeletal development

Molecular regulation of vertebra formation

Vertebral development starts with a **Sonic hedgehog (Shh)**-mediated induction by the notochord on the early somite to form the sclerotome. Under the continuing influence of Shh, causing the expression of *Pax-1*, the ventromedial portion of the somite will ultimately form the body of the vertebra. Formation of the neural arch, the dorsal part of the vertebra, is guided by the expression of different transcription factors. An initial induction from the roof plate of the neural tube results in the expression of *Pax-9* and the homeobox-containing genes *Msx-1* and *Msx-2*, which guide cells of the lateral sclerotome to form the neural arch.

The characteristic regional differences of the vertebrae are specified by the actions of discrete combinations of homeobox-containing genes. Expression of the *Hox* **genes** begins with the first appearance of the presomitic mesoderm and for most genes persists until chondrification begins in the primordia of the vertebrae. Formation of the normal segmental pattern along the craniocaudal axis of the vertebral column is ensured by a unique combination of *Hox* genes for the vertebrae of the different parts of the vertebral column. This has been thoroughly studied in the mouse: for example, the atlas (C-1) is specified by the expression of *Hoxa-1*, *Hoxa-3*, *Hoxb-1*, and *Hoxd-4*. The axis (C-2) is determined by these four genes plus *Hoxa-4* and *Hoxb-4*. Application of **retinoic acid (vitamin A)** can cause shifts in cranial or caudal levels in the overall segmental organization of the vertebrae if applied during specific developmental periods. If, for example, retinoic acid is given early during development, this causes a cranial shift of vertebral development and the last cervical vertebra is transformed into the first thoracic vertebra. Later administration causes a caudal shift, where thoracic vertebrae extend into the levels of the first two lumbar vertebrae. Such shifts in level are called homeotic transformations and are representative of the broad family of homeotic mutations.

Molecular regulation of early limb development

While the limb bud elongates, the mesenchyme within the bud begins to condense and differentiate into **chondrocytes**, establishing first **hyaline cartilage models** of the bones of the extremities. As the limb bud grows, a variation in *Hox* **genes** expression along the proximodistal axis can be observed. Whereas *Hox-9* and *Hox-10* are expressed in the more proximal regions of the limb, *Hox-13* expression appears to be confined to the regions where manus and pes develop. Early in limb bud development, the mesenchymal cells express *Ffg-10* and transcription factors that determine whether a forelimb or a hind limb will develop. Two of these transcription factors are members of the T-box family. *T-box 5* is solely expressed in the forelimb, whereas the expression of *T-box 4* is restricted to the hind limb. Expression of *Pitx-1* is also confined to the hind limb.

Establishment of the limb axis is controlled by interaction of the signalling centres for each of the main axes: **ZPA**, through secretion of Shh, is important in controlling development along the craniocaudal axis, **AER** stimulates the proximodistal outgrowth of the limb by secreting members of the **FGF family**, and organization of the dorsoventral axis begins when the dorsal ectoderm produces the signalling molecule **Wnt-7a** and the signalling factor **radical fringe (r-Fng)**. Wnt-7a stimulates the underlying mesenchymal cells of the limb bud to express the transcription factor **Lmx-1b** which imparts a dorsal character to the mesenchymal cells underlying the dorsal ectoderm. Ventral ectoderm produces **Engrailed-1 (En-1)**, which inhibits the expression of *Wnt-7a* and as a result, the formation of Lmx-1b. The underlying mesenchymal cells become ventral limb mesoderm. The AER marks the border between dorsal and ventral limb mesoderm. The three axial signalling centres interact during the development of the limb bud. The dorsal ectoderm produces Wnt-7a, which stimulates the ZPA. Shh from the ZPA is necessary for the production of FGFs from the AER, which in turn gives additional positive feedback to the ZPA.

At the same time as the ZPA is established, the homeobox containing genes *Hoxd-9* to *Hoxd-13* as well as certain *Hoxa* **genes** are expressed in an orderly sequence along the limb bud. The *Hox*

Continued

genes are important for the patterning along the proximodistal axis of the limb, but the mechanisms, which regulate the expression of the *Hox* genes, are at present not known.

Molecular regulation of face skeleton development

The development of the vertebrate face skeleton is a dynamic multi-step process that starts with the formation of neural crest cells in the developing brain and their subsequent migration to form, together with mesodermal cells, the facial primordia. Signalling interactions coordinate the outgrowth of the facial primordia from buds of undifferentiated mesenchyme into the intricate series of bones and cartilage structures that, together with muscle and other tissues, form the adult face. Some of the molecules that are thought to be involved have been identified through the use of mouse mutants, data from human craniofacial syndromes and by expression studies of signalling molecules during facial development.

The development of the face is critically affected by the following events: (1) the expansion of a subpopulation of **rostral neural crest cells**, (2) the establishment of the **cranial flexure** and subsequent growth of the prosencephalon and eyes, and (3) the elaboration of the **olfactory epithelium**. The lower face (maxillary region and lower jaw) is derived from a greatly expanded first pharyngeal arch. Most of the mesenchyme of the face originates from the neural crest. The tissue components of the early face are products of a unique set of morphogenetic determinants and growth signals. Recent studies have convincingly demonstrated that specific set of molecular signals control the face development along both the proximodistal and rostrocaudal axes.

Structures of the face arise from several primordia that surround the stomodeal depression of the embryo. These primordia consist of the frontonasal prominence, paired nasomedial and nasolateral processes, and paired maxillary and mandibular processes, all being components of the first pharyngeal arch. The frontonasal process is a prominent structure that appears during the earliest phase of facial development. Its formation is the result of a complex signalling system. It begins with

the synthesis of **retinoic acid** in a circumscribed area of ectoderm opposite the forebrain. The retinoic acid maintains the signalling of **fibroblast growth factor-8 (FGF-8)** and **Shh** in both anterior forebrain and overlying frontonasal ectoderm. These two signalling molecules stimulate cell proliferation in the neural-crest-derived mesenchymal cells of the frontonasal process. The frontonasal process is the most dominant structure during early face development. Later, with the subsequent growth of the maxillary process and the nasal processes, it recedes from the oral region. At the tips of the rapidly expanding facial primordia the homeobox-containing gene **Msx-1** is expressed in the proliferating mesenchymal cells. Furthermore, expression of the transcription factor **Otx-2** characterizes the mesenchymal cells of the first pharyngeal arch. In contrast to the more caudal pharyngeal arches, **Hox genes** are not expressed in the first pharyngeal arch.

Molecular regulation of endochondral ossification

The molecular processes during endochondral ossification can be divided into five stages. During the first stage, mesenchymal cells are committed to becoming chondrocytes. This commitment is caused by the transcription factor **Shh**, which induces the nearby sclerotome cells to express the transcription factor **Pax1**. Pax1 induces a cascade of processes that are dependent on external and internal transcription factors.

During the second phase the committed chondrocytes aggregate into compact nodules and differentiate into morphological recognizable chondrocytes. Several **bone morphogenetic proteins (BMPs)** appear to be critical at this stage. They induce the expression of adhesion molecules (N-cadherin, N-CAM), which appear to be important for initiating (N-cadherin) and maintaining of the mesenchymal condensations. They also induce the transcription factor **Sox-9**, which activates genes encoding collagen 2 and agrican.

The third phase of endochondral ossification is characterized by a rapid proliferation of chondrocytes and the formation of the cartilage model of the bone. In the periphery of the cartilage model, the mesenchymal cells flatten and stretch in a longitudinal direction, forming a dense sheet of connective tissue, the later perichondrium, which encircles the cartilage and separates it from the surrounding mesenchyme.

In the fourth stage the chondrocytes at the distal ends continue to proliferate, but chondrocytes in the centre of the cartilage elements stop dividing and increase their volume dramatically. They become hypertrophic chondrocytes. This process is mediated by the transcription factor **Cbfa1**, which is also necessary for the development of intramembranous bone. Cbfa 1 itself is regulated by **histone-deacetylase-4 (HDAC4)**, an enzyme that is solely expressed in prehypertrophic cartilage. The hypertrophied chondrocytes secrete collagen X and fibronectin and enable the extracellular matrix of the cartilage to become mineralized by calcium phosphate. They also secrete **vascular endothelial growth factor (VEGF)**, which can transform mesenchymal cells into endothelial cells. At the same time, when chondrocytes are transformed into hypertrophic chondrocytes, some mesenchymal cells of the perichondrium differentiate into osteoblasts. This process is triggered by the transcription factor **Indian hedgehog**, which is secreted by prehypertrophic chondrocytes.

In the fifth phase, blood vessels from the perichondrium invade the cartilage model of the bone. The metabolism of the hypertrophic chondrocytes is different from normal chondrocytes. During hypertrophy, chondrocytes switch from aerobic to anaerobic respiration and eventually die by apoptosis. The intruding blood vessels bring in both osteoblasts and chondroclasts. The chondroclasts degrade the remnants of the apoptotic hypertrophic chondrocytes. The osteoblasts begin to form osteoid (bone matrix) on the partially degraded cartilage matrix, which later becomes calcified by the deposition of calcium phosphate (hydroxylapatite) on collagen fibrils. Proteoglycans and high-affinity calcium-binding proteins induce this process.

Molecular regulation of myotome development

As described for the sclerotomes, the **myotomes** are induced by at least two distinct signals. The **primordial myoblasts**, which arise from the medial portions of the somites are induced by

factors from the neural tube, probably **Wnt1** and **Wnt3** from the dorsal tube region and low levels of **Shh** from the ventral region. The abaxial myoblasts originating from the lateral edge of the somites appear to be specified by signals from the epidermis (**Wnt** proteins) and **bone morphogenetic protein 4 (BMP4)** from the lateral plate mesoderm. In addition to stimulating signals, inhibitory factors contribute to the determination of myotome cells. For example, Shh not only induces myotome and sclerotome development, but also inhibits BMP4 from the lateral plate mesoderm from expanding too far ventrally and medially. In this way it prevents the conversion of sclerotome cells into muscle cells.

Molecular regulation skeletal muscle development (Fig. 16–23)

The mature skeletal muscle fibre is a complex multinucleated cell that is specialized for contraction. Precursors of most muscle lineages (**myogenic cells**) have been traced to the **myotome of the somite**. Although these cells look like mesenchymal cells that can give rise to many other cell types in the embryo, they have undergone a determination process restricting them to the muscle-forming cell line. The molecular basis for this commitment is the action of members of families of **myogenic regulatory factors (MRPs)** that, acting as master genetic regulators, turn on muscle-specific genes in the premuscle mesenchymal cells.

Myoblasts in the somites express either *Myogenic determination factor (MyoD)* or *Myogenic factor 5 (Myf5)*. They are basic helix-loop-helix (bHLH) transcription factors and their expression is strictly limited to cells committed to the myogenic lineage. Within the myotomes, MRP expression is low and disappears during migration of myoblasts. At the site of muscle formation, MRP expression increases and induces the fusion of **myoblasts** to **myotubes**. **Myogenin**, another member of the MRPs is associated with the final differentiation process of myoblasts. *Muscle regulatory factor 4 (MRF4)* expression is often associated with myofibre maturation. When MRP expression is low the myoblasts are capable of proliferation. However, elevated MRP expression induces *p21* expression, which inhibits CDK4 (cyclin dependent

Continued

kinase 4) activity and prevents karyokinesis of nuclei within the myofibre.

The MRPs are transcription factors, which act to induce expression of other muscle specific proteins such as alpha-actin, myosin heavy chain, tropomyosin, myosin light chain, troponin-C and troponin-I. MRPs dimerize with themselves or more likely with another bHLH protein, constitutively expressed in cells, and then bind to DNA. In myoblasts that are proliferating, growth factors stimulate expression of **HLHId genes**. The HLH protein Id lacks the basic region necessary for DNA binding. Thus, in proliferating myoblasts MRP expression does not cause expression of contractile proteins and this also prevents the myoblasts to enter the final differentiation process: fusion. After dimerization, MRPs bind to DNA at a specific site called the E-box. E-boxes are found only in the promoter region of muscle specific genes. Hence, MRP expression can only enhance the transcription of muscle specific genes.

Muscle growth is negatively controlled, as well. **Myostatin**, a member of the TGF-β family of signalling molecules, arrests muscle growth once a muscle has attained its normal size. In the absence of myostatin function, animals develop a grossly hypertrophic musculature. Breeds of 'double-muscled' cattle (for instance Belgian Blue and Piedmontese cattle) are known to have mutations of the *myostatin* gene.

FURTHER READING

Buckingham M. (2007): Skeletal muscle progenitor cells and the role of Pax genes. C. R. Biol. 330:530–533.

Carlson, B.M. (2004): Human Embryology and Developmental Biology. 3rd edition. Mosby, Philadelphia, USA.

Goldring M.B., Tsuchimochi, K. and Ijiri. K. (2006): The control of chondrogenesis. J. Cell. Biochem. 97:33–44.

Hill R.E. (2007): How to make a zone of polarizing activity: insights into limb development via the abnormality preaxial polydactyly. Dev. Growth Differ. 49:439–448.

Kablar, B., Krastel, K., Ying, C., Asakura, A., Tapscott, S.J. and Rudnicki, M.A. (1997): MyoD and Myf-5 differentially regulate the development of limb versus trunk skeletal muscle. Development. 124:4729–4738.

Kablar, B., Asakura, A., Krastel, K., Ying, C., May, L.L., Goldhamer, D.J. and Rudnicki, M.A. (1998): MyoD and Myf-5 define the specification of musculature of distinct embryonic origin. Biochem Cell Biol. 76:1079–1091.

Pacifici, M., Koyama, E., Shibukawa, Y., Wu, C., Tamamura, Y., Enomoto-Iwamoto, M. and Iwamoto, M. (2006): Cellular and molecular mechanisms of synovial joint and articular cartilage formation. Ann N. Y. Acad. Sci. 2006: 1068:74–86.

Robert, B. (2007): Bone morphogenetic protein signaling in limb outgrowth and patterning Dev. Growth Differ. 49:455–468.

Rüsse, I. and Sinowatz, F. (1998): Lehrbuch der Embryologie der Haustiere, 2nd edn. Parey Buchverlag, Berlin.

Ryan, A.M., Schelling, C.P., Womack, J.E. and Gallagher, D.S. Jr. (1997): Chromosomal assignment of six muscle-specific genes in cattle. Anim. Genet. 28:84–87.

Sadler, T.W. (2006): Langman's Medical Embryology. 10th edition, Lippincott Williams and Wilkins, Baltimore, Maryland, USA.

Shibata, M., Matsumoto, K., Aikawa, K., Muramoto, T., Fujimura, S. and Kadowaki, M. (2006): Gene expression of myostatin during development and regeneration of skeletal muscle in Japanese Black Cattle. J. Anim. Sci. 84:2983–2989.

Simon, Y., Chabre, C., Lautrou and A., Berdal, A. (2007): Known gene interactions as implicated in craniofacial development) Orthod. Fr. 78:25–37.

Tickle, C. (2006): Making digit patterns in the vertebrate limb. Nat. Rev. Mol. Cell Biol. 7:45–53.

Wan, M. and Cao, X. (2005): BMP signaling in skeletal development. Biochem. Biophys. Res. Commun. 328:651–657.

Zakany, J. and Duboule, D. (2007): The role of Hox genes during vertebrate limb development. Curr. Opin. Genet. Dev. 17:359–366.

CHAPTER 17

The integumentary system

Fred Sinowatz

The skin is the largest organ of the mammalian body. It protects the body against dehydration, injury and infection and, moreover, it is constantly renewable.

The **integumentary system** of adult mammals consists of two morphologically and functionally distinct layers and their associated appendages (hairs, glands, hooves, claws, horns). The superficial layer, or **epidermis**, is formed by a stratified squamous epithelium that develops from the surface ectoderm. The deeper layers, the **corium** or **dermis** and **subcutis**, consist of connective tissue originating from the mesoderm.

EPIDERMIS

The epidermis originates from the **ectodermal cells** covering the embryo after completion of neurulation (Figs 17-1, 17-2). This is a single-layered epithelium with its apical plasma membrane, facing the amniotic cavity, possessing occasional microvilli. The cells of this single-layered surface ectoderm start to proliferate in the early embryo and form a second protective layer – the **periderm** or covering layer (Fig. 17-3). The periderm is a temporary covering that is shed once the inner layers differentiate to form a true epidermis. With further proliferation of the cells of the basal layer, a third, intermediate layer is formed. Finally, the epidermis acquires its definitive arrangement and four layers can be distinguished: a) the **basal layer** or germinative layer (stratum basale); (b) the **spinous layer** (stratum spinosum); (c) the **granular layer** (stratum granulosum), and (d) the **cornified layer** (stratum corneum).

Cells in the basal layer sitting on the basal lamina will become the germinative layer, a zone destined to give rise to the stratified epithelium of the epidermis. The **basal layer** contains the **epidermal stem cells that divide mitotically** to continuously replace the upper layers of the epidermis, which cornify and eventually get sloughed off. The stem cells of the epidermis divide asymmetrically: the daughter cell that stays attached to the basal lamina remains a stem cell, whereas the cell that leaves the basal layer and migrates to the surface starts to differentiate. The latter cells produce keratins characteristic of skin and arrange them into dense intermediate filaments. The differentiated epidermal cells are called **keratinocytes**. They are bound tightly together by desmosomes and produce a water-impermeable seal of lipid and protein that minimizes dehydration of the body (Fig. 17-4).

Continuous cell production in the **basal layer** generates cells that **push older cells to the surface** of the epidermis. The movement of epidermal cells from the basal layer is preceded by a loss of adhesiveness to basal membrane molecules, like fibronectin, laminin and collagen types I and IV. These cellular changes can be explained by the loss of several membrane proteins (integrins) from the plasma membrane of basal epidermal cells that mediate the attachment of these cells to basal lamina components. Cells of the **spinous layer** produce prominent bundles of keratin filaments, which converge on desmosomes, binding the cells to each other. During their migration, synthesis of differentiated products, like keratins, ceases in the cells. Keratohyalin granules begin to appear in the cytoplasm of the outer, postmitotic cells of the spinous

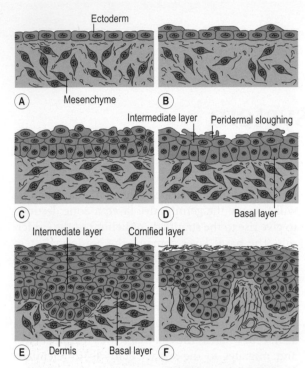

Fig. 17-1: Successive stages in the development of the epidermis and the dermis. **A:** Ectoderm is composed of a single layer of cells with underlying mesenchyme. **B:** Development of a second layer, the periderm. **C** and **D:** Formation of multi-layered epidermis. **E:** Fetal epidermis showing the formation of epidermal papillae. **F:** The epidermis at the late fetal stage displaying the characteristic layers of a stratified sqamous epithelium. Courtesy Sinowatz and Rüsse (2007).

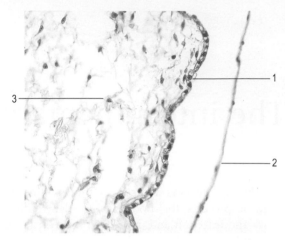

Fig. 17-2: Epidermis of a cat embryo with a CRL of 17 mm. 1: Epidermis; 2: Amnion; 3: Mesenchyme.

layer and become prominent components in the next layer, the **granular layer**. The cells become flattened and their nuclei are pushed to one edge of the cells as they move into the outermost **cornified layer**. There, the cells eventually lose their nuclei and resemble more or less flattened sacs packed with keratin filaments and interconnected by the histidine-rich protein filaggrin. The keratinocytes of the cornified layer are continuously shed. The journey from the basal layer to the sloughed cells takes about 2 weeks in mice, 3 weeks in pigs, and 4 weeks in humans.

The development of the epidermis and its remarkable proliferative activity is stimulated by several growth factors. Transforming growth factor-α is produced by the basal cells and stimulates them by

autocrine mechanisms. Keratinocyte growth factor (KGF, also known as fibroblast growth factor 7, FGF-7), also needed for epidermal development, is made by fibroblasts of the underlying mesenchyme. It is bound by special receptors on the basal cells in the epidermis and probably regulates the differentiation and migration of keratinocytes.

Several other cell types, which are generally termed **epidermal non-keratinocytes**, can be identified in the developing epidermis. Neural crest cells migrate into the dermis and differentiate into **melanoblasts**. They also invade the basal layer of the epidermis. Melanoblasts produce melanosomes containing the brown pigment melanin, which is made by oxidation of L-tyrosine in the presence of the enzyme tyrosinase. Melanosomes are transported to neighbouring keratinocytes and commonly make up the different body colour patterns observed in mammals. **Merkel cells** are intraepidermal mechanoreceptors associated with free nerve terminals. They were once regarded as specialized keratinocytes but new data support the idea that Merkel cells are of neural crest cell origin. Late in prenatal development, the epidermis is invaded by cells of another type, the **Langerhans cells**, which arise from precursors in the bone marrow. These cells are regarded as peripheral components of the immune system and are involved in the

Fig. 17-3: Epidermis of a cat embryo with a CRL of 46 mm. 1: Periderm; 2: Intermediate layer of the epidermis; 3: Basal layer of the epidermis; 4: Epidermal downgrowth; 5: Mesenchyme.

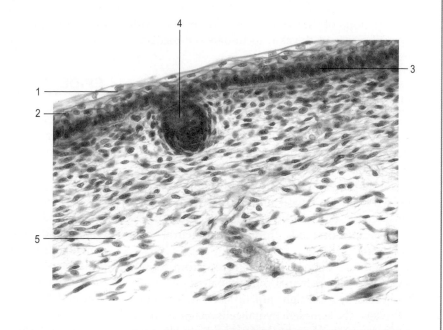

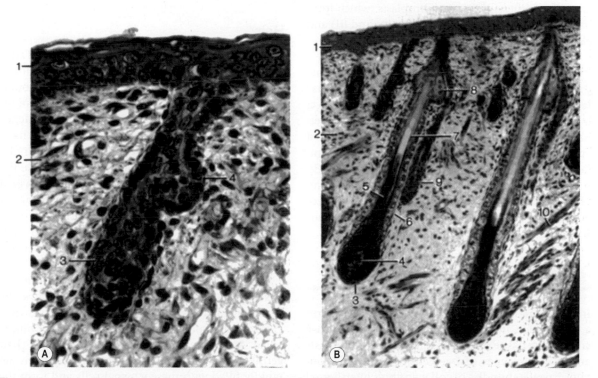

Fig. 17-4: A: Skin of a fetal cat with a CRL of 8 cm. 1: Epidermis; 2: Dermis; 3: Hair bud; 4: Primordium of a sebaceous gland. B: Skin of a fetal cat with a CRL of 10.5 cm. 1: Epidermis; 2: Dermis; 3: Hair bulb; 4: Hair papilla; 5: Hair root; 6: Epithelial hair sheath; 7: Hair shaft; 8: Sebaceous gland; 9: Sweat gland; 10: Arrector pili muscle.

presentation of antigens. They cooperate with T-lymphocytes in the skin to initiate cell-mediated responses to foreign antigens.

DERMIS (CORIUM)

The **dermis** is derived from several sources. In the trunk, dorsal dermis originates from the **dermatomes** of the somites, whereas ventral and lateral dermis as well as the dermis of the limbs are derived from the **lateral mesoderm**. In the head, a considerable part of the cranial skin and anterior neck dermis descends from cranial **neural crest ectoderm**.

The future dermis initially forms from loosely aggregated mesenchymal cells that are tightly interconnected by focal tight junctions on their cellular processes. These mesenchymal cells secrete an intercellular matrix rich in hyaluronic acid and glycogen. Later they differentiate into fibroblasts, which form increasing amounts of collagen (types I and III) and elastic fibres (Fig. 17-1).

When fully developed, the dermis consists of a highly vascularized, fibroelastic connective tissue that can be subdivided into **papillary** and **reticular layers**. Thickenings of the dermis (papillae) project into the basal layers of the epidermis. These alternate with downgrowths of the basal layer, termed epidermal ridges, and are peculiar to the dermoepidermal boundary; they resist shear forces and help maintain the structural integrity of the integument. The papillae contain capillaries and sensory nerve end organs (the Vater-Pacini, Meissner, and Kraus corpuscles).

SUBCUTIS

In most regions of the body mesenchymal cells form a more or less thick layer that gives rise to the **loose connective tissue** of the subcutis. Besides fibroblasts and different types of free cells, the subcutis contains irregular bundles of collagen fibres interspersed with elastic fibres and a varying number of adipocytes. Bundles of skeletal muscle fibres develop in the subcutis in specific regions of the body, such as the thoracic and cervical regions.

EPIDERMAL APPENDAGES

The skin of the domestic animals displays an astounding degree of functional and morphological variety. This is expressed by the presence of highly specialized cutaneous appendages, including a variety of glands (ranging from apo- and eccrine sweat glands and sebaceous glands to mammary glands), hairs, and terminal phalangeal coverings (claws and hooves). The cutaneous epidermal appendages result from a series of reciprocal interactions between the epidermis and the underlying mesenchyme. A complex cascade of proteins in the Wnt and FGF signalling pathway regulate the epithelio-mesenchymal interactions during the formation of epidermal appendages.

Hair

Hairs are specialized epidermal derivatives that arise from the epidermis as the result of inductive stimuli from the dermis. In the smooth bare skin around the lips, periorbita and lower jaws, focal thickenings of the epidermis are the first microscopic evidence of hair development. Later, the primordia of hairs appear in the general integument and, with the exception of some notable anatomical regions, the entire body surface of domestic mammals is covered by closely spaced hairs. Areas that remain devoid of hair include the rhinarium, hooves, digital pads, and muco-cutaneous junctions. Species and even individuals show a marked variation in hair density, type, distribution pattern and colour.

Hairs appear as **solid proliferations from the basal layer** of the epidermis that penetrates the underlying dermis. The basal epidermal cells divide, elongate and penetrate the dermis at an oblique angle. At their terminal ends, these hair buds (hair germs, hair pegs) invaginate. The invaginations are rapidly filled with mesenchymal cells and form the **dermal papillae** which contain blood vessels and nerve endings. Under the continuing influence of

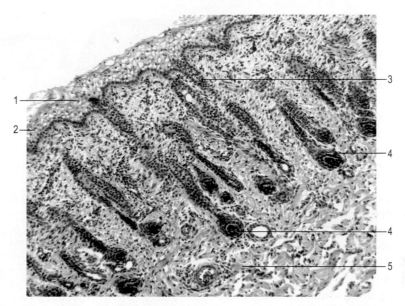

Fig. 17-5: Skin of a bovine fetus with a CRL of 62 cm. 1: Epidermis; 2: Basal layer of epidermis; 3: Epithelial root sheath; 4: Hair papilla; 5: Dermis.

the dermal papilla, the cells of the epidermal down-growth continue to divide and form an early **hair bud**. Soon the cells in the centre of the hair bud become spindle-shaped and keratinized. They form the **hair shaft**, while the peripheral cells remain more cuboidal, giving rise to the **epithelial hair sheath** that later develops into the **internal and external root sheath**. Around the epidermal hair sheath, the surrounding mesenchyme forms a **dermal root sheath** (Fig. 17-5).

In the following weeks the epidermal bud over-grows the dermal papilla, resulting in the shaping of an early hair follicle. At this stage the epithelial wall of the hair follicle shows two bulges penetrating the surrounding mesoderm. The cells of the upper swelling form the **sebaceous glands**, which produce sebum, an oily skin lubricant. During pre-natal development the products of the fetal seba-ceous glands accumulate on the surface of the skin as vernix caseosa. This substance serves as a protec-tive coating for the epidermis while it is continu-ously bathed in amniotic fluid.

The second bulge is the attachment site for a tiny muscle, the **arrector pili muscle**. This bulge induces the adjacent mesenchyme cells to form the smooth muscle cells of the muscle. Its mesodermally-derived smooth muscle fibres can lift the hair to a nearly vertical position in a cold environment. New data show that this lower bulge houses at least two remarkable types of stem cell: the multipotent hair follicle stem cells and the melanocyte stem cells. Melanocyte stem cells are derivatives of the neural crest, produce the pigment melanin, and probably give rise to all pigmented cells of the skin.

Hair follicles can be classified as either **primary** or **secondary**. The bulbs of **primary hair follicles** are located **deep** in the dermis. A single hair (guard hair), which is usually associated both with seba-ceous and sweat glands, emerges from a primary follicle. Primary hair follicles are at first evenly spaced; later, new primary follicles develop between those already established. This leads to a species-specific formation of groups of two, three or four follicles in close proximity to each other (see later).

The spacing of the primary hair follicles involves the influence of several growth and transcription factors. FGF-5, produced by the surrounding mesen-chyme, has a stimulatory effect on the epidermal downgrowth of the hair buds. Counteracting this is an inhibitory influence of BMP-2 and BMP-4, which may regulate the spacing between adjacent hair buds. Soon after its formation, the hair bud begins to express Sonic hedgehog (Shh), which stimulates cell proliferation and growth of the hair follicles.

Secondary hair follicles have a relatively **small diameter** and are located more **superficially** in the dermis. While the hairs emerging from secondary follicles (secondary or under hairs) are usually associated with sebaceous glands, they lack sweat glands and arrector pili muscles.

There is wide variation in the type and surface distribution of hair follicles in domestic animals. In **horses** and **cattle** only primary follicles are present, distributed evenly in rows over the body surface. In **sheep**, wool hair follicles form clusters, each cluster usually consisting of three primary follicles interspersed among secondary follicles. The number of secondary follicles can be up to six times higher than the number of primary follicles, depending on the breed. In the **pig**, primary hair follicles are arranged in clusters of three or four primary follicles per cluster. The skin of **dogs** and **cats** possesses compound follicles (where two or more hairs project through a common pore) that develop postnatally. In cats, single primary follicles are surrounded by several (2–5) compound follicles, which have up to three coarse primary hairs and six to twelve secondary hairs. In dogs, compound follicles occur in clusters of three, with a slightly larger centre follicle.

Sinus hairs

Sinus hairs, which have distinct **sensory** and **tactile functions,** are seen at special locations, primarily in the head region, and predominantly around the lips, cheeks and chin, and above the eyes (Fig. 17-6). During prenatal development, sinus hair follicles appear earlier than do normal hairs. Initially their formation is similar to primary hair follicle development but later the hair bud of sinus hairs enlarges significantly and extends into the subcutis. The characteristic feature of sinus hairs is the development of a **blood filled sinus** within their dermal connec-

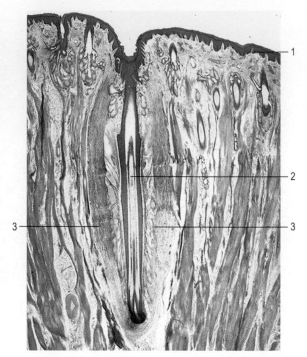

Fig. 17-6: Sinus hair of a horse fetus with a CRL of 78 cm. 1: Epidermis; 2: Hair shaft; 3: Blood sinus.

tive tissue sheath, separating the sheath into an inner and outer layer. In ruminants and horses, trabeculae of connective tissue cross the blood sinus (trabecular type of the sinus hair), whereas in domestic carnivores, no trabeculae are found in the upper third of the sinus. Numerous free nerve endings extending from the inner dermal sheath into the outer epidermal root sheath and are responsible for the enormous tactile sensitivity of sinus hairs.

Skin glands

Sebaceous glands

The development of the sebaceous glands has already been briefly described in the section on hair development. Sebaceous glands arise as **lateral outgrowth of the basal epithelium** of the epithelial hair sheath below the level of sweat gland primordium (Fig. 17-4). The solid swellings become lobulated to form several alveoli that characterize the adult gland. The lumen of the sebaceous gland is formed by breakdown of central sebaceous cells with the resultant oily secretion (sebum) passing into the amnion. Since the sebaceous glands are holocrine (i.e. the secretion consists of disintegrated cells), periodic replacement of secretory cells is required. Sebaceous glands are numerous and well developed in cattle, horses, dogs and cats, but are generally sparse and inconspicuous in pigs.

Sebaceous glands independent of hair follicles are found in the upper eyelids, external genitalia and around the anus. They arise from epithelial buds of the epidermis. In some domestic species especially well developed accumulations of sebaceous glands are found in defined body regions. These include sebaceous glands in the infraorbital and interdigital regions of sheep, base-of-horn glands in goats, and circumanal glands in carnivores.

Sweat glands

Based on their modes of secretion, mammalian sweat glands can be divided into two types: **apocrine** and **eccrine sweat glands**.

Apocrine sweat glands develop in **association with hair follicles** from downgrowths of the basal layer and therefore open into the hair canal above the sebaceous glands (Fig 17-4). The distribution of apocrine sweat glands varies among species. In contrast to the situation in humans, apocrine sweat glands are the principal sweat glands of domestic animals; they are found in all regions of the skin that is covered with hair. Secretions of apocrine sweat glands are relatively viscous and contain a scent that characterizes the individual animal and the species. In humans, apocrine sweat glands are only found in the eyelids, and in the axillary, pubic and perineal regions.

Eccrine sweat glands develop as solid cylindrical downgrowths of the basal layer of the epidermis, each bud penetrating into the underlying mesenchyme. The distal segment becomes coiled to form the secretory portion of the eccrine sweat gland. Lumen formation in the buds is a complex process. The lumen of the intraepithelial portion of the duct forms extracellularly by the separation of cells, while the lumen of the intradermal portion of the duct arises through formation of cytoplasmic vesicles within the cells. These vesicles break through the plasma membranes and coalesce. Epithelial cells of the secretory segment of the gland differentiate into secretory and contractile myoepithelial cells. In humans, eccrine sweat glands are the predominant type of sweat glands. In domestic animals they are found in the footpads of carnivores, the frog of equine hooves, porcine snouts and bovine muzzles.

Hooves and claws

Domestic animals exhibit considerable variation in the morphology of their distal limb integumentary appendages, the result of adaptive development in the evolution of the mammalian limb. Thus, the feet reflect evolutionary changes involving the epidermis, dermis and subcutis as well as bones, tendons and ligaments of the pedal region. The primordium of all of these digital organs is similar but further differentiation varies considerably and leads to digital organs characteristic of the species. During the early development of terminal phalangeal coverings, dermal ridges are found in the feline and canine claw, as well as in the bovine and equine hoof. It is assumed that these dermal ridges are the basic form of a **papillary body** consisting of the epidermis and outer dermis structured in the ridged conformation that is found in all domestic species. Later, the papillary body undergoes species-specific differentiation in forming the hoof and ruminant claws.

During the early fetal period the **equine hoof** (Fig. 17-7) is first foreshadowed by a thickened area of the epidermis on the dorsal and lateral surfaces of the third digit. The thickened epidermis covers a thin layer of dermis up to the end of the second month of gestation. During the third month, an increased growth of the connective tissue at the junction of the presumptive hoof and the hair-bearing skin can be seen, leading to the formation of a proximal, slightly elevated **perioplic cushion** and a more prominent distal elevation, the **coronary cushion**. On the ventral surface of the third digit, the subcutis increases in depth in the areas that will

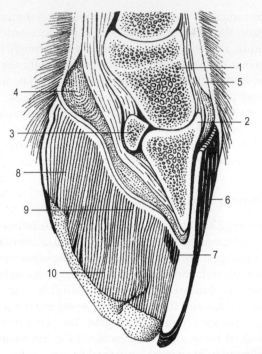

Fig. 17-7: Hoof of an equine fetus at day 266 of pregnancy. 1: Middle phalanx; 2: Distal phalanx; 3: Distal sesamoid bone; 4: Distal cushion; 5: Perioplic corium; 6: Epidermis limbi (Periople); 7: Sole papillae; 8: Bulb; 9: Frog; 10: Eponychium. Courtesy Sinowatz and Rüsse (2007).

become the frog and bulbs, giving rise to shock-absorbing digital cushions. By this stage, the typical hoof-shaped structure of the equine digital end organ, with its **wall**, **bars**, **sole**, **bulbs** and **frog** has already taken shape.

The fetal formation of the papillary body of the hoof in horses shows peculiarities that result in the structure differing somewhat from its counterpart in the hooves of even-toed cattle or pigs, and especially from those in the other homologous digital end organs like claws and the nails. Development of the papillary body in the equine hoof starts with increased mitotic activity of the epidermal basal cells. The epidermal buds, presumably guided by the arrangement of the capillaries in the underlying mesenchyme, invaginate the dermal surface and form a complex dermo-epidermal interface. Then, segment-specific development of the papillary body ensues simultaneously in two different locations: in

the dorsal, distal part of the coronary cushion extending onto the wall, and at the border between the wall and the sole. The papillary body takes the form of **dermal microridges** that are either transformed into individual dermal papillae, arranged in rows, or enlarged to become primary and secondary lamellae. **Dermal papillae** are established in the dermis of the **perioplic** and **coronary cushions** as well as in the dermis of the **sole**, **frog** and **bars**. However, the dermis of the **wall** develops up to 600 **primary folds (laminae)** that run from the coronary groove to the weight-bearing surface of the hoof. Each primary lamina consists of a central core of connective tissue from which between 100 and 200 **secondary laminae** originate at right angles. They are covered by the basal layer of the epidermis. Again, the epidermal buds are presumably guided by the arrangement of the capillaries in the underlying mesenchyme. The dermis of the **coronary cushion** forms cone-shaped dermal papillae covered by epidermis. Growth of the epidermis occurs parallel to the long axis of the third phalanx. At the end of the third month, proliferation of the basal epidermal cells at the apex of the papillae produces **epidermal tubules** that grow distally towards the ventral surface. These epidermal **horn tubules**, round or oval in section, consist of a hollow central medulla containing cellular debris, and an outer dense cortex of keratinized cells. The basal epidermal cells deep in the inter-papillary areas proliferate and form the **intertubular horn**, which fills the space between the horn tubules. The horn from the coronary cushion builds the **intermediate layer of the hoof wall**. During the eighth month of gestation, the epidermal cells on the surface of the **perioplic cushion** proliferate and form the **outer layer of the hoof wall**, also consisting of tubular and intertubular horn and extending distally over part of the surface of the hoof wall. Soft horn originating from the perioplic epidermis also covers the bulbs of the heel. The **internal layer of the hoof wall** is formed by the lamellar horn produced by the epidermis covering the secondary laminae of the wall.

Due to the persistence of the periderm during hoof development, the proliferating epidermis is soft and forms a cushion-like structure covering the tip of each hoof. This soft horn is the **eponychium** which prevents damage to the amnion from fetal movements in late gestation. The eponychium wears off quickly after birth.

The pattern of development of the hooves of even-toed ungulates shows many parallels to that of equine hooves but the main difference is that **ruminant** and **porcine hooves** develop **neither frogs nor bars, and, in the wall segment, no secondary laminae are found**.

In domestic carnivores, the **claw**, too, is composed of a hard, keratinised layer of modified skin that encloses the distal phalanges (Fig. 17-8), but the segment-specific papillary body is poorly developed compared with the most specialized equine form. In the feline claw the development of a distinct papillary body is first seen in the sole segment. This may be due to the higher proliferation rate in the sole epidermis that is characteristic of the feline claw. In the claw, the development of a small papillary body provides a dermo-epidermal contact zone that is only slightly enlarged,

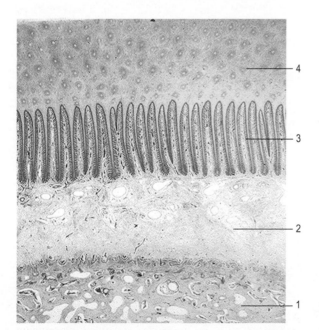

Fig. 17-8: Feline claw: 1: Bone tissue of the distal phalanx; 2: Corium of the distal phalanx; 3: Lamellae of the corium; 4: Horn tubules of the horny wall.

serving mainly to allow for diffusion of nutrients to the epidermal cells; it is not able to transmit tension and compression forces between the claw capsule and the distal phalanx, as the weight-bearing apparatus of the equine hoof has to do.

Horns

In domestic ruminants horns are formed by paired bony **cornual processes**, which are covered by a modified, highly keratinised skin. Bovine horn primordia first appear at the end of the second month of gestation as epidermal thickenings in the frontal region of the head, surrounded by grooves and covered with hair. No significant further development of the horns occurs until after birth. The hairs around the horn primordia are longer than in the surrounding areas and show a whorl-like arrangement postnatally. At approximately one month after birth, the epidermis of the horn primordia proliferates to form conical **horn buds**. Soon afterwards, the **frontal bone develops bony outgrowths** that constitute the osseous core of the developing horns. Over the following month, each solid frontal cornual process becomes hollow and the **frontal sinus extends into the horn cavity**. The dermis covering the cornual process is fused with the periosteum and wears apically directed papillae covered by a highly keratinised epidermis. Proliferation of the epidermis gives rise to keratinised **tubular and intertubular horn**. Soft horn produced at the base of the cornual process is termed **epiceras**. It extends over the tubular and intertubular horn and resembles the external layer of the equine hoof, which is produced by the periople.

Mammary glands

Mammary glands are **specialized sweat glands**. They arise along two lateral lines, the milk lines or **mammary ridges**, on the ventral surface of the developing embryo. The milk lines consist of slightly thickened ridges of epidermis (Fig. 17-9) that appear in most species at a CRL of 12 to 14 mm, slightly later in the horse. Most of each mammary ridge disappears shortly after it forms and the length of

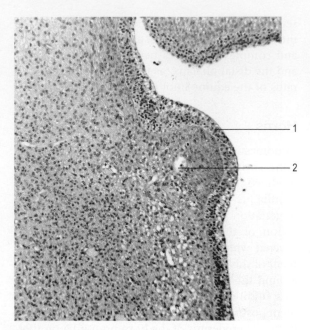

Fig. 17-9: Mammary gland primordium of a bovine embryo, Day 40. 1: Epidermis; 2: Mesenchymal thickening.

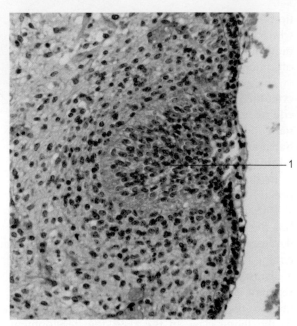

Fig. 17-10: Mammary gland primordium of a bovine embryo, Day 58. An epidermal sprout (1) is protruding into the mesenchyme.

the portion remaining varies with species, corresponding with the number of mammary glands characteristic of the species. In animals like the **dog, cat and pig, groups of glands develop** at predictable positions along the entire path of the mammary ridge on each side, resulting in several papillae with several gland openings in each. In the **cow two single glands**, each with a single papilla, develop in the inguinal region of the mammary ridge on each side. In the **small ruminants, only a single gland develops** on each side of the equivalent area, with one papilla each. In the **horse two glands develop** on each side. However, **both glands open on a single papilla** on each side. Each mammary ridge undergoes a ventral displacement as the dorsal part of the trunk grows.

Focal condensation of the mesenchyme and thickening of the overlying epidermis occur at specific intervals along the mammary ridge. The thickened surface epithelium gives rise to the **primary mammary bud** that pushes into the underlying mesenchyme and forms **secondary mammary buds** as it grows (Figs 17-10, 17-11). These secondary

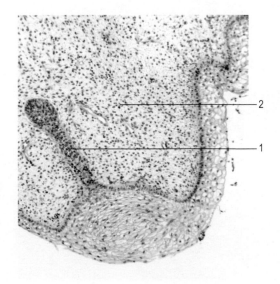

Fig. 17-11: Developing mammary gland of a female bovine fetus at Day 85. 1: Primary epidermal sprout; 2: Mesenchyme.

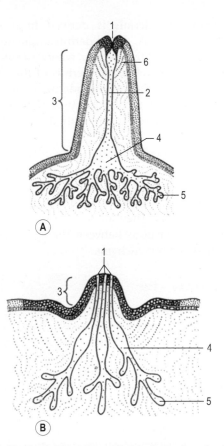

(A)

(B)

Fig. 17-12: Types of teat formation in domestic animals. A: Proliferation type (bovine); B: Eversion type (pig, carnivores); 1: Areolar area; 2: Papillary duct; 3: Teat; 4: Gland sinus; 5: Secondary and tertiary epithelial sprouts. Courtesy Sinowatz and Rüsse (2007).

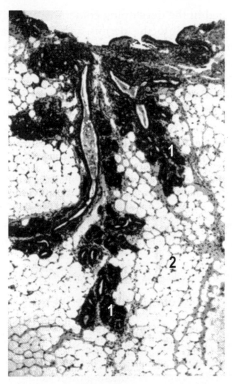

Fig. 17-13: Ovine mammary gland at the beginning of puberty. Epithelial sprouts (1) protrude in a connective tissue rich in fat cells (2). Courtesy Sinowatz and Rüsse (2007).

buds lengthen and branch as embryonic development proceeds. The mammary buds are initially solid cords of epithelial cells but later become patent and form lactiferous ducts that open onto the surface of the developing teats (Fig. 17-12). The **teats** are formed by mesenchymal proliferation that elevates the epidermis surrounding the glandular openings.

Between birth and puberty the mammary gland grows **isometrically** but structural and functional development is not completed until the female has become pregnant and given birth (Fig. 17-13). With the onset of puberty, the mammary gland grows **allometrically** – at a rate that is faster than in the rest of the body. During repeated oestrous cycles, a duct and alveolar framework is established within the mammary gland. Under the influence of oestrogens, growth hormone and prolactin, the ducts begin to branch, and progesterone stimulates the terminal portions of the branches to form alveoli. Further endocrine stimulation during pregnancy is needed for complete mammary gland development.

SUMMARY

The integumentary system of adult mammals consists of two morphologically and functionally distinct layers and their associated appendages (hairs, glands, hooves, claws, and horns).

The superficial layer, or **epidermis**, is formed by a **stratified squamous epithelium** that develops from the surface ectoderm of the embryo and fetus. Besides keratinocytes, several other cell types can be identified in the developing epidermis. Neural crest cells migrate into the dermis and differentiate as **melanoblasts**. They produce melanin, which is transported to neighbouring keratinocytes and commonly make up the different body colour patterns. **Merkel cells** are intraepidermal mechanoreceptors, once regarded as specialized keratinocytes but now believed to be of neural crest cell origin. Late in prenatal development, the epidermis is invaded by cells of another type, the **Langerhans cells**. These arise from precursors in the bone marrow and play an important defensive role in the skin as antigen-presenting cells.

The deeper layers, **dermis** (corium) and **subcutis**, consist of **connective tissue** originating from the mesoderm. The dermis is derived from several sources. In the trunk, dorsal dermis originates from the dermatomes of the somites, whereas ventral and lateral dermis as well as the dermis of the limbs is derived from the lateral mesoderm. In the head, considerable portions of the cranial skin and anterior neck descend from cranial neural crest ectoderm.

The cutaneous epidermal appendages include **hairs**, **glands** (ranging from apo- and eccrine sweat glands and sebaceous glands, to mammary glands) and terminal phalangeal coverings in the form of **claws** and **hoofs**. They all result from a series of reciprocal interactions between the epidermis and the underlying mesenchyme.

Box 17-1 Molecular regulation of the development of the integumentary system

Several growth factors are known to stimulate the development of the epidermis. **Transforming growth factor-α (TGF-α)** for instance, is produced by the cells of the basal layer of the epidermis and is an autocrine stimulant of cell division in the epidermis. Another important growth factor for epidermal differentiation is **keratinocyte growth factor (KGF)**. This paracrine factor is produced by the fibroblasts of the mesoderm-derived dermis and stimulates the migration and differentiation of cells from the basal layer of the epidermis.

In hair formation the establishment of an individual epidermal downgrowth involves the stimulatory influence of **FGF-5** produced by the underlying mesenchyme of the dermal papilla. Counteracting this is an inhibitory influence of **BMP-2** and **BMP-4**, which regulate the spacing between neighbouring hair buds. Soon after its downgrowth the hair bud expresses **Sonic hedgehog (Shh)** which stimulates the proliferation and growth of the hair follicle. Production of **Msx** by the thickened epidermis of the hair bud causes intense proliferation of both the ectoderm and the underlying mesenchyme. Also, the homeobox gene *Hoxc-13* is expressed in all hair follicles and appears to be involved in some aspects of the keratinization process.

During its development, the hair bud develops two swellings on its side. The cells of the upper swelling form the sebaceous glands. The lower swelling (or bulge region) of the hair follicle develops into the arrector pili muscle and houses two populations of stem cells: multipotent hair follicle stem cells and melanocyte stem cells. **Melanocyte stem cells**, located in the lower region of the bulge, are derived from migrating neural crest cells and continuously produce the pigment cells for the skin and its appendages. Differentiation of melanocyte stem cells into melanocytes while they are in the stem cell niche is inhibited by the complicated regulation of the transcription factor **Mitf**, which activates the genes of melanin synthesis. The *Mitf* gene itself is activated by **Sox10** and **Pax3** protein. Sox10 stimulates the enzyme-encoding genes for the melanin pathway and Pax3 competes with Mitf for the enhancer sites of the genes for melanin production. Therefore these genes remain unexpressed as long as the melanocyte stem cells are within their niche. Some of these cells migrate outside the bulge and differentiate into mature melanocytes that pigment the shaft of each new hair as it begins to develop. When the melanin stem cells are outside the niche, **Wnt** signals cause β-catenin to enter their nuclei and to bind with **Lef1**. This transcription factor can remove Pax3 from the binding sites and allow Mitf to bind. With Mitf and Sox10 bound, the genes encoding the melanin-producing enzymes can be transcribed and melanin is produced.

FURTHER READING

Adelson, D.L., Cam, G.R., DeSilva, U. and Franklin, I.R. (2004): Genomics 83:95–105.

Bragulla, H. (2003): Fetal development of the segment-specific papillary body in the equine hoof. J. Morphol. 258:207–224.

Bragulla, H., Ernsberger, S. and Budras, K.D. (2001): On the development of the papillary body in the feline claw. Anat. Histol. Embryol. 30:211–217.

Duboule, D. (1998): Hox is in the hair: a break in colinearity? Genes Devel. 12:1–4.

Fath El-Bab, M.R., Schwarz, R. and Godynicki, S. (1983): The morphogeneis of the vasculature in bovine fetal skin. J. Anat. 136:561–572.

Knabel, M., Kölle, S. and Sinowatz, F. (1998): Expression of growth hormone receptor in the bovine mammary gland during prenatal development. Anat. Embryol. 198:163–169.

Mack, J.A., Anand, S. and Maytin, E.V. (2005): Proliferation and cornification during development of the mammalian epidermis. Birth Defects Res C. Embryo Today. 75:314–329.

Meyer, W. and Gorgen, S. (1986): Development of hair coat and skin glands in fetal porcine integument. J. Anat. 144:201–220.

Monteiro-Riviere, N.A. (1985): Ultrastructure of the integument of the domestic pig (Sus scrofa) from one through fourteen weeks of age. Anat. Histol. Embryol. 14:97–115.

Pispa, J. and Thesleff, I. (2003): Mechanisms of ectodermal organogenesis. Dev. Biol. 262:195–205.

Rabot, A., Sinowatz, F., Berisha, B., Meyer, H.H. and Schams, D. (2007): Expression and localization of extracellular matrix-degrading proteinases and their inhibitors in the bovine mammary gland during development, function, and involution. J. Dairy Sci. 90:740–748.

Robinson, G.W. (2004): Identification of signaling pathways in early mammary gland development by mouse genetics. Breast Cancer Res. 6:105–108.

Robinson, G.W., Karpf, A.B.C, and Kratochwil, K. (1999): Regulation of mammary gland development by tissue interaction. J. Mamm. Gland Biol. Neoplasia 4:9–19.

Rüsse, I. and Sinowatz, F. (1998): Lehrbuch der Embryologie der Haustiere, 2nd edn. Parey Buchverlag, Berlin.

Sinowatz, S., Wrobel, K.H., El Etreby F. and Sinowatz F. (1980): On the ultrastructure of canine mammary gland during pregnancy and lactation. J. Anat. 131:321–332.

Sinowatz, F., Schams, D., Plath, A. and Kölle, S. (2000): Expression and localization of growth factors during mammary gland development. Adv. Exp. Med. Biol. 480:19–25.

CHAPTER 18

Poul Hyttel

Comparative listing of developmental chronology

Table 18-1: Chronological listing of developmental events in cattle in relation to stage of gestation (Days post coitum). Information accumulated from various sources. Open boxes represent lack of data

Day	Event	
1	Fertilization and pronucleus development, minor activation of the embryonic genome	
2	2-cell embryo	
3	6–8-cell embryo	
4	Arrival in the uterus, 8-cell embryo, major activation of the embryonic genome	
5	16-cell embryo developing into morula	
6	Compact morula developing into blastocyst	
7	Blastocyst	
8	Expanded blastocyst around 220µm, hatching from the zona pellucida in some cases	
9	Hatching from the zona pellucida in all blastocysts	
10	Blastocysts, 203–239 µm, hypoblast starts to form	
11	Blastocysts, 145–818 µm	
12	Blastocysts, 0.26–1.42 mm, hypoblast forms a complete lining	
	Complete embryo (conceptus)	**Embryonic disc**
13	Elongation initiated, 0.5–3.1 mm	Circular about 140 µm
14	0.6–40 mm	Circular (200–300 µm) to oval (210x400 µm), primitive streak starts to form
15	1.8–135 mm, maternal recognition of pregnancy by IFN-τ	Amniotic folds start to form
16		Oval up to 450x600 µm, primitive streak with mesoderm and endoderm involution
17	12.5–24 cm	Oval up to 400x750 µm, primitive streak
18	Conceptus elongated to fill pregnant uterus horn and to invade non-pregnant horn	Allantois development initiated
19	Placentation initiated	

Table 18-1: *Continued*

Day	Event	
	Size of the embryo proper/fetus (length or CRL; weight)	**Developmental event**
20	2 mm	Neural groove, first somite pairs
21		Up to 6 somite pairs, neural tube, primitive gut formed by embryo foldings
22		16–20 somite pairs, heart development, first heart beat
23		18–19 somite pairs, first pharyngeal arch, optic and otic placodes, allantois anchor-shaped
24	3.1 mm	Three brain vesicles, second pharyngeal arch, forelimb buds
25	3.5 mm	Third pharyngeal arch, C-shaped embryo
26	5.6 mm	Fourth pharyngeal arch, hind limb buds
30	10–12 mm, 69–280 mg	Nasal placodes, paddle-shaped forelimb buds
34	13 mm	Fusion of facial prominences, forelimb digits
38		Eyelids, genital tubercles, hind limb digits
50	3.9 cm, 5 g	Eyelids partially cover eyes
56	4.8 cm	Secondary palate fused
60	6.6–7.8 cm, 14–19 g	Eyelids fused, differentiation of external genital organs, hoofs and horn primordia
75	10 cm	Tactile hairs, hair follicles on body
83		Cornification of hoofs, development of scrotum
110	24 cm, 550 g	Eruption of first teeth, hairs around mouth and eyes
142	38 cm, 2650 g	Hairs on ears
150	37 cm, 2750 g	Hairs on cheek, colour marks, hard hoofs, descent of testis completed
159	42 cm	Hairs at umbilicus
182		Hairs at tail and horn primordium
187	56 cm, 9.2 kg	Hairs at legs
230	73 cm, 18 kg	Hairs on body
279–290	90 cm, 35 kg (dependent on breed)	Birth

Table 18-2: Chronological listing of developmental events in sheep in relation to stage of gestation (Days post coitum). Information accumulated from various sources. Open boxes represent lack of data

Day	Event	
1	Fertilization and pronucleus development	
2	2-cell embryo	
3	Arrival in the uterus, 8–16-cell embryo, major activation of the embryonic genome	
4	16-cell embryo developing into morula	
5	Compact morula developing into blastocyst around 168 μm	
6	Blastocyst	
7	Expanded blastocyst around 184 μm in diameter	
8	Hatching from the zona pellucida, hypoblast starts to form	
	Complete embryo (conceptus)	**Embryonic disc**
9	Ovoid 0.18 x 0.25 mm	Circular about 45 μm
10	Ovoid 0.4 x 0.9 mm	Complete hypoblast formed
11	Ovoid or elongated up to 6 mm	Oval up to 33 x 260 μm
12	10–22 mm	Primitive streak, mesoderm and endoderm involution
13	32–70 mm, maternal recognition of pregnancy by IFN-τ	Oval up to 370 x 490 μm
14	Up to 35 cm	Oval up to 612 x 1000 μm, development of amniotic folds, giant binucleate trophoblast cells
15	Placentation initiated	Oval from 1.5 x 2 mm to 0.8 x 3.2 mm, neural groove, first somite pairs
	Size of the embryo proper/fetus (length or CRL; weight)	**Developmental event**
16	2.5–4.2 mm, conceptus elongated to fill pregnant uterus horn and invade non-pregnant horn	8–15 somite pairs, neural tube, closure of amnion
17–18	4.0–5.5 mm	25 somite pairs, allantois anchor-shaped, three brain vesicles, first and second pharyngeal arch
19	5.0–7.0 mm	Eye and ear placodes, third pharyngeal arch
20	7.0 mm	Forelimb buds
21		C-shaped embryo, neural tube closed, fourth pharyngeal arch, hind limb buds
22	8.0–9.0 mm	Paddle-shaped forelimb buds, nasal placode
23		Paddle-shaped hind limb buds
24–25	1.4 cm	Lens formation, eye pigmentation
26	1.6 cm	Formation of eye lids, forelimb digits
27	1.4–1.6 cm, 0.9 g	External auditory meatus and auricles
30	1.6–2.2 cm	Fusion of facial prominences, tongue

Table 18-2: *Continued*

Day		Event
34	2.3–3.5 cm	Tactile hairs at eyes
38	2.9–4.4 cm	Tactile hairs at upper lip, secondary palate fused
43	3.3–5.5 cm	Eyelids fused, differentiation of outer genital organs
57		Hairs on head
60–67	11.0–16.5 cm	Hairs on body
70		External genital organs formed
80	19.8–23.7 cm, 340 g	Descent of testis completed
104	27.5–34.3 cm	Colour marks
144–152	47 cm (dependent on breed)	Birth

Table 18-3: Chronological listing of developmental events in the pig in relation to stage of gestation (Days post coitum). Information accumulated from various sources. Open boxes represent lack of data

Day	Event	
1	Fertilization and pronucleus development	
2	Zygote to 2-cell embryo	
3	Arrival in the uterus, 2-, 4- or 8-cell embryo, major activation of the embryonic genome in 4-cell embryo	
4	8–16-cell embryo developing into morula	
5	Blastocyst	
6	Blastocyst	
7	Hatching from the zona pellucida	
8	Blastocyst around 1.2 mm	
9	Blastocyst 0.5–2.4 mm, embryonic disc forming	
10	Blastocyst 2.3–10 mm, embryonic disc established	
11	Elongation, 0.65–4.0 cm, embryonic disc with posterior crescent, maternal recognition of pregnancy by means of oestradiol	
	Complete embryo (conceptus)	**Embryonic disc**
12	Elongation, up to 6 cm	Primitive streak, mesoderm and endoderm involution
13	Elongation	Neural groove, first somite pairs
14–15	Elongation at a rate of 30–35 mm per hour	10–19 somite pairs, neural tube, first aortic arch
15–16	Elongation at a rate of 30–35 mm per hour	28–30 somite pairs, neural tube closed, second and third pharyngeal arch
17–18	Elongation, up to140–150 cm	36 somite pairs, closure of amnion, third, fourth, and sixth aortic arch, fore limb buds, C-shaped embryo, allantois anchor-shaped, otic placode, hind limb buds

Continued

Table 18-3: *Continued*

Day	Size of the embryo proper/fetus (length or CRL; weight)	Developmental event
20–21	14–19 mm, 0.5 g	Eye pigmentation, nasal placode, physiological umbilical herniation, genital tubercles
22	11–13 mm, 0.5 g	Completion of somite formation, mammary line, paddle-shaped fore and hind limb buds
28	21–25 mm	Eylids, tactile hair follicles, differentiation of outer genital organs
34		Secondary palate fused
36	32.5–39 mm	Eyelids cover eyes
44		Prepuce, scrotum, vulva, and clitoris formed
50	66–92 mm, 30.7 g	Eyelids closed, gut returned to abdominal cavity
90	160–227 mm, 411 g	Eyelids open
114–115	Size and weight dependent on breed	Birth

Table 18-4: Chronological listing of developmental events in the horse in relation to stage of gestation (days after ovulation). Information accumulated from various sources. Open boxes represent lack of data

Day	Event	
1	Fertilization and pronucleus development	
2	2–4-cell embryo	
3	8-cell embryo, major activation of the embryonic genome	
4	12–32-cell stage	
5	Morula	
6	Arrival to uterus, morula developing into blastocyst	
6–8	Blastocyst 250–780 µm, formation of capsule, hatching from zona pellucida	
9	Blastocyst 2.0–4.0 mm	
10	Development of yolk sac	
13	Blastocyst 6 mm	
14	Blastocyst 16 mm	
	Complete embryo (conceptus)	**Embryonic disc/embryo proper**
16		Up to 4 somite pairs, neural groove
17–18		5–18 somite pairs, blastocyst ovoid, neural tube
18–19		13–22 somite pairs
20–21	Blastocyst 26–40 mm, loss of capsule	25 somite pairs, closure of amnion, first and second pharyngeal arch, optic vesicles, otic placodes, heart formation, yolk sac with sinus terminalis

Table 18-4: *Continued*

Day	Event	
	Size of the embryo proper/fetus (length or CRL)	**Developmental event**
22	5.7–6.5 mm	Second, third, fourth, and sixth aortic arches
23–24	5–6 mm	C-shaped embryo, fore and hind limb buds, heart beat
25	7–8.5 mm	Lens formation, otic vesicle
26		Eye pigmentation
28	9–9.5 mm	Lens formation, cochlea and vestibulum, pulmonary arteries, complete enclosure of amnion by allantois
30	9–11.5 mm	Genital tubercles
36	15 mm	Complete conceptus about 75 mm ovoid structure, fusion of facial prominences
40	22–25 mm	Placentation
45		Differentiation of outer genital organs
75		Prominent clitoris
80		Scrotum
112		Tactile hairs on lips
120		Fine hairs around mouth, eyes, and on cheek
150		Hairs on eyelids
180		Mane and tail hairs
270		Hairs on body
310–365		Birth

Table 18-5: Chronological listing of developmental events in the dog in relation to stage of gestation (Days post coitum). Information accumulated from various sources. Open boxes represent lack of data

Day	Event
1–3	Completion of meiotic maturation, fertilization, pronucleus development
4	2–8-cell embryo,
5	16–32-cell embryo forming the morula, major activation of the embryonic genome in 8-cell embryo
8	Arrival in the uterus, blastocyst 275–544 µm
11	Blastocyst 500–715 µm
13	Blastocyst up 0.22–1.14 mm
15	Blastocyst up to 0.53–2.0 mm, initial formation of swellings in uterus

Day	Size of the embryo proper/fetus (length or CRL)	Developmental event
16	1.2–1.5 mm	Neural groove, first somite pairs
17	1.3–2.0 mm,	8 somite pairs, placentation, neural tube, three brain vesicles, optic vesicle
18	2.3–5.0 mm	10 somite pairs, allantois starts to form
20		30 somite pairs, first and second pharyngeal arch
21		Amnion closed
22		C-shaped embryo, third pharyngeal arch, fore and hind limb buds
24	7.5 mm	Genital tubercles
25	9–15 mm	49 somite pairs, fourth pharyngeal arch, external acoustic meatus
25–28		Paddle-shaped forelimb buds, eye pigmentation
29	19–21 mm	Differentiation of male gonad
30–33	13–25 mm	Eyelids, tactile hairs on lips, primordia of external genital organs, physiological umbilical herniation, secondary palate fused
35	21–24 mm	Eyelids partially covering eyes, external male genital organs
36–38	29–38 mm	Tactile hairs, regression of mesonephros
40	38–42 mm	Eyelids closed, gut returned to abdominal cavity
43	53–57 mm	Hair follicles on head, fore limb digits well separated
44–46	96–121 mm	Hair on body, colour marking
52–54	124–158 mm	Hair formation completed
62–63 (58–68)	>160 mm	Birth

Table 18-6: Chronological listing of developmental events in the cat in relation to stage of gestation (Days post coitum). Information accumulated from various sources. Open boxes represent lack of data

Day	Event	
2	Ovulation (induced by coitus)	
3	2–8-cell embryo,	
4	16-cell embryo	
5	24–40-cell embryo forming morula	
6	Arrival in the uterus, early blastocyst	
10	Expanded blastocyst	
12	Blastocyst up to 2 mm, hatching from the zona pellucida	
	Size of the embryo proper/fetus (length or CRL)	**Developmental event**
13	2 x 4 mm	5 somite pairs, initiation of placentation, neural plate
14	5.5 x 6 mm	Up to 8 somite pairs, invasion into endometrium, optic vesicles, otic placodes, neural tube
15		20 somite pairs, first, second, and third pharyngeal arch
17	5–6.3 mm	Fourth pharyngeal arch, otic vesicles, optic placodes
18	5–8 mm	Forelimb buds, nasal placodes, lens formation
19	7–11 mm	Hind limb buds
20	8–9 mm	Paddle-shaped forelimb buds
21	10 mm	Eye pigmentation, external auditory meatus, physiological umbilical herniation
22	10 mm	Mammary lines, auricles
24	14–17 mm	Eyelids, forelimb digits, tactile hair follicles on lips
26	20–22 mm	Hind limb digits
27	20–22.5 mm	All digits well separated, tongue, hair follicles on body
28–29	24–26 mm	Eyelids closed
30	26–28 mm	External auditory meatus covered by auricles
32	37–38 mm	Secondary palate fused
37	55 mm	Tactile hairs on head
46	Up to 100 mm	Hair on body, pigmented nose
50	70–98 mm	Colour marks
60–63 (58–65)	>125 mm	Birth

FURTHER READING

Rüsse, I. and Sinowatz, F. (1998): Lehrbuch der Embryologie der Haustiere, 2nd edn. Parey Buchverlag, Berlin.

CHAPTER 19

Fred Sinowatz

Teratology

HISTORY OF TERATOLOGY

Teratology is the study of abnormal development. The idea that extrinsic influences ranging from 'evil spirits' to diet may influence the development of human and animal embryos has been held since Antiquity, but it became more precise in the nineteenth century with Etienne Geoffroy de Saint Hilaire, who studied in great detail several prenatal anomalies like cyclocephalia, anencephaly, and twin monsters and also coined the very term 'teratology'. In the last century two sets of findings strongly influenced the establishment of teratology as a scientific discipline strongly connected to embryology. The first set concerned the deleterious effects of hyper- and hypovitaminosis A on mouse and pig embryos. The second, and more dramatic, set related to the effects of thalidomide, a sedative used to prevent morning sickness during early pregnancy in humans, and which resulted in devastatingly severe limb defects in numerous newborns in Europe during the late 1950s and early 1960s. Since then, the number of known and suspected teratogens has grown tremendously. Recently, the possibility that cloning by somatic cell nuclear transfer can cause severe malformations has caused concern, with developmental defects being attributed to incomplete reprogramming of the somatic cell genome by the oocyte cytoplasm (see Chapter 21).

GENERAL PRINCIPLES

Contrary to the situation in humans, reliable data on the occurrence of congenital defects in domestic animals are not readily available. The frequency of **congenital malformations** varies with species, breed, geographical locations and many other factors. Various studies indicate that approximately **1.5% to 6%** of all live-born domestic mammals show at least one recognizable congenital malformation. Such malformations are comparatively infrequent in cats but occur to an upper limit of 3–4% in sheep, cattle and horses and in up to 6% of newborn dogs and pigs. They range from complex associations of gross anatomical abnormalities to enzyme defects caused by single nucleotide substitution detectable only with molecular diagnostic tools. Traditionally, it has been structural defects that have been emphasized in veterinary embryology textbooks, but it should be kept in mind that congenital malformations really encompass a continuum ranging from purely biochemical abnormalities to gross anatomical defects and include derangements of function, metabolism and behaviour.

The genesis of congenital malformations is best regarded as an interaction between the **genetic constitution** of an embryo and the **environment** in which it develops. The basic instructions for embryonic development are encoded in the genes. As the genetic instructions unfold, the developing structures interact with environmental influences that either are either compatible with normal development or interfere with it; penetration (the degree of manifestation) of an abnormal gene, or of the components of a genetically multifactorial cascade, can be markedly affected by environmental conditions.

CRITICAL PERIODS OF SUSCEPTIBILITY TO ABNORMAL DEVELOPMENT

As we have seen, the developing embryo consists of groups of cells that are growing, differentiating, and undergoing morphogenesis at different rates and over different time periods, but in a strictly controlled sequence of events. Therefore, one of the most important principles of teratology is that the susceptibility to an agent causing malformation – a **teratogen** – varies with the developmental stage of the embryo at the time of exposure. From many studies the following conclusions can be drawn:

- Insults to the embryo during the **first 3 weeks of gestation** (during which the basic body plan is established) are unlikely to result in defective development, because they either kill the embryo or can be compensated by regulatory mechanisms in the early embryo. Agents that disrupt the morula or blastocyst stage, or disturb the normal embryo-maternal communication and interfere with normal apposition of the conceptus to the uterine mucosa, usually induce **early embryonic mortality**.
- The period of **maximal susceptibility** begins when organogenesis is initiated at **three weeks and extends in most organ systems up to the eighth week**. Although most major organs are established during this period, exceptions are the very complex organs like the brain and major sense organs, which show prolonged periods of high susceptibility, and the reproductive organs, which develop comparatively late.
- After **eight weeks** of gestation, **major structural anomalies are unlikely to occur**. At this time, most organs are well-established.

This picture of susceptible periods is rather simplified; it must be remembered that although *exposure* to a teratogen or some other harmful influence might be at an early stage of development, the *expression* of the defects it causes may be seen only at a later stage of embryogenesis. Often, an induced lesion in one system can cause secondary malformation in others. This occurs, for instance, during the development of the heart or the central nervous system.

Not all teratogens act in the same developmental periods. Some are harmful at an early stage of development but not later in pregnancy. Thalidomide is a well-known example, causing malformations of the limbs in humans during a very narrow window of development (considered to be between 34 and 50 days after the beginning of the mother's last menstrual period). Other teratogens affect only later developmental stages; the antibiotic tetracyline, for example, which stains teeth and other bony structures, can only do so after these hard tissues have been formed in the fetus.

Although there are many examples of isolated structural or biochemical defects, it is quite common to find multiple abnormalities in the same individual. This phenomenon can result from a single teratogen acting on the primordia of several organs during their susceptible periods. Another possibility is that a single defective gene affects the structure and metabolism of multiple developing organs.

CAUSES OF MALFORMATIONS

Significance of genotype

Since normal development is controlled by an interaction between the genome of an embryo and its environment, susceptibility to a teratogen depends upon the genotype of the embryo and the manner in which it interacts with adverse environmental factors. This principle is best documented by the fact that some materials that are teratogenic in one species do not cause malformation in other species. A well-known example of this is that cortisone, which when given to mice at a particular developmental stage readily produces cleft palate, does not affect other laboratory species. Furthermore, differences in susceptibility to teratogens have been found even in different strains of mice.

Genetically based malformations result from abnormalities of chromosomal division or mutations of genes. Abnormal genes may either be the direct cause of an anomaly, or may induce the anomaly indirectly by affecting the susceptibility of the embryo to an environmental insult. Thus, the predisposition to an insult may be inherited.

Abnormal chromosome numbers

Quantitative changes in chromosomal numbers result in polyploidy or aneuploidy. In **polyploidy**, the chromosomal number is **more than twice the haploid number of chromosomes** of a given species. Most polyploid embryos are aborted early in pregnancy. Potential causes of polyploidy are fertilization of an egg by more than one sperm (polyspermy) or lack of separation of a polar body during meiosis of the oocyte. Embryos may also display **mixoploidy**, where a group of normal diploid cells is mixed with another portion of polyploid cells. This situation probably results from the lack of cytokinesis during initial mitoses. Interest-

ingly, up to 25% of normal blastocysts recovered from cows are mixoploid and have a low percentage of polyploid cells, most of which become sequestered in the trophectoderm later in development. The incidence of mixoploidy is increased in embryos produced in vitro or by somatic cell nuclear transfer (see Chapter 21).

Numerical **errors in the number of a particular chromosome** result in **aneuploidy**. This is defined as a total number of chromosomes other than the usual haploid set for a given species. Monosomy is the lack of one member of a chromosome pair. In trisomy, a triplet instead of a normal chromosome pair occurs. Both events are typically the result of nondisjunction during meiosis. A number of conditions resulting from monosomy and trisomy are listed in Table 19-1. In most cases, embryos with monosomy of the autosomes and sex chromosomes cannot survive. However, in man as well as in domestic animals, individuals with monosomy of the X-chromosome (XO genotype) are viable. In humans, this condition is called Turner's syndrome, characterized by a female phenotype with sterile ovaries.

Table 19-1: Effects of abnormal karyotypes due to sex chromosome non-disjunction

Species	Normal chromosome number	Abnormal karyotype	Effect
Cattle	60	61XXY	Hypoplastic testes
		61XXX	Hypoplastic ovaries
Horse	64	63XO	Infertility
		63XXY	Hypoplastic ovaries
		65XXX, 66XXXY	Intersex
Pig	38	37X0	Infertility, hypoplasia of external genitalia
		30XXY	Hypoplastic testes
Dog	78	79 XXY	Hypoplastic testes
Cat	38	37X0	Intersex
		39XXY	Intersex
		40XXYY	Intersex

Abnormalities in chromosome structure

Abnormalities in chromosome structure can cause malformations of development. Radiation or certain chemical teratogens can cause chromosome breakages and **deletions** (loss of parts of chromosomes). If a piece of a broken chromosome does not contain a kinetochore, it is lost because it cannot move towards a spindle pole during anaphase. Deletion results in the loss of genetic information. Other common types of structural defects of chromosomes are reciprocal translocation, inversion and **centric fusion**. **Reciprocal translocation** results when two non-homologous chromosomes each break into two segments and then exchange segments. Animals with a reciprocal translocation in their genome are usually of normal phenotype but their fertility is significantly reduced. **Centric fusion** occurs when two acrocentric chromosomes merge to form a metacentric chromosome. Cattle with centric fusion have normal phenotypes but show an increased frequency of monosomy and trisomy in their offspring.

Many **genetic mutations** are expressed as functional or morphological abnormalities. These can affect **recessive** or **dominant genes** and for some of these conditions the molecular and biochemical lesions have been identified. Many of these aberrations are extensively described in textbooks of veterinary genetics and some representative examples will be discussed later in this chapter.

Abnormalities caused by assisted reproductive technologies

Abnormally large offspring, with a body weight increased by 10–50%, are more frequently born following assisted reproductive technologies (see Chapter 21). In cattle and sheep this **large offspring syndrome (LOS)** is often associated with neonatal respiratory distress and perinatal death. The aetiology of LOS is not fully elucidated but it has been proposed that some growth factors in the sera used for embryo culture, co-culture of the embryos with feeder cells, an asynchronous uterine environment, or other unknown factors in assisted reproductive technologies may be involved.

Many aspects of LOS in farm animals, especially the somatic overgrowth, are reminiscent of **Beckwith-Wiedemann syndrome (BWS)** in humans. New data suggest that BWS is induced by loss of imprinting and consequent over-expression of the gene encoding insulin-like growth factor 2 (IGF2). In sheep, a similar mechanism has been elucidated in relation to LOS, a region in intron 2 of the *IGF2 receptor* (*IFG2R*) gene displaying differences in DNA methylation, the mechanism by which the expression of imprinted genes is controlled. This gene is imprinted in the mouse, possibly variably imprinted in humans, and appears to be imprinted in the sheep as well. It has recently been demonstrated that sheep fetuses, developing from embryos cultured under conditions promoting LOS, display loss of maternal *IGF2R* gene methylation and decreased expression of this receptor. This epigenetic aberration is likely to be causally involved in LOS and demonstrates that even subtle manipulations of gametes and embryos may induce epigenetic aberrations that manifest themselves later during embryonic development.

Most studies on LOS have been performed in cattle where the reported abnormalities include increased rates of early embryonic mortality, production of large fetuses and calves (newborn calves weighing up to 80 kg), disproportionate and abnormal organ growth, musculoskeletal deformities, abnormalities of placental vasculature, and hydroallantois. Recently, comparable abnormalities have been reported in mice, sheep and pigs.

The extreme heterogeneity of LOS phenotypes has made it difficult to define the underlying causes and has led to the proposal by Farin et al. (2006) that the term 'abnormal offspring syndrome (AOS)' would more accurately describe the range of abnormal developmental changes following transfer of in vitro produced and cloned embryos in cattle and other species. These authors also proposed the following functional classification system of developmental outcomes resulting from transfer of such embryos:

- Type I AOS: Abnormal development and death of the embryo or early conceptus prior to completion of organogenesis (approximately Day 42 of gestation in cattle).
- Type II AOS: Abnormal development of placenta, fetal membranes, and fetus; fetus dies between completion of organ differentiation and full term (Day 42 to 280 of gestation in cattle).
- Type III AOS: A full term fetus and/or placenta with severe developmental abnormalities and no evidence of compensatory response by the fetus. Parturition is normal (eutocia) or difficult (dystocia). The calves are severely compromised with altered clinical, haematological, or biochemical parameters. Death occurs around the time of parturition or during the neonatal period.
- Type IV AOS: A full term fetus and/or placenta with moderate abnormalities; however, the feto-placental unit compensates and adapts to the compromising genetic or physiological insults and survives. Parturition is normal or difficult. The calves may be normal or abnormal in size for their breed, and they may have clinical, haematological, or biochemical abnormalities.

These abnormal AOS phenotypes resulting from in vitro production of embryos and cloning are stochastic in occurrence. It should also be mentioned that recent reports have documented that cloned animals may display normal fetal development, birth and post-natal development. It is likely that improvement of the technologies employed will alleviate some of the impacts imposed on the gametes and embryos and result in fewer abnormalities.

Environmental factors

Mechanical factors

Several common anomalies, such as clubfoot, congenital hip dislocations, and certain deformations of the skull have been attributed to mechanical factors that impose an abnormal **intrauterine pressure** on the fetus. This phenomenon is often related to a reduced amount of fluid in the amniotic cavity or to uterine malformations in the mother. Amniotic bands may form as the result of tears to the extra-embryonic membranes during pregnancy. If they constrict digits or extremities of the fetus, they may cause intrauterine amputations.

Physical factors

Ionizing radiation is a potent teratogen in all species. The response depends on the dose and the stage of development at which the embryo is exposed to the radiation. As ionizing radiation can cause breaks of DNA strands and is also known to cause mutations, exposure of pregnant animals to radiation should be avoided, although the dose in a diagnostic X-ray examination it usually so small that the risk is minimal. Strong ionizing radiation can result in a variety of congenital defects including microcephaly, cleft palate, and other skeletal malformations. Defects of the central nervous system are also prominent in irradiated embryos.

Chemical factors

Any chemical substance that has the potential to alter cellular function or which is cytotoxic has the potential of being teratogenic. The mechanisms that lead to teratogenesis vary. For example, some drugs can inhibit specific enzyme systems (e.g. carbonic anhydrase), interfere with DNA metabolism, or disturb particular metabolic activities. Retinoic acid, for instance, acts as a potent teratogen when taken orally. This compound produces a wide spectrum of defects, most of which are related to derivatives of the cranial neural crest. These involve facial structures, the heart, and the thymus. As described in Chapter 8, neural crest cells from rhombomeres are instrumental in patterning many structures of the face and neck and contribute to the outflow tract of the heart. Retinoic acid affects the expression of Hox genes in the cranial and pharyngeal regions causing alterations of the anterior rhombomeres and of the neural crest cells derived from them.

It has been shown that at defined exposure levels and at critical stages of development, **several therapeutic drugs** can also be potentially teratogenic (Table 19-2). Special caution should be taken when prescribing cytotoxic drugs such as antimitotic or anthelminthic agents to pregnant animals. For some of these drugs, the teratogenic effects on the developing embryo are well understood. However, for many substances it is still not clear in which species and at what concentrations they might be teratogenic. For instance, the classic teratogen thalidomide is highly teratogenic in humans, rabbits, and some primates, but not in the commonly used laboratory rodents. The use of some antibiotics during pregnancy has been associated with congenital defects: streptomycin in high dose can result in inner ear deafness; tetracycline can cross the placental barrier and cause a yellowish discolouration of teeth (and, in high doses, interfere with enamel formation) when given late in pregnancy.

Many **poisonous plants** containing toxic or teratogenic compounds have been implicated in congenital defects in herbivorous animals. Some of these compounds are listed in Table 19-3. The malformations produced vary widely and include skeletal deformities, limb defects, cyclopia and cleft palate. As with other agents, there are distinct times during development when the embryo or fetus is particularly susceptible to certain plant teratogens. A well-known example is the effect of Veratrum californicum which induces congenital cyclopia if consumed by ewes at around Day 14 of pregnancy.

Table 19-2: Teratogenic drugs

Agent	Function	Species	Affected organs
Androgens	Steroid hormone	All domestic mammals	Masculinization of female embryos
Benzimidazole compounds	Anthelmintic	Ewes	Skeletal, renal and vascular anomalies
Corticosteroids	Steroid hormone	Rodents	Palate, limbs, oedema
Cyclophosphamide	Antimitotic	Rodents	Embryotoxic
Diethylstilboestrol	Steroid hormone	Rodents	Genital tract anomalies
Phenylhydantoin	Anticonvulsant	Cats	Cleft palate
Folic acid antagonists	Antimitotic	Dogs, sheep	Embryotoxic
Griseofulvin	Antifungal	Cats, dogs, horses	Head, brain, skeleton, palate, bone marrow
Metrifonate	Antiparasitic	Pig	Cerebellar hypoplasia
Methallibure	Oestrus synchronization	Pig	Limb and cranial defects
Streptomycin	Antibiotic	All domestic mammals	Deafness, ototoxicity
Tetracycline	Antibiotic	All domestic mammals	Teeth, skeleton
Thalidomide	Sedative	Nonhuman primates, rabbit, dog, pig	Growth retardation, Intestinal defects
Valproic acid	Anticonvulsant	Rodents, nonhuman primates	Neural, cranial-facial, skeletal and cardiovascular defects

Table 19-3: Common teratogenic plants

Plant	Common name	Species	Affected system/ Defects
Quercus species	Acorns	Cattle	Shortened limbs, overdistension of distal joints
Astralagus lentigus	Locoweed	Cattle, sheep, horses	Skeletal malformation
Conium maculatum	Poison hemlock	Cattle, pigs, horses, sheep	Skeletal malformations, cleft palate
Lathyrus species	Pea		Limbs
Leucaena leucocephala	Mimosine	Pigs	Multiple
Lupinus species	Lupin	Cattle	Limbs: arthrogryposis
Nicotiana tabacum	Tobacco	Pigs, cattle, sheep	Arthrogryposis, brachygnathia, cleft palate
Oxytropus species	Locoweed	Cattle	Limbs
Prunus serotina	Wild black cherry	Cattle	Limbs, vertebrae
Sophora sericea	Silky sophora	Cattle	Limbs, vertebrae
Thermopsis monatan	False lupin	Cattle	Limbs, vertebrae
Veratrum californicum	False hellibore	Sheep, goats	Craniofacial malformations, cleft palate, limb malformations
Vicia faber	Common vetch	Cattle	Limbs, vertebrae

Infectious agents

Most infectious diseases that cause birth defects are **viral**. The pathogenicity of a virus, the stage of gestation at which infection occurs, and the immunological competence of the fetus determines the outcome of in utero viral infections. A summary of infectious virus diseases that can cause birth defects in domestic animals is given in Table 19-4. During early development, the **zona pellucida is protective against viral infections**, but when the blastocyst hatches from the zona pellucida, the embryo becomes vulnerable to attack by viruses. Many viral infections are toxic and/or lethal to the embryo. Later, the placental barrier prevents viral infections to some degree but **many viruses can cross the placental barrier**. Therefore maternal viral infections at critical stages of development can be a serious cause of malformations. Infection of pregnant sheep, cattle, and goats with Akabane virus causes teratogenic defects (e.g. arthrogryposis; hydranencephaly) that are closely related to fetal age at time of infection.

CLASSIFICATION OF MALFORMATIONS

The major types of developmental disturbances found in domestic animals include:

Agenesis or aplasia

This is a developmental **failure of an organ or part of an organ to form**. It results in the **absence** of the involved structure. Absence of the lens (aphakia) or a kidney (renal agenesis) can be due to absent or abnormal inductive tissue interactions during development.

Table 19-4: Common teratogenic viruses

Virus	Species affected	Effects
Akabane virus	Cattle, sheep, goat	Brain defects (hydranencephaly, porencephaly), limb defects (arthrogryposis)
Bluetongue virus	Sheep, cattle, goats	Brain, spinal cord, limb defects
Border disease virus	Sheep, goats	Wide range of embryonic and fetal changes, skeletal growth retardation, cerebellar dysplasia
Bovine rhinotracheitis	Cattle	Embryotoxic
Bovine viral diarrhoea	Cattle	Embryonic death; abnormalities of the central nervous system and ocular abnormalities
Classical swine fever	Pigs	Malformation of the central nervous system (cerebellar and spinal hypoplasia)
Equine rhinopneumonitis	Horses	Embryotoxic
Equine encephalitis	Horses	Limb defect
Feline panleukopaenia	Cats	Cerebellar defects, retinal dysplasia
Herpesvirus 2	Dogs	Eye, brain defects
Japanese encephalitis	Pigs, sometimes horses	Hydrocephalus, cerebellar hypoplasia, hypomyelinogenesis
Porcine herpesvirus 1	Pigs	Abortion, stillborn or mummified piglets
Porcine parvovirus	Pigs	Abortion, stillborn or mummified piglets
Rift valley fever virus	Sheep, cattle, goat	Arthrogryposis, hydranencephaly, cerebellar hypoplasia, microcephaly
Rubella	Monkey, rabbit	Heart, eye, brain and skeletal defects

Hypoplasia and hyperplasia

The normal formation of organs requires a precise control of cellular proliferation. If cellular proliferation in developing organs is reduced, the organ becomes **too small** (hypoplastic). Increased proliferation results in hyperplasia, where organs become **too large**. Even relatively minor growth changes can cause severe problems in complex regions of the body such as the face.

Failure to fuse or close

Fusion is a basic morphogenic process involved in the formation of many structures (Fig. 19-1). Therefore, failure of completion of a fusion process is one of the more important types of developmental defects. Examples are cleft palate, defects in the diaphragm, and various septal defects in the heart. A classic case is the failure of tube formation in spina bifida anomalies, in which fusion of the neural tube is incomplete.

Absence of normal cell death

Genetically or epigenetically controlled cell death in the form of apoptosis is an important mechanism in forming certain structures of the body. For instance, syndactyly (webbed digits) occurs when normal cell death fails to occur in the interdigital areas.

Disturbances in tissue resorption

Some structures present in the early embryo must be resorbed for normal development. Examples

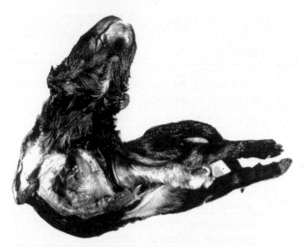

Fig. 19-1: Failure of a fusion process is one of the more important types of developmental defects. In the example here, the body wall of the thorax and abdomen of a puppy has failed to fuse. Courtesy Sinowatz and Rüsse (2007).

include the resorption of the oro-pharyngeal membrane and the cloacal membrane that cover the future oral and anal openings. Anal atresia is a common anomaly in piglets.

Failure of migration

Failure of migration can occur at the level of cells or entire organs. An important example is the migration of cells of the neural crest. Disturbances in migration cause malformations in any of the structures in which the participation of neural crest cells is important, for example the thymus, outflow tracts of the heart, and the adrenal medulla. At the organ level, the kidneys normally ascend from their origin in the pelvic region to the upper part of the abdominal cavity. If migration fails, the result is pelvic kidneys. Other examples are ectopic cordis, in which the heart is located outside of the thoracic cavity, and cryptorchidism, in which the testes are not in the scrotum.

Developmental arrest

Some malformations are characterized by the persistence of structures in a state that was normal at

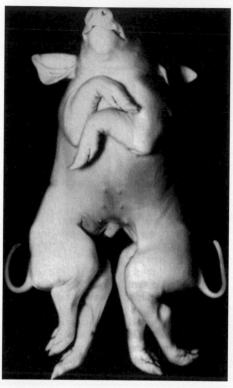

Fig. 19-2: These twin pigs are conjoined at the thorax and head, resulting in a cephalothoracopagus. Courtesy Sinowatz and Rüsse (2007).

an earlier state of development. An example is the persistence of a thyroglossal duct in which persisting epithelial cells mark the path of the thyroid gland as it migrates from the base of the tongue to its normal position.

Duplication and reversal of asymmetry
(Figs 19-2, 19-3, 19-4, 19-5)

Under normal circumstances, both members of a twin pair are completely separated. Sometimes the separation is not complete and the twins remain conjoined to various degrees and at almost any site of their bodies. In the extreme, one member of the pair is more or less normal whereas the other has a much smaller body, often consisting of just the torso and limbs (parasitic twins).

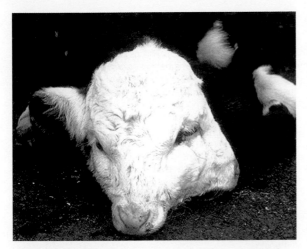

Fig. 19-3: Cephalopagus of a bull calf. Courtesy Sinowatz and Rüsse (2007).

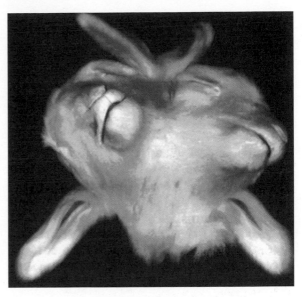

Fig. 19-5: Dicephalus in a goat. Courtesy Sinowatz and Rüsse (2007).

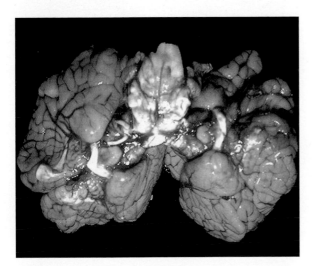

Fig. 19-4: The brain of the calf shown in Fig. 19-3 shows a doubling of the hemispheres but only one brain stem.

ORGAN MALFORMATIONS

The following descriptions of major malformations in the organ systems should be read in conjunction with former chapters that describe their normal development.

CONGENITAL MALFORMATIONS OF THE CARDIOVASCULAR SYSTEM

Congenital heart malformations
(Fig. 19-6)

Heart defects represent the **most common class of congenital malformation**. Cardiac malformations are more frequently encountered in dogs and cattle than in horses and cats. Clinically, heart malformations are typically classified as cyanotic or acyanotic, depending on whether they are associated with cyanosis in postnatal life. In animals with acyanotic malformations the body receives sufficient oxygenated blood to maintain life-sustaining levels of activity. In cyanotic malformation the body receives insufficient oxygenated haemoglobin in the peripheral capillary bed. Cyanosis is readily diagnosed by the purplish to bluish tinge in tissues with a dense superficial capillary circulation, most easily seen in the oral mucosa and gums.

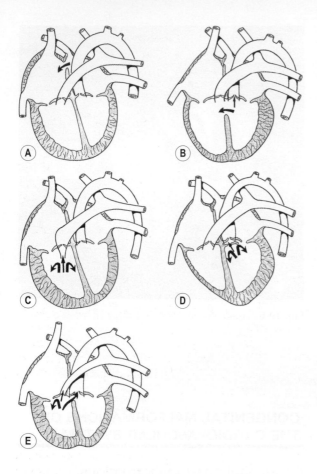

Fig. 19-6: Schematic representation of cardiac malformations (modified according to Noden and De Lanhunta, 1985).
A: Atrial septal defect (ASD). The blood is shunted from left to right, because of the higher pressure in the left atrium. The right heart becomes overloaded and overworked from the additional volume of blood it receives. The result is dilatation and hypertrophy of the right atrium and ventricle.
B: Ventricular septal defect (VSD) is characterized by the presence of a small opening at the dorsal part of the interventricular septum. The physiological consequences are determined by the size and the relative resistance in the systemic and pulmonary vascular beds.
C: Pulmonary stenosis (PS) is one of the most common cardiac defects in dogs. It can be present as a single defect or associated with other heart defects. Obstruction of the right ventricular outflow tract cause increased resistance to ejection, leading to right ventricular hypertrophy and septal flattening.
D: Aortic stenosis, obstruction of the left ventricular outflow (LVOT) is caused by a proliferative thickening encircling the aortic outlet immediately below the aortic valves. It results in a ventricular overload, which causes hypertrophy of the left ventricle.
E: Tetralogy of Fallot. It is characterized by a large ventricular septal defect, an aorta that overrides the left and right ventricles, obstruction of the right ventricular outflow (pulmonary stenosis) and right ventricular hypertrophy. (Courtesy Sinowatz and Rüsse (2007).

Ectopia cordis

Ectopia cordis, the condition in which the **heart does not attain its expected position in the thorax,** is most frequently reported in cattle. Often, the heart remains in the neck region (ectopia cordis cervicalis). The initial position of the cardiogenic area is anterior to the oro-pharyngeal membrane and the neural plate. With the anteroposterior folding of the embryo proper in conjunction with the closure of the neural tube and growth of the brain vesicles, the cardiogenic field and the developing heart with the future pericardial cavity is brought to a cervical location. Later, further migration into the thorax is accomplished. A delay in the onset of cardiac descent can trap the heart at, for example, a cervical location. Occasionally, the paired sternal bars that form the sternum do not fuse and the heart may be located outside the thorax. This condition is called ectopia cordis thoracis.

Dextrocardia

Dextrocardia is a malformation in which the heart lies more to the **right side of the thorax** than to the left. This condition is caused early in development, when the heart tube loops to the left instead of the right. Dextrocardia may be associated with **situs inversus**, a complete reversal of asymmetry in all organs. In this anomaly the chambers normally on the left and right are reversed in position and the ductus arteriosus, aortic arches and pulmonary veins form on the right. The condition can be compatible with normal life. In other cases sidedness is random and only some organs show a reversed position. This condition is called heterotaxy and is associated with an increased incidence of other malformations, especially heart defects.

Acyanotic heart malformations

Acyanotic malformations are the most commonly encountered congenital heart anomalies, especially in dogs, and include the following.

Obstruction of the left ventricular outflow (aortic stenosis)

Obstruction of the left ventricular outflow tract (LVOT) is **one of the most common congenital heart defects** and is usually caused by a proliferative thickening that forms a fibromuscular ring around the aortic outlet immediately below the aortic valve. It is quite frequently detected in large breed of dogs (e.g. Golden Retrievers, Rottweilers, Boxers, German Shepherds and Samoyeds). Although supravalvular and valvular forms of aortic stenosis have been recognised, fibromuscular subaortic stenosis, causing a fixed form, is the most common form in the dog. In cats aortic stenosis is uncommon but valvular and supravalvular forms of LVOT have been reported and the incidence of subaortic stenosis is somewhat higher in Siamese cats.

Three different grades of severity of LVOT obstruction have been described:

- Grade 1: The lesion consists of small, raised nodules of thickened endocardium of the interventricular septum below the aortic valve.
- Grade 2: The lesion forms a narrow ridge of thickened fibrous endocardium that partially encircled the LVOT below the aortic valve.
- Grade 3: The lesion forms a fibrous band, ridge or collar completely encircling the LVOT just below the aortic valve.

The most severe effects are generally found in dogs older than six months but pups of just a few weeks of age may be affected by severe forms of stenosis.

LVOT obstruction results in a ventricular pressure overload which requires higher systolic pressure to maintain adequate stroke volume. The ventricle hypertrophies, increasing the demand for myocardial blood flow. Aortic pressures are normal but left ventricular luminal pressures are higher than normal, so that the coronary driving pressure may be inadequate and coronary flow may sometimes be in a reversed direction during systole. Papillary muscles and subendocardial regions are the areas most commonly affected by syncope. Although cardiac output is normal at rest, the fixed obstruction makes it difficult to increase the stroke volume in response to the exercise as would occur normally. This lowers exercise tolerance and may induce syncope. Eventually a poststenotic dilation develops in the ascending aorta distal to the valve. Clinically signs vary considerably, from none at all to characteristic left heart failure (with characteristic pulmonary congestion and oedema, panting, coughing, and dyspnoea). Until recently, surgery on this malformation has not been successful and most patients are managed medically.

Pulmonary stenosis

Uncomplicated pulmonary stenosis (i.e. without other heart anomalies) is **one of the most common cardiac defects in dogs** of breeds predisposed to the condition (English Bulldogs, Mastiffs, Fox Terriers, Samoyeds, miniature Schnauzers, Cocker Spaniels, and West Highland White Terriers are particularly susceptible). An hereditary form of pulmonary valve dysplasia has been found in the Beagle (with a polygenetic mode of transmission) and Boykin Spaniel.

Pulmonary stenosis consists of a **narrowing of the pulmonary outflow** and can occur at several possible sites. Although subvalvular and supravalvular forms of pulmonary stenosis have been reported, the most common form of the right ventricular obstruction in dogs is **pulmonary valve dysplasia** which can be present as a single defect or associated with other heart defects. A pulmonary artery atresia represents the extreme form of obstruction of the right ventricular tract. The nature of the obstruction can be diagnosed by echocardiography.

When valvular fusion exists, the semilunar cusps are fused towards the tips of the leaflet, resulting in doming of the valves. When hypoplastic type of pulmonary stenosis is present, the valve appears thickened and immobile and the annulus may be narrow and hypoplastic. The main haemodynamic effects of pulmonary stenosis can be visualized as concentric right ventricular hypertrophy, paradoxical septal motion, and reduced size of the left atrium and left ventricle in moderate to severe pulmonary stenosis. Dilatation of the main pulmonary artery can be seen distally to the obstruction, close to the bifurcation. Spectral Doppler echocardiography of pulmonary stenosis will record increased peak pulmonary artery velocity (>1.6 m/s) and often prominent pulmonary insufficiency. A Doppler gradient across the stenosis of <50 mm Hg is considered as mild pulmonary stenosis. Gradients between 50 and 100 mm Hg are moderate in severity and higher gradients are associated with severe pulmonary stenosis.

Obstruction of the right ventricular outflow tract causes increased resistance to ejection and a proportional increase in ventricular systole pressure leading to right ventricular hypertrophy, leftward septal flattening, and a systolic gradient across the pulmonary valve. Clinical signs may not occur in puppies, but the onset of right heart failure are usually seen between 6 months and 3 years of age. Typical symptoms of right heart failure include fatigue, weakness, dyspnoea, and venous congestion.

Ventricular septal defects

Ventricular septal defects are characterized by the presence of a **small opening at the dorsal part of the interventricular septum**. Depending on the location, ventricular septal defects are classified as: (a) membranous/perimembranous (the most common type in dogs), (b) outflow (infundibular/supracristal), (c) inflow (atrioventricular canal), and (d) muscular (trabecular). They are caused by a deficient growth of one or more of the septa that normally close the interventricular foramen (ventricular septum, conu-truncal cushions). Ventricular septal defects can appear as isolated lesions or in associa-

tion with other heart defects such as pulmonary stenosis, pulmonary atresia, truncus arteriosus, and double-outlet right ventricle. Some defects can predispose the animal to prolapse of the aortic valve into the defect.

The physiologic consequences of a ventricular septal defect depend on the size of the defect and the relative resistance in the systemic and pulmonary vascular beds. If the defect is small ('restrictive' ventricular septal defect), there is little or no functional disturbance, since pulmonary blood flow is increased only minimally. In fact, many bovine hearts have small ventricular septal defects. In contrast, if the defect is large ('non restrictive' ventricular septal defect), right ventricular dilatation and hypertrophy occur. Often, a ventricular septal defect is accompanied by other cardiac malformations, some of which probably arise secondarily and can produce cyanotic signs. Ventricular septal defects have been reported in all domestic species. Among dogs it is more common in English Bulldogs, Keeshonds (in which a genetic basis has been documented), English Springer Spaniels, and Beagles.

Atrial septal defects

Atrial septal defects, characterized by an **opening in the interatrial septum**, have been described in all domestic species. In dogs, they are more common in Boxers and Samoyeds. Atrial septal defects occur when the foramen ovale of the septum secundum overlies one (or more) openings in the septum primum. Functionally the blood is shunted from left to right, because of the higher pressure in the left atrium. The right heart becomes overloaded and overworked from the additional volume of blood it receives. The result is dilatation and hypertrophy of the right atrium and ventricle. The left heart also frequently undergoes hypertrophy.

Dysplasia of the atrioventricular valves

Dysplasia of the atrioventricular valves is caused by an abnormal development of the atrioventricular cushions that lead to the formation of **valve cusps that are too short to fully close** the atrioventricular orifice. The condition has been reported in all domestic species. A wide spectrum of lesions has been identified in dogs and cats with atrioventricular valve malformations, including anomalies in valve leaflets, chordae tendineae and/or papillary muscles. Dysplasia of the atrioventricular valves may appear as an isolated lesion or in association with others defects such as subvalvular aortic stenosis (SAS), ventricular septal defects, or atrial septal defects. Cats, and the following dog breeds show a predisposition to mitral dysplasia: Great Danes, German Shepherds, Bull Terriers, Golden Retrievers, Newfoundlands, Dalmatians, and Mastiffs. Tricuspid dysplasia has also been reported in cats. Regurgitation of blood occurs upon systole. This condition is often called left atrioventricular valve insufficiency and usually leads to left heart failure.

Cyanotic heart malformations

Two deviations from normal cardiac blood flow characterize most cyanotic heart malformations: a venoatrial shunt, that allows the blood flow between the right and left sides of the heart; and an impediment to pulmonary tract outflow. Two conditions that include these deviations are the Tetralogy of Fallot and the Eisenmenger syndrome.

Tetralogy of Fallot

Tetralogy of Fallot is the most common cyanotic congenital heart defect in domestic animals and is characterized by the following four lesions: a large **ventricular septal defect**, an **aorta that overrides the left and right ventricles**, **obstruction of the right ventricular outflow tract** (pulmonary stenosis), and **right ventricular hypertrophy**. These anomalies are produced by a failure of the conutruncal cushions and septum to align properly. **Pulmonary** stenosis causes resistance to flow from the right ventricle, which consequently dilates and hypertrophies. This is aggravated by the left-to-right flow of left ventricular blood and results in right ventricular hypertrophy, the fourth lesion characteristic of the Tetralogy of Fallot. As a result of the right ventricular outflow tract obstruction and elevated right ventricular systolic pressure, desaturated blood

is shunted through the ventricular septal defect to mix with blood entering the left ventricle. Chronic hypoxaemia may result in polycythaemia by increasing renin production and release of erythropoietin. Signs of this heart defect usually occur in young animals. Even limited exercise often causes marked cyanosis. Other symptoms are fatigue, poor growth, dyspnoea on exercise and occasionally episodic syncope.

Eisenmenger syndrome

This malformation is **similar to the Tetralogy of Fallot** except that **no pulmonary stenosis** is found. The primary defects consist of a slight dextro-aorta and a large interventricular septal defect. This condition arises from hypoplasia of the proximal portions of the cushions of the bulbus cordis during heart development. Eisenmenger syndrome is characterized by an elevated pulmonary vascular resistance and right-to-left shunting of blood through a systemic-to-pulmonary circulation connection such as a patent ductus arteriosus, ventricular septal defects, atrial septal defects, and aortico-pulmonary septal defects. This additional source of blood induces the right ventricle to dilate and hypertrophy.

With substantial left-to-right shunting, the exposure of the pulmonary vasculature to increased blood flow as well as increased pressure often results in pulmonary vascular obstructive disease, leading to increased pulmonary vascular resistance. As the pulmonary vascular resistance approaches or exceeds systemic resistance, the shunt is reversed and cyanosis appears. The right ventricle becomes hypertrophied because it must eject against a high pulmonary vascular resistance. Perfusion of the kidneys with hypoxaemic blood leads to secondary polycythemia.

Transposition of great vessels

Reversal of systemic and pulmonary outflows is a rare event. On rare occasions the conu-truncal cushions fail to spiral as they divide the outflow tract into two channels. This causes the fourth aortic arches to connect with the right ventricles and the sixth aortic arches with the left ventricle. This results in two totally independent circulatory arcs, with the right ventricle emptying into the aorta and the left ventricles into the pulmonary artery. In such a condition the ventricles are of the same size and generate comparable pressure. Since the systemic and the pulmonary circulations are separate and closed, the presence of left-right shunts in the heart is necessary for postnatal survival. This anomaly is compatible with life only if an atrial and ventricular septal defect and an associated patent ductus arteriosus accompany it, but even with these anatomical compensations, the quality of the blood reaching the body is poor.

Congenital malformations of the vascular system

Patent ductus arteriosus

In the fetus, the ductus arteriosus allows pulmonary arterial blood to bypass the unexpanded lungs and enter the descending aorta for oxygenation in the placenta. At birth, closure of the ductus arteriosus must occur so that the lungs will receive an adequate flow of unoxygenated blood from the pulmonary trunk. The increase in oxygen tension at birth leads to inhibition of local prostaglandins and causes functional closure of the ductus, followed by anatomic closure during the ensuing weeks of life.

If the ductus fails to close, blood shunts from the descending aorta to the pulmonary artery. **Patent ductus arteriosus** is the **most common cardiovascular malformation in dogs**, with a breed disposition in Poodles, German Shepherds, Collies, Pomeranians, Cocker Spaniels, Maltese, English Springer Spaniels, Keeshonds, and Yorkshire Terriers making them particularly afflicted.

The consequences of a patent ductus arteriosus depend primarily on the diameter of the duct and the pulmonary vascular resistance. When pulmonary vascular resistance is normal, blood will shunt from the descending aorta to the pulmonary artery because the aortic pressure exceeds that of the pulmonary artery during all phases of the cardiac cycle. This results in increased pulmonary flow and

increased venous return to the left atrium and left ventricle. Volume overloading of the left side of the heart causes left atrial dilatation, left ventricular eccentric hypertrophy and mitral insufficiency. Left-sided congestive heart failure may develop from volume overload. When pulmonary vascular resistance increases, left-to-right shunting decreases and right-to-left shunting develops.

Symptoms of patent ductus arteriosus are extremely variable. The most common sign found by physical examination is a continuous murmur often accompanied by a thrill at the craniodorsal cardiac base in an otherwise normal dog. The abnormal sound most frequently found with patent ductus arteriosus is referred to as 'machinery murmur' since it is heard continuously through all phases of the cardiac cycle. The point of maximal intensity of the murmur is over the main pulmonary artery, high on the left base, from where it radiates cranially to the manubrium of the sternum and to the right base of the heart. Frequently, a systolic murmur is evident over the left apex if mitral incompetence is present. As a rule the left side (aortic) pressure is greater than that of the right (pulmonary) side. The strong blood flow from the higher pressure system (aortic) circulation into the pulmonary circulation overloads the vasculature of the lungs, resulting in pulmonary hypertension and ultimately heart failure.

Surgical ligation of the patent ductus arteriosus is recommended in all cases of left-to-right shunting as soon as possible after diagnosis. Without ligation, at least 50% of the cases are expected to die within a year of diagnosis. Some dogs, presumably with small shunts, may live for many years. A less invasive surgical correction of the ductus is coil embolization via transcatheter delivery of thin metal coils.

Persistent right aortic arch

Persistent right aortic arch results from a **failure of the right dorsal aorta to degenerate** between the seventh dorsal intersegmental artery and the point of fusion of the paired aortae. Persistence of the right aortic arch has been found in cattle, pigs, horses, and cats, and it is fairly common in dogs. It is responsible for 95% of the vascular ring defects in dogs and is most frequently seen in larger breeds (e.g. German Shepherds, Weimeraners, and Irish Setters). This malformation can appear under different phenotypes: in one form, the right arch connection persists and the left one disappears, resulting in the arch of the aorta being on the right instead on the left side; in a second form, both connections persist, but the right one is only a fibrous remnant without a vascular lumen; in a third form, both connections possess the characteristics of a vessel, which results in a double aortic arch.

A clinical consequence of the persistence of the right aortic arch is a **complete or partial vascular ring being formed around the oesophagus and trachea**. This vascular ring is made up of the right aortic arch, the ligamentum arteriosum (the remnant of the ductus arteriosus), and the pulmonary trunk. It surrounds and compresses the oesophagus and the trachea. Signs of a vascular ring formation are found typically when the animal begins to consume solid foods. After eating, regurgitation of undigested food occurs. As a consequence, the oesophagus secondarily dilates cranial to the stricture producing a megaoesophagus cranial to the base of the heart.

Anomalous origin of the right subclavian artery

Although an anomalous origin of the left subclavian artery is found occasionally (as a sequel to a persistent right aortic arch), anomalies more usually involve the right subclavian artery; an anomalous origin of the right subclavian artery is one of the more common vascular malformations in dogs. In such cases, the **right subclavian artery arises directly from the aorta** instead of from the brachiocephalic trunk. The anomaly develops when the right dorsal aorta, between the fourth aortic arch and the seventh dorsal intersegmental artery, disappears while the part caudal to it (which normally regresses) remains. As a consequence, the right subclavian artery consists of the remnant of the right dorsal aorta caudal to the seventh dorsal intersegmental artery and the intersegmental artery itself. The anomalous origin of the right subclavian artery

can cause a vascular ring around the oesophagus, causing the same symptoms as described for a persistent right aortic arch. Sometimes the condition remains asymptomatic and is found only at necropsy.

Coarctation of the aorta

Coarctation of the aorta consists of a local **narrowing of the aorta** distal to the origin of the left subclavian artery and usually near, but distally to, the ductus arteriosus (postductal coarctation). It is caused either by a lack of growth of the aorta at the affected point or by an abnormal proliferation of connective tissue in the wall of the vessel resulting in a narrowing of the lumen. Coarctation of the aorta develops during embryological development, when an abnormally high amount of ductus arteriosus material is incorporated into the wall of the aorta. The ductus wall has a higher content of collagen compared to the aorta and so an excessive contribution of ductus material could result in a contraction of the aortic wall. Preductal coarctation (which occurs in less than 5% of the cases of aortic coarctation) causes a narrowing of the aorta upstream of the ductus arteriosus. In this case the ductus arteriosus must remain patent to compensate for the coarctation and to sustain life. It is related to inadequate expression of MFH-1, and the ductus arteriosus typically remains open after birth.

Malformations of the veins

Malformation of the venae cavae. The complex mode of formation of veins cause a wide range of malformation in the venous system. Common variants are **duplications of the cranial and caudal venae cavae** or persistence of the left instead of the right segments of these vessels along with the absence of the normal vessels. In most cases, these anomalies cause no symptoms, but sometimes deep venous thrombosis occurs.

Portal-caval shunt. This malformation is a venous anomaly of clinical significance. Portal-caval shunts have been frequently reported in cats and dogs but are only rarely seen in other domestic species. In this condition a **shunt exists between the portal** circulation (or sometimes the mesenteric veins) and the caudal vena cava. The shunt can take different forms, but the most common ones are a persistent ductus venosus, mesenteric veins entering the caudal vena cava directly, or a direct shunt between the portal vein and the caudal vena cava. As a result, blood from the intestinal tract bypasses the liver sinusoids and so materials in the blood cannot be processed by the liver. As a consequence, metabolic toxins that are normally detoxified in the liver build up to the point where they affect brain functions.

Malformations of the lymphatic system

Minor anatomical variations of the lymphatic vessels are common in domestic animals but malformations that cause clinical symptoms are rare. The latter typically appear in the form of swellings caused by dilatation of major lymphatic vessels, like the cystic hygroma which manifests as a large swelling, most commonly in the head and neck.

CONGENITAL MALFORMATIONS OF THE NERVOUS SYSTEM

The central nervous system (CNS) is very susceptible to congenital malformations because of the nature of its complex development. In both humans and domestic animals, CNS anomalies are a comparatively common birth defect, surpassed in frequency only by congenital cardiovascular abnormalities.

Myelodysplasia

Myelodysplasia is the general term for a malformation of the spinal cord. Such conditions can be classified into the following major categories:

- **Aplasia** is the absence of the development of one or more segments of the spinal cord.
- **Hypoplasia** is the reduced development of segments of the spinal cord.
- **Hydromyelia** is characterized by a dilatation of the central canal due to an excess accumulation of cerebrospinal fluid.

- **Syringomyelia** means abnormal cavitation of several segments of the spinal cord. It is considered as a specialized condition of spina bifida, because an occult form of spina bifida often accompanies syringomyelia. Syringomyelia is generally rare, but it is inherited in Weimaraner dogs and in tailless Manx cats.
- **Diplomyelia** describes the situation where two spinal cords exist beside each other. Usually they are covered by only one set of meninges and are contained within one vertebral canal.

Neural tube defects

Neural tube defects comprise a group of heterogeneous and complex congenital malformations of the CNS. They range from severe structural anomalies resulting from incomplete closure of the neural tube to functional defects without any obvious structural basis. Commonly included in this group are **spina bifida**, **anencephaly**, and **encephalocoeles**. Failures of the neural tube to close occur most commonly in the cranial and caudal neuropores, but failure to close at other locations is not uncommon. A closure defect of the brain is called **cranioschisis**, whereas a closure defect of the spinal cord is termed **rachioschisis**.

It has been suggested that neural tube defects may also occur due to excessive production of cerebrospinal fluid, leading to reopening of an already closed neural tube. As outlined in Chapter 8, development of the neural tube is a multi-step process strictly controlled by genes and modulated by a host of environmental factors. The process involves gene-to-gene, gene-to-environment, and gene-to-nutrient interactions.

Spina bifida

Spina bifida (Fig. 19-7), which is the most severe of the neural tube defects, includes all abnormalities in which the **vertebral arches fail to close** dorsal to the spinal cord to form the vertebral canal. In its simplest form the defect is called spina bifida occulta referring to a 'hidden' occurrence of the phenomenon. The spinal cord and meninges remain in place,

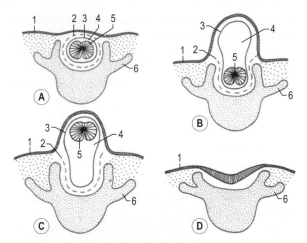

Fig. 19-7: Different form of dysraphia.
Dysraphia includes congenital defects of closure of one or more vertebral arches, which may be associated with malformations of the spinal cord and nerve roots. These malformations range from mild (A: spina bifida occulta) to severe (B: meningocoele; C: meningomyelocoele), including rachischisis (D) where there is complete failure of neural tube and spinal cord fusion, resulting in exposure of the spinal cord at the surface. 1: Epidermis; 2: Dura mater; 3: Arachnoid; 4: Subarachnoideal space; 5: Spinal cord; 6: Transverse process. Courtesy Sinowatz and Rüsse (2007).

but the vertebral arch of one or more vertebrae is incomplete. The meninges may also be distended by fluid (myelomeningocoele, see later), in which case the phenomenon is referred to as a spina bifida cystica. In many such cases, the spinal cord bulges or is entirely dislocated into the protruding subarachnoidal space. The dislocation causes problems associated with displaced spinal roots; consequently, neurological symptoms are commonly associated with this condition.

Spina bifida is a vertebral anomaly, and the defect can go unnoticed for years. During normal development, the neural arches are induced by the roof plate of the neural tube via the mediation of *Msx-2*. Thus spina bifida is caused by a local defect in induction.

Meningocele

The next most severe category of neurotubal defects of the spinal cord is **meningocoele** in which the meninges herniate and become distended by fluid accumulation. The dura mater may be missing in the area of the defect, and the arachnoidea bulges prominently beneath the skin. The spinal cord, however, remains in place and neurological symptoms are usually minor.

Rachioschisis

Rachioschisis refers to a situation when any **part of the posterior portion of the neural tube completely fails to close** resulting in a permanent cleft (schisis). As a consequence, the vertebral arches cannot form and fuse normally. This malformation resembles a primitive neural plate before neural tube closure. Rachioschisis has been reported in ruminants, horses, dogs and cats.

Congenital malformations of the brain

Dysraphia of the anterior neural tube
(Fig. 19-7)

A spectrum of malformations, similar to those mentioned for the posterior portion of the neural tube, is associated with defects affecting the most anterior portion of the tube. Many of these conditions are based on **dysraphia** where the **cranial neuropore fails to fuse properly or even remains open**. This malformation is commonly expressed as one of the following conditions. In a mild form, dysraphia results in a cranial **meningocoele** where the meninges protrude through a small defect in the skull. At a more severe level, the protrusion involves both meningeal and brain tissue (**meningoencephalocoele**) or brain tissue containing part of the ventricular system (**meningohydroencephalocoele**) and is combined with the existence of a larger opening in the skull. An even more severe variation of these conditions is **exencephaly**, characterized by a complete failure of the cephalic part of the neural tube to close. In this condition, the vault of the skull does not form, leaving the malformed brain exposed. The most extreme cases of cranial dysraphia result in the absence of the telencephalon and much of the diencephalon, and are termed **anencephaly**, although the brainstem remains intact. Some evidence of eye formation is usually present, because the primordia arise from the diencephalon. Anencephaly is rare, but it is most commonly reported in ruminants.

Hydrocephalus (Figs 19-8, 19-9, 19-10)

Hydrocephalus is an **abnormal accumulation of cerebrospinal fluid within the ventricular system**

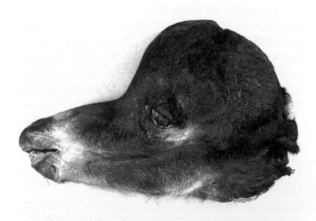

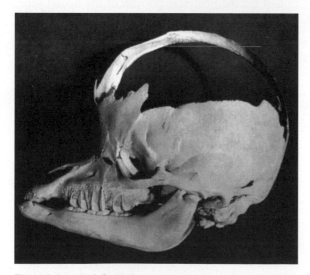

of the brain. In most cases, hydrocephalus in newborn domestic animals is due to an obstruction of the aquaeductus mesencephali. This prevents the cerebrospinal fluid of the lateral and third ventricles from passing into the fourth ventricle and from there into the subarachnoid space, where it is normally resorbed. This type of hydrocephalus is called 'non-communicating'. Other common areas of blockage are the interventricular foramina and the lateral foramina of the fourth ventricles. Hydrocephalus can also result from excessive cerebrospinal fluid production or impaired fluid resorption from the subarachnoid space.

The increase in cerebrospinal fluid exerts an increasing pressure on the brain tissue. In severe cases, the accumulated fluid expands the volume of the brain ventricles so much that the sutures of the skull cannot close. In extreme cases, brain tissue and bones become thin and the head is grossly enlarged and malformed.

Hydrocephalus is probably **one of the most common congenital anomalies of the nervous system**. It has been described most often in dogs and cattle, but it is found in all domestic species. In dogs it is most common in small brachycephalic breeds, where the stenosis of the aquaeductus mesencephali is correlated to the retarded develop-

Figs 19-8 and 19-9: Hydrocephalus of a foal. An abnormal amount of cerebrospinal fluid has accumulated within the ventricular system of the brain. The increased amount of fluid expands the volume of the brain vesicles so much that the sutures of the skull cannot close, resulting in a malformation of the skull. Courtesy Sinowatz and Rüsse (2007).

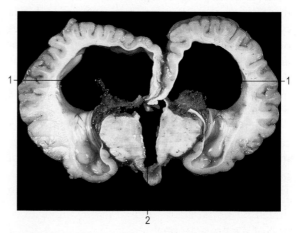

Fig. 19-10: Hydrocephalus of a bovine calf. Note the dilatation of the ventricular lumen. 1: Lateral ventricle; 2: Third ventricle. Courtesy Sinowatz and Rüsse (2007).

ment of the cartilaginous base of the skull. In cattle, achondroplastic dwarfs are frequently hydrocephalic.

Arnold-Chiari malformation

Arnold-Chiari malformation is a condition characterized by **caudal displacement and herniation of cerebellar structures** through the foramen magnum into the cranial cervical vertebral canal. Arnold-Chiari malformation is often accompanied by spina bifida, meningomyelocoele, and hydrocephalus.

Microcephaly

Microcephaly, an **abnormally small brain**, has been reported in calves, lambs, and piglets. Since the size of the cranium depends on the development of the brain, the cranial vault is considerably smaller than normal. External features of microcephaly include a narrow and flattened frontal area of the cranium. Cranial bones appear thicker than normal. The cause of the condition may be genetic or a prenatal insult such as an infection or exposure to a teratogen.

Hydranencephaly

In **hydranencephaly**, the **cerebral hemispheres are replaced by two fluid-filled sacs**. The brain stem is usually not affected, but some degree of cerebellar hypoplasia may be observed. In domestic animals this condition is most commonly caused by an in utero viral infection (blue tongue virus in ruminants and panleukopaenia in cats) or, more rarely, by an interruption of the blood supply to the telencephalon.

Holoprosencepaly

Holoprosencepaly comprises a group of congenital malformations of the brain and face that is characterized by **impaired or incomplete midline division of the prosencephalon**. Holoprosencepaly has been associated with chromosomal abnormalities, such as trisomy, various deletions, and other chro-

mosomal rearrangements, but environmental causes have also been proposed. In humans, it is often associated with a characteristic dysmorphic face, resulting secondarily from the brain malformation. Holoprosencepaly has been described in calves and may represent a failure of the neural tube to separate from the surface ectoderm at its most rostral extent (rostral neuroporus) that prevents the normal development of the telencephalic vesicles. The brain stem and the cerebellum are present although their shape is altered. In calves, where holoprosencepaly has been reported, the development of the face, the nasal openings and oral cavity appears normal.

Cerebellar hypoplasia

Cerebellar hypoplasia (Fig. 19-11) describes a situation where **an insufficiency of neurons causes hypoplasia of the granular layer** of the cerebellum. In severe cases, the Purkinje neurons will also be destroyed. The condition is most frequently found in kittens and calves, most commonly caused by prenatal or perinatal viral infections. The specific viruses are the feline panleukopaenia virus and the bovine virus diarrhoea (BVD) virus. These viruses exert their maximal effect if the infection occurs during the time of rapid cerebral growth and differentiation of the external germinal layer at midgestation (from the end of first trimester to the beginning of last trimester).

Cerebellar abiotrophy

Cerebellar abiotrophy is characterized by the **degeneration of the Purkinje cells** in the already formed cerebellar cortex. It occurs postnatally or, occasionally, prenatally and has been observed in many domestic species. The primary defect that causes the degeneration is not known.

Functional anomalies of the central nervous system

The abnormalities of the CNS described above are the most serious ones found in domestic animals and many of them are incompatible with life.

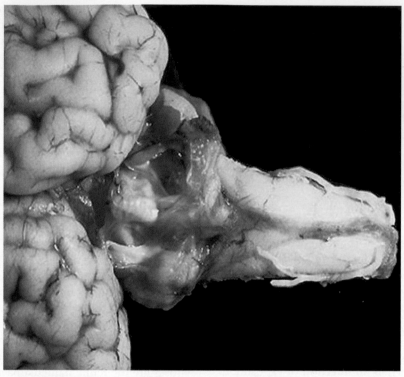

Fig. 19-11: Cerebellar hypoplasia is most frequently found in kittens and calves. The most common cause is prenatal or perinatal viral infections. Courtesy Sinowatz and Rüsse (2007).

A great number of other defects of the CNS may occur without much morphological manifestation. The most common examples of these disorders are **congenital idiopathic epilepsy** and **kinetic disorders**. Congenital idiopathic epilepsy is quite common in dogs and has been also observed in cats and horses. Hyperkinetic disorders have been reported in cattle and dogs (Scottish Terriers). This anomaly is probably caused by disorders of neurotransmitters.

On the other hand, morphologic malformations are not always associated with functional disturbances. For example, the corpus callosum can be partially absent without severe functional disturbance and even the partial absence of the cerebellum may result in only a slight disturbance of coordination. Contrary to the situation in domestic animals, minor congenital defects are often of great importance in human medicine.

Congenital malformations of the peripheral nervous system

Aganglionic large instestine

Aganglionic large intestine, which is manifested by **great dilatation of certain segments of the colon**, has been reported in several species including horses and mice. In humans it is called 'Hirschsprung's disease'. The basis of this syndrome is the **absence of enteric ganglia** in the wall of the affected segments of the colon. Aganglionic large intestine arises from both dominant and recessive mutations. It has been shown that human patients, in whom only a small region of the colon or rectum is usually affected, do not express the c-RET oncogene along with a co-receceptor, Gfra-1, which is a receptor for glia-derived neurotrophic factor (GDNF). Other mutations underlying aganglionic megacolon could involve defects in the migration or proliferation of neural crest precursor cells. Apoptosis of precursor cells before or after they reach their final position in the hindgut reduces the number of enteric ganglia considerably. An alternative hypothesis is that changes in the local environment prevent the successful migration of neural crest cells into the colon. Evidence from mutant mice supports this idea. Experiments have shown that neural crest cells from mutant mice were capable of colonizing normal gut, but normal crest cells could not enter gut segments of mutant mice because an accumulation of laminin in the gut wall, resulting from an overproduction of endothelin-3, blocked their migration.

In domestic animals, aganglionic large intestine has been reported in white foals, born from crossings of Overo horses. Overo is a spotting pattern in Painted and Pinto ponies in which melanocyte-free, white skin areas appear preferentially in the ventral midline of the trunk and the distal parts of the limbs and snout. The condition starts with signs of colic within one day of birth and the affected foals die shortly thereafter. Necropsy shows that there is no meconium present in the bowel. Histological examination reveals a complete absence of ganglia of the myenteric plexus in the terminal ileum, caecum, and colon.

Congenital defects affecting Schwann cells

Contrary to the more common incidence of abnormalities of CNS myelin production by oligodendrocytes, only a few **abnormalities affecting the myelin production by Schwann cells in the peripheral nervous system** have been reported in domestic animals. Abnormal production with eventual loss of myelin sheath around peripheral nerve fibres results in a hypertrophic neuropathy that has been found in Tibetan Mastiff dogs. A similar condition has been described in certain inbred mice carrying a gene called Trember. Several cases of a congenital bovine neuropathy have been reported in which peripheral nerves show 'sausage-shaped' thickenings of the myelin sheaths at different sites of the internodes. Clinical signs of dysphagia and chronic ruminal bloat developed after weaning, which were attributable to bilateral vagus nerve degeneration. Trunks of the sciatic nerves and brachial plexuses were similarly affected resulting in a weak shuffling gait.

Malformations of the eye

Congenital malformations of the eye have been reported six times more frequently in the **dog** than in all other domestic animal species combined. Therefore, the following discussion focuses mainly on eye anomalies in the dog.

Anophthalmos and microphthalmos

Anophthalmos, the absence of an eye, results from the failure of formation of an optic vesicle. Since the optic vesicle acts as an inductive trigger for subsequent developmental processes, the formation of an eye fails to occur. In **microphthalmos**, which can range from an **eyeball only slightly smaller than normal to one that is only vestigial**, the growth of the optic cup is more or less severely inhibited. It can be associated with genetic defects or various other causes, including intrauterine infections. In dogs, pigs and cattle, microphthalmos often results from vitamin A deficiency. Microphthalmos has been observed in kittens exposed to griseofulvin during gestation as part of craniofacial malformation in kittens. Hereditary microphthalmos has been reported in all domestic species. In dogs, Collies, Schnauzers, Australian Shepherds, and Great Danes appear to be most frequently affected. In Guernsey cattle microphthalmos is sometimes associated with cardiac malformation and a missing tail.

Coloboma

Coloboma results from the **optic fissure failing to close properly or at the proper times**. Although this cleft-like defect is usually in the iris only (**coloboma iridis**), it may extend into the ciliary body, the retina, the choroid, and the optic nerve. Coloboma is a common eye malformation frequently associated with other eye defects such as microphthalmos. Mutations in the PAX2 gene have been linked with coloboma of the optic nerve and may play a role in other types of coloboma as well.

Collie eye syndrome

Collie eye syndrome is regarded as one of the most common eye anomalies. A large percentage of Collie dogs show this malformation. In its full form, the syndrome consists of **microphthalmos, focal thinning of the choroid and sclera** resulting in ecstasia and retinal detachment. The aetiological basis of the Collie eye syndrome is a defect in the growth of the optic cup.

Retinal dysplasia

Retinal dysplasia is defined as an **abnormal growth and differentiation of the retina** and has been reported mainly in dogs. This malformation results from an abnormal development of the inner or outer layer of the optic cup. Retinal dysplasia occurs when the two primitive layers of the retina do not interact properly. In most cases retinal dysplasia is hereditary. The condition may appear mono-symptomatically, involving only the eye, or as complex disorders with multisystemic anomalies. Retinal dysplasia is reported in 25 of the 100 breeds of dogs listed in the 1996 edition of the Canine Eye Registration Foundation (CERF) book 'Ocular Disorders Presumed to be Hereditary in Purebred Dogs. Twenty-four of these breeds had retinal folds reported, and 11 had localized areas of dysplasia and/or retinal detachment. Simple autosomal recessive inheritance has been suspected in Akitas, American Cocker Spaniels, Australian Shepherds, Bedlington Terriers, Beagles, Dobermans, English Springer Spaniels, Labradors, Rottweilers, Old English Sheepdogs, Sealyham Terriers, and Yorkshire Terriers. However, the mechanism of inheritance has not been determined in many breeds. In Labradors and Samoyeds a combination of retinal dysplasia and skeletal defects has been described. In kittens, retinal dysplasia can also result from in utero infections with feline panleukopaenia virus.

Progressive retinal atrophies

The **progressive retinal atrophies** are a group of inherited retinal dystrophies that share a similar phenotype. They cause a **progressive loss of vision usually leading to blindness**. Initially, rod photoreceptor vision is affected, causing night blindness, and this is followed by a progressive loss of cone photoreceptors with a resultant deterioration in daytime vision. In all the breeds that have been investigated in sufficient detail, the mode of inheritance has turned out to be a single recessive gene. Recent data suggest that in the dog the rcd2 locus represents a novel retinal degeneration gene.

The onset of the condition can begin prenatally or up to several years after birth. Different breeds of dogs actually suffer from different forms of progressive retinal atrophies, but the end result is the same: the rod and cone cells eventually degenerate and the affected dogs become totally blind. There are two different types of progressive retinal atrophies in the dog: rod/cone dysplasia and rod/cone degeneration. Breeds like the Irish Setter and the Miniature Longhaired Dachshund suffer from rod/cone dysplasia. In this case the rod and cone cells develop abnormally and begin to degenerate even before they are fully mature, leading to a very early age of onset in affected dogs, usually within the first few months of life. In breeds that suffer from rod/cone degeneration, like the Labrador, the Golden Retriever, and the Cocker Spaniel, the rod and cone cells develop normally and only begin to degenerate later in life leading to a much later age of onset of the disease, usually anywhere from 3 to 4 years of age onwards.

Congenital cataract

Cataracts are defined as loss of **loss of clarity in the lens or lens capsule**. It is a leading cause of blindness in both dogs and humans. Mutation in the HFS4 genes have been associated with inherited forms of cataract in several dog breeds (e.g. Staffordshire Bull Terriers, Boston Terriers, and Australian Shepherds). Congenital cataracts are also occasionally seen in cattle, but rarely in cats and horses.

Congenital primary glaucoma

Congenital primary glaucoma results from an abnormal development of the anterior chamber of the eye. The trabecular meshwork in the iridocorneal angle is particularly affected. The trabecular spaces fail to form correctly and to enlarge. Therefore the **resorption of aqueous humour from the anterior chamber is reduced** and glaucoma develops. This defect is inherited in Cocker Spaniels, Beagles, and Basset Hounds. Familial glaucoma secondary to congenital lens luxation has been found in Fox Terriers and Sealyhams.

Persistent pupillary membrane

Persistent pupillary membrane describes a situation in which the **pupillary membrane**, which regresses during normal develoment, **fails to disappear**. This is especially common in the Basenji dogs, in which this anomaly is inherited.

Persistent hyaloid artery

Usually the distal portion of the hyaloid artery regresses, whereas the proximal part forms the central artery of the retina. Sometimes also the distal portion persists and forms a cord or cyst.

Cyclopia (Figs 19-12, 19-13)

Cyclopia (single eyes) is a defect in which the **eyes are partially or completely fused**. The anomaly is caused by a loss of midline tissue and occurs early in development. The lack of midline tissue results in underdevelopment of the forebrain and fronto-nasal prominence. These defects are usually associated with cranial defects. Cyclopia is characterized by a single, centrally located orbit, which contains a normal or rudimentary eye. In several cases various degrees of fusion of two eyeballs have been reported. The eyelids are rudimentary or completely absent.

Malformations of the ear

The ear is subject to a wide variety of genetically based defects. They range from defects of the hair

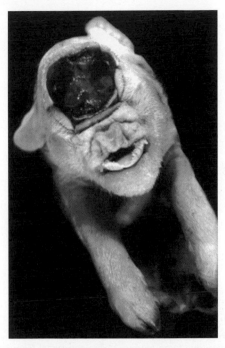

Fig. 19-12: Cyclopia incompleta (single eye) in a piglet. The anomaly results from a loss of midline tissue causing a partially (cyclopia incompleta) or total fusion (cyclopia completa) of the eyes. Courtesy Sinowatz and Rüsse (2007).

cells of the inner ear to gross malformation of the middle and external ear.

Congenital deafness

Congenital deafness occurs infrequently in dogs and cats and is rare in other domestic animals. Dalmatians have been reported to have the highest incidence of congenital deafness, followed by English Setters, Australian Shepherds and Boston Terriers. In 54 breeds, occasional congenital deafness has been described. It can be caused by an abnormal development of the membranous or bony labyrinths, or malformations of the auditory ossicles and eardrum. In extreme cases the tympanic cavity and external meatus can be completely absent. In most dog and cat breeds, inherited congenital sensorineural deafness results from perinatal degeneration of the stria vascularis, the vascular bed of the outer wall of the cochlear duct, which

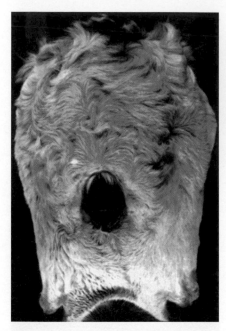

Fig. 19-13: Diprosopus, calf. Diprosopus is a craniofacial duplication and is an extremely rare congenital disorder whereby part or all of the face is duplicated on the head. In this case, the diprosopus shows a common orbita. Courtesy Sinowatz and Rüsse (2007).

leads to hair cell degeneration. The strial degeneration appears to result from the absence of melanocytes, but their precise function in this structure is unknown. Accordingly, congenital deafness in cats is correlated with an absence of pigmentation in the skin and eyes.

Abnormalities of the middle ear ossicles or ligaments are associated with anomalies of the first and second pharyngeal arches. The interference with sound transmission results in middle ear deafness.

External ear malformations

In humans, all frequently occurring chromosomal syndromes and many of the less common ones have ear anomalies as one of their characteristics. Malformations of the auricles have occasionally been reported in dogs and cats but their genetic basis is unknown.

CONGENITAL MALFORMATIONS OF THE URINARY SYSTEM

Congenital anomalies of the urinary system are quite common, but many of them remain asymptomatic or manifest only later in life.

Renal agenesis

Renal agenesis is a condition in which **one or both kidneys fail to develop**. Bilateral agenesis is lethal after birth. In unilateral agenesis the opposite kidney usually undergoes compensatory hypertrophy. Renal agenesis results from a faulty inductive interaction between the ureteric bud and the metanephrogenic mesenchyme. Failures in the expression of molecules like PAX2, WT-1, or Wnt-e, which play a significant role in early metanephrogenic development, is a likely cause of at least some cases of renal agenesis.

Renal hypoplasia

Renal hypoplasia is an **intermediate condition** between a normal kidney and renal agenesis. One, or more rarely, both kidneys are distinctly smaller than normal. Usually the cortex of the kidney appears underdeveloped. Renal cortical hypoplasia has been reported as an hereditary condition in Cocker Spaniels and in several other dog breeds (e.g. Norwegian Elkhounds, Samoyeds, Keeshonds, Bedlington Terriers). The congenital hypoplasia causes secondary renal hypoparathyroidism, which in turn induces fibrosis of the kidney. Although a specific cause for renal hypoplasia has not yet been identified, deficiencies in growth factors and their receptors, active during critical stages of metanephrogenesis, may be involved in the pathogenesis of this anomaly.

Renal duplications

The spectrum of **renal duplication** ranges from **duplication of the renal pelvis to the production of a complete supernumerary organ**. This condition can be asymptomatic, although the incidence of renal infection may be increased. Several variants of duplications of the ureters have also been described. Duplication anomalies of the urinary system are mostly attributed to excessive splitting of branches of the ureteric bud. A kidney that develops from an extra ureteric bud may be fused to, or separate from, the normal kidney.

Anomalies of renal migration

Ectopic kidneys are typically seen in the **pelvic region** either normally shaped, having failed to ascend normally to the lumbar region, or as a horseshoe kidney, comprising two kidneys typically fused at their caudal poles. Horseshoe kidneys cannot ascend, because their way is blocked by the caudal mesenteric artery. Pelvic kidneys often also show a malrotation, with the hilus of each facing cranially instead of medially.

Ectopic ureters have been reported in all domestic species but are most common in dogs. A high risk for this anomaly exists in Siberian Huskies, West Highland Terriers, and small Poodles. Ectopic ureters cause clinical problems when the ureter enters the urethra distal to the sphincter in the neck of the bladder. In most cases ectopic ureters open into the urethra or even into the vagina. This condition is a common cause of incontinence and results in a continous slow dripping of urine from the vulva. Hydroureter and hydronephros can accompany this defect. In males, an ectopic ureter usually opens into the urethra proximal to the sphincter of the bladder and so incontinence does not occur. This difference in position between female and male has been explained by the retention of the mesonephric duct in the male.

CONGENITAL MALFORMATIONS OF THE GENITAL SYSTEM

Abnormalities of sexual differentiation

Genital malformations are common birth defects in man and domestic animals and occur **most frequently in males**, since many genes are required to take sexual differentiation in the male direction. The need of a precise dose, timing, and coordination of their expression adds to the proneness of various stages in male sex differentiation to be disturbed (Fig. 19-14). The identification of genes involved in the sex differentiation cascade is making it clear that over 85% of sex anomalies in human and domestic animal populations are attributable neither to chromosome aberrations nor to mutations in a known gene. Rather, the high rates of abnormalities of sexual differentiation are more likely to result from either new mutations or from aberrant interactions between environmental and genetic factors. Increases in genital malformations in domestic animals often indicate an increased concentration of 'liability genes' brought together in the conceptus by inbreeding.

Abnormalities of chromosomal sex

XO Genotype (Turner's syndrome in humans)

An **XO genotype** is most prevalent in horses, but has been also reported in pigs and cats. It results in an **infertile, anoestrous female** with hypoplastic ovaries, a small uterus, and underdeveloped external genitalia. From the observation that YO is always lethal, it can be conclude that at least one X-chromosome must be present to keep a mammal viable.

XXY Genotype (Klinefelter's syndrome in humans)

As an extra female sex chromosome interferes with male gonad development, the **XXY genotype** produces **infertile males with hypoplastic or aplastic testes**. The XXY syndrome has been found in tortoiseshell and tricolour (calico) cats (karyotype of 2n = 39,XXY). The tortoiseshell cat has orange and black patches; the calico cat has the same with varying amounts of white. The orange gene is a dominant sex-linked gene on the X-chromosome. The black gene is either a co-dominant allele of the orange gene, or is autosomal with its expression being masked by the orange gene. The white genes are autosomal and are expressed independently of the other colour genes.

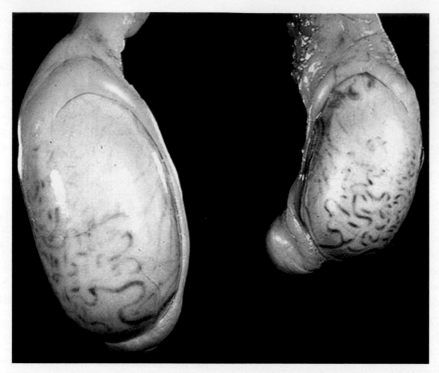

Fig. 19-14: Hypoplasia of a bovine testis (right), with a normal testis on the left side. Courtesy Sinowatz and Rüsse (2007).

Early during embryogenesis at blastulation or gastrulation, one of the X-chromosomes is inactivated in each cell, except in the primordial germ cells. X-inactivation occurs randomly and, therefore, in some cells the maternally derived X-chromosome is active, while in others the genes of the paternal X-chromosome are expressed. If the active X-chromosome carrying the orange or black gene is expressed in the epidermal cells of the cat, the hair colour will be orange or black, respectively. If none of the genes are expressed, the white colour will result.

Abnormalities of gonadal sex

Sex reversal

A large number of genes participate in the masculinization of the embryo and fetus. Consequently, absence or alteration of any one of these genes has

the potential to disrupt male sex differentiation. Several genes with stage-specific expression in the sex differentiation pathway have been identified through the genetic analysis of individuals with abnormal sex phenotype in human and domestic animal populations. Mutations in the open reading frame of the *SRY* gene, with or without any influence on the DNA-binding and -bending property of its HMG domain, account for a substantial proportion of XY gonadal dysgenesis. Other mutations causally related to sex reversal in humans include a base pair substitution in the DNA-binding domain of *SF1* which, even in the heterozygous state, causes feminization of XY individuals due to haplo-insufficiency for *SF1* transcript. Similarly, absence of functional *WT1*, which normally codes for various transcription factors, causes failure of gonad and kidney development in homozygotes and XY sex reversal in heterozygotes. Also, duplication or mutation in the *SOX9* gene causes XY sex reversal and skeletal defects in humans. Another factor that affects males more profoundly than females is the variety of missense and nonsense mutations in an androgen receptor gene. While severe mutations in this X-linked intracellular androgen receptor gene cause complete androgen insensitivity, less severe mutations cause compromised masculinization often with impaired fertility since both testosterone and 5α-dihydrotestosterone require functional androgen receptors for their action. In the absence of a normal androgen receptor gene, the primary male sexual development before birth and the development of secondary sex characteristics after birth (at puberty) are all affected. A considerable proportion of XY males displaying a spectrum of female characteristics are androgen-insensitive since the rates of de novo mutations of androgen receptor gene, leading to complete androgen insensitivity (in cases of nonsense mutations) or partial insensitivity (in cases of missense mutations), are relatively high. Females carrying androgen receptor mutations are not affected to the same degree since androgens, although essential, are required only around puberty and for sexual function in the adult state. This, coupled with the inactivation of one of the two X chromosomes, leads to the diminished expression of X-linked genes in female mammals and allows these mutations to be transmitted through the female line.

Sex reversal of (XY) male domestic animals is not uncommon although rigorous selection in animal husbandry generally tends to keep the prevalence low. Cases of male sex reversal in cattle have been identified in various countries. Similar cases in other domestic animals including goats, sheep, and dogs have been reported. The incidence of male sex reversal in domestic animals is generally lower than that for female sex reversal with the exception of horses in which sex reversal of the genetic (XY) male is relatively common. XY mares generally possess small abdominal gonads (in the ovarian position) and small uteri. The affected horses appear phenotypically female, and often the only clues to their status as sex-reversed 'mares' are their total lack of oestrous behaviour, including interest in males, during the breeding season, their XY karyotype, their low plasma testosterone concentration, and indications of gonadal dysgenesis.

Abnormalities of phenotypic sex

Pseudohermaphroditism

Pseudohermaphroditism is the most common form of intersex, especially in dogs. In pseudohermaphrodites, the chromosome constitution and gonadal sex are in agreement, yet the internal or external genitalia are ambiguous. Affected individuals are either male or female pseudohermaphrodites, with gonads of one sex and genital organs with some characteristics of the other. The type of pseudohermaphroditism (male or female) is defined by the gonadal sex. Canine female pseudohermaphrodites are 78,XX and have bilateral ovaries. Müllerian or paramesonephric duct derivatives develop normally, forming oviducts, a uterus, and a cranial vagina. Androgen-responsive organs are, however, masculinized during development. Masculinization ranges from mild clitoral enlargement to nearly normal male external genitalia with an internal prostate. Iatrogenic causes include androgen or progestagen administration during gestation. To prevent this disorder, steroid hormone administration should be avoided during gestation, particularly during the period that canine internal and external genitalia normally develop (Days 34 to 46 of gestation, counting from the serum LH peak (Day 0) of the dam. Male pseudohermaphroditism is more common than female; most affected dogs have undescended testes, a female duct system, and male external genitalia.

True hermaphrodites

Animals with **true hermaphroditism**, which is an extremely rare condition, possess **both ovarian and testicular tissue** either separately or in combination. In cases of genetic mosaicism, both an ovary and a testis can be present separately. In other cases, ovarian and testicular tissues form a single organ called an **ovotestis**. Most true hermaphrodites have two X-chromosomes and the external genitalia are basically female with a hypertrophied clitoris.

Testicular feminization syndrome (androgen insensitivity syndrome)

Animals with **testicular feminization syndrome** are genetic males and possess internal testes, but they typically display a normal female external phenotype. Thus, the condition is a form of pseudohermaphroditism. This condition is especially prevalent in pigs (up to 0.4% of individuals in some populations). The testes typically produce testosterone, but because of a deficiency in androgen receptors caused by a mutation in the X-chromosome, the testosterone is unable to act on the appropriate androgen-dependent tissues. Because Müllerian inhibiting substance is produced by the testis, the uterus and upper part of the vagina do not develop.

Intersexuality in goats (horned goats) has been found in several breeds, for instance in Canarian goats, and the association among intersexuality, polledness and gonadal development has been firmly established. Horned intersex goats are rare and usually present a 60XX/T0XY karyotype.

Vestigial structures from the embryonic genital ducts

Vestigial structures are **remnants from incomplete regression of the embryonic genital ducts**. They are quite common and are not always considered to be malformations, although they can become cystic and interfere with normal functions.

Mesonephric ducts abnormalities

Mesonephric duct abnormalities include **stenosis or aplasia of the epididymis or ductus deferens**. In males, aplasia of the mesonephric duct may be associated with a blind cranial end of the mesonephric duct appearing as an appendix of the epididymis. Persistent mesonephric tubules caudal to the efferent ductules are referred to as a **paradidymis**. In females, remnants of the cranial part of the mesonephros can persist as the **epoophoron** or **paroophoron**. The epoophoron consists of vestiges of the mesonephric tubules and a segment of mesonephric duct between the ovary and the uterine tube. The paroophoron is formed by remnants of mesonephric tubules medial to the ovary. Nonfunctional remnants of the caudal part of the mesonephric duct are constantly found in the cow, sow, and cat, and are referred to as Garner's ducts. In the cow, these are found as openings into the vestibule adjacent to the urethral opening. In the sow, they are either tubular cords in the wall of the uterine horns or in the wall of the vagina. In dog and cat they are usually located in the wall of the vagina.

Paramesonephric duct abnormalities
(Fig. 19-15)

Paramesonephric duct abnormalities are expressed as remnants of the duct, lack of proper fusion of the ducts, or lack of development of part of the ducts.

In the male, **remnants of the paramesonephric duct** often appear as small appendices of the testis. The fused caudal ends of the paramesonephric duct are commonly seen in the prostate, where they form the small midline prostatic utricle. This is regarded a rudimentary uterine primordium. In some cases of male pseudohermaphroditism, the prostatic utricle is enlarged to a uterus-like structure. This phenomenon may be referred to as the **persistent Müllerian duct syndrome**, which is characterized by the formation of a uterus and uterine tubes. This condition has been reported in male Miniature Schnauzers and the Basset Hound. Affected dogs have bilateral oviducts, a complete uterus with cervix, and a cranial portion of the vagina. An intersex condition that may be a parallel to the persistent Müllerian duct syndrome has also been reported in Persian cats.

In females a small part of the cranial tip of the paramesonephric duct may persist at the fimbriated end of the uterine tube as the hydatid of Morgagni. If the **more anterior portions of the paramesonephric ducts fail to join and fuse**, a **duplex uterus (uterus didelphys)** is formed where each duct enters the vagina separately. Failure of proper fusion of the **more caudal portions of the paramesonephric ducts** may result in a **double vagina**.

Unilateral uterine aplasia refers to **absence of one uterine tube and horn (uterus unicornis)**. This

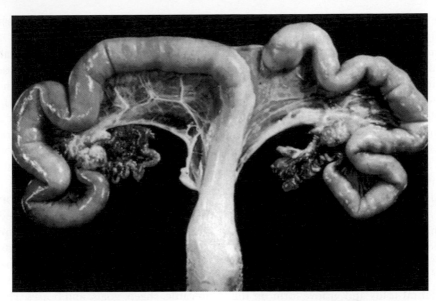

Fig. 19-15: Partial hypoplasia of a uterine horn in a pig. Courtesy Sinowatz and Rüsse (2007).

condition is often associated with unilateral renal agenesis. Local defects in the development of the paramesonephric duct cause segmental aplasia or stenosis of the uterine tube or horn. Uterine aplasia is an hereditary disease of Shorthorn cattle, where it occurs in conjunction with the inheritance of white coat (white heifer disease).

Abnormalities of testicular descent (cryptorchidism)

Cryptorchidism is a **failure of one or both testicles to descend into the scrotum**. It is seen in all domestic mammals, is **common** in stallions and boars, and is the most common disorder of sexual development in dogs (13%). Predisposing factors include testicular hypoplasia, oestrogen exposure in pregnancy, breech birth compromising blood supply to the testes, and delayed closure of the umbilicus resulting in an inability to increase abdominal pressure.

Descent of the testes requires the activity of the *Insl-3* gene and androgens, but how disturbances in these molecules lead to cryptorchidism has not been established. In most cases, the intra-abdominal descent is normal, and the testes are usually found in, or at the internal opening of, the inguinal canal. Non-descended testes are infertile because spermatogenesis does not occur, but they do produce normal amounts of androgens. Isolated cryptorchidism is the most common disorder of the reproductive tract reported in dogs. Canine testes normally descend by 10 days after birth, although they are not easily palpable at this age. However, both testes should certainly be palpable within the scrotum by 6 to 8 weeks of age, and the diagnosis of cryptorchidism is warranted if they are not. Dogs with bilateral cryptorchidism are sterile, while those with unilateral cryptorchidism can be fertile. However, the recommended treatment for both is bilateral castration because there is an increased risk of a Sertoli cell tumour in cryptorchid testes. Isolated cryptorchidism is also clearly a familial trait in several breeds, and is very likely to be inherited. Both unilateral and bilateral cryptorchidism are inheritable in pigs, but there is no convincing evidence for single-locus inheritance.

Malformation of the external genitalia

Hypospadia. In **hypospadia**, the most common malformation of the penis, the **urethra opens onto the** ventral surface of the penis rather than at the end of the glans. It results from a complete or partial failure of the urethral folds to close in the male. The causes of this disorder are unknown, but could be teratogens or inherited traits that affect androgen production or receptor binding. It has been reported as an inheritable defect in some dog breeds. If hypospadia is accompanied by scrotal abnormalities or retention of Müllerian duct derivatives, inherited defects such as XX sex reversal should be considered in the differential diagnosis. Although dogs with mild hypospadia may be able to breed normally, they are not recommended as breeding stock, because they may transmit the defect.

Epispadia. In epispadia, the urethra opens onto the dorsal surface of a shortened penis. This may be due to the malpositioning of the phallus, or because the urethral folds and groove form on the dorsal instead of on the ventral surface of the phallus. This rare defect is accompanied by a failure of the caudal ventral abdominal wall to develop properly. In this case the dorsal wall of the bladder and pelvic urethra are exposed ventrally (extroversion of the bladder).

CONGENITAL MALFORMATIONS OF THE DIGESTIVE SYSTEM

Facial cleft, cleft lip (harelip), and cleft palate complex

Failure of the maxillary and lateral nasal process to fuse produces an oblique facial cleft running from the medial corner of the eye to the oronasal cavity, accompanied by secondary asymmetries of the face.

Cleft lip (cheiloschisis) results from the lack of fusion of the maxillary and medial nasal prominences during embryonic development. Cleft of the lower lip is rare and usually occurs on the midline. Clefts of the upper lip, usually at the junction of the premaxilla and maxilla, may be unilateral or bilateral, complete or incomplete, and often are associated with clefts of the alveolar process and palate. Developmental anomalies affecting other organ systems are seen in approximately 8% of dogs and cats with cleft palate or lips.

Cleft palates (palatoschisis) usually result from partial or complete failure of apposition and fusion of the palate processes resulting in an open connection between oral and nasal cavities. The frequent occurrence of cleft palate in domestic animals is due to the fact that for correct palate formation, which happens comparatively late in development, several relatively independent tissues must interact precisely and synchronously. In large animals, cleft palate or lip is seen with other malformations, such as arthrogryposis, which is inherited in a simple autosomal recessive manner in Charolais cattle. In small animals, brachycephalic breeds can have up to a 30% increased risk of cleft palate. In large animals, cleft palate/lip complex has been reported in cattle, sheep, goats, and horses. The primary aetiology is hereditary, although maternal nutritional deficiencies, drug or chemical exposure, mechanical interferences with the fetus, and some viral infections during pregnancy may also play a role. Many teratogens have been implicated as causes of the defects, including those of toxic plants; maternal ingestion of lupins (lupinus sericeus and lupinus caudatus) during the second and third months of gestation in cattle, for example, can result in 'crooked calf disease', (Fig. 19-14) of which cleft abnormalities may be a component.

Initial signs reflect the extent of the malformation but may include difficulty in sucking, dysphagia, and evidence of milk dripping from the nostrils when the newborn attempts to nurse. Respiratory infection due to aspiration of food is common. Examination of the oral cavity generally reveals the defect, except that it may be difficult to see in foals having a cleft of the soft palate only.

Cleft lip and cleft palate may occur separately or together.

Occlusal abnormalities

Embryonic abnormalities of the lower jaw include mandibular agnathia, which is the complete absence of the lower jaw, and mandibular brachygnathia, also referred to as short lower jaw or 'overshot' or parrot mouth in horses, where the mandible is **shorter than the maxilla**. Such abnormalities, of varying severities and incidence, have been reported in all domestic species. In cattle, lower jaw problems are inherited as a polygenetic factor and can be associated with other abnormalities such as impacted molar teeth and osteopetrosis in Angus calves and Simmental calves, or with chromosomal aberrations such as trisomy, which is lethal. In small animals, mild forms may be of no clinical significance. However, more severe forms may result in trauma to the hard palate or the restriction of normal mandibular growth secondary to erupting adult mandibular canine teeth.

Maxillary brachygnathia, also referred to as prognathia or 'undershot' in horses, is found when the **mandible is longer than the maxilla**. It is identified on oral examination by finding the mandibular incisors in contact with, or rostral to, the maxillary incisors or dental pad. In brachycephalic dogs and Persian cats, it is considered a normal breed characteristic. In ruminants, it is often seen to minor degrees at birth, and it corrects spontaneously as the animal grows. More severe anomalies can impair the ability to graze and masticate and therefore have more serious repercussions.

A range of occlusal defects in sheep, from brachygnathia to mandibular aplasia and agnathia, is reportedly inherited as a simple autosomal recessive.

Craniofacial dysplasia of Limousin cattle is characterized by a convex profile of the nose, short lower jaw, deficient ossification of frontal sutures, exophthalmos, and a large tongue. It is probably caused by homozygosity of a simple autosomal recessive gene.

Tongue abnormalities

The most common malformation of the tongue is **ankyloglossia**, in which the tongue is **incomplete or abnormally developed**. It is caused by a deficient regression of the frenulum, the thin midline tissue that connects the ventral surface of the tongue to the floor of the mouth. It is often referred to as 'bird tongue' in dogs and may be a component of the fading puppy syndrome. Affected puppies have difficulty nursing and do poorly. Oral examination reveals missing or underdeveloped lateral and rostral thin portions of the tongue that result in prehensile and motility disturbances. The condition is generally lethal.

Less common malformations are **macroglossia**, enlargement of the tongue, and **microglossia**, an abnormally small tongue. Macroglossia is seen in Belted Galloway cattle but is rarely clinically significant.

Epitheliogenesis imperfecta, or 'smooth tongue', is a condition of **incomplete development of the lingual filiform papillae**. It is transmitted as an autosomal recessive trait in Holstein, Friesian, and Brown Swiss cattle and causes excessive salivation and an unthrifty condition.

Abnormalities of teeth

Abnormal number

Abnormalities in the number of teeth are common. In most species, a reduction in the number of teeth is rare, although in dogs, molars and premolars may fail to develop or erupt. A complete absence of teeth is termed anodontia, and results from disturbances in the interaction between the dental lamina and neural crest mesenchyme.

Extra teeth (supernumerary teeth) may be found within the jawbone or, in cases referred to as heterotopic polydontia, in other areas of the head. Supernumerary teeth are occasionally found in the incisor or molar regions of horses. In dogs, they occur usually unilaterally and most often in the upper jaw. In the dog, rarely, improper germination of the permanent dental arcade may lead to splitting of the tooth bud to form two teeth. The result may be crowding and subsequent rotation of the teeth necessitating extraction to prevent or correct occlusal abnormalities. In horses extra teeth are occasionally found near the external ear cartilage ('ear teeth').

Apparent supernumerary teeth are also seen if a deciduous tooth is retained. This happens when the permanent tooth bud is not positioned directly under the deciduous tooth and therefore does not cause erosion of the root of the deciduous tooth.

The permanent tooth erupts either behind or in front of the retained deciduous tooth. Retention of deciduous teeth is most often found in toy breeds, where it usually involves incisor or canine teeth.

Abnormalities in position, shape, and direction

Abnormalities in shape and position of teeth have been reported in various species and breeds. Clinical significance is variable and based on severity, with most being incidental findings. In horses, this may affect the incisors and result in long-axis rotation or overlapping of adjacent teeth. In brachycephalic dogs, the upper third premolar and occasionally other premolar or molar teeth may rotate. Usually, this is of no clinical significance but may require extraction of some involved teeth if crowding or occlusal abnormalities occur.

Enamel lesions

Hypoplasia or disruption in enamel formation can occur in both large and small animals and is due to a defective differentiation or development of the inner epithelial layer of the enamel organ. This can be caused by pyrexia, trauma, malnutrition, toxicosis (e.g. fluorosis in cattle), and infections (e.g. distemper virus in dogs). Lesions vary, depending on the severity and duration of the insult, from pitted enamel to the absence of enamel with incomplete tooth development. Affected teeth are prone to plaque and tartar accumulation and subsequent bacterial penetration and formation of caries.

Enamel may also develop discolouration. In small animals, administration of tetracyclines to pregnant females or to puppies younger than 6 months old may result in a permanent brownish yellow discolouration of the teeth. In ruminants, the enamel of some teeth may demonstrate flecks of varying colour. The condition is thought to have a genetic aetiology but is generally of no clinical significance.

Malformations of the oesophagus

Malformations of the oesophagus, which are found predominantly in small animals, can be classified as congenital stenosis, megaoesophagus, vascular ring entrapment anomalies, and achalasia.

Stenosis and atresia

Stenosis (narrowing) or **atresia (closure)** of the oesophagus can occur singly or in association with a tracheo-oesophageal fistula. Hypoplasia of the muscular wall of the oesophagus can cause a focal weakness leading to an evagination called oesophageal diverticulum.

Megaoesophagus

Congenital megaoesophagus, which is an **abnormal dilation of the oesophagus**, results from developmental anomalies in oesophageal neuromuscular innervation. Its incidence is increased in Chinese Shar-Peis, Fox Terriers, German Shepherds, Great Danes, Irish Setters, Labrador Retrievers, Miniature Schnauzers, Newfoundlands, and in Siamese cats. In Fox Terriers, it is an autosomal recessive trait, whereas in Miniature Schnauzers, it is an autosomal dominant. Megaoesophagus may also be a component of a more diffuse congenital neuropathy.

Vascular ring entrapment anomalies

Vascular ring entrapment anomalies most commonly result from **persistence of the right fourth aortic arch** during embryonic development, which results in oesophageal entrapment at the base of the heart by the right fourth aortic arch, left atrium, pulmonary artery, and the ligamentum arteriosum. This condition obstructs food passage and results in food retention and subsequent oesophageal dilation anterior to the anomaly. Boston Terriers, German Shepherds, and Irish Setters are especially prone to the anomaly.

Cricopharyngeal achalasia

Cricopharyngeal achalasia is a **failure of the cricopharyngeus muscle to relax during swallowing**, thereby preventing the normal passage of a food bolus from the caudal pharynx to the cranial oesophagus. It has been mainly identified in toy dog breeds and rarely in cats. Lower oesophageal sphincter achalasia is now considered to be a component of a more generalized oesophageal motor disturbance (i.e. megaoesophagus) and no longer a distinct entity.

Malformations of the gut

Stenosis and atresia of the gut

Stenosis (narrowing) or **atresia (closure)** of the gut lumen are common malformations of the digestive tract and can be found at any part of the gut. In the domestic species, intestinal atresia occurs with greater frequency at particular locations. For instance, atresia of the colon is found only in kittens and foals, whereas atresia of the small intestine and rectum occurs predominantly in puppies. In calves, intestinal atresia is most common in the jejunum, the colon and the rectum. **Atresia ani** has been reported in sheep, pigs, and cattle; it results when the cloacal membrane fails to rupture. Clinical signs are apparent at birth and include tenesmus, abdominal pain and distension, retention of faeces, and the absence of an anal opening. Surgical removal of the membrane is indicated.

Duplications

Colonic and rectal duplications are **rare malformations** of the gut. The affected animals generally show signs of large-bowel disease. Diagnosis is by contrast colonography. Correction is via surgical removal of the duplication.

Urorectal fistula

Urorectal fistula is a condition in which the **rectum and the urogenital tract communicate openly**. The malformation results from an abnormality in the development of the urorectal septum that permits communication between the rectum and a derivative of the urogenital sinus. Depending on the exact site of communication, the fistula is termed **recto-vesicular**, **recto-urethral**, **recto-vaginal**, or **recto-vestibular**.

Rectourethral fistula has been reported in English Bulldogs and is manifest clinically as simultaneous urination from both the urogenital and anal orifices along with a history of chronic urinary tract infections. If the fistula is large, faecal material may pass through the urogenital system

Rectovaginal fistula is a fistulous tract that connects the vagina and rectum and usually is seen in conjunction with atresia ani. Passage of faeces through the vulva or signs of colonic obstruction are diagnostically suggestive.

Neuromuscular disorders

Neuromuscular disorders of the gut have been discussed to some extent under malformations of the peripheral nervous system. They may result in many of the same clinical signs that stenosis produces. Aganglionic large intestine has been reported in white foals produced by mating of Overo horses to each other (see 'Congenital malformations of the peripheripheral nervous system').

CONGENITAL ABNORMALITIES OF THE MUSCULOSKELETAL SYSTEM

Normal muscle development and intrauterine activity of the fetus are essential for normal bone, joint, and tendon development. It is often difficult to determine whether a given skeletal anomaly is primary, or secondary to abnormal morphogenesis of the attached muscles. This is especially true of anomalies of the limbs, in which musculoskeletal defects in domestic animals are most common. Until recently, most classifications of musculoskeletal anomalies have been based upon morphology alone. However, during the past decade, it has become possible to assign genetic or molecular causes to some of the more common limb malformations. Much less is known in domestic animals, and, although an increasing number of limb malformations can be attributed to genetic causes, the ways in which many gene mutations are translated into defective limb development are mostly unknown.

Abnormalities of the limbs

In many malformations of the extremities, specific parts of the limbs have been lost. They are named using the particular defect as a descriptive prefix, indicating the affected location, and 'melia' (Greek melos: limb) or 'dactyl' (Greek dactylos: digit) as a suffix.

Amelia is a **complete absence of a limb**. **Meromelia** (Greek meros: part) means the **absence of one or more parts of a limb**. For instance, in crural meromelia the tibia and fibula are absent. The **reduced size of a limb** is called **micromelia**; all parts of the limb are present but significantly smaller than usual. **Partial or complete duplication of one limb** is termed **bimelia**.

Syndactyly indicates that the **digits are fused** and in **brachydactyly** they are **shorter than normal**. Syndactyly or mule foot is the partial or complete fusion of the digits of one or more feet and has been reported in numerous cattle breeds, especially Holsteins in which it is inherited as a simple autosomal recessive condition. The right forelimb is most frequently affected. Syndactyly is due to the fusion of adjacent digital primordia.

Polydactyly is the presence of **one or more extra digits** resulting from a supernumerary primordium. It is a genetic defect of cattle, sheep, pigs, and occasionally horses. Polydactyly in cattle appears to be polygenic with a dominant gene at one locus and a homozygous recessive at another. Polydactyly is also inherited in some breeds of dogs.

Contracted tendons

Contracted tendons usually involve the **digital flexor tendons** and the joint capsule. Although they occur in all ungulates, they are most often reported in foals, where contracted flexor tendon is probably the most prevalent abnormality of the musculoskeletal system.

An autosomal recessive gene causes this condition. In utero positioning may also affect the degree of disability. At birth, the pastern and fetlocks of the forelegs and sometimes the carpal joints are flexed to varying degrees due to shortening of the deep and superficial digital flexors and associated muscles. In many cases involving joint contraction, the major factor restricting the joint movement is a thickened and tight joint capsule. This may be due to thickenings in the mesenchyme forming the joint capsule and ligaments. A cleft palate may accompany this condition in some breeds. Slightly affected animals bear weight on the soles of the feet and walk on their toes. More severely affected animals walk on the dorsal surface of the pastern and fetlock joint. If not treated, the dorsal surfaces of these joints become damaged, and suppurative arthritis develops.

Arthrogryposis

Arthrogryposis can be considered to be a form of contracture (Figs 19-17, 19-18). It has been reported in horses, cattle, sheep and pigs but most frequently in cattle, particularly the Charolais. At birth, affected calves exhibit **joints fixed in abnormal positions**, frequently have scoliosis and kyphosis, and are usually unable to stand or nurse. Muscle changes, notably atrophy, have also been seen. In the spinal cord, necrosis of neurons and lesions of the white matter may be seen. Contraction of tendons is regarded as secondary to the primary neuromuscular malformation.

Arthrogryposis has more than one aetiology and pathologic entity and deviations in basic processes such as development of motor neurons or establishment of motor pathways in the spinal cord may be involved in causing the condition. An autosomal recessive gene causes the arthrogryposis syndrome in Charolais with complete penetrance in the homozygous state. Teratogens identified as causing arthrogryposis include plants such as lupins (anagyrine being the toxic agent) that are ingested by pregnant cows between days 40 and 70 of gestation ('crooked-calf' disease, Fig. 19-17). Prenatal infections with the Akabane or bluetongue viruses can also cause the condition.

Arthrogryposis is also found in horses and is referred to as contracted foal syndrome. Distal limb segments are usually affected; pastern and fetlocks of the forelegs, and sometimes the carpal joints, are twisted and flexed. Inheritance, influenza virus, and ingestion of toxic plants (locoweed) have been implicated in causing equine arthrogryposis.

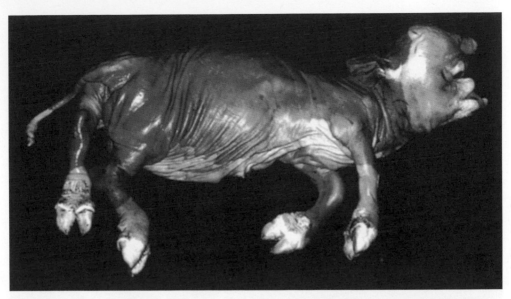

Fig. 19-16: Bulldog calf with a short muzzle and brachycephalic skull, usually resulting from chondrodysplasia. Associated with this condition are shortened limbs and anomalies of the vertebrae. Courtesy Sinowatz and Rüsse (2007).

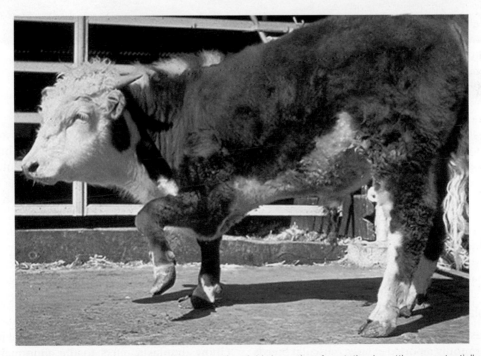

Fig. 19-17: Crooked calf disease. Lupins during the second and third months of gestation in cattle can potentially result in 'crooked calf disease', of which malformation of the limbs may be an important component. Courtesy Sinowatz and Rüsse (2007).

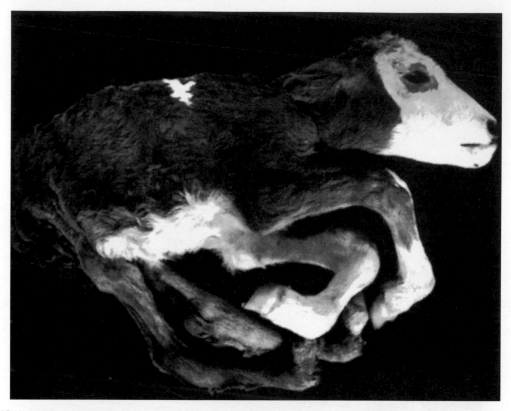

Fig. 19-18: In arthrogryposis, affected calves exhibit joints fixed in abnormal positions and frequently have scoliosis and kyphosis. They are usually unable to stand or nurse. Muscle changes, notably atrophy, have also been seen. Courtesy Sinowatz and Rüsse (2007).

A form of hereditary arthrogryposis has been reported in young Swedish Lapland dogs. This autosomal recessive disease becomes clinically manifest at 5 to 7 weeks after birth and results in rapidly progressive muscle atrophy accompanied by contractions of the tendons, causing fixation of joints and limb deformities. The observed clinical symptoms are due to cell death of neurons in the central nervous system, especially in the ventral grey horns of the spinal cord.

Hip dysplasia

Hip dysplasia occurs in most domestic animals but is most commonly reported in large muscular breeds of dog like the German Shepherd, Golden Retriever, or Mastiffs. In these breeds, the condition, which is characterized by abnormal maturation of the hip joint, is assumed to be inherited. The hip joint of affected animals has a **shallow acetabulum** and a **malformed femoral head**. Although the hip joints of affected dogs appear normal at birth, onset of clinical signs may occur at 3–5 months after birth or not until the dog is fully grown. Initial signs include stiffness and pain upon movement. About 75% of dogs that develop hip dysplasia can be identified radiographically at one year of age and 95% at two years.

Elbow dysplasia

Elbow dysplasia refers to the abnormal development of certain parts of the elbow joint during the growing phase of a dog's life. Some areas of the joint may have a **disruption of normal cartilage development** or fusion failure (in the anconeal or coronoid processes, for instance) during growth. This leads to uneven joint surfaces, inflammation, joint swelling, lameness and arthritis. In some dogs it results from a failure of the anconeal process of the ulna to ossify. Osteochondrosis may also be involved in the pathogenesis.

The exact cause of elbow dysplasia is not known, but it is probably due to a combination of genetic, nutritional (over-nutrition with rapid postnatal growth), traumatic and hormonal factors. Affected dogs are usually from large breeds, including Labrador Retrievers, Golden Retrievers, Rottweilers, Bernese Mountain Dogs, Newfoundlands, German Shepherds, and Chow Chows. Signs usually begin between 5 and 12 months after birth.

Abnormalities of the body wall

Occasionally the opposing sides of the body fail to fuse as the embryo assumes its cylindrical shape. A quantitatively minor defect in closure is manifested as **failure of sternal fusion**. In severe cases, the growth of the two sides of the thoracic wall is strongly inhibited, resulting in ectopia cordis, where the heart develops outside the thoracic cavity.

Umbilical hernias are also a result of **failures in closure of the muscular body wall**. They occur in all species but are by far most common in pigs. The abdominal organs protrude through the umbilicus under the skin; in cats and dogs it is usually the small intestine that protrudes whereas in calves it is the abomasum that is dislocated.

An **omphalocoele** is a **hernia that occurs in the embryo.** The abdominal contents that protrude through the umbilicus remain within the umbilical stalk and are therefore covered by the amniotic epithelium. This malformation probably results from a failure of the normal withdrawal of the developing intestinal loop during its physiological herniation. A complete absence of the ventral abdominal wall is called gastroschisis and causes the viscera to lie externally.

General skeletal anomalies

Chondrodysplasia

Chondrodysplasia results in a **general retardation of growth and ossification** of endochondral bone. In domestic animals, the long bones of the limbs are much more severely affected than are the bones of other parts of the skeleton. Chondrodysplasia of genetic origin is seen in many breeds of cattle and range from the so-called Dexter 'bulldog' (Fig. 19-19), in which the calf is invariably stillborn, to animals that are only mildly affected. Brachycephalic calves are usually dwarfs with short faces, bulging foreheads, prognathism, large abdomens, and short legs.

Chondrodysplasia of the appendicular and axial skeletons also is seen in dogs; the former in Poodles and Scottish Terriers, the latter in Alaskan Malamutes, Basset Hounds, Dachshunds, Poodles, and Scottish Terriers. A tendency toward chondrodysplasia is considered a normal breed characteristic in Dachshunds, Pekinese, and Bassets.

Osteopetrosis

In osteopetrosis bone resorption and remodelling of the bones, a major morphogenic mechanis in skeletal development, is disturbed. This can cause gross skeletal malformation with thickened bones throughout the skeletal system (Fig. 19-20). In long bones, medullary cavities are reduced or absent and the amount of bone marrow appears significantly reduced. In osteopetrotic cattle, the cranial vault shows a decreased size and causes pressure on the developing brain. Also the sinus frontalis is usually absent due to lack of bone remodelling and the cranium retains its prenatal rounded shape. Osteopetrosis has also been reported in some breeds of dogs and laboratory animals.

Anomalies of the vertebral column

Malformations of the vertebral column

Severe malformations of the vertebral column **compromise the prenatal development of the**

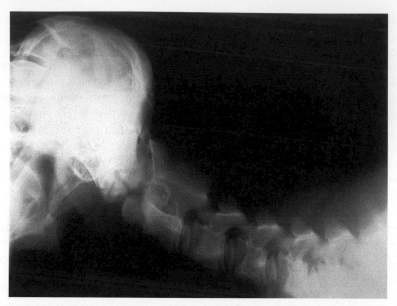

Fig. 19-19: Malformation of the articulatio atlanto-occipitalis. In this condition, which occurs as an autosomal recessive inherited disease in Arabian horses, the atlas is unilaterally or bilaterally fused to the occipital bone and its transverse processes are significantly reduced in size. The marked narrowing of the foramen magnum and the vertebral canal at the atlanto-axial level can cause a spinal cord compression. The affected foals either cannot get up at birth or are paretic and ataxic. Courtesy Sinowatz and Rüsse (2007).

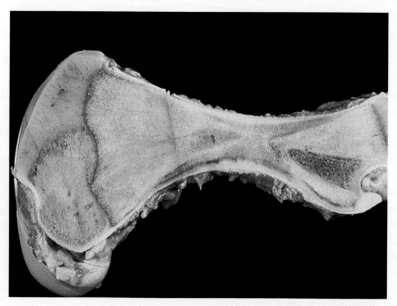

Fig. 19-20: Osteopetrotic humerus from a calf (longitudinal section). Osteopetrosis is a genetic defect of osteoclasts, which fail to reabsorb the primary spongiosa. Osteopetrosis causes an increased density of trabecular bone with corresponding reduction of the medullary cavity. Although bone density is increased, there is an abnormal fragility of bones often leading to pathological fractures. Courtesy Sinowatz and Rüsse (2007).

spinal cord. Vertebral anomalies often result from disruption of normal development and regression of the embryonic notochord, segmentation of meso-derm into somites, or vascularization and ossifica-tion of the vertebrae. Clinical signs are present at birth or, in precocious species, when the animal begins to walk. The term 'complex congenital verte-bral anomalies' denotes the presence of several vertebral malformations occurring in an animal.

Many malformations of the vertebral column are **less severe** and **affect the spinal cord only later during postnatal development**. In these cases neurological signs may not appear until the animal is a few months old.

Block vertebrae

Block vertebrae are **fused vertebrae**, which, in radi-ographs, give the appearance of a more or less solid bony mass like that seen normally in the sacrum. This condition can involve vertebral bodies, arches, or the entire vertebra in any spinal region. It results from disturbed somite segmentation.

Hemivertebrae

In **hemivertebrae only a portion of the vertebral body is present**. Hemivertebrae may be caused by so-called hemimetameric displacement of somites, resulting in right and left (or lateral) hemivertebrae, or it may be due to altered vascularization and ossi-fication of vertebrae. While the majority of cases do not produce any obvious clinical signs, hemiverte-brae are more often associated with neurological deficits than any other congenital vertebral anomaly. Neurological signs may result from a progressive, severe angulation of the spine from kyphosis (asso-ciated with dorsal hemivertebra), lordosis (associ-ated with ventral hemivertebra), or scoliosis (most often associated with lateral hemivertebra). Neuro-logical problems can also originate from narrowing of the spinal canal (spinal stenosis) or instability of the involved segments that ultimately produces spinal cord compression, vertebral luxation, or frac-ture at the site of hemivertebrae following a sudden jump, fall or trauma.

Butterfly vertebrae

Butterfly vertebrae result from persistence of the notochord or sagittal cleavage of notochord produc-ing a **sagittal cleft of the vertebral body** that extends through the body dorsoventrally. The cranial and caudal vertebral end-plates are funnel shaped and this produces a butterfly shape when viewing a dorso-ventral radiograph. Butterfly vertebrae are most often detected in brachycephalic, screw-tailed breeds. This anomaly is rarely clinically significant.

Spina bifida

Spina bifida is a developmental vertebral anomaly characterized by the presence of a **midline cleft in the vertebral arch of a single or several vertebrae**. The cleft may involve most of the vertebral arch or only the dorsal spinous process. It is often an inci-dental finding, but sometimes severe neurological signs ensue with involvement of the spinal cord or cauda equina. There is a high incidence of spina bifida in young English Bulldogs and in Manx cats with sacrocaudal dysgenesis.

Transitional vertebrae

Transitional vertebrae are abnormal vertebrae occurring at cervicothoracic, thoracolumbar, lum-bosacral or sacrocaudal junctions that possess **char-acteristics of other vertebral spinal regions** (e.g. a rib present on the transverse process of C7 or an isolated transverse process present on the first sacral vertebra). Of these malformations only the transi-tional lumbosacral vertebral anomalies appear to be clinically significant, presumably by affecting the size, shape, and plane of the vertebral body, verte-bral canal, and intervertebral disc. Transitional lum-bosacral vertebral anomalies are considered to be inherited in German Shepherd dogs and a possible cause of cauda equina syndrome associated with degenerative lumbosacral stenosis.

Deviation of the vertebral column

The terms for deviation of the vertebral column are **torticollis** (twisted neck, wryneck) **kyphosis** (dorso-ventral deviation, humpback; abnormal curvature and dorsal prominence of the vertebral column), **lordosis** (ventrodorsal deviation, curvature of the spinal column with a ventral convexity), and **scoliosis** (lateral deviation). As mentioned above, scoliosis may develop in animals with hemivertebrae. It also occurs in cats with hypervitaminosis A. In severe cases of these alignment defects of the vertebral column, the vertebral canal is compromised and the spinal cord compressed, resulting in paresis and ataxia in the limbs caudal to the site of the lesion.

An important association between developmental anomalies of the spinal cord, including Weimeraners with spinal dysraphism, and vertebral anomalies, such as scoliosis, has been noted. In particular, there are increasing numbers of reports of scoliosis occurring in animals with congenital or acquired cystic lesions involving the spinal cord, especially with cervical hydrosyringomyelia, (distension of the central canal of the spinal cord, with the formation of cavities and degeneration) in which the spinal curvature often presents itself clinically as torticollis. A direct causal relationship between scoliosis and hydrosyringomyelia has been suggested via progressive destruction of grey matter by the hydrosyringomyelic cavitation resulting in denervation and atrophy of epaxial muscles unilaterally, followed by asymmetrical lateral muscle tension and subsequent vertebral deviation.

Many minor vertebral malformations occur with greater frequency in certain species and breeds and at a particular axial level. The most well-known are the following:

Occipito-atlanto-axial malformations. Occipito-atlanto-axial malformations (Fig. 19-19) result from abnormal segmentation and development of the caudal occipital and cranial cervical sclerotomes. In this condition, which occurs as an autosomal recessive inherited disease in Arabian horses, the **atlas is unilaterally or bilaterally fused to the occipital bone** and its transverse processes are significantly reduced in size. The marked narrowing of the foramen magnum and the vertebral canal at the atlanto-axial level can cause a spinal cord compression and affected foals either cannot get up at birth or are paretic and ataxic.

Hypoplasia of the dens axis. Hypoplasia of the dens axis with concomitant subluxation of the atlanto-axial joint is most commonly found in puppies of toy breeds. This can cause spinal cord compression that occurs either suddenly (sometimes associated with a mild trauma) or progressively.

Malformations of midcervical vertebrae. Malformations of midcervical vertebrae is seen in young, rapidly growing foals of most breeds, mostly involving 3rd and 4th cervical vertebrae. The size of the cranial or caudal opening of the vertebral foramen appears reduced leading to a focal compression of the spinal cord. The resulting paresis and ataxia are referred to as cervical stenotic myelopathy which causes an unsteady gait in the affected horses, often called 'wobblers'.

Malformations of caudal cervical vertebrae. Malformations of the caudal cervical vertebrae, in which the **vertebral foramina are relatively reduced in diameter**, have been recognized in several breeds of dogs, most commonly in Great Danes and Dobermans. Midsagittal and interpedicular diameters of the cranial and caudal aspects of cervical vertebral foramina (C3–C7) were found to be significantly larger in small breeds than in these two large breeds and Dachshunds. This condition increases the risk of spinal cord compression resulting from relative stenosis of the cervical vertebral foramina.

Malformations of thoracolumbar vertebrae. A relatively common malformation of the thoracolumbar part of the vertebral column in dogs involves **hypoplasia and incomplete ossification** of one or more vertebrae. The vertebral bones are shaped like inverted wedges (hemivertebrae), resulting in a marked kyphosis. The spinal cord can become compressed causing paresis or ataxia of the pelvic limbs. In horses, hypoplasia of the articular processes of midthoracic (T2–T10) vertebrae results in congenital lordosis.

Anomalies of the skull
(Figs 19-21, 19-22, 19-23)

Although many of the observed malformations of the skull are true congenital malformations, others fall into the class of deformities that can be

Fig. 19-21: Cleft palate in a calf. Cleft palate usually results from incomplete or absent apposition and fusion of the lateral palatine processes resulting in an open connection between oral and nasal cavities. Courtesy Sinowatz and Rüsse (2007).

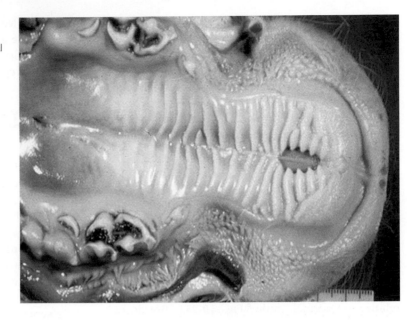

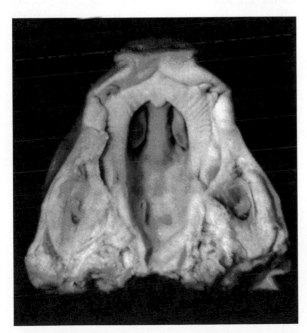

Fig. 19-22: Extensive cleft palate in a piglet. Courtesy Sinowatz and Rüsse (2007).

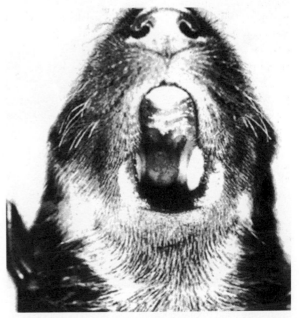

Fig. 19-23: Cleft palate in a Doberman pup. Courtesy Sinowatz and Rüsse (2007).

attributed to mechanical stress during intrauterine life or birth. The development of the skull involves the interaction of many head structures. Some malformations of the skull are, therefore, secondary to disturbances in the development of the brain (e.g. acrania and ancencephaly, microcephaly, hydrocephalus) and eyes (cyclopia). Anomalies of the facial skeleton (e.g. brachygnathia, facial cleft, cleft lip, cleft palate) have been described earlier in this chapter.

Muscular hypertrophy in cattle

The muscular hypertrophy (mh), or double-muscle phenotype, is a heritable condition in cattle that primarily results from an increase in the number of muscle fibres (hyperplasia) rather than the enlargement of individual muscle fibres (hypertrophy), relative to normal cattle (Fig. 19-24). Breeds of

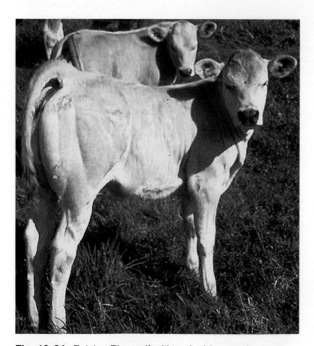

Fig. 19-24: Belgian Blue calf with a double muscle phenotype (hind limb). Double muscle, an abnormal increase in muscular tissue, is caused by enlargement of existing cells (hypertrophy).

'double muscled' cattle, like Belgian Blue and Piedmontese cattle are known to have mutations of the myostatin gene, a member of the TGF-family, which is a negative regulator of muscle growth.

SUMMARY

Teratology is the study of abnormal development. Contrary to the situation in humans, reliable data on the occurrence of congenital defects in domestic animals are not readily available. The frequency of congenital malformations varies with species, breed, geographical locations and many other factors. According to different studies, approximately 1.5% to 6% of all live-born domestic mammals show at least one recognizable congenital malformation.

The genesis of congenital malformations can be regarded as an interaction between **genetic endowment of the embryo** and the **environment** in which it develops. From many studies the following four conclusions can be drawn: (1) Insults to the embryo during the first 3 weeks of embryogenesis (during which the basic body plan is established) are unlikely to result in defective development, because they either kill the embryo or can be compensated by regulatory mechanisms of the early embryo. (2) The period of maximal susceptibility to teratological deviations begins with the onset of organogenesis at 3 weeks and extends in most organ systems up to the 8th week. This is the period, when most major organs are first being established. (3) After 8 weeks of pregnancy, major structural anomalies are unlikely to occur. At this time, most organs have become well established. (4) Not all teratogens act in the same developmental periods. Some cause malformations if the embryo is exposed to them at an early stage of development, but are not harmful at later periods of pregnancy.

Since normal development is controlled by an interaction between the genome of an embryo and its environment, susceptibility to a teratogen depends upon the genotype of the embryo and the manner in which it interacts with adverse environmental factors. Genetically based malformations result from abnormalities of chromosomal division or mutations of genes, causing abnormalities of chromosome structure or gene imprinting. Abnormal genes may be the direct cause of an anomaly, or cause it indirectly by affecting the susceptibility of the embryo to an environmental insult.

Environmental factors causing abnormalities of embryos and fetuses include physical factors, chemical and biological teratogens and infectious agents (mostly viruses). The chief types of developmental disturbances found in domestic animals include:
- Agenesis or aplasia
- Hypoplasia and hyperplasia
- Failure to fuse or close
- Absence of normal cell death
- Disturbances in tissue resorption
- Failure of cell migration
- Developmental arrest, and
- Duplication and reversal of asymmetry.

FURTHER READING

Batista, M., González, F., Cabrera, F., Palomino, E., Castellano, E., Calero, P. and Gracia, A. (2000): True hermaphroditism in a horned goat with 60XX/60XY chimerism. Can. Vet J. 41:562–564.

Brent, R.L. and Beckman, D.A. (1999): Teratogens. In: Encyclopedia of Reproduction, Vol. 4. Eds. Knobil, E. and Neill, J.D. Academic Press, San Diego, 735–749.

Butterworth, C.E. and Bendich, A. (1996): Folic acid and the prevention of birth defects. Annu. Rev. Nutr. 16:73–97.

Chetboul, V., Tran, D., Carlos, C., Tessier, D. and Pouchelon, J.L. (2004): Congenital malformations of the tricuspid valve in domestic carnivores: a retrospective study of 50 cases. Schweiz. Arch. Tierheilkd. 146:265–275.

Cornillie, P. and Simoens, P. (2005): Prenatal development of the caudal vena cava in mammals: review of the different theories with special reference to the dog. Anat. Histol. Embryol. 34:364–372.

David, L.E. (1983): Adverse effects of drugs on reproduction in dogs and cats. Mod. Vet. Pract. 1:960–974.

Finnell, R.H., Gellineau-Van Waes, J., Eudy, J.D. and Rosenquist, T.H. (2002): Molecular basis of environmentally induced birth defects. Ann. Rev. Pharmacol. Toxicol. 42:181–208.

Gallagher, D.S. Jr., Lewis, B.C., De Donato, M., Davis, S.K., Taylor, J.F., Edwards, J.F. and Hansen, D.K. (1999):

Autosomal trisomy 20 (61,XX,+20) in a malformed bovine fetus. Vet. Pathol. 36:448–451.

Hiraga, T. and Dennis, S.M. (1993): Congenital duplication. Vet. Clin. North Am. Food Anim. Pract. 9:145–161.

Huston, K. (1993): Heritability and diagnosis of congenital abnormalities in food animals. Vet. Clin. North Am. Food Anim. Pract. 9:1–9.

Keeler, R.F. and van Balls, L.D. (1978): Teratogenic effects in cattle of Conium maculatum and conium alkaloids and analogs. Clin. Toxicol. 12:49–64.

Lee, E., Halina, W., Fisher, K.R., Partlow, G.D. and Physick-Sheard, P. (2002): Single ventricle, total transposition, and hypoplastic aorta in a calf. Vet. Pathol. 39:602–605.

Navarro, M., Cristofol, C., Carretero, A., Arboix, M. and Ruberte, J. (1998). Anthelmintic induced congenital malformations in sheep embryos using netobimin. Vet. Rec. 142:86–90.

Oberst, R.D. (1993): Viruses as teratogens. Vet. Clin. North Am. Food Anim. Pract. 9:23–31.

Rieck, G.W. (1968): Exogene Ursachen embryonaler Entwicklungsstörungen beim Rind. Z. Tierzüchtung Züchtungsbiol. 84:251–261.

Ruść, A., and Kamiński, S. (2007): Prevalence of complex vertebral malformation carriers among Polish Holstein-Friesian bulls. J. Appl. Genet. 48:247–252.

Rüsse, I. and Sinowatz, F. (1998) Lehrbuch der Embryologie der Haustiere, 2nd ed. 1998, Paul Parey, Berlin, Hamburg.

Saperstein, G. (1993): Congenital abnormalities of internal organs and body cavities. Vet. Clin. North Am. Food Anim. Pract. 9:115–125.

Scott, F.W., DeLahunta, A., Schultz, R.D., Bistner, S.I. and Riis, R.C. (1975): Teratogenesis in cats associated with griseofulvin therapy. Teratology 11:79–86.

Smith, K.C., Parkinson, T.J., Pearson, G.R., Sylvester, L. and Long, S.E. (2003): Morphological, histological and histochemical studies of the gonads of ovine freemartins. Vet. Rec. 152:164–169.

Spencer, T.E. and Gray, C.A. (2006): Sheep uterine gland knockout (UGKO) model. Methods Mol. Med. 121:85–94.

Szabo, K.T. (1989): Congenital Malformations in Laboratory and Farm Animals. Academic Press, San Diego.

Viuff, D., Rickords, L., Offenberg, H., Hyttel, P., Avery, B., Greve, T., Olsaker, I., Williams, J.L., Callesen, H. and Thomsen, P.D. (1999): A high proportion of bovine blastocysts produced in vitro are mixoploid. Biol. Repod. 60:1273–1278.

Viuff, D., Greve, T., Avery, B., Hyttel, P., Brockhoff, P.B. and Thomsen, P.D. (2000): Chromosome aberrations in in vitro-produced bovine embryos at Days 2–5 post-insemination. Biol. Reprod. 63:1143–1148.

Viuff, D., Hendriksen, P.J.M., Vos, P.L.A.M., Dieleman, S.J., Bibby, B.M., Greve, T., Hyttel, P. and Thomsen, P.D. (2001): Chromosomal abnormalities and developmental kinetics in in vivo-developed cattle embryos at days 2 to 5 after ovulation. Biol. Reprod. 65:204–208.

Viuff, D., Palsgaard, A., Rickords, L., Lawson, L.G., Greve, T., Schmidt, M., Avery, B., Hyttel, P. and Thomsen, P.D. (2002): Bovine embryos contain a higher proportion of polyploid cells in the trophectoderm than in the embryonic disc. Mol. Reprod. Dev. 62:483–488.

Woollen, N.E. (1993): Congenital diseases and abnormalities of pigs. Vet. Clin. North Am. Food Anim. Pract. 9:163–181.

Young, L.E., Fernandes, K., McEvoy, T.G., Butterwith, S.C., Gutierrez, C.G., Carolan, C., Broadbent, P.J., Robinson, J.J., Wilmut, I. and Sinclair, K.D. (2001): Epigenetic change in IGF2R is associated with fetal overgrowth after sheep embryo culture. Nature Gen. 27:153–154.

CHAPTER 20

Palle Serup (chicken) and Ernst-Martin Füchtbauer (mouse)

The chicken and mouse as models of embryology

EARLY DEVELOPMENT OF THE CHICK EMBRYO

The three-week long development of a chicken embryo was first documented by Aristotle in the 4th Century B.C. Since then the domestic chicken (*Gallus gallus*) has been a **favourite model organism in embryological studies**. Today, modern hatcheries provide year round access to vast numbers of cheap and easily reared eggs. As the developmental stage can be accurately predicted at any given temperature, large numbers of embryos at defined stages can be obtained. Another advantage of the chick embryo is that it can be experimentally manipulated in a number of ways, from the surgical techniques used by John Saunders and Nicole Le Douarin in their classical experiments to current molecular techniques which, assisted by the nearly completed sequencing of the chick genome, allows forced expression and knock-down of genes via electroporation and/or use of retroviral vectors. Since both germ layer development (gastrulation) and subsequent organ formation is orchestrated by genes and cell movements similar to those of mammalian embryos, the chick embryos provide an important experimental system in which one can address fundamental questions about vertebrate development.

Fertilization, cleavage, and blastulation

Fertilization of the egg occurs in the oviduct **prior to the secretion of albumen** ('egg white') and the deposition of the shell. As with other eggs rich in yolk, **cleavage occurs only in the blastodisc**, a small disc of cytoplasm 2–3 mm in diameter. The horizontal cleavages create a single layered **blastoderm** where the cells are continuous with one another and with the yolk at their bases (Fig. 20-1). Later cleavages divide the blastoderm into a 5–6 cell layer thick tissue.

Between the blastoderm and the yolk is a space called the **subgerminal cavity** or space (Fig. 20-2A) which is created when the blastoderm cells absorb water from the albumen and then secrete it between themselves and the yolk. At this stage, the deep cells in the centre of the blastoderm are shed and die, leaving behind a one-cell-thick area pellucida which is the part of the blastoderm that forms most of the embryo proper (Fig. 20-1). The peripheral blastoderm cells retain their deep cells and constitute the area opaca. Between the area pellucida and the area opaca is a narrow layer of cells called the marginal zone some of which become very important in later development.

Gastrulation

Development of the hypoblast

By the time the egg is laid, the blastoderm contains approximately 20 000 cells. Most of the area pellucida cells stay on the surface and form the epiblast. A number of area pellucida cells delaminate and migrate into the subgerminal cavity where they form the **primary hypoblast**, a loose collection of cell groups containing 5–20 cells each (Fig. 20-2B). Next, a sheet of cells originating from a local thickening at the posterior margin of the blastoderm (**Koller's sickle**) migrate anteriorly and push the primary hypoblast cells in front of them (Fig.

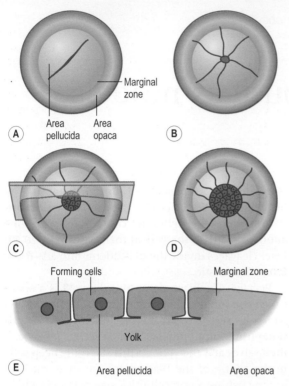

Fig. 20-1: Discoidal meroblastic cleavage in a chick embryo. Four stages (A-D) viewed from the animal pole. **E:** An early-cleavage embryo viewed from the side. Modified from Gilbert (2003). Reprinted with permission of Sinauer Associates Inc.

20-2C), thereby forming the **secondary hypoblast**, or **endoblast**. The resulting **two-layered blastoderm** (**epiblast** and **hypoblast**) is joined together at the marginal zone of the area opaca, and the space between the layers makes up the **blastocoel**. The hypoblast does not contribute any cells to the actual embryo; those cells come exclusively from the epiblast. Instead, the hypoblast cells form parts of the extraembryonic membranes, particularly the yolk sac and the vitelline duct – the stalk linking the yolk mass to the digestive tube. Hypoblast cells also provide chemical signals that direct the behaviour of epiblast cells.

Development of the primitive streak

The chief structural feature of amniote (avian, reptilian, and mammalian) gastrulation is the **primitive streak**. Dye-marking experiments, which allow cells

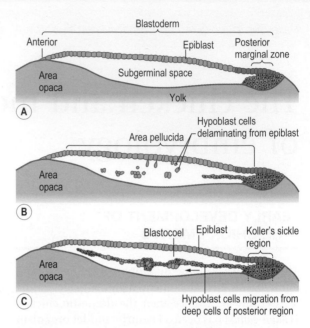

Fig. 20-2: Formation of the two-layered blastoderm of the chick embryo. Modified from Gilbert (2003). Reprinted with permission of Sinauer Associates Inc.

to be traced as development progresses, suggest that primitive streak cells arise in the posterior marginal region. The streak is first visible as cells gather in the middle layer, followed by a thickening of the epiblast at the posterior marginal zone, just anterior to Koller's sickle (Fig. 20-3A). The surrounding cells, which will later join the streak, become globular and motile, and they digest away the extracellular matrix beneath them. As the streak cells ingress they undergo **convergent-extension**. This process is responsible for the progression of the streak – a doubling in streak length is accompanied by a concomitant halving of its width. Those cells that initiated streak formation appear to migrate anteriorly and appear to comprise an unchanging cell population that directs the movement of epiblast cells into the streak.

As cells come together to form the primitive streak, a depression called **the primitive groove** forms within the streak. The primitive groove serves as an opening through which migrating cells pass into the blastocoel. The primitive groove is thus equivalent to the amphibian blastopore. At the anterior end of the streak is a thickening of the cells known as **Hensen's node**. The centre of Hensen's

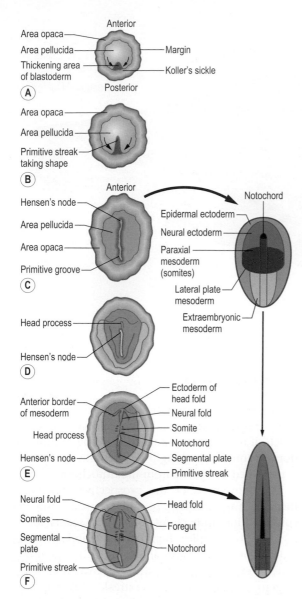

Fig. 20-3: Cell movements of the primitive streak of the chick embryo. Drawings to the right show fate maps of the epiblast in 'B' and 'F'. Modified from Gilbert (2003). Reprinted with permission of Sinauer Associates Inc.

node has a funnel-shaped indentation through which cells migrate into the blastocoel. Hensen's node is the functional equivalent of the dorsal blastoporal lip (also known as Spemann's organizer) in amphibians.

The first cells to enter the primitive streak are endodermal progenitors (endoblast cells) from the epiblast (Fig. 20-3B). These cells go through an **epithelio-mesenchymal transition** and the underlying basal lamina breaks down. As these cells migrate into the streak, the streak extends in an anterior direction. Mitosis adds to the length generated by convergent-extension, and a number of the cells from the anterior part of the epiblast contribute further to the node. Simultaneously, the endoblast cells maintain their anterior migration away from the posterior edge of the blastoderm. The extension of the primitive streak appears to follow the anterior movement of the endoblast cells, and these are believed to direct the movement of the streak. In the end, the primitive streak will grow to ~70% of the length of the area pellucida.

When the primitive streak is formed it **defines the axes** of the avian embryo. It stretches from anterior to posterior; gastrulating cells ingress from its dorsal side and move to the ventral side; and it divides the left part of the embryo from the right.

Fate of cells ingressing through the primitive streak

As soon as the streak has developed, epiblast cells begin to move through it into the blastocoel to form mesoderm and endoderm (Fig. 20-4). Thus the primitive streak is formed by an always changing cell population. With respect to mesodermal components, the **anterior** end of the **streak** (Hensen's node) gives rise to **prechordal plate mesoderm, notochord,** and **rostral somites.** Cells that migrate through the **middle** part of the **streak** give rise to **somites, heart,** and **kidneys.** Cell coming from the **posterior** part of the **streak** make the **lateral plate** and **extraembryonic mesoderm** (Fig. 20-3C–F).

The first cells that migrate through Hensen's node form the **pharyngeal endoderm** of the foregut. These endodermal cells migrate rostrally and thereby displace the hypoblast, confining the hypoblast cells to the anterior part of the area pellucida. There they form the germinal crescent which does not form any of the embryonic structures but does contain germ cell precursors derived from the epiblast. The next

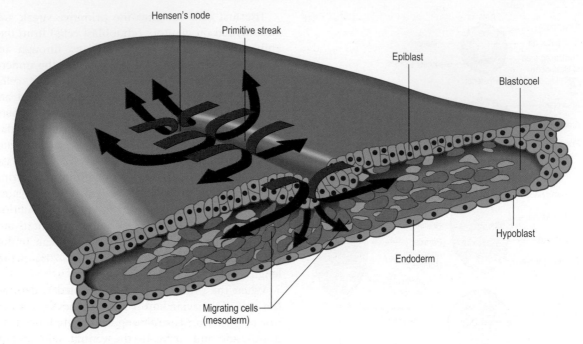

Fig. 20-4: Migration of endodermal and mesodermal cells through the primitive streak.

cells moving through Hensen's node also migrate rostrally, but they do not progress as far ventrally as the future foregut endoderm. Instead, these cells take up a location between the epiblast and the endoderm and form a portion of the **head mesenchyme** and **the prechordal plate mesoderm**. The head mesenchyme will later be enriched by contributions from the neural crest cells. The next cells to move through the node form the **chordamesoderm**. The chordamesoderm has two parts: the head process, which is formed by the medial mesodermal cells moving rostrally behind the prechordal plate mesoderm, and the notochord. The head process will underlie those cells that form the fore- and midbrain. When the primitive streak begins to regress, the cells migrating through Hensen's node will lay down the second part of the chordamesoderm, the **notochord**. The notochord begins at the level where the ears and the hindbrain form, and extends caudally, where it will emit signals that instruct progenitor cells in adjacent tissues to adopt a specific cellular fate depending on the distance between the notochord and the responding progenitor cells. In fact, studies using chick embryos have delivered much of today's detailed understanding of how the dorsal-ventral axis along the vertebrate spinal cord is patterned by signals from the notochord.

The movement of the prospective mesoderm through the anterior primitive streak and its condensation into chordamesoderm seems to be regulated by complex chemoattractive and chemorepulsive processes, both involving FGF signalling. FGF8 is expressed in the primitive streak and repels migrating cells away from the streak, while the same cells are attracted to FGF4 secreted from the developing chordamesoderm. The experiments leading to the elucidation of these chemotaxic actions of different fibroblast growth factors could most likely only be performed in a model like the chick embryo and further illustrates the usefulness of this model in developmental studies.

As the epiblast cells continue to move through the more posterior lateral parts of the streak they separate into two layers as they enter the blastocoel.

The lower layer intercalates into the hypoblast and displaces its cells to the sides. These lower cells give rise to **endoderm** and will later form all of the embryo's endodermal organs, as well as most of the extraembryonic membranes (with the hypoblast forming the rest). The other layer spreads between the epiblast and the endoderm forming a loosely connected layer of **mesoderm**. This mesodermal layer of cells gives rise to organs such as kidneys, heart, and vasculature as well as connective tissue parts of the endodermal organs. Also, the mesoderm lining the extraembryonic membranes is derived from these ingressed cells. The movement of these cells away from the streak is also controlled by FGF8 but a putative chemoattractive signal that can attract the cells towards the caudal end of the embryo has not yet been identified. By the end of the first day of incubation most of the future endodermal cells are located within the embryo but future mesodermal cells continue to move through the streak.

Now a transition of gastrulation occurs. While mesodermal cells continue to ingress, **the primitive streak begins to regress**, changing the position of Hensen's node from near the centre of the area pellucida to a more posterior location (Fig. 20-5). The regressing streak generates the posterior dorsal axis of the embryo, including the notochord. As the node moves posteriorly, the caudal part of the notochord is laid down from precursors located in the node. Eventually, the node regresses to its most caudal position, forming the anal section. At this time, all the future meso- and endodermal cells have migrated into the embryo, and the remaining epiblast has gradually been transformed into the **ectoderm**.

As a result of the order in which the head mesoderm and the notochord are formed, avian (as well as fish, reptilian, and mammalian) embryos show a marked **anterior-to-posterior grade of developmental progression**. As cells of the posterior part of the embryo are undergoing gastrulation, cells at the anterior end are already beginning to form organs. For the next several days, development has progressed further in the anterior part of the embryo than in the posterior part.

As the future meso- and endodermal cells are moving into the embryo, the ectodermal progenitors divide and migrate to enclose the yolk by **epiboly** (the expansion of a sheet of cells over other cells). The encircling of the yolk by the ectoderm takes almost four days to complete. It includes the constant production of cellular material and the movement of the future ectodermal cells along the underside of the vitelline envelope (an extracellular envelope that forms a fibrous mat around the egg). Notably, only the cells at the periphery of the area opaca attach tightly to the vitelline envelope. These cells are intrinsically different from other blastoderm cells, as they can send out enormous (> 500 µm) cytoplasmic filopodia onto the vitelline envelope. These elongated processes appear to be responsible for the locomotive force by which the marginal cells pull other ectodermal cells around the yolk. The filopodia bind to fibronectin, a basal lamina protein present in the chick vitelline envelope. If the contact between the marginal cells and the fibronectin is disrupted experimentally, the filopodia retract and ectodermal epiboly ceases.

Thus, as gastrulation concludes, the ectoderm has encircled the yolk, the definitive endoderm has replaced the hypoblast, and the mesoderm has been placed between these two layers. Although many of the processes involved in avian gastrulation have been identified, we are only just beginning to comprehend the mechanisms responsible for carrying out these processes.

Axis formation

Although the formation of the chick body axes is accomplished during gastrulation, axis specification occurs earlier, during the cleavage stage.

The **dorso-ventral axis** is set up when the blastoderm creates a barrier between the basic albumin above the blastodisc and the acidic subgerminal cavity below it. Water and sodium ions are transported from the albumin to the subgerminal cavity, creating a potential difference across the epiblast. The side facing the negative and basic albumin will become the dorsal side, and the side facing the positive and acidic subgerminal cavity fluid will become

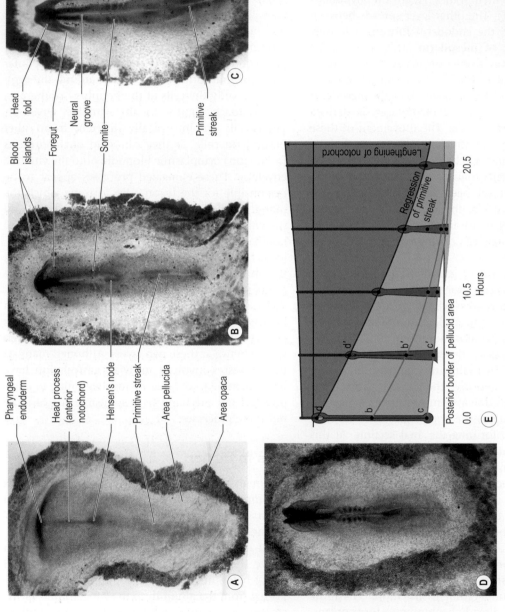

Fig. 20-5: Chick gastrulation 24–28 hours after fertilization. **A:** The primitive streak at full extension (24 hours). The head process (anterior notochord) can be seen extending from Hensen's node. **B:** Two-somite stage (25 hours). Pharyngeal endoderm is seen anteriorly, while the anterior notochord pushes up the head process beneath it. The primitive streak is regressing. **C:** Four-somite stage (27 hours). **D:** At 28 hours, the primitive streak has regressed to the caudal portion of the embryo. **E:** Regression of the primitive streak, leaving the notochord in its wake. Various points of the streak (represented by letters) were followed after it achieved its maximum length. The x axis (time) represents hours after achieving maximum length (the reference line is about 18 hours of incubation). Modified from Gilbert (2003). Reprinted with permission of Sinauer Associates Inc.

the ventral side. This orientation of the axis can be switched around experimentally by reversing either the pH gradient or the potential difference across the cell layer.

The establishment of a bilaterally symmetrical structure, exhibiting an **anteroposterior axis**, from an initial radially symmetric blastoderm is determined by gravity. Before the egg is laid, it rotates in the shell gland. This rotation shifts the yolk such that its lighter components end up beneath one side of the blastoderm. This tips up that part of the blastoderm, which will become the posterior region of the embryo, the part where primitive streak formation begins.

The mechanism that causes this portion of the blastoderm to become the posterior margin and to initiate gastrulation is still unclear but recent work has begun to reveal its nature. The entire marginal zone has the ability to initiate primitive streak formation, and if the blastoderm is separated into parts, each having its own marginal zone, each part will form its own primitive streak. Yet, once a **posterior marginal zone (PMZ)** has formed, it regulates the other areas of the margin. Not only do these PMZ cells initiate gastrulation, they also prevent other parts of the margin from initiating the formation of primitive streaks.

However, recent studies indicate that *Nodal* expression is required to initiate primitive streak formation, and that secretion of Cerberus (a Nodal antagonist) by the primary hypoblast prevents primitive streak initiation all through the margin. As the primary hypoblast cells move away from the PMZ, the resulting loss of Cerberus allows Nodal protein to be active in the PMZ and induce primitive streak formation there. It is tempting to speculate that the lighter components of the yolk, which tip up and define the posterior blastoderm, push away the hypoblast and thereby the action of Cerberus. Nodal also induce the expression of *Lefty* (another antagonist of its own activity) in the streak cells and thereby prevent the development of additional primitive streaks.

The above observations suggest that the PMZ contains cells that act as the equivalent of the amphibian Nieuwkoop centre. When grafted to the anterior marginal zone, PMZ tissue is able to initiate the formation of a primitive streak, including Hensen's node, without itself contributing any cells to these structures. Like the amphibian Nieuwkoop centre, this region is thought to be the place where Wnt signalling (or at least nuclear localization of β-catenin) and a TGF-β family signal coincide. The specific expression of the TGF-β family member *Vg1* in the PMZ is consistent with this is hypothesis. Also, supporting a critical role of Wnt and Vg1/Nodal signalling for primitive streak formation, is the observation that beads soaked in Wnt8c as well as beads soaked in Vg1 can induce ectopic primitive streaks when placed in the anterior marginal zone.

The **'organizer'** of the chick embryo forms just rostral to the PMZ, where the epiblast and middle layer cells in the anterior part of Koller's sickle form **Hensen's node**. The posterior part of Koller's sickle contributes to the posterior part of the primitive streak (Fig. 20-6). As mentioned above, Hensen's node is considered to be the avian equivalent of the dorsal blastoporal lip in amphibians, since they are located at equivalent positions and share many properties. Thus, the cells of both can organize a second embryonic axis when transplanted into other locations of the gastrula (Fig. 20-7) and both are destined to become the chordamesoderm.

Gene expression in the chick organizer can be regarded as being comprised of two separate sets of genes. The first set contains genes that are first expressed in the posterior region of Koller's sickle and which probably exert their action during the formation of the Nieuwkoop centre-like part of the PMZ cells. These genes, which include *Vg1* and *Nodal*, then appear all through the primitive streak (Figs 20-8, 20-9). As hinted above, recent studies have shown that Vg1 plays an important role in forming the primitive streak, and that if Vg1 is ectopically expressed in the anterior marginal zone, Nodal will be induced and a secondary axis will form there. The second set of genes comprises those whose expression is confined to the anterior portion of the primitive streak, and finally to Hensen's node (Figs 20-8, 20-9). These genes include *Chordin* and *Sonic hedgehog*.

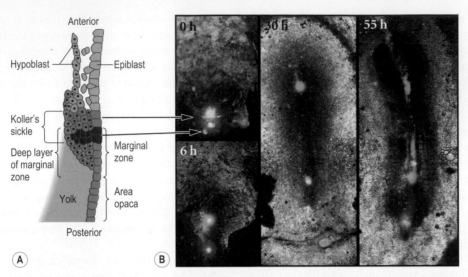

Fig. 20-6: Formation of Hensen's node from Koller's sickle. **A**: Diagram of the posterior end of an early (pre-streak) embryo, showing the cells labeled with fluorescent dyes in the photographs. Modified from Gilbert (2003). Reprinted with permission of Sinauer Associates Inc. **B**: Just before gastrulation, cells in the anterior end of Koller's sickle (the epiblast and middle layer) were labeled with green dye. Cells of the posterior portion of Koller's sickle were labeled with red dye. As the cells migrated, the anterior cells formed Hensen's node and its notochord derivatives. The posterior cells formed the posterior region of the primitive streak. The time after dye injection is labeled on each photograph. Reproduced with permission from Bachvarova (1998).

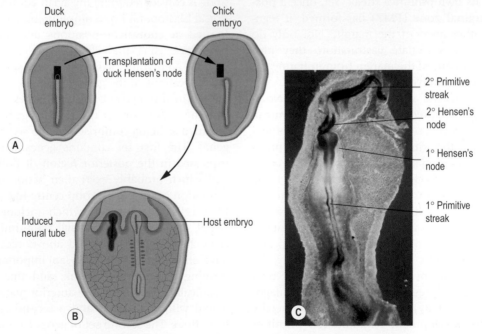

Fig. 20-7: Induction of a new embryo by transplantation of Hensen's node. **A**: A Hensen's node from a duck embryo is transplanted into the epiblast of a chick embryo. **B**: A secondary embryo is induced (as is evident by the neural tube) from host tissues at the graft site. **A**, **B** modified from Gilbert (2003). Reprinted with permission of Sinauer Associates Inc. **C**: Graft of Hensen's node from one embryo into the periphery of a host embryo. After further incubation, the host embryo has a neural tube whose regionalization can be seen by in situ hybridization. Probes to *otx2* (red) recognize the head region, while probes to *hoxb1* (blue) recognize the trunk neural tube. The donor node has induced the formation of a secondary axis, complete with head and trunk regions. Reproduced with permission from Boettger (2001).

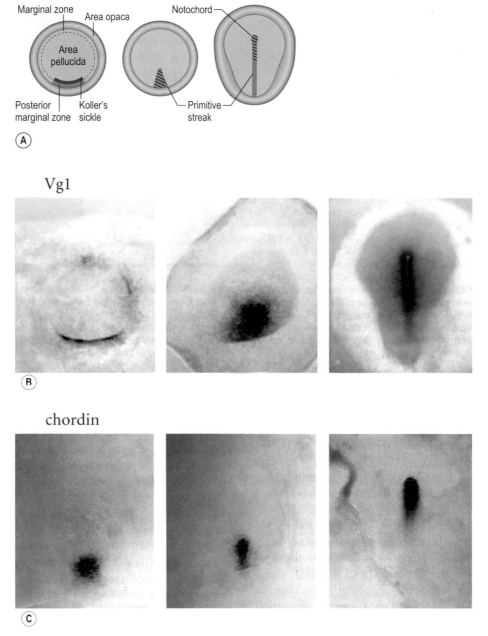

Fig. 20-8: Gene expression in the primitive streak. **A**: Schemata of the two general gene expression patterns. The early chick epiblast (left panel) shows the area opaca, area pellucida, marginal zone, Koller's sickle (red), and posterior marginal zone (blue). At a slightly later stage (middle panel), cells expressing both the Nieuwkoop center genes and organizer genes extend into the primitive streak. At later stages (right panel), the Nieuwkoop center genes are expressed throughout the streak, while the organizer genes are expressed in the most anterior region. Modified from Gilbert (2003). Reprinted with permission of Sinauer Associates Inc. **B**: Expression of Vg1 protein as the primitive streak forms. **C**: Expression of chordin as the primitive streak forms. Photographs courtesy of Professor G Schoenwolf.

Schlesinger, A.B. (1958): The structural significance of the avian yolk in embryogenesis. J. Exp. Zool. 138:223–258.

Seleiro, E.A., Connolly, D.J. and Cooke, J. (1996): Early developmental expression and experimental axis determination by the chicken Vg1 gene. Curr. Biol. 6:1476–1486.

Shah, S.B., Skromne, I., Hume, C.R., Kessler, D.S., Lee, K.J., Stern, C.D. and Dodd, J. (1997): Misexpression of chick Vg1 in the marginal zone induces primitive streak formation. Development 124:5127–5138.

Skromne, I. and Stern, C.D. (2002): A hierarchy of gene expression accompanying induction of the primitive streak by Vg1 in the chick embryo. Mech. Dev. 114:115–118.

Smith, J.L. and Schoenwolf, G.C. (1998): Getting organized: new insights into the organizer of higher vertebrates. Curr. Top. Dev. Biol. 40:79–110.

Spratt, N.T., Jr. (1946): Formation of the primitive streak in the explanted chick blastoderm marked with carbon particles. J. Exp. Zool. 103:259–304.

Spratt, N.T., Jr. (1947): Regression and shortening of the primitive streak in the explanted chick blastoderm. J. Exp. Zool. 104:69–100.

Spratt, N.T., Jr. (1963): Role of the substratum, supracellular continuity, and differential growth in morphogenetic cell movements. Dev. Biol. 7:51–63.

Spratt, N.T., Jr. and Haas, H. (1960): Integrative mechanisms in development of early chick blastoderm I. Regulated potentiality of separate parts. J. Exp. Zool. 145:97–138.

Stern, C.D. (2004): Gastrulation. Cold Spring Harbor Laboratory Press, Cold Spring Harbor.

Stern, C.D. (2006): Neural induction: 10 years on since the 'default model'. Curr. Opin. Cell. Biol. 18:692–697.

Stern, C.D. and Canning, D.R. (1988): Gastrulation in birds: a model system for the study of animal morphogenesis. Experientia 44:651–657.

Storey, K.G., Goriely, A., Sargent, C.M., Brown, J.M., Burns, H.D., Abud, H.M. and Heath, J.K. (1998): Early posterior neural tissue is induced by FGF in the chick embryo. Development 125:473–484.

Streit, A., Berliner, A.J., Papanayotou, C., Sirulnik, A. and Stern, C.D. (2000): Initiation of neural induction by FGF signalling before gastrulation. Nature 406:74–78.

Vakaet, L. (1984): The initiation of gastrula ingression in the chick blastoderm. Am. Zool. 24:555–562.

Waddington, C.H. (1933): Induction by the primitive streak and its derivatives in the chick. J. Exp. Zool. 10:38–46.

Waddington, C.H. (1934) Experiments on embryonic induction. J. Exp. Zool., 11:211–227.

Yang, X., Dormann, D., Munsterberg, A.E. and Weijer, C.J. (2002): Cell movement patterns during gastrulation in the chick are controlled by positive and negative chemotaxis mediated by FGF4 and FGF8. Dev. Cell. 3:425–437.

THE MOUSE AS A MODEL IN EMBRYOLOGY

Because of its short generation time, small size, and large litter size, the mouse is the **primary mammalian model organism** for functional genetics – the study of the phenotypic consequences of mutations. Many of the genetic and molecular explanations of embryonic and fetal development given in this book originate from observations made in the mouse. Furthermore, many techniques used in preimplantation embryology, including the production of chimaeric animals and the generation of embryonic stem (ES) cells, were pioneered in mice. This chapter will focus on the few differences in mammalian embryo development between mice and 'normal' large domestic species and will give a very short introduction to the burgeoning studies of murine ES cells. The differences in initial embryonic development have also resulted in a slightly different set of terms applied to mouse embryos.

The litter size of laboratory mice depends on the genetic background, but is typically between **8 and 10 pups**. Female mice have a short **sexual cycle of 4–5 days**. Normal **gestation time** in mice is around **19 days**. However, in lactating females, this period is prolonged by 4–5 days, to the time when pups are normally weaned. The decreased speed of development is achieved by **delayed implantation** (or **diapause**), and is biologically necessary because female mice are in oestrus a few hours post partum and will copulate if a male is present.

Mating and fertilization

In mice, copulation is indicated by the presence of a **vaginal plug**, which is composed of coagulated secretions from the coagulating and vesicular glands of the male. This makes it much simpler to achieve timed matings in mice than in many other small mammals in which post partum matings or the presence of sperm in vaginal smears are used to confirm copulation. As mice are nocturnal animals, copulation normally occurs around midnight, so noon of the day the plug is found is normally defined as Day 0.5 of gestation. However, matings in the early afternoon also happen. The age of embryos is often abbreviated either as '**dE**', day of embryonic development or '**days p.c.**', days post coitum. The oocytes and the preimplantation embryos are surrounded by a glycoprotein envelope, the **zona pellucida**, which protects the oocyte from polyspermic fertilization and the embryos from attaching to the wall of the oviduct and to each other. As in all mammals, **fertilization** occurs in the oviduct close to the ovary. The morning after copulation, the zygotes can be found in the ampulla, a transparent widening at the distal end of the oviduct close to the infundibulum. It is at this stage that zygotes may be isolated for the **generation of transgenic mice by pronucleus injection**, because the (smaller) maternal and the (larger) paternal pronuclei have not yet dissolved and can be identified under the microscope.

Cleavage stages and compaction

By about dE 1, the embryo has undergone the **first cleavage division**. At this time, the **embryonic genome undergoes a major activation** and the maternally contributed messenger RNAs start to be degraded. This is earlier than in many other mammals and might explain why cloning by transfer of somatic cell nuclei proved more difficult in mice than in many larger mammals; if the new nucleus has to sustain development after only one division, there is very little time for reprogramming.

The cleavage divisions in mice are not truly synchronous and embryos with an uneven number of blastomeres can be found. However, in general, the embryo consists of four cells at dE 1.5–2, and eight cells at dE 2.5. At this stage, the first morphological signs of differentiation become apparent in the form of increased cellular adhesion between the blastomeres. This adhesion overcomes the surface tension of the individual cells and results in a more spherical embryo in which the single blastomeres no longer protrude; a process referred to as **compaction**. Compaction is caused by the expression of *E-cadherin* (originally called uvomorulin), a

Ca^{2+}-ion-dependent cell adhesion molecule; removal of Ca^{2+}, or incubation with antibodies that inhibit E-cadherin, can prevent or reverse compaction. Blocking of compaction for an extended time period will inhibit further development of the embryo. The outer blastomeres of the compacted embryo form tight junctions and a seal between the interior and exterior of the embryo. Even though all the cells remain pluripotent for a short time, this outside-inside distinction creates the first 'visible' inequality amongst the cells of the developing embryo.

Blastulation

After another two to three cell divisions, at dE 3–3.5, the outer cells begin to form an epithelium in which cells are asymmetrical and express Na^+/K^+-ATPase on their basolateral membranes facing the inside of the embryo. This Na^+/K^+-ATPase pumps Na^+ ions into the intercellular space inside the embryo and brings about a passive water influx into the space. As the outer epithelial cell layer is sealed by tight junctions, the water cannot escape and creates an inner cavity, the **blastocyst cavity**. This process of **blastulation** results in development of the **blastocyst** and presses the outer cells to the zona pellucida. The affinity of the inner cells of the embryo for each other is higher than for the outer cell layer and so they group together forming the **inner cell mass (ICM)** which is attached to the outer cell layer, now referred to as the **trophectoderm**. The trophectoderm over the ICM is referred to as polar trophectoderm whereas that around the blastocyst cavity is referred to as mural trophectoderm.

Whether there is any axis pre-determination in the murine embryo is still controversial. From its beginning the embryo is not completely radially symmetrical, and the polar bodies might be used as a landmark giving positional information. Using this measure, it has been proposed that the dorsoventral and anteroposterior axis can already be predicted before the first cell division. However, other investigators have argued that the polar bodies themselves are not fixed and therefore cannot serve as a positional landmark. Furthermore, it has been argued that the blastomeres, at least up to the 8- to

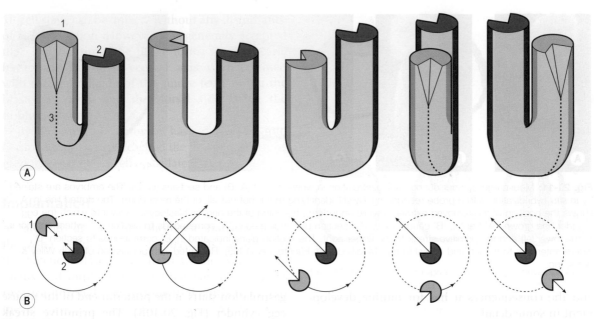

Fig. 20-12: Schematic model of turning of the mouse embryo. **A:** Three dimensional view of the embryo. 1: Ventral side of the posterior end of embryo (blue); 2: Dorsal side of the anterior end of embryo (red); 3: Neural axis. **B:** Sections of the schematic embryo. 1: Transverse section through the caudal end of the embryo; 2: Transverse section through the cranial end of the embryo. The straight arrows point to dorsal, the curved arrows indicate direction of turning. Modified from Kaufman (1992).

around its anterior end (Fig. 20-12). The invagination of the egg cylinder had originally placed the embryo inside the blastocyst cavity and, thus, in the **yolk sac** instead of on top of the yolk sac as in other species. As a consequence of the rotary movement during turning, the embryo stays in the yolk sac which thus becomes a prominent structure that covers the developing embryo and fetus until birth. This is in contrast to other mammals in which the yolk sac is a relatively small and more or less involuted 'appendix' during later fetal development. In order to get access to post-implantation mouse embryos, one has therefore to open two layers of tissue: the opaque and vascularized yolk sac and the thin and transparent yet quite stable amnion in which the embryo develops. Fig. 20-13 shows three embryos before, during and after turning.

After the turning of the embryo, murine development is similar to that of other mammalian embryos without significant mouse-specific variations.

Embryonic stem (ES) cells

Under suitable cell culture conditions, blastocysts will hatch from the zona pellucida and attach to the substrate, which often consists of mitotically inactive feeder cells such as embryonic fibroblasts. Eventually, the trophoblast cells will form a monolayer while the cells of the ICM will form a three dimensional colony. Certain signalling peptides, like LIF or BMP4, can prevent the ICM cells from differentiating and keep them in their original pluripotent stage as **embryonic stem (ES) cells** (Fig. 20-14). If re-introduced into a murine blastocyst by microinjection (Fig. 20-15), they have the potential to form any tissue of an adult mouse including germ cells. The resulting mouse, which is made up of a mixture of cells derived from the ICM of the recipient blastocyst and cells derived from the ES cells, is referred to as a **chimaera** (Figs 20-15, 20-16). However, the ES cells cannot contribute to

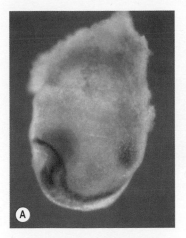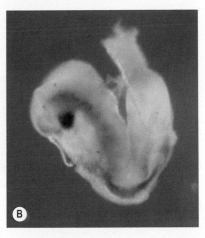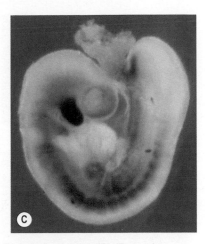

Fig. 20-13: Mouse embryos dE 8.0 before turning (A), dE 9.0 during turning (B) and dE 9.5 after turning (C). The embryos are stained by *in situ* hybridization with a probe recognizing *Twist1* identifying head mesenchyme and most, but not all, mesoderm. Modified from Füchtbauer (1995). Reprinted with permission of John Wiley & Sons, Inc.

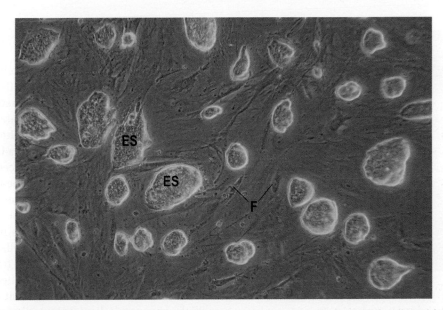

Fig. 20-14: Mouse ES cells form three dimensional colonies (ES) which are grown on mitotically inactivated feeder (F) cells, in this example primary mouse embryonic fibroblasts.

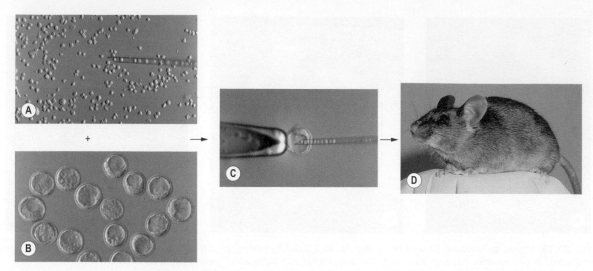

Fig. 20-15: Production of chimaeric mice from ES cells (A) and host blastocysts (B). ES cells are injected into the blastocyst cavity (C), blastocysts are than transferred into a pseudopregnant foster mother. Chimaeric offspring (D) can be recognized in this case by the presence of two coat colour genotypes: the agouti (brownish) colour originates from ES cells while the non-agouti (black) colour originates from the recipient blastocyst.

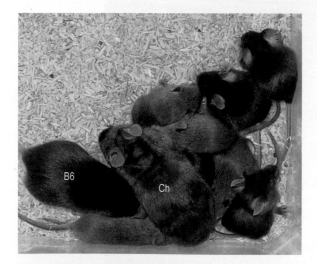

Fig. 20-16: A male mouse chimaera (Ch) developed from agouti (brownish, dominant) ES cells inserted into a non-agouti (black, recessive) blastocyst. The male was mated with a black C57Bl/6 female (B6). Sperm cells originating from host blastocyst cells will result in homozygous non-agouti black pups while sperm cells originating from ES cells will produce heterozygous agouti/ non-agouti pups that are phenotypically agouti.

extra-embryonic tissues like the placenta, for which the trophectoderm is required.

The scientific importance of ES cells lies in their dual character. As fast growing cells that can be **cultured indefinitely**, they can be **easily genetically manipulated** and selected for rare events like **homologous recombination**. As pluripotent stem cells, they can be re-introduced into a blastocyst and give rise to a chimaera consisting of cells originating from both the host blastocyst and the introduced ES cells. If the ES cells participate in germ cell formation, the chimaera can be used for breeding and result in pure genetically modified animals. It should be mentioned that, so far, no ES cells from species other than mice, and since 2008 from rat, have shown germ line competence. It has been speculated that the reason for this may be that diapause (by which mice can delay implantation of blastocysts, and which is missing in other species for which germline competent ES cells have not so far been established) is a physiological equivalent to the protracted lifespan of pluripotent ES cells. In recent years, ES cells have also gained a lot of attention as pluripotent stem cells that can be differentiated in culture and potentially used for regeneration or replacement therapies in a wide variety of diseases. In an aging society, this aspect of ES cell research can be expected to become of increasing interest and importance.

FURTHER READING

Copp, J. and Cockroft, D.L. (eds.) (1990): Postimplantation Mammalian Embryos: A Practical Approach. Oxford University Press, USA.

Füchtbauer, E.-M. (1995): Expression of *M-twist* during postimplantation development of the mouse. Dev. Dynamics 204:316–322.

Hedrich, H. (2004): The Laboratory Mouse. Academic Press, USA.

Kaufman, M.F. (1992): The Atlas of Mouse Development. Academic Press, USA.

Kaufman, M.F. and Bard, J.B.L. (1999): The Anatomical Basis of Mouse Development. Academic Press, USA.

Nagy, A., Gertsenstein, M., Vintersten, K. and Behringer, R. (eds.) (2003): Manipulating the Mouse Embryo: A Laboratory Manual. Cold Spring Harbor Laboratory Press, USA.

Rossant, J. and Tam, P. (2002): Mouse Development, Patterning, Morphogenesis, and Organogenesis. Academic Press, USA.

Theiler, K. (1989): The House Mouse. Springer-Verlag, New York, USA.

CHAPTER 21

Gábor Vajta, Henrik Callesen, Gry Boe-Hansen, Vanessa Hall and Poul Hyttel

Assisted reproduction technologies

Over thousands of years, mankind has slowly altered the traits of domestic animals to meet the needs of production. Over recent decades, more and more complicated manipulations of gametes and embryos have emerged as a means to that end. Collectively, these techniques are referred to as **assisted reproduction technologies (ARTs)**.

Assisted reproduction technologies are widely used in domestic animals, experimental animals (notably mice), and in man. However, it is important to stress that the goals of using the techniques in these three groups differ enormously. In the **mouse**, the technologies are used as a research tool, including the production of genetically modified animals; the production of 'knock-out' mice, for example, has been an extremely important tool in the analysis of gene function. In **man**, solving infertility problems is the focus, although recent research suggests that the therapeutic use of embryonic stem (ES) cells is likely to become an increasingly important application of the techniques in future.

The goals of reproduction technologies in the **domestic species** have gradually changed over the years. **Increased productivity** (especially milk yields and growth rates) and the elimination of venereal diseases were the first objectives; now the aims have been extended to encompass the achievement of **better health** in animals. Moreover, in recent years some of the technologies (genetic modifications mediated through cloning by somatic cell nuclear transfer, for example) have to some degree turned to the production of valuable experimental **animal models** for biomedical research. The emphasis placed on these different goals varies greatly in different parts of the world. Hence, in the Western

countries with their plentiful food supplies and high standards of living, technologies such as cloning and genetic modification are applied only to biomedical goals. This is because of public concern over safety and ethical issues when biotechnology is proposed for use in food production. On the other hand, in the Far East (China especially) the technologies are more openly accepted not only as research tools, but as potential means of improving the quantity and quality of food. At present, we are in a delicate balance between Western and Eastern technological development; the exponential phase of development in the East includes the reproduction technologies, and it will be very exciting to see what the coming years bring.

This chapter will focus on the applications of ARTs in the domestic species, but with a brief mention of some of the more medically oriented technologies used in the treatment of human infertility.

ARTIFICIAL INSEMINATION

Artificial insemination (AI) is the oldest ART. It was refined in cattle during the 1930s and 1940s and gradually became the most valuable breeding tool so far developed. Discovery in 1949 of the cryoprotective properties of glycerol during the freezing and thawing of sperm cells revolutionized the practical use of AI in cattle reproduction. The technology has been, and remains, of enormous significance in **improving production and health** traits through an effective use of superior male animals, as well as in **eliminating certain venereal diseases**.

The procedural steps of AI will be described for cattle, with the peculiarities of pig, horse, small ruminant, and dog and cat AI discussed subsequently. Basic parameters of the semen of each of these species are presented in Table 21-1.

Artificial insemination in cattle

Semen collection

Characteristics of the ejaculate vary greatly between species with respect to **semen volume** and **concentration**, the number of **fractions** in which it is delivered, and the duration of the ejaculation process. The techniques employed for semen collection vary correspondingly. The male is normally allowed to mount a phantom during the procedure. In cattle, an **artificial vagina** is used. This comprises a lubricated rubber cylinder, warmed by a water jacket, with a funnel leading to a vial into which the semen is collected. Semen from bulls may alternatively be collected through stimulation of the urethra and accessory genital glands using an electric rectal probe (electroejaculation) or by transrectal massage. When collected, the ejaculate should be quickly transported to the laboratory (with minimal exposure to light and abrupt temperature changes) where a primary dilution in an **extender** – a special medium that is well suited for preserving the viability of the spermatozoa – is performed. After this primary dilution, the semen is ready for evaluation and further processing, including secondary dilution and packaging.

Semen evaluation

Evaluating the semen is an extremely important step in preparing it for further processing. If the semen is to be used to inseminate many females, it needs to be divided and packaged into doses. This division, based on the evaluation results, provides a constant number of viable spermatozoa per dose. The most simple semen evaluation includes examination of the **concentration**, **progressive motility** and **morphological normality** of the spermatozoa.

Table 21-1: Characteristics of normal ejaculates in domestic animals

	Stallion	Bull	Ram	Boar	Dog
Duration of ejaculation	30–60 sec	1 sec	1 sec	5–25 min	1–45 min
Normal site of deposition of semen	Vagina and uterus	Vagina	Vagina	Uterus	Vagina
Volume of ejaculate	30–100 ml	5–10 ml	0.5–2 ml	30–300 ml	0.5–50 ml
Fractions	Three	One	One	Three	Three
Concentration of spermatozoa	$100–800 \times 10^6$/ml	$500–3,000 \times 10^6$/ml	$3,000–6,000 \times 10^6$/ml	$100–500 \times 10^6$/ml	$4–400 \times 10^6$/ml
Progressive motility (%)	>50	>70	>90	>80	>60
Recommended number of viable spermatozoa per semen dose					
– Fresh	500×10^6	5×10^6	300×10^6	2000×10^6	150×10^6
– Cryopreserved	250×10^6	15×10^6	400×10^6	5000×10^6	200×10^6

The concentration of spermatozoa in an ejaculate is a major quality characteristic and determines how many doses can be produced from a particular semen collection. The concentration is normally assessed by photometry, microscopy, or flow cytometry.

The motility of the spermatozoa can be evaluated by phase contrast light microscopy using a heated microscope stage. It is expressed as the percentage of spermatozoa displaying progressive motility, i.e. directed movement. This parameter can also be assessed by **computer assisted sperm analysis (CASA)** in which special software calculates ratios of linearity and progressive motility based on microscopic real-time image recording.

The morphology of the spermatozoa is normally assessed by traditional light microscopy from a smear subjected to simple negative staining, with Eosin Nigrosin or Giemsa stain for example. This is adequate to reveal defects of the sperm head, neck and middle and principal piece of the tail – defects that, in the worst cases, can render the semen sample useless.

The qualities required of a spermatozoon if it is to fertilize an oocyte and initiate early embryonic development go well beyond its motility and morphology. Consequently, additional ways of assessing the quality of individual spermatozoa are being developed. These include measures of the integrity of the sperm membrane, acrosome, mitochondria and DNA, as well as competence for sperm-oocyte interaction. Sperm membrane integrity (presumed to be a measure of viability) may be evaluated by double staining of the spermatozoa in suspension with two DNA staining dyes, one that is permeating and therefore stains DNA in live as well as dead spermatozoa (e.g. Hoechst and SYBR) and a second (often propidium iodide) that stains only dead cells because it cannot penetrate live cell membranes. The stained spermatozoa are then examined by fluorescence microscopy or **flow cytometry**, using appropriate excitation wavelengths, to determine the proportions of live and dead spermatozoa.

Other potential indicators of sperm quality and fertilizing capability that are under investigation include: the measurement of sperm energy metabolism; damage to sperm DNA (by the **sperm chro-** matin structure assay (SCSA), TUNEL, and Comet assays, for example); and the ability to undergo the acrosome reaction (e.g. by the **in vitro acrosome reaction, IVAR**). To detect DNA damage by the SCSA, spermatozoa are stained with acridine orange, which stains double-stranded DNA to emit green fluorescence and single-stranded DNA to emit red fluorescence. By flow cytometry using the appropriate laser excitation wavelength, a dot plot indicating the proportion of spermatozoa with intact double-stranded DNA can be produced. These plots can apparently be related to the potential of the sperm sample to fertilize and initiate embryonic development. In the IVAR test, spermatozoa are chemically induced (by treatment with calcium ionophores, for example) to undergo the acrosome reaction in vitro. The proportion of acrosome-reacted spermatozoa can be assessed by flow cytometry after staining by certain fluorochrome-coupled lectins that bind only to the inner acrosomal membrane and therefore do not stain spermatozoa that remain acrosome-intact. Again, there is apparently a relationship between the IVAR dot plots and the fertilizing capability of the sperm sample. However, further research is needed in order to standardize these and other advanced techniques before they become practical for routine semen evaluation.

Semen dilution, packaging and freezing

After evaluation, the semen is ready for **dilution** and **packaging**. There are species-specific requirements of the storage medium for spermatozoa; factors of importance for the survival of the spermatozoa include the ionic strength, pH, osmolality and presence of antimicrobial compounds in the medium. If the semen is to be frozen in liquid nitrogen, cryoprotectants such as glycerol must also be added.

The extent to which a semen sample can be diluted depends upon parameters determined during its evaluation. In cattle, the frozen semen doses are normally produced to contain between 15 and 20×10^6 progressively motile spermatozoa.

After packaging, the semen doses must be stored properly until used for insemination. In cattle, this is usually by **cryopreservation.** The doses are prepared by dilution of the semen sample with a cryoprotective extender, usually so that each dose can be packed into a plastic straw containing 0.25 ml. The straws are then frozen, either by suspension in the vapour above liquid nitrogen for 10 min or by using a microprocessor-controlled freezer, and stored in liquid nitrogen until used. Thawing (which should immediately precede insemination) needs to be rapid; slow thawing leads to extensive crystallization of water and consequent damage to sperm membranes.

Insemination

It is crucial that insemination be performed **when the female is receptive for copulation**, i.e. when she is in **oestrus**. Oestrus detection requires both a trained eye and regular observations several times per day. This is labour intensive and therefore expensive and so several mechanical and electronic devices have been produced to assist in heat monitoring; none of them, however, fully replaces the accuracy of a teaser male or the devoted stockperson's eye.

In cattle, just one insemination per oestrus is normally used. Insemination is performed by guiding the end of the insemination catheter, loaded with one straw of semen, per vaginam to the interior os of the cervix uteri by rectal palpation. The cow or heifer presents a prominent portio vaginalis of the cervix, and the cervical canal is characterized by numerous circular plicae facing caudally. To negotiate these anatomical obstacles it is necessary to maintain a firm grip of the cervix per rectum while passing the catheter. The semen is deposited in the uterus.

Artificial insemination in the pig

A phantom is used for support of the boar during ejaculation, and the semen collection is performed using the gloved-hand technique, which involves a steady firm pressure applied to the spiral-shaped portion of the penis. The ejaculate of the boar is fractionated, and so collection is normally done through a filter cloth to avoid mixing the more gelatinous portion with the sperm-rich fraction (Fig. 21-1).

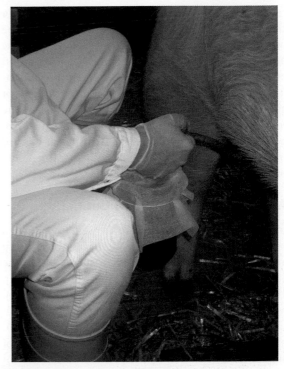

Fig. 21-1: Collection of semen from a boar through a filter cloth.

Artificial insemination has become gradually more widespread in countries with intensive pig production. The major drawback has been the relatively **poor survival of boar spermatozoa after cryopreservation**; they survive much more poorly after freezing than after storage at 16–18°C. Thus, diluted fresh semen is generally used and this poses logistical problems for both its production and distribution. The poor survival of cryopreservation by boar spermatozoa is primarily due to their high susceptibility to cold shock, which may be related to the lipid composition of their membranes and their relatively high content of cholesterol. Insemination doses from the boar are usually packaged in tubes or plastic bags containing about $2–3 \times 10^9$ spermatozoa in 70–80 ml.

Insemination of the sow or gilt is easy because the porcine cervix presents neither a portio vaginalis nor circular plicae. Instead, the vagina gradually leads into the cervix through a funnel and, in the cervical canal, the pulvini cervicales create a softer closure. This allows the insemination catheter to be positioned with its tip firmly interlocked with the pulvini cervicales, just as the spiral-shaped portion of the penis would be during copulation. Interestingly, it is now clear that stimulation of the sow or gilt by massage and riding on the back improves the results of insemination by helping the uterus transport semen to the oviducts. Often, a repeat insemination is performed if oestrus is sufficiently prolonged (see Chapter 2).

Artificial insemination in the horse

In the horse, the stallion is allowed to mount a phantom or teaser mare and semen is collected using an artificial vagina. The gel fraction and debris of the ejaculate should be removed using a nontoxic filter. The collected semen can be used fresh, cooled (5°C), or frozen-thawed, using appropriate extenders. Typically, an insemination dose contains $250-500 \times 10^6$ progressively motile spermatozoa in a volume of 10–25 ml. For frozen semen, straws of 0.5–4.0 ml are used and insemination doses should contain a minimum of 250×10^6 progressive motile sperm post thawing. The lower number of spermatozoa used for frozen semen allows for production of more straws per ejaculate. Successful use, however, requires that insemination is performed close to the time of ovulation. The semen is normally deposited by catheter in the corpus uteri, using a lubricated gloved finger in guiding the tip of the insemination catheter into the cervical lumen. For specialized purposes (e.g. when using sex-sorted semen) low-dose insemination close to the ostium tubae uterinae can be accomplished through a hysteroscope. The wide opening and lumen of the cervix in the mare provides easy passage of an insemination catheter or hysteroscope into the uterus.

Artificial insemination in small ruminants

In the ram and buck, semen is collected through an artificial vagina as from the bull and stallion. A female, preferably in oestrus, or a phantom can be used for the male to mount. Ejaculation is com-pleted within seconds and the ejaculate is low in volume, but high in concentration of sperm, in both species. Semen can also be collected by electro-ejaculation. The collected semen can be used either fresh or frozen-thawed using appropriate extenders. Typically, an insemination dose contains $300-500 \times 10^6$ progressive motile spermatozoa for intravaginal insemination, $100-200 \times 10^6$ progressively motile spermatozoa for intracervical insemination, or 50×10^6 sperm for intrauterine insemination. In the ewe the semen is deposited either in the cranial part of the vagina or in the cervical canal. The method of direct intrauterine insemination using laparoscopy has been developed to overcome some of the difficulties of intravaginal and intracervical insemination, especially by reducing the number of spermatozoa required. In the goat the semen may be deposited either intracervically or into the uterus, with less difficulty than in the ewe.

Artificial insemination in the dog and cat

In the dog, semen is collected into a wide-mouth glass or plastic vial or a disposable semen collection cone by digital manipulation. The penis is massaged through the prepuce until an erection of the bulbus glandis and pars longa glandis occurs. The prepuce is then moved caudally so that both the bulbus and pars longa glandis of the penis are exposed. Tightening the grip, the penis is then rotated 180° caudally, keeping the dorsum of the penis dorsal. Only the second fraction of the ejaculate is collected; the first and third fractions consist of prostatic fluid and are discarded. The semen is collected in the presence of a teaser bitch, preferably in oestrus. At insemination, the semen can be placed into either the vagina or the uterus. Intravaginal insemination is uncomplicated and is most commonly used. However, with cryopreserved semen intrauterine insemination is preferred. This can be done either transcervically using a vaginoscope, or surgically through the uterine wall by laparoscopy or laparotomy. Surgery may become necessary due to problems caused by the dorsal position of the portio vaginalis and difficulties in immobilizing the cervix.

Collection of semen from a tomcat requires extensive training and patience, and the presence of a receptive female. Semen can be collected in a tiny artificial vagina customized for rabbits. Alternatively, semen can be collected using electro-ejaculation after sedation. Insemination is intravaginal.

Sex sorting of spermatozoa

Livestock owners have for years sought methods for predetermining and controlling the sex of offspring in their herds for economic reasons. The obvious example is in the dairy industry, where heifer calves are far more valuable than bull calves.

The ability to separate and sort functional spermatozoa according to whether they carry the **X**- or the **Y-chromosome** became a reality in the 1990s, based on their different DNA contents (Fig. 21-2). When stained with the DNA-binding dye Hoechst 33342, X-chromosome-bearing spermatozoa absorb more of the dye than do Y-chromosome-bearing. As a consequence, the X-chromosome-bearing spermatozoa will emit more light than will the Y-chromosome-bearing when excited by a laser in a flow cytometer. In the flow cytometer, this difference is measured extremely rapidly in individual stained spermatozoa, each in its separate micro-droplet formed by pumping the semen sample through a special nozzle at high pressure. An electromagnetic charge (positive, negative, or no charge) is then applied to each micro-droplet depending on the DNA content of the spermatozoon within the droplet, and these can then be directed to one side or the other depending on charge. Furthermore, selection of only viable, membrane-intact spermatozoa is made possible by staining with a food dye. Two defined populations of spermatozoa are therefore achieved after flow cytometric sorting using this method; one vial primarily containing viable X-chromosome-bearing spermatozoa, and another primarily containing viable Y-chromosome-bearing spermatozoa. The method has provided a means of determining the efficacy of any sperm sex-sorting enrichment approach, and is the basis for the sperm sexing system that is now used commercially to predetermine the sex of offspring in several species,

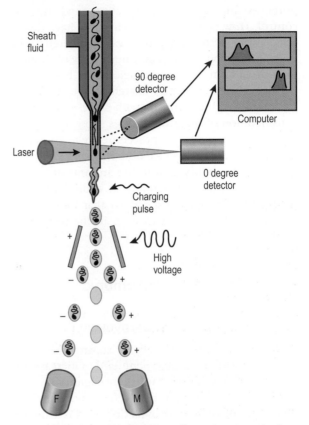

Fig. 21-2: Sorting of X- and Y-bearing spermatozoa by flow cytometry.

primarily cattle. Flow cytometric sex-sorting of spermatozoa according to their DNA content is patented and is sub-licensed for mammals (non-human) to XY Inc., through Colorado State University. Species variation in factors such as DNA content and sperm head size make it necessary to optimize sorting conditions species by species to achieve acceptable results. In cattle, the sperm sexing efficiency is about 90% in a commercial setting.

MULTIPLE OVULATION AND EMBRYO TRANSFER

It has been the detailed knowledge of embryonic development and reproductive biology that has made it possible to use embryos for commercial purposes in breeding, production, and disease control. How embryo-based techniques have developed varies with species because of differences in the anatomy, physiology, and husbandry of domestic animals but the technologies have been most widely applied in cattle. Therefore, the following paragraphs will deal mostly with cattle, with briefer consideration of the other species subsequently.

The basic steps in the procedure are to stimulate a **donor** female to produce desirable embryos, then to **collect** the embryos from her and **transfer** them to unmated **recipient** females at equivalent post-ovulatory reproductive stages so that the donor's embryos will be carried to term in the recipients' uteri.

Multiple ovulation and embryo transfer in cattle

Multiple ovulation ('superovulation')

Multiple ovulation results from superovulation or superstimulation – a treatment used to increase the number of ovulations (and thence embryos) in a donor above the norm for a given species. For cattle this means three or more ovulations, and is achieved in three steps. First, the donor is injected with a **drug with FSH or FSH-like activity** once, or over a period of days, in the mid-luteal phase. Second, **oestrus is induced** by causing luteolysis with an injection of prostaglandin-$F_{2\alpha}$ or its analogue approximately 3 days after beginning the FSH treatment. Third, during the induced oestrus, the donor is **inseminated**, usually once or twice, so that she will provide multiple embryos. **Embryo recovery** is usually practised **6–7 days** after the onset of standing heat.

Methods for inducing superovulation. One of the first hormones used to induce superovulation in cattle was the placental gonadotropin Pregnant Mare's Serum Gonadotropin (PMSG) or, more correctly, **equine chorionic gonadotrophin (eCG)**. This is a glycoprotein produced by the endometrial cups around Days 50–80 of pregnancy in mares and can be isolated from their serum. Because eCG has a long half-life (about 5 days) following its injection into cattle, it only has to be injected once. However, residual amounts of eCG remain in the circulation throughout the subsequent periods of ovulation and early embryonic development and this may adversely affect the environments (follicles, oviducts and uterus) in which the oocytes, zygotes, and early embryos develop. **Follicle stimulating hormone (FSH)** is one of the pituitary gonadotropins and is currently the substance most widely used for superovulating cattle. In contrast to eCG, FSH has a short half-life (about 5 h), and therefore has to be injected repeatedly, normally twice daily for 3–4 days, to maintain stimulatory levels in the circulation. FSH is available in various commercial preparations derived mainly from pituitary glands of pigs or sheep.

Timing of superovulation in the oestrous cycle. The start of the **superovulation treatment must be co-ordinated with the ovarian follicular waves**. The follicles most responsive to the treatment are those in their growing or plateau phase of the wave, or possibly in their early atretic phase. The first gonadotropin injection is most often given on Day 8–12 of the oestrous cycle. Giving several FSH injections over a period of days is laborious and stresses the donor animals, especially those not used to being handled. Reducing the number of FSH injections to a single daily injection given for 4, 3 or 2 days, or even for 1 day, has therefore been tried. In spite of the short half-life of FSH, the results have been good, but reducing the number of injections seems to increase the variability in the superovulatory response.

Insemination of the donor cow. The prostaglandin (or analogue) given to induce oestrus is injected either once, or twice at a 12 h interval, starting approximately 3 days after initiation of the eCG or FSH treatment. Following the prostaglandin injection, the donor has to be observed closely for external signs of heat. Superovulated cows often do not show oestrous behaviour as clearly as untreated cows do, and it may occur at irregular intervals. The first insemination is usually carried out approximately 12 h after the onset of standing oestrus, and a second about 12 h later. In instances of prolonged heat, three and even four inseminations may be required.

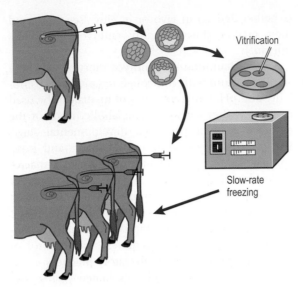

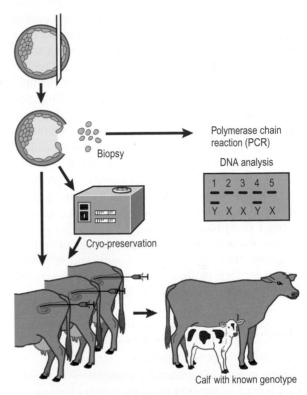

Fig. 21-3: Embryo transfer in cattle. Embryos at the morula to blastocyst stage are collected from a donor cow and transferred to synchronized recipients after cryopreservation by either slow-rate freezing or vitrification.

Fig. 21-4: Isolation of a sample of trophectoderm by biopsy of a bovine blastocyst for PCR detection of its Y-chromosome content. The embryo may be transferred directly or cryopreserved while the analysis is performed.

Selection of potential donor cows. Because the superovulatory treatment stresses the donor's endocrine system, selecting a potential donor should include minimization of other stressful factors. A donor should show regular oestrous cyclicity, be in a good **nutritional state**, not have calved recently or be recovering from a **disease**, and have **normal genital organs** upon a thorough clinical examination.

Embryo recovery

Embryos are recovered 6–8 days after the onset of oestrus (Fig. 21-3). At this stage most embryos will have passed through the oviduct and entered the uterine horns, still surrounded by the zona pellucida. They are therefore accessible for collection through a **non-surgical flushing of the uterine cavity**. At this stage the embryos are fairly tolerant to handling, not only during their recovery but also in additional procedures such as **cryopreservation** (see later) or **biopsy** to isolate cells for sex determination (Fig. 21-4).

The procedure for embryo recovery. Embryos are collected by flushing, either both uterine horns at one time or each horn separately, using a special transcervical catheter with an inflatable cuff to occlude the lumen of the horn. The most commonly used **flushing medium** is modified phosphate-buffered saline (PBS) that contains glucose and pyruvate, substrates that are beneficial for post-compaction bovine embryonic development. The phosphate buffer helps keep the pH of the medium stable under practical conditions. Other additions are usually serum or bovine serum albumin (BSA) to provide nutrients and to prevent the embryos from sticking to plastic surfaces during the flushing and handling, and some form of antibiotic to minimize the risk of uterine infection. **Epidural analgesia** is routinely used during the non-surgical collection; it facilitates rectal manipulations of the genital tract and the collection catheter, and makes the animal stand more quietly both by reducing her discomfort and because she senses reduced control of her hind legs. Flushing fluid is introduced into the uterine cavity until, by rectal palpation, the uterus is judged to be sufficiently distended, at which point the fluid is drained into a collection vessel. The filling and emptying is repeated several times with additional fluid to ensure that the cavity is properly flushed. The combined flushes are filtered through a mesh that retains the embryos but allows debris and blood cells to pass. After this filtration, the reduced volume of flushing fluid above the mesh (and appropriate rinses) must be searched for embryos, using a stereomicroscope.

The results of embryo recovery. The rates of embryo recovery after superovulation vary widely, influenced by factors already described. However, the overall results can be summarized as follows:

- Approximately 5% of the treated donors are not flushed due to a poor response to the superovulatory treatment.
- No transferable embryos are recovered from 20–30% of the flushed donors either because no ova/embryos were recovered, or because none of those recovered were transferable.
- The average total number of ova/embryos per flushed donor is 8–10.
- The average total number of transferable embryos per flushed donor is 5–6.

Embryo handling

Most embryos are transferred at the **late morula or blastocyst stage**; stages that, in vivo, are obtained by flushing donors about 6–7 days after insemination. After collection the embryos need to be handled for evaluation and transfer, and possibly for other procedures such as biopsy or cryopreservation for long-term storage.

Embryo handling requires that they be kept under in vitro conditions outside an incubator, and the handling conditions are crucial with respect to both time and the medium used. The length of the handling period should be as short as possible. The tolerance of the embryos depends on their origin

(whether derived in vivo or in vitro; see later) and their quality (lower quality embryos being less tolerant).

During handling the embryos must be kept in a sterile medium with controlled temperature, osmolality and pH. Different types of media can be used as long as they satisfy the metabolic needs of the embryos at their particular developmental stage. For cattle embryos at the compaction and post-compaction stages, PBS with addition of a macromolecule such as BSA or serum is adequate. All materials with which the embryos will be in contact (glassware, disposable plastic filters, dishes, pipettes etc.) must meet stringent standards of quality, cleanliness and sterility. This requires strict control of both manufacturing and laboratory practices.

Embryos are normally evaluated using the **grading system** proposed by the International Embryo Transfer Society (IETS); each is evaluated under a microscope at a magnification of at least 50× and is classified under two codes of description, one for stage of development, and one for quality. The stages described are the main ones from the unfertilized oocyte to the expanding hatched blastocyst. Four measures of quality are used: from excellent to dead, based on the number and appearance of the cells in relation to the embryo's developmental stage.

Embryo transfer

When ready for transfer, the embryo is aspirated into a small **plastic straw** (of the type used for bovine insemination) in a small volume (usually 0.25 ml) of the handling medium.

Selection of recipients is based on whether they had exhibited external signs of heat at about the same time as the donor, and a thorough gynaecological examination including evaluation of the consistency of the uterine horns and location (left or right ovary) of a palpable protruding corpus luteum.

Synchrony between the embryo and the recipient is optimal when the embryo is transferred to a recipient at exactly the same post-ovulatory stage as the donor. However, for good-quality embryos, pregnancy rates are not affected by asynchronies of as much as 36 hours; embryos of poorer quality, on the other hand, seem less tolerant of asynchrony.

The actual transfer is usually done via a catheter passed **non-surgically through the cervix** (with the aid of rectal palpation) to deposit the embryo in the uterine cavity. Normally a single embryo is transferred to the uterine horn ipsilateral to the ovary containing the corpus luteum.

After non-surgical transfer under good field conditions, it is possible to obtain an overall pregnancy rate of 50–70%. Again, this outcome is variable and depends on many factors. One important consequence of this variability is that a considerable proportion of flushed donors fail to provide any calves.

After pregnancy has been confirmed (i.e. at approximately Day 40–50 after transfer), the calving rate is similar to that obtained after artificial insemination, with an abortion rate of approximately 5%. At late gestation or at birth the congenital defects are within the normal range, i.e. 0.2–2%.

Practical uses of multiple ovulation and embryo transfer

Embryo transfer is used to its best advantage in specialized breeding programmes in which it can **increase the number of calves originating from donor cattle of high genetic value**. Similar exploitation of genetically valuable bulls has been possible for 50 years through the use of artificial insemination.

Although embryo transfer is a relatively simple technology, requiring only simple equipment, it does require efficient infrastructure and management, especially the reproductive management of both the donors and recipients. It is because of these expenses and investments that the value of each embryo/calf produced has to be rather high, limiting the application of embryo transfer primarily to donors of high genetic and monetary value. Nevertheless, although embryo transfer is used much less than artificial insemination in cattle production, its impact is disproportionately high because most of the bulls used as semen donors for artificial insemination are produced from transferred embryos.

Embryo transfer has other uses, too. From a **sanitary** point of view it is a safer, cheaper, simpler and more efficient way to transport genetic quality than is the shipment of live animals; disease control at the level of embryos rather than live animals is much easier and, after transplantation, the native recipient can provide the offspring with passive immunity to local diseases. Thus, for **conservation of farm animal genetic resources** embryo transfer is a good means of exchanging genetic material and maintaining genetic diversity. Whereas frozen semen has long facilitated this on the male side, embryo transfer offers the possibility of storing the entire genetic makeup of a given strain. It must be remembered, however, that such conservation is not in line with all objectives of conservation because banked genetics do not contribute actively to improvement programmes.

A systematic application of embryo transfer is in the so-called **MOET breeding programmes** in which young females are genetically selected and multiplied by using multiple ovulation (MO) and embryo transfer (ET). In contrast to traditional progeny testing, MOET schemes use embryo transfer to create large full-sib or half-sib families from which information is gathered on a bull's sisters rather than on his daughters before deciding whether the bull should be culled or retained as a sire. Through MOET, the decision can be made approximately two years earlier than by a progeny test. Several MOET programmes were designed and tested in different countries with the first practical trials appearing in the mid-1980s on national, regional or breed scales, or within a company. The genetic advantages were demonstrated and evidenced by the large number of top bulls obtained in this way. However, the schemes also underlined the limitations of embryo transfer, notably the variability of the superovulation response, and the expense of operating recipient herds, as discussed earlier.

Multiple ovulation and embryo transfer in pigs

Hormonal stimulation to increase the number of ovulations is **not often used** because the inherently high ovulation rate in pigs makes it unnecessary. Hormonal interventions are, however, used for synchronization purposes in timing embryo collection. This is especially true when young pigs (gilts) are used; in sows, the natural synchronization following weaning is often adequate.

Embryos are recovered **surgically**, under full anaesthesia and using a flank or midline approach to the uterus. The uterine horns are flushed through a flared tube or cuffed catheter inserted through an incision or bluntly made puncture, and the embryos are collected and handled as described for cattle.

Pig embryos are generally considered to be much more sensitive to handling than are cattle embryos. This limits the number of treatments that they will tolerate. However, the last decade has brought about significant improvements in this situation, especially in cryopreservation (see later).

The transfer of embryos is also performed surgically under full anaesthesia but instruments for non-surgical transfer are under development.

The naturally high reproductive capacity of the pig has dampened the interest in developing embryo transfer technology in pigs compared to cattle. Still, the technology is of considerable usefulness, both industrially and for research, for reasons similar to those explained for cattle. These include allowing movement of genetic resources with enhanced animal welfare, minimal risk of disease transmission and reduced transportation costs in comparison with transport of live animals. However, it is only during the last decade that application of the technology has started to expand, thanks to several technical advances, and also stimulated by the increasing use of pigs in medical research as a model animal for certain human diseases.

Multiple ovulation and embryo transfer in horses

Horses are very **difficult to superovulate**, for both physiological and anatomical reasons; the anatomy of the ovaries may hinder ovulation of larger numbers of follicles than usual over a short time period. Therefore, most embryo recoveries are from normally cycling mares.

Embryo collection, handling and transfer are basically as described for the cow because of the similarities in animal size and anatomy of the reproductive organs.

The rejection of all modern breeding techniques in some of the most prominent horse-breeding societies has limited the acceptance and practice of equine embryo transfer. However, that situation is changing and, in recent years, the numbers of transferred embryos have increased, though they remain much lower than in cattle. It is expected that this expansion will continue, fuelled by various breakthroughs in other reproductive technologies.

Multiple ovulation and embryo transfer in small ruminants

Superovulation is performed according to the same principles as for the cow, with synchronization often accomplished with intravaginal sponges or plastic devices that release progesterone.

Embryo collection and transfer are currently done **surgically** because of the small size of the animals. However, attempts are being made to develop non-surgical embryo transfer methods.

In sheep and goats, multiple ovulation and embryo transfer has been an established technology for many years. It is an essential component of the international trade of genetic resources, facilitates the conservation of endangered species or breeds, and provides an additional genetic tool for dairy breeders owning highly productive flocks that are near the limit of genetic gain attainable through the use of artificial insemination.

Multiple ovulation and embryo transfer in carnivores

Though not used very much in these species, embryo transfer has been applied successfully under special circumstances of commercial interest, for experimental purposes and for preserving endangered species (tigers, for example). In spite of these successes, all aspects of the procedures still require much improvement to make them more practicable.

IN VITRO PRODUCTION OF EMBRYOS

Among the domestic species, it is in **cattle that in vitro production of embryos has been most successful**. Porcine embryos can also be produced in vitro, but their viability is severely compromised as compared to embryos produced naturally. Although it is now possible to produce bovine embryos in vitro with viabilities comparable with those produced naturally (in vivo), the technology has not found widespread practical use. One reason may be that, at least during the optimization of these technologies, transfer of in-vitro-produced bovine embryos, particularly those cloned by somatic cell nuclear transfer (see later), led to an increased frequency of fetal overweight at calving, associated decreased labour activity in recipients, and consequent calving problems. Collectively, this condition became known as the **large offspring syndrome (LOS),** although the increased birth weight is not the only feature of the syndrome and sometimes does not occur at all. Very recently, it has been discovered that LOS is probably associated with aberrant expression of imprinted genes (such as the IGF2 receptor) that are of great importance for fetal growth and, in particular, placental development. The vastly improved techniques of embryo culture in recent years have now resolved most of the problems of LOS. While the practical potential of in vitro embryo production in animal husbandry remains to be realized, the technology has been and still is a valuable tool in embryological research, allowing direct observation and investigation of fertilization and embryonic development up to the blastocyst stage.

In vitro production of embryos in the domestic species is normally performed in three steps: **oocyte maturation, fertilization** and, finally, **embryo culture** (Fig. 21-5). Each will be described briefly, using cattle as an example.

In vitro production of embryos in cattle

Oocyte collection and in vitro maturation

The objective of in vitro maturation of the oocyte is to mimic the natural preovulatory maturation of the

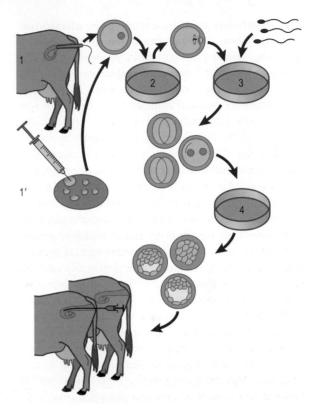

Fig. 21-5: In vitro production of embryos in cattle. Immature oocytes are aspirated from live animals by ultrasound-guided ovum pick up (1) or from abattoir ovaries (1'). Immature oocytes at prophase I are submitted to in vitro maturation (2) resulting in progression of meiosis to metaphase II, in vitro fertilization (3) resulting in pronucleus formation, and in vitro culture (4) to the morula or blastocyst stage, at which time they can be transferred to recipients.

oocyte in the follicle in vivo, as stimulated by the preovulatory LH-surge. This is when the oocyte completes its nuclear (meiotic) and cytoplasmic maturation preparing it for fertilization. As long ago as the 1930s it was discovered that oocytes released from the inhibitory environment of the follicle (which keeps meiosis blocked at the diplotene stage of prophase I) spontaneously resume meiosis and complete nuclear maturation to metaphase II. Later it was found that the maturation was not only nuclear but also cytoplasmic, and could be mimicked in vitro.

Oocytes used for in vitro embryo production may originate from **ovaries collected at the** slaughterhouse or may be retrieved by **ultrasound-guided ovum pickup** from genetically valuable animals. Most laboratories producing bovine embryos in vitro routinely collect ovaries at the slaughterhouse several times per week. At the laboratory, the contents of follicles larger than 2–3 mm are aspirated by means of a needle and vacuum pump and the oocytes are isolated from the follicular fluid by stereomicroscopy. This, of course, provides an extremely **mixed population of oocytes** for further culture: some oocytes come from healthy antral follicles, others from follicles that are more or less atretic. Therefore, oocytes without a cumulus investment (generally from atretic follicles) are discarded, having lost their developmental competence. In the case of ovaries from genetically valuable animals, oocytes may be more efficiently harvested by slicing the ovary with a set of several razor blades mounted in parallel about 1 mm apart; this chopping releases more oocytes from more follicles at various stages of development, including oocytes in their growth phase in secondary and small tertiary follicles. The oocyte's growth phase ends, and its active transcription ceases, at a diameter (inside the zona pellucida) of around 110 μm, corresponding to the time when the oocyte becomes fully competent to mature to metaphase II and to sustain initial embryonic development.

After washing in an appropriate medium, the oocytes are allowed to **mature in vitro** in a medium supplemented with hormones with FSH and LH activity for 24 hours. At the end of this maturation, between 80 and 90% of the oocytes have extruded the first polar body and reached metaphase II. Moreover, the cumulus investment has expanded and formed a loose layer in which the cells are embedded in a matrix of hyaluronic acid.

In vitro fertilization

For **in vitro fertilization**, the oocytes are co-cultured with spermatozoa separated from fresh or commercially available frozen semen, depending on the species. Efforts to establish new evaluation methods for sperm quality and ability to induce normal embryo development have not become very practical and, in most laboratories, post-thaw motility is still the only test used routinely; the quality of a particular batch of semen is generally judged from the rates of embryo production that it gives.

Various techniques are used to prepare the **spermatozoa**, most commonly centrifugation of the spermatozoa in a percol gradient followed by the so-called 'swim-up' separation: progressively motile spermatozoa are capable of swimming up into the more superficial layers of the fluid columns, away from their inactive counterparts. Capacitation of spermatozoa in the uterus and oviduct is, of course, not possible in vitro. Hence, to **promote capacitation in vitro**, some laboratories treat the spermatozoa with Ca^{++} ionophore, but most use heparin treatment before and/or after addition of spermatozoa to the oocytes. To stimulate sperm motility, a mixture of penicillinamine, hypotaurine and epinephrine is commonly added to the fertilization medium, although the efficacy of such treatment has been questioned.

Two features in particular underline how markedly different are fertilization in vitro and fertilization in the oviduct: first, the spermatozoa/oocyte ratio is approximately 10^3–10^4 times higher in vitro than in vivo; second, the oocytes usually remain surrounded by cumulus cells in vitro whereas in the large domestic species these cells are largely shed during or shortly after ovulation in vivo. The seemingly feasible explanation that the high number of spermatozoa is needed to overcome the cumulus barrier has not really been substantiated because similarly high spermatozoa/oocyte ratios are required to fertilize cumulus-denuded oocytes. Indeed, removing the cumulus cells from the zona pellucida may actually *decrease* the percentage of penetrated oocytes without increasing the rate of polyspermic fertilization. Attempts to mimic, in vitro, the much lower spermatozoa/oocyte ratio and the cumulus cell investment that prevail in vivo have generally resulted in decreased rates of fertilization and blastocyst formation. The reasons for this are not clear; however, it is hardly surprising that fertilization in the two locales should differ considerably, and that abnormalities in the process should be frequently encountered in vitro.

The suggested length of the co-culture of gametes varies from 5 to 30 hours. Many laboratories opt for a period of about 20 hours which, from a practical point of view, allows for convenient incubation from one day to the next.

In vitro embryo culture

For practical reasons, cattle embryos produced in vitro are most conveniently **cultured for about 7 days** by which time they have become blastocysts, the stage they would be at in the uterus. This makes them suitable for simple non-surgical transfer to the uterus, as described earlier for embryo transfer in general. If earlier embryonic stages need to be transferred after shorter culture in vitro, they have to be placed in the oviduct in order to survive. Oviduct transfer of embryos is a much more complicated procedure that demands surgical or laparoscopic intervention.

Recently, great efforts have been made to **improve the in vitro culture systems** for bovine embryos. Extensive studies of the environment in the oviduct and uterus have shown that complex combinations of autocrine, paracrine (including oviduct-specific proteins) and other environmental factors regulate embryonic growth. Most of these are produced by the embryos themselves or by the oviductal epithelium. To create an analogous environment in vitro, co-culture of embryos with oviduct epithelial cells was tried, and was found to support embryo development. However, it was then found that cells from other sources in the reproductive tract (cumulus and granulosa cells, uterine fibroblasts), other organs (liver, kidney) or even other species were equally beneficial in co-culture, suggesting a non-specific effect of the additional somatic cells. This benefit is now attributed mainly to a reduction in the levels of free oxygen radicals, an effect that can also be achieved without co-culture by decreasing the level of the atmospheric oxygen.

The development of simplified, defined media for embryo culture is probably the biggest single advance for practical in vitro production of bovine embryos. Complex media with plentiful components and supplements may provide many components needed by the embryos, but they also contain detrimental components. Among several media tested for their efficacy in sustaining initial embryonic development in cattle, **synthetic oviduct fluid (SOF) medium** with amino acid supplementation is one of the most effective. Protein supplementation by albumin or serum is frequently used on the grounds that it promotes and stabilizes embryonic development over time, but it also contributes undefined components that may cause subcellular abnormalities. Serum itself has a biphasic effect on the development of cattle embryos: while inhibiting the first cleavage division, it stimulates peri-compaction development, morula-blastocyst transformation, blastocyst development, and hatching from the zona pellucida.

As it grows, the pre-hatching embryo creates a microenvironment around itself that promotes its own development in an autocrine manner. One particular embryo culture system, the so-called 'well of the well' (WOW) exploits this phenomenon by placing each embryo in a small subcompartment formed by pressing a needle into the bottom of the culture well. In these microwells the embryos are able to build up high concentrations of autocrine factors that allow them to survive better than in the usual culture systems.

Improvement of culture media has minimized the problems of LOS; in the best laboratories, in cattle, it is possible to achieve a blastocyst rate of up to 50% of the oocytes subjected to in vitro maturation.

In vitro production of embryos in the pig

Production of embryos in vitro has not reached the level of perfection in pigs that it has in cattle; it is used in fewer laboratories and is currently still 'under development'. Basically, the in vitro production technique is comparable to that described for cattle. The media, however, are specially designed for the pig, and the in vitro maturation culture period needs to be longer (up to 30–40 hours) because the natural preovulatory maturation of the porcine oocyte takes longer. A high rate of polyspermic fertilization hampers the use of the technique, and the in vitro culture of pig embryos also remains problematic, resulting in blastocysts with significantly fewer cells than they have in vivo. World-wide, only a few piglets have so far been born from embryos produced in vitro.

CRYOPRESERVATION OF OOCYTES AND EMBRYOS

As described by Kuwayama (2007), in the 20th century we dealt more or less successful with three of the four dimensions: we can reach practically any point on the globe within 36 hours by flying 10 km above its surface. Time, however, the fourth dimension, has resisted our mastery; we cannot speed it up or slow it down, nor can we travel backwards or forward in time. The only real success in this field has been to arrest biological time in certain organisms by cooling them to extremely low temperatures such as −80°C (the temperature of solid carbon dioxide) or, preferably, −196°C (the boiling point of liquid nitrogen).

Generally, the **smaller the object, the easier is its cryopreservation**. Of course there are many exceptions to this rule but it is still broadly applicable to mammals: suspensions of single mammalian cells can be cryopreserved relatively simply; small tissue fragments (ovarian tissue, for example) are more sensitive to damage; and only limited success has been achieved in the preservation of large, complicated parts of the body (such as whole organs) or whole animals. According to this principle, reproductive biology is in a privileged situation: gametes and preimplantation embryos are good candidates for cryopreservation. Experience has justified the hypothesis, and provided additional evidence for size-related sensitivity: success was first achieved with spermatozoa, then with blastocysts consisting of cells resembling those of a monolayer culture in size. The larger cells of early cleavage stage embryos, and relatively enormous oocytes, are prone to more serious damage during cooling and warming.

Cellular injuries during cryopreservation

A low temperature environment is far from normal for mammals and so it is not surprising that it damages mammalian cells. However, oocytes and embryos have a formidable ability to regenerate after loss of as much as half of their cell mass. The purpose of all cryopreservation methods is to **minimize the injury and to promote the regeneration**. There are two general approaches to achieving this: addition of **cryoprotective additives (cryoprotectants)**, and regulation of **the rate of cooling and warming**.

Cryoprotectants are heterologous groups of compounds with the common effect of promoting survival of cryopreservation. Some permeate the plasma membrane of cells (ethylene glycol, DMSO and glycerol for example) and their main effect is to minimize intracellular ice formation. Others (including sucrose and trehalose) remain in the extracellular space and decrease intracellular ice formation by their osmotic effect, i.e. by removing water from the cells. Cryoprotectants also have (or are thought to have) other effects, including membrane stabilization and support or prevention of some intracellular processes.

During cooling and warming, different kinds of injuries may develop.

- The first usually occurs around physiological temperatures and results from the effort to prevent later injury: the addition of cryoprotectants inflicts considerable **toxic and osmotic shock** on the cells. A careful selection of the cryoprotectant solution (combining up to four cryoprotectants to decrease their separate, individual toxicities) or adding them stepwise may help to decrease this injury.

- The second type of damage, **chilling injury**, is related to initial cooling and occurs between +15 and −5°C. It damages lipid droplets, lipid-rich membranes and microtubules. So far, there are very few strategies to eliminate the problem. One is to remove the particularly sensitive lipid droplets from the cytoplasm by high-speed centrifugation, usually followed by mechanical removal of the separated lipids by micromanipulation. The other possibility is to ensure that oocytes and embryos traverse this temperature zone very quickly to minimize their exposure to the danger. However, this can only be applied in certain types of cryopreservation methods (see later).

- The third potential injury, which occurs between −5 and −30 to 40°C, is probably the most dangerous one: **intracellular ice crystal formation** may mechanically destroy the structures of organelles. The two strategies used to prevent this are slow-rate freezing and vitrification (see later).

- Between −50 and −150°C (approximately) **fracture damage** may occur: the solidified solution may crack, and scissor-like movement of its plates can cut the oocytes or embryos. Careful handling, especially during warming, can prevent this type of injury.

- Surprisingly, **storage at −196°C** is probably the least dangerous phase of the cryopreservation procedure. Potential causes of damage are mostly external and are not strictly related to the process. There is a theoretical possibility of cross contamination between stored samples, mediated by the liquid nitrogen and leading to disease transmission. In practice, however, such an eventuality has never been proved. More dangerous is warming caused by accidental loss of liquid nitrogen. Finally, the mutagenic effect of background (cosmic) radiation is probably less harmful than previously thought.

Methods for cryopreservation

From the many approaches to mammalian oocyte and embryo cryopreservation over the past three decades, two main categories have emerged: **slow-rate freezing** and **vitrification**.

Slow-rate freezing aims to establish a balance between the various potential injuries by using relatively low concentrations of cryoprotectant and a highly controlled cooling rate in the temperature zone where ice formation may occur. Careful cooling of solutions to subzero temperatures, then induc-

tion of ice formation remote from the embryo or oocytes (so-called seeding) followed by very slow cooling can result in stepwise ice formation and slowly increasing concentrations of cryoprotectants in and around the specimen, thereby decreasing the size and quantity of ice crystals in that region. Finally, inside the oocytes and embryos and in their microenvironment, solidification happens almost without ice, the result of a phenomenon known as vitrification (vitreus: glass; ice-free solidification of solutions, that can also be defined as an extremely increased viscosity at subzero temperatures).

However, in cryobiology the term '**vitrification**' is reserved for a different cryopreservation approach: the strategy of not minimizing, but totally eliminating, all ice crystal formation from the whole solution containing the biological sample. The considerable benefit of this approach is that the main source of injury (damage due to ice crystal formation) is also eliminated. However, the price is high: vitrification depends upon high concentrations of cryoprotectants (all with potential toxic and osmotic effects) and high cooling and warming rates. The higher the cooling rate, the lower the concentration of cryoprotectant needed, and vice versa, within certain limits. Another advantage of vitrification is that it can considerably reduce chilling injury by shortening the time over which the sample is held between +15 and −5°C.

Because it was slow-rate freezing that was introduced first, and has produced acceptable results in commercially important cattle and sheep as well as in human embryos, most practitioners use this approach exclusively, despite its disadvantages which include the need for an expensive controlled-rate freezing machine and a freezing process that can take up to 2 hours. Although vitrification was first used successfully with mouse embryos more than 20 years ago, its practical application remains very limited; only recently has its usefulness for special purposes been acknowledged. These include the cryopreservation of lipid-rich and chilling-sensitive pig embryos, oocytes (bovine and human), and the more fragile in-vitro-produced embryos in several species. The advantages of vitrification include its speed, the low cost of equipment (a foam box filled with liquid nitrogen!), and its practicability in relatively unskilled hands. On the other hand, to achieve high cooling and warming rates, most vitrification methods require direct contact between the solution containing the embryo or oocyte and the liquid nitrogen. The potential for disease transmission through this contact may be overemphasized but it cannot be disregarded. Recent vitrification methods offer safe ways to minimize or eliminate this potential danger, decreasing the chance of contamination to a level that is lower than that in traditional slow-rate freezing. In general, for most biological specimens vitrification is more efficient than traditional slow-rate freezing and no scientific paper in the last 5 years has claimed otherwise for oocytes or embryos.

Size and developmental stage are just two of the factors that influence the efficiency of cryopreservation. There are considerable **differences between species**. Some of these may be due to structure (chilling sensitivity of the lipid-rich pig oocytes and embryos, for example) but others are not yet clarified.

In summary, both slow-rate freezing and vitrification can provide biologically acceptable survival rates and commercially/medically applicable methods for bovine, ovine, murine and human embryo cryopreservation. Porcine embryo cryopreservation is only possible with vitrification, and is still in the experimental phase. Cryopreservation of oocytes is difficult in all species and, until recently, only reliable in the mouse. New vitrification methods may result in breakthroughs in this field and are likely to be key to the future of cryopreservation, the rate of progress depending principally on the rate at which specialists accept this likelihood.

CLONING AND GENETIC MODIFICATIONS OF EMBRYOS BY SOMATIC CELL NUCLEAR TRANSFER

Part of the road towards the birth of the first cloned mammal has been described in Chapter 1. It should be emphasized that the term 'cloning' refers to artificially induced asexual reproduction – a procedure used in plants since the earliest days of civilization. In mammals, the process is more complicated, but artificial twinning by bisection of embryos has been used in cattle for decades, although perpetually at the borderline of commercial feasibility.

Nowadays, cloning in mammals refers to the use of the **nuclear transfer technology**, initially developed for the rapid propagation of superior animals. In the first experiments of Steen M. Willadsen, cells of early morula-stage embryos were fused with enucleated oocytes. Unfortunately this technically brilliant method never produced sufficiently reproducible results for practical use and, for more than a decade, it was regarded as being interesting but basically a dead end. Retrospectively, it is hard to understand why all scientists engaged in cloning felt that the donor cells could only be derived from preimplantation stage mammalian embryos, before their so-called 'irreversible' differentiation. The lamb Dolly, in fact, resulted from almost the first serious attempt to use adult, differentiated somatic cells as donors (somatic cell nuclear transfer). The slight technical change that was originally regarded as key to that success, namely 'starving' the somatic cells by culturing them in medium with very low serum concentration, was proved later to be insignificant; the most important factor was apparently the research group's courage to break the psychological barrier of scientific dogma.

Since that success, somatic cell nuclear transfer has slowly but steadily advanced as evidenced by the numbers and species of cloned animals (Table 21-2), the tissue origins of donor somatic cells, and the efficiency of the technology.

The method of somatic cell nuclear transfer

The principles of somatic cell nuclear transfer are simple, as summarized in Fig. 21-6. Key factors for the success of the method are:

- *The developmental stage of the recipient cell.* So far, only **mature oocytes** have proved appropriate for producing the cytoplast that receives the somatic cell nucleus and reprogrammes its

Table 21-2: List of mammalian species cloned by somatic cell nuclear transfer

Sheep	Wilmut et al 1997
Mouse	Wakayama et al 1998
Cattle	Cibelli et al 1998a
Goat	Baguisi et al 1999
Pig	Poleajeva et al 2000
Gaur	Lanza et al 2000
Mouflon	Loi et al 2001
Rabbit	Chesné et al 2002
Cat	Shin et al 2002
Mule	Woods et al 2003
Horse	Galli et al 2003
Rat	Zhou et al 2003
Deer	Westhusin 2003 (press release)
African wildcat	Gomez et al 2004
Dog	Lee et al 2005
Ferret	Li et al 2006
Buffalo	Shi et al 2007
Wolf	Kim et al 2007

genome. No clones have been born after using cytoplasts made by enucleating immature oocytes or zygotes. Furthermore, apparently the oocyte only possesses the reprogramming ability during a rather short time.

- *The origin and cell cycle phase of the somatic donor cell.* So far, for unknown reasons, only about a dozen of the approximately 230 mammalian somatic cell types have proved suitable for nuclear transfer. The cell cycle phase of the donor cell is also important; it should be synchronized to that of the recipient oocyte, at the **G1 or the quiescent G0 phase**, to avoid problems arising from chromosome ploidy.
- *The technique for oocyte enucleation and somatic cell nuclear transfer.* Rapid, relatively harmless, efficient and repeatable enucleation and nuclear transfer procedures are crucial.
- *The technique for activation of the reconstructed embryo.* After the fusion of the somatic cell and

the cytoplast, the reconstructed embryo must be activated to initiate its development. At fertilization, the sperm induces activation. During nuclear transfer, electro-fusion is in most cases insufficient to activate the reconstructed embryo, and an additional activation step is required. The method of choice varies with species and among laboratories and may be chemical, electrical or a combination of the two.

- *The surrounding supportive technologies.* An excellent reproductive infrastructure that provides good quality oocytes, optimal in vitro culture conditions and efficient embryo transfer is crucial.

Problems associated with somatic cell nuclear transfer

Unfortunately, the cellular and molecular biology of cloning are extremely complicated and poorly understood. The literature is extensive, controversial and correspondingly difficult to summarize. Anybody interested in details can find the latest updates in the regularly published reviews.

The birth of Dolly occasioned extremely harsh reactions from various segments of society: political, legislative, ethical, religious, and even entertainment. While not entering the debate in this summary, it must be stated that the mainly hostile atmosphere surrounding the handful of scientists working in the field, and the consequent legal and financial restrictions to the work, have seriously impeded progress, especially since the requirement for sophisticated equipment and a skilled workforce has made cloning research rather expensive. A vicious circle has resulted: society asks for evidence that domestic animal cloning is potentially useful, but reacts against the research that is necessary to get that evidence. Thus, developmental abnormalities, low success rates and the early death of Dolly receive much attention, while the fact that most cloned animals are healthy, normal, and have a normal life span (the second cloned mammal, the mouse Cumulina, has lived much longer than the average mouse) is ignored. Slowing the research has delayed

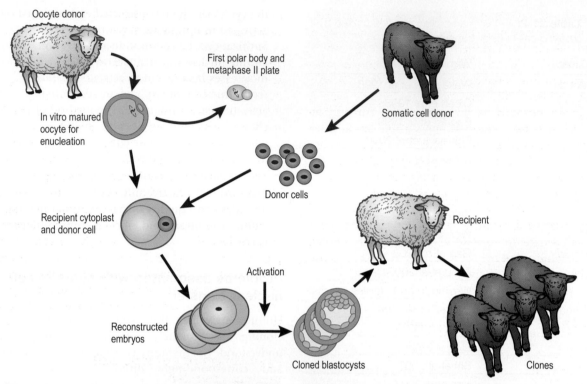

Oocyte donor

First polar body and
metaphase II plate

In vitro matured
oocyte for
enucleation

Somatic cell donor

Recipient cytoplast
and donor cell

Donor cells

Recipient

Activation

Reconstructed
embryos

Cloned blastocysts

Clones

Fig. 21-6: Cloning by somatic cell nuclear transfer. Oocytes are collected from a donor, matured in vitro to metaphase II, and enucleated (usually by micromanipulation) to remove the first polar body and the portion of the oocyte containing the metaphase plate. The resulting cytoplast is combined with a donor cell (e.g. a cultured fibroblast cell) originating from the animal to be cloned. The cytoplast and donor cell are submitted to electrofusion resulting in production of reconstructed embryos in which the oocyte cytoplasm is mixed with the donor cell cytoplasm and carries the donor cell nucleus. The reconstructed embryos are activated in order to initiate embryonic development and, after culture for about one week to the blastocyst stage, can be transferred to recipients for development into cloned offspring. Modified after an unpublished drawing by Hamish Hamilton.

both the elimination of initial problems, and the gathering of evidence for or against cloning's usefulness in practical applications. Accordingly, the **overall success rate has remained low** (between 0.5 and 5% of reconstructed embryos result in live offspring, depending on the species) and will only improve if the vicious circle can be broken.

The reasons for the low success rates are not fully understood, but, in addition to the **methodological factors** enumerated above, it is likely that **epigenetic factors** associated with the reprogramming of the somatic cell genome are involved.

Epigenetic reprogramming of the somatic cell genome appears to be of central importance in cloning biology. At sexual reproduction, the genome is 'reset' to a totipotent state during gametogenesis (formation of oocytes and spermatozoa) by the eradication of the existing epigenetic marks and the establishment of new ones. These marks are defined by various molecular changes to the DNA, but one of the most important in relation to embryonic development is the **methylation of cytosine** (see Chapter 2); highly methylated regions of the genome are not expressed. Upon fertilization, the paternal component of the embryonic genome is actively demethylated whereas the maternal component is demethylated more slowly and passively, though this phenomenon varies with species. One set of genes is not included in this round of demethylation: the imprinted genes, i.e. those that are marked to be expressed from either the maternal or the paternal allele specifically. During subsequent development, the embryonic genome is remethylated as cell differentiation occurs, requiring silencing of certain portions of the genome. In somatic cell nuclear transfer embryos, the demethylation is less pronounced than in normally fertilized embryos. Thus, the 're-setting' of the somatic cell genome to a totipotent state is apparently not as efficient as during sexual reproduction. Simply put, there may be a conflict between closing the epigenetic programme of the somatic cell and opening the epigenetic programme that drives embryonic development – a conflict that may cause losses and abnormalities during embryonic and fetal development.

Problems associated with somatic cell nuclear transfer cloning begin early and continue postnatally. The most frequent anomalies include:

- Low cleavage and embryo developmental rates in vitro.
- Low pregnancy rates, early and late losses of fetuses.
- Placental abnormalities.
- Fetal overgrowth and prolonged gestation.
- Stillbirth, hypoxia, respiratory failure, circulatory problems, and lack of post-natal vigour.
- Increased body temperature at birth.
- Malformations of the urogenital tract (hydronephrosis and testicular hypoplasia for example).
- Malformations of the liver and brain.
- Immune dysfunction, lymphoid hypoplasia, anaemia and thymic atrophy.
- Bacterial and viral infections.

However, in the past few years the results of somatic cell nuclear transfer have improved remarkably thanks to cumulative but unheralded worldwide research efforts. Thus, **partial or almost total elimination of the developmental problems** has been achieved. Another positive aspect is that the *offspring* **of cloned animals do not show any increase in developmental problems** compared to control animals, showing that the epigenetic problems inherent to somatic cell nuclear transfer is transient, expressed only in the cloned generation and not its successors. Yet another advance is the introduction of **new, simple techniques for somatic cell nuclear transfer**, for example so-called 'hand-made cloning' which has eliminated the need for micromanipulation equipment for the production of cytoplasts and for their fusion with somatic cells. This innovation has radically decreased the costs of equipment and the need for a skilled workforce, and therefore promises to minimize the production costs of healthy live clones. Finally, in cattle and pigs, the overall efficiency of cloning, as measured in terms of live offspring, has increased considerably, making direct scientific and commercial application a realistic perspective in these economically important species.

Application of somatic cell nuclear transfer

Some of the potential applications are based on using the technology just to produce cloned animals, but the major applications are likely to be based on **nuclear transfer from genetically modified** donor cells so that the cloned embryos and offspring carry the same modifications (Fig. 21-7). This may even allow for targeted genetic modifications (where the genome is modified at specific sites) during culture of the donor cells, making somatic cell nuclear transfer the most powerful technique for production of genetically modified large domestic species. The areas of application can be summarized as follows:

- *Basic research*. Somatic cell nuclear transfer may provide deeper insight into cell differentiation, and into epigenetic reprogramming including imprinting, inheritance and the roles of environmental versus genetic factors in the process. Additionally, cloned animals may provide more uniform animals (with variation restricted to the mitochondrial genes) for

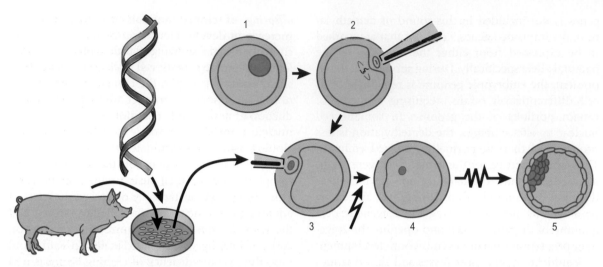

Fig. 21-7: Production of genetically modified blastocysts by somatic cell nuclear transfer. Cultured fibroblasts are genetically modified and used as donor cells for nuclear transfer. An immature oocyte at prophase I (1) is matured to metaphase II in vitro (2) and enucleated (3) to receive the genetically modified donor cell. Electrofusion results in generation of a reconstructed embryo (4) which, during culture, develops into a blastocyst (5) that can be transferred to a recipient to produce genetically modified offspring.

constituting experimental groups in any field, thereby lowering the number of animals required.

- *Disease models*. Certain human diseases are genetically well characterized and caused by rather simple changes in the genome. Insertion of selected human genes into porcine nuclear donor cells can result in the birth of **pigs carrying the genetic potential of developing human diseases**. Such animal models may help unravel the pathogenesis and consequences of these diseases and provide an opportunity to test therapies for their treatment or prevention.

- *Living bioreactors*. Tailored genetic modification may similarly result in **domestic animals producing pharmaceutically or commercially important proteins** in accessible fluids including milk, blood, seminal plasma or even urine. Just a few such animals may be enough to decrease radically (10–100-fold) the costs of some proteins needed in human medicine, and consequently make them more accessible in poor countries. Examples of such proteins include blood clotting factors for the treatment of haemophilia, and alpha-1 anti-trypsin for the treatment of cystic fibrosis. For unknown reasons none of these proteins have yet reached the market.

- *Xenotransplantation*. In Europe alone, around 250,000 individuals are alive as a result of receiving a transplanted organ, and more than 45,000 patients are on waiting lists. The demand for organ transplantation continues to grow by 15% per year, and an estimated 15–30% of candidates for a liver or heart transplant will die before the appropriate organs become available. Approximately 2,000 heart transplants are performed every year in the United States, but 500 patients die before a heart becomes available. On the other hand, the number of brain-dead donors remains constant world-wide. These data show that a radical solution to the problem is required. One possibility is to use **animal organs for xenotransplantation** into humans. Pigs are excellent potential donors as their organ sizes and metabolism are similar to those of humans. However, the problem of immune rejection, the potential danger of infections (zoonoses), ethical concerns, and public aversion hamper progress. While the latter two factors may disappear soon when the first scientific successes are presented, the problem of zoonoses should be carefully investigated, although recent data support the view that the actual risk is much lower than was supposed earlier. The greatest barrier at present is the need to obtain genetic modifications to delete antigens and/or to enable the transplanted organ to defend itself successfully against the immune attacks of the human body. To achieve either the first or the second modification (or preferably both) careful tailoring of the genetic material is required and the only system that seems suitable for producing piglets carrying the modified genes is somatic cell nuclear transfer. As mentioned above, the efficiency of cloning in pigs (a bottleneck until recently) has now increased dramatically, leaving the success of xenotransplantation to depend mostly on the efficiency and creativity of genetic engineers.

- *Agricultural applications.* Used alone or together with genetic modification of the donor cells, somatic cell nuclear transfer can perhaps be used to produce animals that will increase **productivity, animal welfare** (for example by increasing resistance to diseases) and the **quality of food products**. However, the idea of using genetically modified animals for human consumption is very **far from acceptable by the authorities and public** in Europe, and probably in the United States, Canada, Australia and Japan. Without genetic modification, however, there is a good chance of seeing products of cloned animals on supermarket shelves in the foreseeable future, first in the United States, and soon after in most developed countries outside the more conservative Europe. Cloning is so far regarded as an expensive technology, and mass production of cloned animals seems to be commercially less likely than the cloning of a few, excellent quality animals for breeding purposes. On the other hand, with improving techniques and decreasing costs, countries with livestock of low average quality may use cloning to rapidly improve its overall quality.

Unfortunately, most of these countries are unable to cover the costs of even the less expensive technologies. Probably the only two exceptions are Brazil and China. In China, there are fewer legal and public concerns about new embryo technologies and it may be there that cloning and genetic modification first become part of breeding strategies, especially in the large domestic species.

- *Special purposes: pets, endangered species, etc.* For many, the cloning of pet cats, dogs, racehorses or racing camels poses serious **ethical questions**. Nevertheless, the exploitation of this area will probably be determined by commercial considerations or, in racing for example, by the rules of governing bodies. Cloning individuals from endangered species or breeds to increase populations is an unlikely application; the cost is too high when even simpler ways to save these species or breeds are impossible to finance.

From this list it is clear that only the future can reveal what benefits will be realized from somatic cell nuclear transfer technology. Animal cloning certainly has great theoretical potential but, at its current level of efficiency, its role in the near future is likely to remain within basic research and bio-medicine where the value of each animal is very high. Whether the technology will spread into agri-cultural applications remains to be seen and scien-tists are divided as to that likelihood.

STEM CELLS

Several human diseases including Alzheimer's, Parkinson's, diabetes, hepatitis, arthritis and stroke, are caused by a loss of function of particular cell populations in the body. Consequently, the poten-tial of **cell replacement therapy**, in which diseased or lost cells are replaced by new healthy cell popula-tions, has created a new and quickly developing platform for biotechnology. Stem cells are thought to be an excellent tool for cell replacement therapy and are at the focus of immense research activity.

The stem cell principle

Stem cells have the capacity for **indefinite self-renewal**. Thus, when a stem cell divides, it produces either two daughter stem cells (symmetrical division), as seen in embryonic stem cells for example, or it divides into one stem cell and another cell destined for differentiation (asymmetrical division), as seen in haematopoietic stem cells and spermatogenic stem cells for example (Fig. 21-8). Another feature of stem cells is that they are able to **differentiate into other cell types** (to varying degrees) when given specific cues in vitro.

Stem cells can be categorized according to their origin: **embryonic stem (ES) cells** which are derived from the early embryo (from the inner cell mass of the blastocyst); **fetal stem cells** from the fetus (e.g. umbilical cord blood stem cells); and **adult stem cells** from various adult tissues (e.g. haematopoietic stem cells and mesenchymal stem cells from the bone marrow). The term 'adult stem cell' is poorly defined and fetal and adult stem cells are better con-

sidered as **somatic stem cells**. ES cells have the highest ability to differentiate into other cell types and are termed **pluripotent cells** (see later). Somatic stem cells of fetal origin are thought to have an intermediate capacity for differentiation into other cell types although this is poorly understood. Somatic stem cells differentiate only into a finite number of cell types (usually concordant with the tissue type from which they are derived) and are thus termed **multipotent**. Interestingly, mesenchymal stem cells are considered by some researchers to be pluripotent, however, this research has been difficult to replicate in many labs and remains controversial.

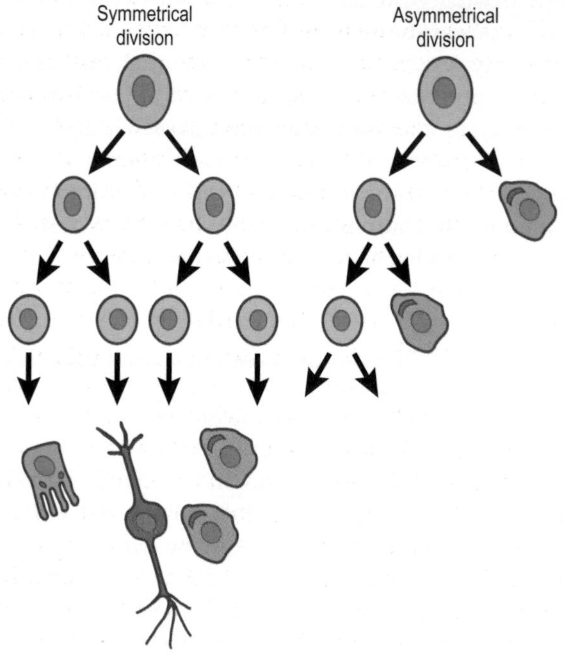

In the present context, emphasis will be on ES cells because their origin and biology are strongly related to embryological and fetal development. Although ES cells *originate* from the inner cell mass or epiblast, they can no longer be considered inner cell mass or epiblast cells. Thus, whereas the state of pluripotency in the inner cell mass and epiblast is short and measured in days in vivo, pluripotency of ES cells cultured in vitro is retained as an artifact and maintained for months or years. How this transformation occurs is poorly understood and awaits further insight into the mechanisms that regulate pluripotency.

At least in the mouse, there are two additional avenues through which pluripotent stem cell lines can be established: the formation of **embryonic germ (EG) cells** and **embryonic carcinoma (EC) cells** (see below).

Fig. 21-8: Symmetrical and asymmetrical division of stem cells.

Embryonic stem (ES) cells

ES cells were first described in the **mouse** but later cells with similar characteristics were described in **man**, and most recently ES cells have been derived in the **rat**. There have been numerous attempts to establish ES cell lines in other species, so far without authenticated success. Very rigorous characterization of ES cell lines is required for this authentication; many reports have been published on the culture of cells with 'ES-like' features, but which fall short of full characterization.

It is not surprising that ES cells were first described in the mouse as it is the most commonly used and best understood mammalian species. Furthermore, the mouse blastocyst can enter into diapause (see Chapter 20), a period of developmental quiescence in the uterus. Diapause depends upon the presence of leukaemia inhibitory factor (LIF), an important signalling molecule for which the mouse embryo possesses receptors. The fact that the inner cell mass is arrested in an undifferentiated pluripotent state (in other words much like ES cells) during diapause explains why mouse ES cells require LIF in the culture medium in order to remain pluripotent and undifferentiated.

Characteristics of ES cells

Precise characterization of ES cells is vital. Both mouse and human ES cells can undergo **indefinite self-renewal**. This capacity depends to some degree on their possession of the enzyme telomerase, which is necessary for rebuilding the chromosome telomeres that are shortened during each S-phase of the cell cycle.

ES cells are also characterized by the presence of a long list of **molecular markers** (Table 21-3). Some of these markers, including the transcription factors Oct3/4, Sox2 and Nanog, have well defined cell biological roles. These crucial transcription factors are involved in maintaining cell pluripotency (see Chapter 6). The roles of other factors are poorly

understood. Interestingly, although these markers are expressed in both mouse and human ES cells, there is a longer list of characterization markers that are not totally conserved between these two species. For example, cell surface marker SSEA1 is detected in mouse ES cells but not in human ES cells. In contrast, human ES cells express surface markers SSEA3, SSEA4, TRA-1-60 and TRA-1-81, which are not observed in mouse ES cells (see Table 21.3). Furthermore the cell signalling pathways that govern the pluripotent state differ between these two species. Notably, Leukaemia Inhibitory Factor (LIF) is required to maintain mouse ES self-renewal in vitro. This is added into medium as a supplement to maintain LIF-dependent activation of STAT3. Thus, variations differ between ES cells derived from these two species and more research is needed to standardize and characterize their profiles. Recently, the International Stem Cell Initiative has published a comprehensive study on the standardization of human ES cell markers in which they have compared human ES cell lines from many laboratories from all over the world.

One of the most intriguing characteristics of ES cells is their **ability to differentiate** into varying cell types; spontaneous differentiation into cells with fibroblast and neural morphology are often observed in culture, especially after long periods of growth without passage into new culture dishes. It is also possible to direct their differentiation in vitro by stimulation with various combinations of growth factors into specific cell types of interest (into dopaminergic neurons for example). This is well described as **directed differentiation**. In addition, ES cells are able to **differentiate spontaneously**. This can be induced by removing key factors (such as LIF or bFGF for mouse and human ES cells, respectively) from the culture medium and feeder cells that ES cells may be grown on. If cells are cultured in these conditions of deprivation and kept in suspension culture (e.g. in hanging droplets) they form characteristic **embryoid bodies**. An embryoid body is a mass of cells typically derived from all three embryonic germ layers, ectoderm, endoderm and mesoderm. This is a unique composition that only pluripotent cell types may be able to produce.

Table 21-3: Expression of stem cell markers in ES cell lines or ES-like cell lines (cow) derived from different species

Marker	Human	Monkey	Mouse	Cow
Oct3/4	+	+	+	+
Nanog	+	+	+	+
Sox2	+	+	+	?
SSEA1	–	–	+	–
SSEA3	+	+	–	?
SSEA4	+	+	–	+
TRA-1-60	+	+	–	+
TRA-1-81	+	+	–	+

Another way of testing the pluripotency of ES cells is to inject them into well-defined locations in immune-deficient mice where they develop into **teratomas**, tumours comprised of various differentiated tissues, representative of all three embryonic germ layers.

The ultimate verification of the pluripotent nature of mouse ES cells is to prove that they contribute to the formation of **chimaeric offspring.** These are produced by injection of labelled ES cells (usually genetically modified, so that they constitutively express Green Fluorescent Protein, GFP) into blastocysts, followed by transfer of these mosaic embryos into surrogate foster-mothers. Typically in chimaerism, the ES cells colonize the inner cell mass and contribute to multiple organs and tissues of resultant offspring (detectable under ultraviolet light in the case of ES cells expressing GFP). Full pluripotency is demonstrated when the ES cells also give rise to a portion of the primordial germ cells of the chimaeric embryos and form oocytes or spermatozoa in the adult chimaeric animal. Because of ethical constraints, contribution of ES cells to the germline in mammals has so far only been demonstrated in the mouse.

Derivation and culture of ES cells

ES cells are derived from the inner cell mass or the epiblast of blastocysts in one of two ways: either the whole blastocyst is cultured and allowed to attach after collapse, which renders the inner cell mass or epiblast distinct; or the intact blastocyst is subjected to microsurgical or immunosurgical isolation of the inner cell mass or the epiblast. For **immunosurgical isolation**, the blastocyst is treated with an antiserum against the donor species, and this incubation is followed by treatment with complement, resulting in lysis of the trophectoderm exclusively (the only cells reached by the antiserum and complement) and allowing the inner cell mass or the epiblast to be unperturbed and ready for culture (Fig. 21-9).

To provide optimal conditions for the inner cell mass or epiblast cells to undergo the enigmatic **transformation into ES cells**, the blastocysts, isolated inner cell masses or epiblasts are cultured on feeder cells (usually mouse embryonic fibroblast cell lines) where they form small colonies. After one to two weeks these colonies can be passaged to new feeder cells in order to keep the cells growing in an undifferentiated, pluripotent state. Subsequently, the ES cells are generally passaged each week and samples may be cryopreserved for later use.

Most murine ES cell lines tolerate passage by trypsinization, and so it is possible to establish clonal ES cell lines from single cells. Certain human ES cell lines do not withstand trypsination and must be passaged manually (using ultrasharp blades or needles) by excising undifferentiated parts of the colonies into small clumps that are transferred to the new dishes containing feeder cells.

In an attempt to culture ES cells in more defined conditions, many researchers have developed protocols for growing cells in the absence of feeder cell lines and in completely defined culture medium. This is particularly important if human ES cells or, rather, their derived counterparts, are to be considered safe to transfer into human patients. Elimination of both mouse feeder cells

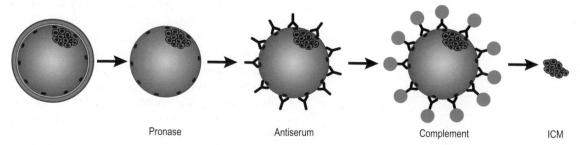

Pronase   Antiserum   Complement   ICM

Fig. 21-9: Immunosurgical isolation of the ICM from a blastocyst. After removal of the zona pellucida by pronase treatment, the blastocyst is subjected to antiserum and complement treatment to release the ICM.

and reagents derived from non-human species from these cultures has already been achieved for some human ES lines.

In vitro differentiation of ES cells

Several media and culture protocols have been developed for stimulating ES cells to undergo controlled differentiation in vitro but exactly how they do so is not well defined. In the embryo, molecular signalling pathways govern sequential differentiation of cells from a pluripotent, down to a multipotent and then to a **unipotent** state. In vitro, external or paracrine signalling is absent; thus control of the differentiation pathway from the required signals/factors is lost. In other words, in the developing embryo the controlled sequential differentiation results in about 230 cell types that form the body, whereas, in vitro, an unrestricted number of intermediate cell types may arise in the absence of proper molecular signalling. These facts have prompted discussion of whether differentiation of ES cells in vitro has to follow the same sequential pattern as in the embryo, or whether simpler differentiation protocols could be equally effective. Ongoing research indicates that the only successful avenue to controlled in vitro differentiation is a sequential recapitulation of the in vivo developmental events. In general, it seems easiest to make ES cells differentiate towards an **ectodermal fate**, and most difficult to obtain **endodermal differentiation**, with differentiation towards a **mesodermal fate** being of intermediate difficulty. Thus, neurons of different types can be produced from ES cells relatively easily whereas differentiation into insulin-producing β-cells, for example, is less efficient. Complex protocols that may take days or weeks to complete are being developed. By following the addition or removal of specific proteins/factors to the medium at specific days during the protocol, it is possible to obtain some of the desired cell types. However, the end population is often heterogeneous and may contain residual non-differentiated ES cells or other specific cell types. Studies continue in attempts to improve the specificity of the protocols and/or sorting the end cell population so that a single cell type is obtained. Unfortunately, there is still a great lack of reproducible in vitro differentiation protocols and this obstacle is probably the most critical to overcome before the therapeutic potential of ES cells can be realized.

Animal models for human ES cell therapy

Currently, the only validated animal model for human ES cell therapy is the mouse. It is evident, however, that the anatomy, physiology and life span of the mouse are considerably different from those of humans. It is clear that alternative non-human models are needed. Transplanting ES-cell-derived cell populations into the body poses certain risks that may not be appropriately analyzed using the mouse model. If the therapeutic cell populations are polluted by undifferentiated ES cells, what is the risk of producing teratomas in the recipient? The growth of teratomas or other benign or malign tumours has already been demonstrated following transplantation of differentiated mouse or human ES cells into mice and remains a huge issue to be overcome. To test such **safety concerns,** as well as to evaluate the **potentials** of ES cell therapy, an ES cell model in a large **domestic species** such as the pig would be of great value. The pig is a large mammal with similar sized organs to the human. In addition, its physiology is more closely parallel to that of the human than is mouse physiology. Current efforts aim at establishing such a model (Fig. 21-10). However, world-wide efforts have clearly demonstrated that the technology of establishing and culturing ES cells in the mouse cannot directly be transferred to the pig and, so far, stable validated ES cell lines have not been established in this species. One issue that still remains is the concern of long-term immunosuppression. The transplantation of non-human cells or non-compatible human cells requires a patient to take life-long immunosuppressive drugs. The alternative is to develop transplanted cells that are not recognized by the host, but this has yet to be achieved. Irrespective of the hurdles required to take ES cells to the clinic, there is much hope that the hurdles will be cleared and that ES cells will form a large part of future treatments of disease.

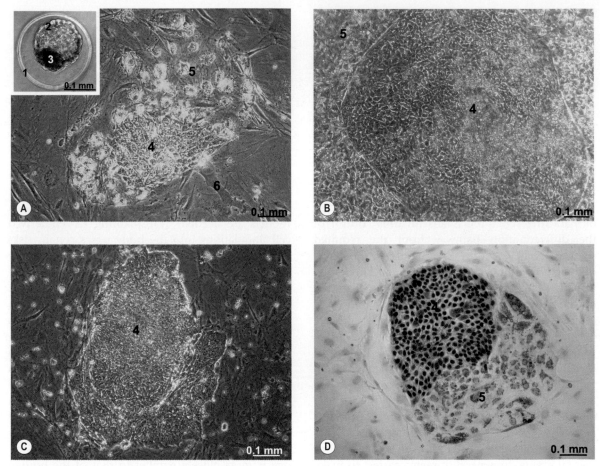

Fig. 21-10: Different stages in the isolation and culture of porcine ES-like cells. **(A)** Outgrowth colony on Day 4 after immunosurgical isolation of the ICM. Note the ES-like cells (4) and the putative trophectoderm cells (5) together with the mouse embryonic fibroblasts (6). Insert: Unhatched porcine blastocyst showing the zona pellucida (1), trophectoderm (2), and inner cell mass (3). **(B)** Outgrowth colony on Day 6. Note the ES-like cells (4) and the putative trophectoderm cells (5). **(C)** ES-like cell colony (4) on Day 4 after the first manual passage (passage 1) at, in total, 10 days after ICM isolation. **(D)** Immunocytochemical staining for Oct4 of porcine outgrowth colony on Day 7 after ICM isolation. Note the reddish stained nuclei of the ES-like cell area (4) as opposed to the unstained nuclei of the potential trophectoderm (5).

Alternative avenues to pluripotent stem cells

Besides ES cells, there are at least two other types of pluripotent stem cell lines in the mouse: **embryonic germ (EG) cells** and **embryonic carcinoma (EC) cells** (Fig. 21-11).

EC cells are also derived from the inner cell mass. Thus, if inner cell masses are transplanted into mice, they can develop into specific tumours, called **tera-**

tocarcinomas. These consist of differentiated cells derived from the pluripotent inner cell mass cells, but they also contain a smaller proportion of undifferentiated cells. The latter cells can be isolated and cultured in vitro as EC cells that display pluripotent characteristics. Analogous authenticated EC cells have not been developed in any domestic animal, although EC-like cells have been reported in the pig.

EG cells are derived from the **primordial germ cells** of the embryo during their migration from the

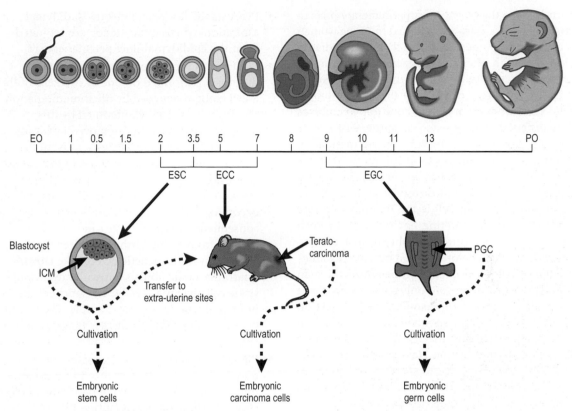

Fig. 21-11: Production of ES cells (ESC), EC cells (ECC), and EG cells (EGC) in the mouse. The time axis depicts embryonic development from embryonic Day 0 (E0) to postnatal Day 0 (P0). ESC are harvested from the ICM of blastocysts. If the ICM is transplanted ectopically into another mouse, teratocarcinomas may develop from which ECCs can be harvested. EGCs are harvested later from the primordial germ cell population of the genital ridge.

yolk sac to the genital ridge after gastrulation. The primordial germ cells can be cultured in vitro as EG cells that are pluripotent. Again, definite EG cells have not been developed in any domestic animal although EG-like cells have been reported in the pig.

Most recently, a new type of embryonic-like stem cell has been derived, called **induced pluripotent stem cells (iPS cells)**. These cells are reprogrammed from adult somatic cells by viral transduction of different pluripotency genes. Mouse iPS cells were first produced by transduction of *Oct4*, *Sox2*, *c-Myc* and *klf4* and human iPS cells were later produced by viral transduction using either a combination of *Oct4*, *Sox2*, *klf4*, and *c-Myc* or *Oct4*, *Sox2*, *Nanog* and *Lin28*. These cells allow for **patient-specific stem**

cell lines to be produced and may be an exciting stem cell tool used for future cell therapy.

ASSISTED REPRODUCTION TECHNOLOGIES IN MAN

The main purposes of using assisted reproduction technologies in human medicine are to bypass **infertility problems** and to perform **preimplantation genetic diagnosis**.

In vitro production of embryos is usually referred to as **in vitro fertilization (IVF)** in humans because the concomitant in vitro phases (oocyte maturation and embryo culture) are generally shorter than in the domestic species. Following **ovarian stimulation**, which leads to the growth of supernumerary preovulatory follicles, oocytes are collected from the woman by **ultrasound-guided ovum pick up** immediately before ovulation. They are **fertilized in vitro**, cultured only to the 2- to 4-cell stage and then **non-surgically transferred** (or reinserted) into the uterine lumen of the same woman. In general, one to two embryos are transferred, but transfer of single embryos is becoming the standard. In vitro oocyte maturation and culture of the embryos to the blastocyst stage are used on some occasions but, in general, the in vitro periods are shorter than those used in animals. Key to the success of human IVF is the unusual tolerance of an asynchronous uterine environment by such early cleavage stage primate embryos, first demonstrated in monkeys before IVF had become possible.

If the infertility problem is inherent to the man rather than the woman, and only a few spermatozoa are available, **intracytoplasmic sperm injection (ICSI)** is used; a single spermatozoon is picked up from the ejaculate and mechanically injected into the oocyte through a fine glass pipette. The same procedure may be applied to spermatozoa collected from the epididymis or even the testicle. There are even reports of the birth of babies from ICSI of round spermatids from the testis.

In human assisted reproduction technology, **numerous abbreviations** are used which may be confusing for other scientists and the general public. Some of the more commonly used abbreviations, in an alphabetic order, are:

- AHA stands for 'assisted hatching' where the escape of the blastocyst from the zona pellucida is facilitated by rupturing the zona by micromanipulation.
- GIFT stands for 'gamete intra-fallopian transfer.' The gametes, the oocyte and the spermatozoa, are washed and, with a catheter, placed directly into the woman's oviduct (Fallopian tube) where fertilization and initial embryonic development take place in vivo.
- MESA stands for 'microsurgical epididymal sperm aspiration' where spermatozoa are aspirated from the epididymal duct by a surgical procedure.
- PESA stands for 'percutaneous epididymal aspiration' where spermatozoa are aspirated from the epididymal duct percutaneously.
- PGD stands for 'preimplantation genetic diagnosis' performed on one or two cells of the 8-cell embryo removed by micromanipulation. The embryo is usually unharmed by this procedure and the cell(s) removed by biopsy can be subjected to genetic analysis. Most of the twenty-five thousand or so genes in the human genome have now been identified and their DNA sequenced. Molecular analysis of genes is becoming simpler and more efficient. As a consequence, PGD with IVF can now prevent couples from giving birth to children with almost any of the genetic defects like Down's syndrome, cystic fibrosis, muscular dystrophy, sickle cell anaemia, Tay-Sachs, Gaucher's disease, or mental retardation, for example. The fine line between using PGD for disease prevention versus positive selection is a current ethical issue.
- PROST stands for 'pronuclear stage tubal transfer' where zygotes fertilized in vitro are transferred back to the woman's oviduct before cleavage, allowing initial embryonic development to take place in vivo.
- SUZI stands for 'subzonal sperm injection' where a spermatozoon is injected into the perivitelline space by micromanipulation.
- TESE stands for 'testicular sperm extraction' where spermatozoa for in vitro fertilization are harvested from the testis.
- TET stands for 'tubal embryo transfer' where early IVF embryos are transferred back to the woman's oviduct.
- ZIFT stands for 'zygote intrafallopian transfer' where an oocyte is fertilized in vitro and then transferred back to the woman's oviduct at the zygote stage.

SUMMARY

The assisted reproduction technologies (ARTs) comprise numerous manipulations of gametes and embryos to control and/or improve reproduction. One of the oldest ARTs is **artificial insemination** in which semen collected from superior males is used to inseminate many females. Artificial insemination is often combined with **cryopreservation of the diluted semen** and, recently, especially in cattle, sometimes with **sex sorting of spermatozoa** by flow cytometry. Artificial insemination is still the ART that has had the most significant influence on domestic animal breeding. Another ART that has found practical use, particularly in cattle, is **multiple ovulation and embryo transfer (MOET)** in which superior females are superovulated in order to induce multiple ovulations, inseminated with selected semen, and used as donors of embryos at the blastocyst stage for transfer to recipient animals. More recently, **in vitro production of embryos** has become practicable. This comprises maturation of the oocyte, fertilization, and culture of the resultant embryos to the blastocyst stage, all in vitro before transfer. Embryo transfer and in vitro production of embryos have called for **cryopreservation** of oocytes and embryos, to which end both **slow-rate freezing** and **vitrification** techniques have been developed. **Cloning by somatic cell nuclear transfer** is a particularly remarkable technique in which a differentiated cell's genome is reprogrammed by an oocyte. The oocyte's nucleus containing its DNA is first removed, leaving the so-called cytoplast. The cytoplast is then fused with a somatic donor cell. The differentiated genome in the nucleus of the donor cell is reprogrammed to a totipotent state by the cytoplasm of the oocyte's cytoplast and embryonic development is initiated upon activation of the reconstructed embryo. Combined with the use of genetically modified cells as nuclear donors, somatic cell nuclear transfer can be used to produce **genetically modified animals**, which has prompted research into the use of such modified domestic animals as models of human disease and, in the case of pigs, as organ donors for xenotransplantation. In human medicine, stem cells are envisioned as being useful in future for so-called cell-based therapy in which stem cells are differentiated into therapeutically relevant cell populations. **Embryonic stem cells**, which are pluripotent and, hence, can differ-entiate into all cell types of the mammalian body, are of special interest for such purposes – purposes which would benefit greatly from improved (domestic) animal models in which important issues such as safety can be investigated.

REFERENCES AND FURTHER READING

Allen, W.R. (2005): The development and application of the modern reproductive technologies to horse breeding. Reprod. Dom. Anim. 40:310–329.

Anderson, G.B., Choi, S.J. and Bondurant, R.H. (1994): Survival of porcine inner cell masses in culture and after injection into blastocysts. Theriogenology, 42:204–212.

Baguisi, A., Behboodi, E., Melican, D.T., Pollock, J.S., Destrempes, M.M., Cammuso, C., Williams, J.L., Nims, S.D., Porter, C.A., Midura, P., Palacios, M.J., Ayres, S.L., Denniston, R.S., Hayes, M.L., Ziomek, C.A., Meade, H.M., Godke, R.A., Gavin, W.G., Overstrom, E.W. and Echelard, Y. (1999): Production of goats by somatic cell nuclear transfer. Nature Biotech. 17:456–461.

Bavister, B.D. (2002): Early history of in vitro fertilization. Reproduction 124:181–196.

Bo, G.A., Baruselli, P.S., Chesta, P.M. and Martins, C.M. (2006): The timing of ovulation and insemination schedules in superstimulated cattle. Theriogenology 65:89–101.

Brevini, T.A., Tosetti, V., Crestan, M., Antonini, S. and Gandolfi F. (2007): Derivation and characterization of pluripotent cell lines from pig embryos of different origins. Theriogenology, 67:54–63.

Callesen, H. and Greve, T. (2002): Management of reproduction in cattle and buffaloes – embryo transfer and associated techniques. In: Animal Health and Production Compendium. Wallingford, UK: CAB International. 41 pp.

Campbell, K.H., McWhir, J., Ritchie, W.A. and Wilmut, I. (1996): Sheep cloned by nuclear transfer from a cultured cell line. Nature, 380:64–66.

Chambers, I., Colby, D., Robertson, M., Nichols, J., Lee, S., Tweedie, S., and Smith, A. (2003): Functional expression cloning of Nanog, a pluripotency sustaining factor in embryonic stem cells. Cell, 113:643–655.

Chen, L.R., Shiue, Y.L., Bertolini, L., Medrano, J.F., Bondurant, R.H. and Anderson, G.B. (1999): Establishment of pluripotent cell lines from porcine preimplantation embryos. Theriogenology, 52:195–212.

Chesné, P., Adenot, P.G., Viglietta, C., Baratte, M., Boulanger, L. and Renard, J.P. (2002): Cloned rabbits produced by nuclear transfer from adult somatic cells. Nature Biotech. 20:366–369.

Chew, J.L., Loh, Y.H., Zhang, W., Chen, X., Tam, W.L., Yeap, L.S., Li, P., Ang, Y.S., Lim, B., Robson, P. and Ng, H.H.

(2005): Reciprocal transcriptional regulation of Pou5f1 and Sox2 via the Oct4/Sox2 complex in embryonic stem cells. Mol. Cell. Biol., 25:6031–6046.

Cibelli, J.B., Stice, S.L., Golueke, P.J., Kane, J.J., Jerry, J., Blackwell, C., Ponce de Leon, F.A. and Robl, J.M. (1998a): Cloned transgenic calves produced from nonquiescent fetal fibroblasts. Science 280:1256–1258.

Cibelli, J.B., Stice, S.L., Golueke, P.J., Kane, J.J., Jerry, J., Blackwellm, C., Ponce de Leon, F.A. and Robl, J.M. (1998b): Transgenic bovine chimeric offspring produced from somatic cell-derived stem-like cells. Nat. Biotechnol., 16:642–646.

Di Berardino, M.A. (2001): Animal cloning – the route to new genomics in agriculture and medicine. Differentiation 68:67–83.

Durocher, J., Morin, N. and Blondin, P. (2006): Effect of hormonal stimulation on bovine follicular response and oocyte developmental competence in a commercial operation. Theriogenology 65:102–115.

Evans, M.J. and Kaufman, M.H. (1981):. Establishment in culture of pluripotential cells from mouse embryos. Nature, 292:154–156.

Evans, M.J., Notarianni, E., Laurie, S. and Moor, R.M. (1990): Derivation and preliminary characterization of pluripotent cell lines from porcine and bovine blastocysts. Theriogenology, 33:125–128.

Evenson, D.P. and Wixon, R. (2006): Clinical aspects of sperm DNA fragmentation detection and male infertility. Theriogenology 65:979–991.

Galli, C., Lagutina, I., Crotti, G., Colleoni, S., Turini, P., Ponderato, N., Duchi, R. and Lazzari, G. (2003): Pregnancy: a cloned horse born to its dam twin. Nature 425:680

Gerfen, R.W. and Wheeler, D.A. (1995): Isolation of embryonic cell-lines from porcine blastocysts. Anim. Biotechnol., 6:1–14.

Ginis, I., Luo, Y., Miura, T., Thies, S., Brandenberger, R., Gerecht-Nir, S., Amit, M., Hoke, A., Carpenter, M.K., Itskovitz-Eldor, J. and Rao, M.S. (2004): Differences between human and mouse embryonic stem cells. Dev. Biol., 269:360–380.

Gjorret, J.O. and Maddox-Hyttel, P. (2005): Attempts towards derivation and establishment of bovine embryonic stem cell-like cultures. Reprod. Fertil. Dev., 17:113–124.

Golos, T.G., Pollastrini, L.M. and Gerami-Naini, B. (2006): Human embryonic stem cells as a model for trophoblast differentiation. Semin. Reprod. Med., 24:314–321.

Gomez, M.C., Pope, C.E., Giraldo, A., Lyons, L.A., Harris, R.F., King, A.L., Cole, A., Godke, R.A. and Dresser, B.L. (2004):Birth of African Wildcat cloned kittens born from domestic cats. Cloning Stem Cells 6:247–258.

González-Bulnes A, Baird DT, Campbell BK, Cocero MJ, Garcia-Garcia RM, Inskeep EK, López-Sebastián A, McNeilly AS, Santiago-Moreno J, Souza CJH, Veiga-López A (2004) Multiple factors affecting the efficiency of multiple ovulation and embryo transfer in sheep and goats. Reprod Fert and Develop 16:421–435.

Greve, T. and Callesen, H. (2005): Embryo technology: implications for fertility in cattle. Revue Scientifique et Technique-Office International des Epizooties 24:405–412.

Hall, V.J., Stojkovic, P. and Stojkovic, M. (2006): Using therapeutic cloning to fight human disease: a conundrum or reality? Stem Cells 24:1628–1637.

He, S., Pant, D., Schiffmacher, A., Bischoff, S., Melican, D., Gavin, W. and Keefer, C. (2006): Developmental expression of pluripotency determining factors in caprine embryos: novel pattern of NANOG protein localization in the nucleolus. Mol. Reprod. Dev., 73:1512–1522.

Hochereau-de Reviers, M.T. and Perreau, C. (1993): In vitro culture of embryonic disc cells from porcine blastocysts. Reprod. Nutr. Dev., 33:475–483.

Hoffman, J.A. and Merrill, B.J. (2007): New and renewed perspectives on embryonic stem cell pluripotency. Front. Biosci. 12:3321–3332.

Iwasaki, S., Campbell, K.H., Galli, C. and Akiyama, K. (2000): Production of live calves derived from embryonic stem-like cells aggregated with tetraploid embryos. Biol. Reprod., 62:470–475.

Johnson, L.A. (2000): Sexing mammalian sperm for production of offspring: the state-of-the-art.Anim. Reprod. Sci. 60–61:93–107.

Johnson, L.A, Weitze, K.F., Fiser, P. and Maxwell, W.M. (2000): Storage of boar semen. Anim. Reprod. Sci. 62:143–172.

Keefer, C.L., Pant, D., Blomberg, L. and Talbot, N.C. (2007): Challenges and prospects for the establishment of embryonic stem cell lines of domesticated ungulates. Anim. Reprod. Sci., 98:147–168.

Kim, H.S., Son, H.Y., Kim, S., Lee, G.S., Park, C.H., Kang, S.K., Lee, B.C., Hwang, W.S. and Lee, C.K. (2007a): Isolation and initial culture of porcine inner cell masses derived from in vitro-produced blastocysts. Zygote, 15:55–63.

Kim, M.K., Jang, G., Oh, H.J., Yuda, F., Kim, H.J., Hwang, W.S., Hossein, M.S., Kim, J.J., Shin, N.S., Kang, S.K. and Lee, B.C. (2007b): Endangered wolves cloned from adult somatic cells. Cloning Stem Cells 9:130–137.

Kirchhof, N., Carnwath, J.W., Lemme, E., Anastassiadis, K., Scholer, H. and Niemann, H. (2000): Expression pattern of Oct-4 in preimplantation embryos of different species. Biol. Reprod., 63:1698–1705.

Kutzler, M.A. (2005): Semen collection in the dog. Theriogenology 64:747–754.

Lanza, R.P., Cibelli, J.B., Diaz, F., Moraes, C.T., Farin, P.W., Farin, C.E., Hammer, C.J., West, M.D. and Damiani, P. (2000): Cloning of an endangered species (Bos gaurus) using interspecies nuclear transfer. Cloning 2:79–90.

Lee, B.C., Kim, M.K., Jang, G., Oh, H.J., Yuda, F., Kim, H.J., Hossein, M.S., Kim, J.J., Kang, S.K., Schatten, G. and Hwang, W.S.. (2005): Dogs cloned from adult somatic cells. Nature 436:641.

Levick, S.E. (2007): From Xenopus to Oedipus: 'Dolly', human cloning and psychological and social clone-ness. Cloning Stem Cells 9:33–39.

Li, M., Zhang, D., Hou, Y., Jiao, L., Zheng, X. and Wang, W.H. (2003): Isolation and culture of embryonic stem cells from porcine blastocysts. Mol. Reprod. Dev., 65:429–434.

Li, M., Li, Y.H., Hou, Y., Sun, X.F., Sun, Q. and Wang, W.H. (2004a): Isolation and culture of pluripotent cells from in vitro produced porcine embryos. Zygote, 12:43–48.

Li, M., Ma, W., Hou, Y., Sun, X.F., Sun, Q.Y. and Wang, W.H. (2004b): Improved isolation and culture of embryonic stem cells from Chinese miniature pig. J. Reprod. Dev. 50:237–244.

Li, Z., Sun, X., Chen, J., Liu, X., Wisely, S.M., Zhou, Q., Renard, J.P., Leno, G.H. and Engelhardt, J.F. (2006): Cloned ferrets produced by somatic cell nuclear transfer. Dev. Biol. 293:439–448.

Li, P., Tong, C., Mehrian-Shai, R., Jia, L., Wu, N., Yan, Y., Maxson, R.E., Schulze, E.N., Song, H., Hsieh, C., Pera, M.F. and Ying, Q. (2008): Germline competent embryonic stem cells derived from rat blastocysts. Cell 135:1299–1310.

Loi, P., Ptak, G., Barboni, B., Fulka, J. Jr., Cappai, P. and Clinton, M.. (2001): Genetic rescue of an endangered mammal by cross-species nuclear transfer using post-mortem somatic cells. Nature Biotech. 19:962–964.

Long CR, Walker SC, Tang RT, Westhusin ME (2003) New commercial opportunities for advanced reproductive technologies in horses, wildlife, and companion animals. Theriogenology 59:139–149.

Luvoni GC, Chigioni S, Beccaglia M (2006) Embryo production in dogs: from in vitro fertilization to cloning. Reprod. Dom. Anim. 41:286–290.

Mapletoft, R.J. and Hasler, J.F. (2005): Assisted reproductive technologies in cattle: a review. Revue Scientifique et Technique-Office International des Epizooties 24:393–403.

Martinez EA, Vazquez JM, Roca J, Cuello C, Gil MA, Parrilla I, Vazquez JL (2005) An update on reproductive technologies with potential short-term application in pig production. Reprod. Dom. Anim. 40:300–309.

Mitalipova, M., Beyhan, Z. and First, N.L. (2001): Pluripotency of bovine embryonic cell line derived from precompacting embryos. Cloning, 3:59–67.

Mitsui, K., Tokuzawa, Y., Itoh, H., Segawa, K., Murakami, M., Takahashi, K., Maruyama, M., Maeda, M. and Yamanaka, S. (2003): The homeoprotein Nanog is required for maintenance of pluripotency in mouse epiblast and ES cells. Cell, 113:631–642.

Miyoshi, K., Taguchi, Y., Sendai, Y., Hoshi, H. and Sato, E. (2000): Establishment of a porcine cell line from in vitro-produced blastocysts and transfer of the cells into enucleated oocytes. Biol. Reprod., 62:1640–1646.

Mueller, S., Prelle, K., Rieger, N., Petznek, H., Lassnig, C., Luksch, U., Aigner, B., Baetscher, M., Wolf, E., Mueller, M. and Brem, G. (1999): Chimeric pigs following blastocyst injection of transgenic porcine primordial germ cells. Mol. Reprod. Dev., 54:244–254.

Munoz-Sanjuan, I. and Brivanlou, A.H. (2002): Neural induction, the default model and embryonic stem cells. Nat. Rev. Neurosci., 3:271–280.

Nichols, J., Zevnik, B., Anastassiadis, K., Niwa, H., Klewe-Nebenius, D., Chambers, I., Scholer, H. and Smith, A. (1998): Formation of pluripotent stem cells in the mammalian embryo depends on the POU transcription factor Oct4. Cell, 95:379–391.

Pelican KM, Wildt DE, Pukazhenthi B, Howard J (2006) Ovarian control for assisted reproduction in the domestic cat and wild felids. Theriogenology 66:37–48.

Piedrahita, J.A., Anderson, G.B. and Bondurant, R.H. (1990a): Influence of feeder layer type on the efficiency of isolation of porcine embryo-derived cell lines. Theriogenology, 34:865–877.

Piedrahita, J.A., Anderson, G.B. and Bondurant, R.H. (1990b): On the isolation of embryonic stem cells: Comparative behavior of murine, porcine and ovine embryos. Theriogenology, 34:879–901.

Piedrahita, J.A., Moore, K., Oetama, B., Lee, C.K., Scales, N., Ramsoondar, J., Bazer, F.W. and Ott, T. (1998): Generation of transgenic porcine chimeras using primordial germ cell-derived colonies. Biol. Reprod., 58:1321–1329.

Polejaeva, I.A., Chen, S.H., Vaught, T.D., Page, R.L., Mullins, J., Ball, S., Dai, Y., Boone, J., Walker, S., Ayares, D.L., Coman, A. and Campbell, K.H. (2000): Cloned pigs produced by nuclear transfer from adult somatic cells. Nature 407:86–90.

Rodda, D.J., Chew, J.L., Lim, L.H., Loh, Y.H., Wang, B., Ng, H.H. and Robson, P. (2005): Transcriptional regulation of nanog by OCT4 and SOX2. J. Biol. Chem., 280:24731–24737.

Saito, S., Sawai, K., Ugai, H., Moriyasu, S., Minamihashi, A., Yamamoto, Y., Hirayama, H., Kageyama, S., Pan, J., Murata, T., Kobayashi, Y., Obata, Y., Kazunari, K. and Yokoyama, K. (2003): Generation of cloned calves and transgenic chimeric embryos from bovine embryonic stem-like cells. Biochem. Biophys. Res. Commun., 309:104–113.

Schenke-Layland, K., Angelis, E., Rhodes, K.E., Heydarkhan-Hagvall, S., Mikkola, H.K. and MacLellan, W.R. (2007): Collagen IV induces trophoectoderm differentiation of mouse embryonic stem cells. Stem Cells, 25:1529–1538.

Shi, D., Lu, F., Wei, Y., Cui, K., Yang, S., Wei, J. and Liu Q. (2007): Buffalos (Bubalus bubalis) cloned by nuclear transfer of somatic cells. Biol. Reprod. 77:285–291.

Shim, H., Gutierrez-Adan, A., Chen, L.R., Bondurant, R.H., Behboodi, E. and Anderson, G.B. (1997): Isolation of pluripotent stem cells from cultured porcine primordial germ cells. Biol. Reprod., 57:1089–1095.

Shin, T., Kraemer, D., Pryor, J., Liu, L., Rugila, J., Howe, L., Buck, S., Murphy, K., Lyons, L. and Westhusin, M. (2002): A cat cloned by nuclear transplantation. Nature 415:859.

Silva, P.F and Gadella, B.M. (2006): Detection of damage in mammalian sperm cells. Teriogenology 65:958–978.

Simpson, J.L. (2007): Could cloning become permissible? Reprod Biomed Online; 14 S1:125–129.

Smukler, S.R., Runciman, S.B., Xu, S. and van der Koy, D. (2006): Embryonic stem cells assume a primitive neural stem cell fate in the absence of extrinsic influences. J. Cell Biol., 172:79–90.

Squires, E.L., Carnevale EM, McCue PM, Bruemmer JE (2003) Embryo technologies in the horse. Theriogenology 59:151–170.

Stice, S.L., Strelchenko, N.S., Keefer, C.L. and Matthews, L. (1996): Pluripotent bovine embryonic cell lines direct embryonic development following nuclear transfer. Biol. Reprod., 54:100–110.

Strelchenko, N.S. (1996): Bovine pluripotent stem cells. Theriogenology, 45:131–140.

Strojek, R.M., Reed, M.A., Hoover, J.L. and Wagner, T.E. (1990): A method for cultivating morphologically undifferentiated embryonic stem cells from porcine blastocysts. Theriogenology, 33:901–913.

Strong, C.(2005): The ethics of human reproductive cloning. Reprod. Biomed. Online 10 S1: 45–49.

Takahashi, K., Tanabe, K., Ohnuki, M., Narita, M., Ichisaka, T., Tomoda, K. and Yamanaka, S. (2007): Induction of pluripotent stem cells from adult human fibroblasts by defined factors. Cell 131:861–872.

Takahashi, K. and Yamanaka, S. (2006): Induction of pluripotent stem cells from mouse embryonic and adult fibroblast cultures by defined factors. Cell 126:663–676.

Talbot, N.C., Rexroad, C.E. Jr., Pursel, V.G., Powell, A.M. and Nel, N.D. (1993): Culturing the epiblast cells of the pig blastocyst. In Vitro Cell Dev. Biol. Anim., 29A:543–554.

Talbot, N.C., Powell, A.M. and Garrett, W.M. (2002): Spontaneous differentiation of porcine and bovine embryonic stem cells (epiblast) into astrocytes or neurons. In Vitro Cell Dev. Biol. Anim., 38:191–197.

The International Stem Cell Initiative (2007): Characterization of human embryonic stem cell lines by the International Stem Cell Initiative. Nature Biotech., 25:803–816.

Thomson, J.A., Itskovitz-Eldor, J., Shapiro, S.S., Waknitz, M.A., Swiergiel, J.J., Marshall, V.S. and Jones, J.M. (1998): Embryonic stem cell lines derived from human blastocysts. Science, 282:1145–1147.

Vajta, G. and Nagy, Z.P. (2006): Are programmable freezers still needed in the embryo laboratory? Review on vitrification. Reprod. Biomed. Online 12:779–796.

Vajta, G., Zhang, Y. and Machaty, Z. (2007): Somatic cell nuclear transfer in pigs: Recent achievements and future possibilities. Reprod. Fert. Dev. 19:403–423.

Vejlsted, M., Avery, B., Gjorret, J.O. and Maddox-Hyttel, P. (2006a): Effect of leukemia inhibitory factor (LIF) on in vitro produced bovine embryos and their outgrowth colonies. Mol. Reprod. Dev., 270:445–454.

Vejlsted, M., Avery, B., Schmidt, M., Greve, T., Alexopoulos, N. and Maddox-Hyttel, P. (2006b): Ultrastructural and immunohistochemical characterization of the bovine epiblast. Biol. Reprod., 72:678–686.

Vejlsted, M., Du, Y., Vajta, G. and Maddox-Hyttel, P. (2006c): Post-hatching development of the porcine and bovine embryo–defining criteria for expected development in vivo and in vitro. Theriogenology, 65:153–165.

Vejlsted, M., Offenberg, H., Thorup, F. and Maddox-Hyttel, P. (2006d): Confinement and clearance of OCT4 in the porcine embryo at stereomicroscopically defined stages around gastrulation. Mol. Reprod. Dev., 73:709–718.

Wakayama, T., Perry, A.C.F., Zuccoti, M., Johnson, K.R. and Yamagimachi, R. (1998): Full term development of mice from enucleated oocytes injected with cumulus cell nuclei. Nature 394:369–374.

Wang, L., Duan, E., Sung, L.Y., Jeong, B.S., Yang, X. and Tian, X.C. (2005): Generation and characterization of pluripotent stem cells from cloned bovine embryos. Biol. Reprod., 73:149–155.

Wheeler, M.B. (1994): Development and validation of swine embryonic stem cells: a review. Reprod. Fertil. Dev., 6:563–568.

Wheeler, M.B. (2003): Production of transgenic livestock: promise fulfilled. J. Anim. Sci. 81 Suppl. 3:32–37.

Willadsen, S.M. (1976): Deep freezing of sheep embryos. J. Reprod. Fertil. 46:151–154.

Williams, R.L., Hilton, D.J., Pease, S., Willson, T.A., Stewart, C.L., Gearing, D.P., Wagner, E.F., Metcalf, D., Nicola, N.A. and Gough, N.M. (1988): Myeloid leukaemia inhibitory factor maintains the developmental potential of embryonic stem cells. Nature, 336:684–687.

Wilmut, I. and Rowson, L.E. (1973): The successful low-temperature preservation of mouse és cow embryos. J. Reprod. Fertil. 33:352–353.

Wilmut, I., Schnieke, A.E., McWhir, J., Kind, A.J. and Campbell, K.H. (1997): Viable offspring derived from fetal and adult mammalian cells. Nature 385:810–813.

Woods, G.L., White, K.L., Vanderwall, D.K., Li, G.P., Aston, K.I., Bunch, T.D., Meerdo, L.N. and Pate, B.J. (2003): A mule cloned from fetal cells by nuclear transfer. Science 301:1063.

Wu, D.C., Boyd, A.S. and Wood, K.J. (2007): Embryonic stem cell transplantation: potential applicability in cell replacement therapy and regenerative medicine. Front. Biosci. 12:4525–4535

Yuan, H., Corbi, N., Basilico, C. and Dailey, L. (1995): Developmental-specific activity of the FGF-4 enhancer requires the synergistic action of Sox2 and Oct-3. Genes Dev., 9:2635–2645.

Yu, J., Vodyanik, M.A., Smuga-Otto, K., Antosiewicz-Bourget, J., Frane, J.L., Tian, S., Nie, J., Jonsdottir, G.A., Ruotti, V., Stewart, R., Slukvin, II. and Thomson, J.A. (2007): Induced pluripotent stem cell lines derived from human somatic cells. Science 318:1917–1920.

Zhou, Q., Renard, J.P., Le Friec, G., Brochard, V., Beaujean, N., Cherifi, Y., Fraichard, A. and Cozzi, J. (2003): Generation of fertile cloned rats by regulating oocyte activation. Science 302:1179